Chronic Fatigue and its Syndromes

Chronic Fatigue and its Syndromes

PROFESSOR SIMON WESSELY

Academic Dept of Psychological Medicine,
Guy's, King's and St. Thomas' Medical School and Institute of Psychiatry,
Honorary Consultant Psychiatrist, King's College and Maudsley Hospitals

DR MATTHEW HOTOPF

Senior Lecturer,
Academic Dept of Psychological Medicine,
Guy's, King's and St. Thomas' Medical School and Institute of Psychiatry

DR MICHAEL SHARPE

Senior Lecturer in Psychological Medicine,
University of Edinburgh,
Honorary Consultant to the Royal Infirmary
and Western General Hospital Trusts of Edinburgh

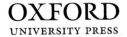

OXFORD
UNIVERSITY PRESS

*This book has been printed digitally and produced in a standard specification
in order to ensure its continuing availability*

OXFORD
UNIVERSITY PRESS

Great Clarendon Street, Oxford OX2 6DP

Oxford University Press is a department of the University of Oxford.
It furthers the University⊙ objective of excellence in research, scholarship,
and education by publishing worldwide in

Oxford New York

Auckland Bangkok Buenos Aires Cape Town Chennai
Dar es Salaam Delhi Hong Kong Istanbul Karachi Kolkata
Kuala Lumpur Madrid Melbourne Mexico City Mumbai Nairobi
S‹o Paulo Shanghai Taipei Tokyo Toronto

Oxford is a registered trade mark of Oxford University Press
in the UK and in certain other countries

Published in the United States
by Oxford University Press Inc., New York

ISBN 0-19-263046-6

Printed in Great Britain by

Antony Rowe Ltd., Eastbourne

Preface

Fatigue is the Central Africa of medicine, an unexplored territory which few men enter

Thus begins George Beard's now classic account of neurasthenia, the Victorian illness of chronic fatigue*. What was true in 1869 remains largely true today. If the subject of chronic fatigue syndrome is rarely absent from our media, this is in part because of the scarcity of professional and scientific exploration of the topic of chronic fatigue. What is it, what causes it?

In this book we attempt an ambitious, some might say too ambitious, visit to that unexplored territory. We present a comprehensive review of the problem of chronic fatigue, mixing medical, psychological, social, and historical perspectives. We know there will be those who criticize all of these approaches. One school of thought, influential in reductionist medical circles, is that there is no medical basis to chronic fatigue, and hence it is a waste of time to talk of one. Others will be equally vehemently opposed to the introduction of any psychological perspective on what is obviously a physical problem, and will take the mere mention of any alternative thesis as an insult. Both camps may be sceptical of any social analysis. Both camps, committed as they are to a reductionistic, ever optimistic, view of the potential of medical science and progress, may wonder what history has to offer. Whilst we know we can never answer all criticisms, we hope to convince our readers of the cumulative richness of medical, social, and psychological thought on the problem of chronic fatigue.

Our thesis is that chronic fatigue and its various syndromes cannot easily be pigeon-holed into physical or psychiatric categories, whatever those terms may mean. We locate it in the grey area that lies between those two concepts. It is because of its ambiguous nature that chronic fatigue provides such an opportunity to examine modern attitudes to sickness and health, an opportunity that would be absent from better defined or characterized disorders.

Chronic fatigue is thus a conceptual challenge to both medical and psychological orthodoxy. But it is more than that – it is also a tangible problem and challenge to patients and practising doctors alike. We also wish this book to be of practical benefit. For that reason we end the book with three chapters aimed with the generalist, and indeed the patient, very much in mind. These include an overview of the assessment, investigation, and management of chronic fatigue, a review of the evidence on treatment, and a practical guide to treatment based on our own clinical practice.

* Beard G. Neurasthenia, or nervous exhaustion. *Bost. Med. Surg. J.* 1869; **3**: 217–221.

The stimulus for our interest, and our publisher's interest, was the emergence of the latest fatigue illness, chronic fatigue syndrome (CFS), and hence this makes up a substantial proportion of the book. We have pursued a biopsychosocial approach to the problem of CFS by reviewing the evidence from a variety of perspectives, and attempted to be as comprehensive as possible. Given the recent upsurge of publications on the subject, a book such as this must draw out general themes and concepts in order to assist the reader in interpreting new findings in their appropriate scientific and historical contexts. Nevertheless, now that the medical community has at long last shown signs of wakening from its professional slumber on the subject it is probable that a second edition, should our wives, partners, and publishers permit one, would require considerable revision of some sections of the text. We have thus made every effort to draw wider conclusions wherever possible. For example, we hope that our observations on the relationships between viral agents and illness will survive the appearance of new data on the subject. Similarly, we hope that our thoughts on the origins of CFS and its social meanings will not be outdated by further research. For that reason throughout this book we have attempted to use a broad brush, and in particular to emphasize the place of CFS in the wider context of the subject of chronic fatigue, and the history of illness.

Many people have contributed to the book in more ways than they know. Anthony David and Antony Pelosi began Simon Wessely's interest in the subject, and have remained a constant source of support, assistance, and well deserved criticism ever since. Trudie Chalder has played a similar role over the years. Michael Sharpe entered the field by accident after being invited into an infectious disease clinic by Geoff Pasvol. This began an interest in unexplained fatigue – a common passion with Simon Wessely that is the basis of this book. His researches have been guided and supported by Keith Hawton, Michael Gelder, and Tim Peto. More recently Alison Clements has helped him to keep his feet on the ground. Matthew Hotopf's earliest exposure to the field was personal. As a medical student at Barts he suffered glandular fever and was enrolled into Peter White's study*. This experience was an insight into the rigours of well conducted research. At the Maudsley he met Simon Wessely and was encouraged to develop a professional interest in the field. Glyn Lewis has since helped broaden and deepen his research interests and critical faculties.

The globalization of medical research has permitted us to meet and talk to a range of colleagues across the world. There are too many individuals to mention all by name, but traces of our travels from Brussels, Bethesda to Boston, from the Netherlands to New Jersey, and from Seattle to Sydney, can all be found in the pages of the book. We are particularly grateful to our Australian colleagues Andrew Lloyd and Ian Hickie, who have shown that it is possible to combine professional argument with personal friendship. From America we are indebted to Wayne Katon, Dedra Buchwald, Mark Demitrack, Susan Abbey, Stephen Straus, and Norma Ware, who have influenced our thinking in different ways, whilst Edward Shorter has constantly reminded us of the central historical issues.

---

* White P, Thomas J, Amess J, Grover S, Kangro H, Clare A. The existence of a fatigue syndrome after glandular fever. *Psychol. Med.* 1995; **25:** 907–916.

We are also grateful to the many patients who have tolerated our lengthy interviews, painstakingly completed seemingly endless questionnaires and submitted with good grace to time-consuming laboratory investigations. Some have welcomed our attempts to understand their illness. Others have passionately disagreed with us. All have influenced our thoughts and ideas.

Anthony Cleare, Phil Cowen, Elena Garralda, John Gow, Rachel Jenkins, Russell Lane, Andrew Lloyd, Rona Moss Morriss, Ben Natelson, Leonie Ridsdale, Edward Shorter, Ann Sharpley, Caroline Swanink, Frederick Wolfe, and Adam Zeman have all commented on various aspects of the manuscript, particularly in areas unfamiliar to us. We appreciate their efforts to keep us on the straight and narrow scientific path, but where we stray the fault remains ours.

Finally, our long-suffering partners have had to live with our obsession. Without the support of Claire, Elizabeth, and Emma there would be no book. We also thank our young children Alex and Benjamin Wessely and Joseph Sharpe on learning to sleep at night so allowing their fathers to finish the manuscript.

Edinburgh and London   M.S.
October 1997   S.W.
                                                                             M.H.

Contents

Section II: The history of chronic fatigue

Section III: Chronic fatigue syndrome

**Section IV: Assessment and management of chronic fatigue
and chronic fatigue syndrome**

Section V: Overview

Abbreviations

ACTH	Adrenocorticotrophic hormone
ADP	Adenosine diphosphate
AIDS	Acquired immune deficiency syndrome
ATP	Adenosine triphosphate
CANTAB	Cambridge automated neuropsychological test battery
CBT	Cognitive behaviour therapy
CDC	Centers for diseases Control
CFIDS	Chronic fatigue and immune dysfunction syndrome
CHF	Chronic heart failure
CMV	Cytomegalovirus
CNS	Central nervous system
CPAP	Continuous positive airway pressure
CRH	Corticotrophin releasing hormone
DSM	Diagnostic and Statistical Manual
DST	Dexamethasone Suppression Test
EBV	Epstein–Barr virus
ECG	Electrocardiogram
EEG	Electroencephalogram
EMG	Electromyogram
FM	Fibromyalgia
GHQ	General Health Questionnaire
HIV	Human immunodeficiency virus
HHV	Human herpes virus
HLA	Human leucocyle antigen
HPA	Hypothalamo–pituitary–adrenal
HRSd	Hamilton rating scale for depression
HSV	Herpes simplex virus
IBS	Irritable bowel syndrome
ICD	International Classification of Diseases
IgG	Immunoglobulin G
IL	Interleukin
LMN	Lower motor neurone
MCS	Multiple chemical sensitivity
ME	Myalgic encephalomyelitis
MG	Myasthenia gravis
MHC	Major histocompatibility complex

MMPI	Minnesota Multiphasic Personality Inventory
MRC	Medical Research Council
MRI	Magnetic resonance imaging
MS	Multiple sclerosis
MSLT	Multiple sleep latency test
NIH	National Institutes of Health
NK	Natural killer
NMJ	Neuromuscular junction
NSAID	Non-steroidal anti-inflammatory agent
OA	Osteoarthritis
PASAT	Paced Auditory Serial Attention Test
PCR	polymerase chain reaction
PET	Positron emission tomography
PHA	Phytohaemagglutinin
PTSD	Post-traumatic stress disorder
PVFS	Post-viral fatigue syndrome
RA	Rheumatoid arthritis
rCBF	Regional cerebral blood flow
RCT	Randomized controlled trial
REM	Rapid eye movement
RNA	Ribonucleic acid
RPE	Rating of perceived effort
SD	Somatization disorder
SF-36	Medical Outcomes Survey: 36-item short form questionnaire
SLE	Systemic lupus erythematosus
SWS	Slow-wave sleep
TNF	Tumour necrosis factor
VAS	Visual analogue scale

Section I:

The nature and extent of fatigue

1. The nature of fatigue

1.1 What is fatigue?

Fatigue is a convenient but problematic concept. We all 'know' what it means in common parlance, but when attempts have been made to define it for the purpose of more precise discourse, the essential meaning can seem vague, elusive, and difficult to operationalize. This problem has vexed many previous writers on fatigue and has even led to the suggestion that the term 'fatigue' be abandoned altogether[1]. We are, as the title of this book suggests, less nihilistic. In our view, the problem with the definition of fatigue has arisen because of a failure to differentiate between its various meanings. This chapter will outline those specific meanings of fatigue and will briefly review the history, definition, and method of measurement of each. In this way we aim to prepare the reader for the chapters that follow. Before we begin a review of the literature we would like to suggest that you try the following four thought experiments:

Thought experiments

1. You are asked to run five miles. Then to climb a steep hill. Think how you might feel at each stage. Before starting you feel daunted and even weak in anticipation. Once you have been going for a while you feel hot, breathless, achey, and very, very tired. When you hit the hill you will feel a great sense of effort and a desire to stop . . . As you climb you notice that you are finding it hard to maintain the pace and you get slower and slower . . . You stop. You feel exhausted. Your legs feel weak, the muscles tremble, like jelly. You don't want to do much at all, just to lie down. The very idea of running any further is aversive. The feeling lasts for a while perhaps until the next day when you still feel weary and stiff.

2. Flick through this book. We want you to carefully check all the references. There are a large number – a very large number! You feel daunted, suddenly weary (but you haven't started yet and you felt fine five minutes ago). How much are we going to pay you? Nothing. No enthusiasm. But we insist. Somebody has to do it. OK, we will pay you a hundred pounds to do it. You start, but two hours later you feel weary, your eyes are uncomfortable (are you getting eyestrain?). You are bored. We are monitoring your work, and you have been getting slower, making mistakes, distracted by noises outside. You really want to do something else – almost anything else (even go for a run!). Your head aches. You feel that you can't do any more. After six hours we let you stop . . . You feel thick-headed for hours. Even the next day you feel a little weary, lacking energy.

3. A runny nose, sore throat, a cough. Your legs ache. It's the flu. You go down stairs to get the paper. Its hard to go back up. No motivation. No power in the legs. You can't concentrate to read it. You just want to sleep.

4. You have been up all night. You feel weak, hot, and cold. You just want to go to bed.

So, what did you observe? You may have noticed one or more of the following phenomena:

- You can feel fatigued before starting a task, even by just *thinking* about it.
- Fatigue associated with a task is influenced not only by the *physical factors* of magnitude and duration but also by *psychological factors* such as how interesting (and rewarding) it is.
- Whilst performing the task fatigue manifests as a sensation of *effort*.
- The feeling of fatigue is *aversive* largely because it competes with the desire to continue with a task.
- Both *physical and mental* tasks can make you feel tired.
- As well as a feeling, fatigue manifests in *behaviour* as a decrement in performance. When fatigued you are more likely to make errors and to be distracted.
- The feeling of acute fatigue lasts for a while after completing the task, presumably because of some *internal process*.
- Illness, stress, and sleep deprivation may be accompanied by similar but more pervasive feeling of *chronic fatigue*.

All of these phenomena can be described as fatigue, illustrating the tremendous breadth of the concept. They also hint at how fatigue may usefully be subdivided, a topic we will pursue further from an historical perspective.

1.2 History and fatigue

The origins of research into fatigue

Whilst the history of interest in fatigue is no doubt longer, concern with fatigue as a problem, both scientific and medical, came into its own around the middle of the last century. Why then? It has been argued that fatigue came into prominence as a result of the convergence of a number of social and cultural influences[2]: earlier philosophical ideas of 'man as machine' and notions of the immorality of inactivity, exemplified by the saying 'the devil makes work for idle hands', set the scene for a concern with activity and the factors that limited it. But it was the rise of science and technology that brought fatigue to centre stage. Industrialization had placed a new kind of demand on workers; the pressure to perform consistently for long periods of time. In fact the need to work not only with machines, but like machines. Fatigue became a key limitation of 'man the machine' and a barrier to be overcome if the full potential of the 'human motor' was to be realized[2]. The quest was on to understand fatigue and, if possible, to conquer it.

Science and the deconstruction of fatigue

Some landmarks in the history of fatigue are illustrated in Table 1.1.

Table 1.1 Historical landmarks in fatigue

1869	Beard establishes the concept of neurasthenia – the fatigue illness
1884	Mosso invented the 'ergograph' to measure fatigue in muscle function
1890	Fatigue laboratories established
1914	First World War
1918	Sir Thomas Lewis describes 'effort syndrome' in soldiers
1921	Muscio recommends that the term fatigue be abandoned[1]
1939	Second World War
1943	Fatigue laboratories closed
1947	Bartley and Chute distinguish between aspects of fatigue[4]
1988	Chronic fatigue syndrome defined

The early scientific work on the nature of fatigue by Marley in France and Kronecker in Germany culminated in a classical work by the Italian physiologist Mosso. His book *Fatigue*, published in 1904, became the intellectual focus of a new 'science of fatigue'[3]. Mosso's work focused on only one of the various fatigue phenomena we noted above; the measurable decrement in performance occurring with the repetition of a simple task. His book describes a series of experiments using an instrument that he developed to measure this aspect of fatigue. This device, which he named the 'Ergograph' (shown in Fig. 1.1) made multiple graphical records ('fatigue curves') of the travel of a man's middle finger whilst repeatedly lifting a weight.

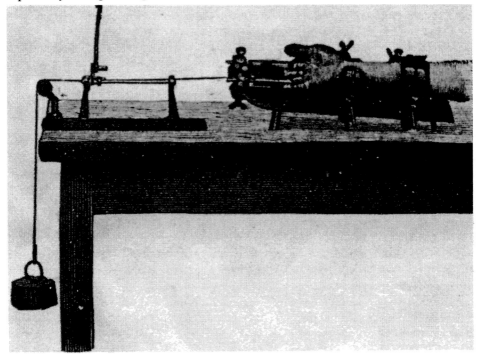

Fig. 1.1 Mosso's ergograph (reproduced from Rabinbach).

The components of fatigue

From these experiments Mosso was able to draw four conclusions. First, that the work a person is able to do (their *behaviour* as measured by the ergograph) shows evidence of a decline over time. Second, that there was a poor correlation between the *feeling* of fatigue and fatigued *behaviour*, as measured by the decrement in work output. Third, that there must be a *mechanism* or process underlying fatigue which he conceived of as a substance produced by work. Fourth, that fatigue could be affected by a number of *contextual* factors including other demands and stresses in the person's life at the time. In this early work we can see the beginnings of the separation of the global concept of fatigue into measurable components. Forty years later Bartley and Chute[4] offered a similar analysis. The main components of fatigue are listed in Table 1.2.

Table 1.2 The components of fatigue

Behaviour (decrement in performance)
Feeling state
Mechanism or intervening variable
Context

Fatigue as behaviour

Consistent with the concerns of the time, much of the early interest in fatigue focused on behaviour, and especially on the inability to maintain work output for long periods. Tasks affected by fatigue can be broadly divided into those requiring the performance of physical work and those that emphasize mental demands such as decision-making.

Physical performance decrement

By 1900, laboratories devoted to the study of fatigue had been established in most European countries. Indeed, it is reported that at the turn of the century the journals of the German, French, and Belgian scientists 'overflowed with literature' on fatigue[2]. Josefa Ioteyko was a prominent women amongst those contributing to them. In 1904 she named the new science of fatigue 'Ergography', after Mosso's instrument, thereby defining the emphasis of the early research[5]. Interest in fatigue as inability to maintain physical work continued into the First World War, during which time the output of workers in munitions factories became a major concern and subsequently led to the setting up of the British Industrial Fatigue Research Board[6]. As time passed, the demands technology made on people changed; interest in fatigue as physical work output was replaced with an emphasis on mental performance. None the less, fatigue as a limitation on physical performance remained a major concern, especially to those concerned with sport and athletics[7].

Mental performance decrement

Mental or intellectual fatigue as exhibited by a decrement in mental performance hit the headlines as long ago as the 1880s when there was widespread concern about intellectual fatigue in French and German school children[2,8] (a topic to which we return later). Research on mental fatigue began in earnest during the Second World War. The increase in the technology of war led to greater demands being placed upon those called on to operate the increasingly sophisticated war machines. Concern was expressed about how fatigue affected the vigilance of those operating radar[9], and the decision-making of those flying aircraft[10]. These concerns led to the setting up in Cambridge of an early version of the flight simulator and to a famous series of experiments known as the Cambridge cockpit experiments[10]. These investigations examined the ability of pilots to complete complex and stressful tasks over long periods[11]. One conclusion was that an important aspect of mental fatigue was a deterioration in not only the amount of mental work but in its quality, a change manifest as skimping on routine tasks and an increasing numbers of mistakes[10]. Interest in fatigue as decrement in mental performance has continued to the present day, especially in relation to the demands placed on pilots by long-distance flight[12] and by a desire to reduce fatigue-related vehicle accidents[13].

Fatigue as a feeling state

Mosso's original work[3] demonstrated the independence of the feeling of fatigue from the behavioural aspects of performance decrement, a finding confirmed by Iotekyo[5]. Kraepelin elaborated this distinction using the German word *Ermüdung* to indicate performance decrement and *Müdigkeit* for the feeling of fatigue[2]. The feeling of fatigue is itself a broad concept, covering a range of nuances. These may be approached via the many synonyms for fatigue[14], some of which are listed in Table 1.3.

Table 1.3 Verbal concepts of fatigue

Lack of energy
Weakness
Fatiguability
Effort – in relation to task
Sleepiness
Tiredness
Desire for rest
Lack of motivation
Lassitude
Boredom

Despite the large number of synonyms, attempts to discern important dimensions of subjective fatigue have been few[14]. In the absence of any generally agreed scheme, we suggest the following: it is based in part on that used for pain[15] and highlights distinctions that we believe are of clinical importance.

Sensory quality of fatigue

Perhaps the most common meaning of fatigue is of a feeling of lack of energy, weariness[16], and aversion to (further) effort[17]. Weakness (fatigue preventing performance of a task) and effort (fatigue when performing a task) have distinct meanings[18] but are closely related. As long ago as 1891, Augustus Waller[19] linked the sense of effort with the feeling of fatigue: 'the sense of effort and the sense of fatigue are sensations – the first with action, the second after action'[19]. This increased sense of effort became the defining characteristic of the effort syndromes described by Lewis in 1918 (see Chapters 6, 8, and 14), which were important precursors of modern chronic fatigue syndromes[20]. The feeling of sleepiness also overlaps with the feeling of fatigue described above[6] but is important to distinguish between them. This is because prominent sleepiness suggests problems with sleep and may be a pointer to treatable sleep disorders[21] (see also Chapter 3). Similarly, weakness that is local rather than general in nature should also be distinguished from an overall feeling of fatigue as it may point to a specific problem with that part of the body[18].

Affective and motivational aspects of fatigue

Fatigue is also strongly associated, especially in its chronic form, with the emotional states of irritability, depression, pain, frustration[6,14,22,23], and, in the experimental literature on fatigue, especially with anxiety[11,24]. Fatigue is also an active aversion to (further) activity, and in that sense is a motivational concept[25], an aspect of fatigue much emphasized by Bartley and Chute[17]. Again, there are important distinctions to be made. The clinical analysis of fatigue suggests a division between fatigue in which the emphasis is on a 'paralysis of initiative' and fatigue in which desire persists but there is 'inadequate peripheral effectiveness'[26]. A lack of desire for action associated with a general lack of interest or pleasure is of clinical relevance; when described as anhedonia[27] it is central to the concept of depressive disorder, an important and potentially treatable cause of chronic fatigue (See also Chapter 10).

Cognitive and evaluative aspects of fatigue

Although there is little systematic research into the cognitions associated with acute fatigue, simple observation suggests that it is typically accompanied by self-statements about bodily feelings and the need to stop what one is doing. Studies of patients with chronic fatigue reveal that as well as similar self-statements, others may be present that have a more 'catastrophic' quality, for example: 'I'll run out of energy, and 'I'll harm myself'[28,29].

We tend to take it for granted that the sensation of fatigue has a negative connotation, although a moment's reflection will reveal that this is not always the case. Fatigue can be pleasant when no work has to be done. Indeed Rabinbach points out that in medieval writings fatigue was often depicted in a positive light as a welcome 'sign of limit, of the point of rest, even of spiritual awakening'[2]. These observations indicate how context and culture can influence the individual's labelling of, and experience of, fatigue (see below).

Fatigue as mechanism

Fatigue may also be conceived of as a hypothetical internal state of the person, like hunger, that manifests as both a feeling and as a tendency to certain types of behaviour[30]. Since the earliest days of fatigue research one of its aims has been to discover the 'mechanism' underlying this state. This search has been an essentially reductionist one, each investigator seeking to find the mechanism of fatigue from within their own discipline and using the measures most readily available to them. Although we believe that an adequate explanation of fatigue will only come from an approach that integrates biological, psychological, and contextual factors, we have followed the literature and summarized the reports of these studies according to the discipline of their authors (see also Chapter 3).

Biochemistry and physiology of fatigue

The study of the biochemistry of fatigue goes back to the turn of the century when Mosso[3] concluded that fatigue was caused by the accumulation of a chemical within the fatigued person. This idea was pursued by Weichardt who claimed to have identified the 'fatigue toxin'. He called it 'kenotoxin'. The application to the problem of the moment, fatigue amongst school children, followed with indecent haste. Rabinbach reports 'On the 30th June 1909 armed with sprayers containing "anti-kenotoxin" solution, Weichardt and an assistant appeared in a Berlin secondary school where they sprayed a classroom with the chemical'. Remarkably, the initial results were positive, and we are told that 'The speed of students' calculation increased by 50 per cent'. Perhaps not surprisingly further evaluations revealed the substance to be ineffective[2]. Subsequent attempts to isolate biochemical factors implicated in fatigue have involved the measurement of plasma cortisol[31], neurotransmitters[32], amino acids[33], and immune factors[34] – themes to which we will return later.

The physiology of physical fatigue in terms of performance of a task has been pursued using neurophysiological techniques. Recording and stimulation experiments have investigated the mechanism of muscle fatigue and led to the distinction between such *peripheral* mechanisms of fatigue and the rest of the nervous system or *central* factors[35]. These are elaborated in Chapter 3. Other strands of physiological investigation have concerned the pattern of rest and sleep. Although acute fatigue has been typically construed as following activity and being relieved by rest, somewhat paradoxically there is a considerable literature concerning the role of *inactivity* in producing chronic fatigue[36,37]. This is an association which we will also return to later (see Chapter 3). The failure of sleep to achieve its usual restorative role has long been considered to be cause of fatigue[38]. It has been studied by both recordings of sleep patterns using the polysomnograph[39] and experimental manipulation of duration and pattern of sleep (see Chapter 3).

Psychological mechanisms in fatigue

Psychologists have understandably focused on fatigue as manifest by reduced performance on mental tasks. These studies have often been linked to a particular theoretical approach to fatigue. For example, one strand of research has focused on errors in vigilance tasks and linked these to the concept of 'arousal'[6,40]. Measures of arousal included the critical function frequency (CFF) – the rate of flicker at which the individual is no longer able to distinguish a flickering light from a continuous light[41]. This approach had the potential advantage of a unifying theory that linked the effect of sleep deprivation with other forms of fatigue. Unfortunately the concept of arousal is not without its own problems of definition and measurement. Another strand of fatigue research has used information-processing theory to explore the hypothesis that the limited capacity of the human nervous system can explain fatigue[42]. Despite a considerable body of research, neither theory seems able to provide a complete explanation of even this limited aspect of fatigue.

More recently, cognitive behavioural theories of fatigue have emphasized the role of psychological variables such as belief and expectation, the focus of attention onto bodily sensations, and of mood and motivation. There is evidence that the beliefs that a person holds about fatigue influence how it is perceived. For example, the effect of expectancies on the experience of acute fatigue was demonstrated experimentally by giving subjects inaccurate feedback about how long they had been doing a rotor pursuit tracking task. The task involved the subject following a small spot with a stylus whilst it rotated on a turntable. The severity of the subjects, reported fatigue was found to be more closely related to the *perceived* (and false) duration to the *actual* duration of the task[43]. Fatigue may also be caused by a conflict between the perceived demands of a task and the estimate of available resources[4]. In a clinical setting persons with chronic fatigue who believe that fatigue is dangerous are more disabled by fatigue[28]. Beliefs that portray fatigue as threatening may also increase its apparent magnitude by increasing the attention paid to it, a process that has been called somatosensory amplification[44]. The effect of attention of fatigue has been investigated experimentally by Pennebaker. He found that subjects asked to run on a treadmill became more fatigued if given auditory feedback of the sounds of their exertion, and less fatigued if distracted from them[45].

Finally, both depressed and anxious moods are important contributors to fatigue. They are associated not only with increased fatigue at rest, but also with a greater sense of effort when performing physical tasks[46,47].

The function of fatigue

What function does fatigue have? The obvious suggestion, and one that was made by Ioteyko for acute fatigue, is that fatigue is 'a defence against the dangers of a work pursued to the extreme'[2]. A similar suggestion made from a different perspective is that fatigue acts as a 'stop signal' for activity that gives rise to emotional conflict[48]. But what of chronic fatigue? It has been suggested that chronic fatigue may represent a general behavioural inhibition occurring as part of a stress response[6], and also that it is defensive against the emotional consequences of chronic conflict and feelings of inadequacy[49]. Although speculative, these ideas serve to remind us of the importance of the context of the fatigued person.

Fatigue in context

The fatigued person does not exist in isolation but in a temporal, physical, and social context. Their fatigue is often considered in relation to specified activities or tasks.

The duration of fatigue

When considering the cause of fatigue it is most important to specify whether the fatigue is acute or chronic. The importance of this distinction has not always been appreciated. In fact one of the major shortcomings of much of the aforementioned experimental work on fatigue is its almost exclusive focus on acute fatigue. In the 'real world', and in medical practice, the principal problem is more often one of chronic fatigue[50].

The physical environment

In laboratory studies the effect of the environment is controlled. Naturalistic studies of fatigue have drawn attention to the fact that fatigue is influenced not only by work done and time spent, but also by many psychological and environmental factors[51]. For example, it is a common experience to feel fatigued in hot humid conditions. During the Second World War studies were made of fatigue in troops who had been stationed in tropical climes. Interestingly, a careful analysis of the factors contributing to their fatigue suggested that the psychological and social consequence of being stationed overseas were as important as the temperature in making them fatigued[52].

The social environment

Another aspect of chronic fatigue is the accumulation of life stresses over a period of time prior to the manifestation of the fatigue. This contribution to chronic fatigue has been repeatedly highlighted by those investigating the problem in real-world settings[24,53], but often underestimated.

Demands on the fatigued person

As we have noted, fatigue is essentially a negative feeling when it is in *relation to* an actual or anticipated task (although the actual performance of a task is not a prerequisite for the feeling). Many characteristics of the task may be relevant to both the severity of the feeling of fatigue and to the actual performance. Boring tasks are more prone to produce fatigue[54]. Incentives may both reduce the feeling of fatigue and improve the performance. This latter phenomenon was illustrated in an experiment which required a group of hapless subjects to hang from a bar by their arms for as long as they could; those who were offered a five dollar reward hung onto a bar almost twice as long as subjects who were not[55]. Analogous findings in industrial research highlight the importance of work attitudes and satisfaction as influences on workers' fatigue[56].

Summary of analysis of fatigue

The main findings of our analysis of fatigue is that it is best considered in terms of a number of components, the principal ones being fatigue as behaviour, fatigue as a feeling, and fatigue as an internal state or mechanism, in addition to which the environment of the fatigued person and the demands upon them must always be specified. The delineation of these components of fatigue allows for more precise definition and measurement. We have also shown how the main components of fatigue may, in turn, be divided further into the elements listed in Table 1.4.

Table 1.4 The dimensions of fatigue

Behaviour	Work output, error rate, endurance Relation to rest
Feeling state	Mental and physical Severity and quality Associated symptoms
Affective and evaluative	Pleasant/unpleasant Associated anxiety and depression
Cognitive/motivational	Enthusiasm Aversion
Mechanism	Physiology and biochemistry Psychology
Context	Physical factors: temperature and noise Social stressors Cultural context

1.3 Medicine and fatigue

The reconstruction of fatigue

Having 'deconstructed' fatigue into its component parts we find that the clinical problem of fatigue requires we reconstruct it. This is because patients rarely visit a doctor simply because of the symptom of fatigue but rather, because other factors have led to the fatigue becoming a cause for concern[57,58]. Concern is more likely when fatigue is chronic, severe, and unrelieved by rest; accompanied by disability or preventing the performance of important duties; or causing distress because of a real or imagined association with disease (see Chapter 2). Furthermore, the symptom of fatigue always has to be considered within the person's physical and social context. Typically therefore, a complaint of fatigue to a doctor is complex and includes many, if not all, of the separate aspects of fatigue described above. Fatigue as symptom is therefore a complex phenomenon.

Fatigue as illness

The last century saw an explosion of interest not only in acute fatigue as a factor limiting work but also in chronic fatigue as a medical illness[59]. Physicians then, as now, appreciated that fatigue could be the accompaniment of a considerable range of medical diseases (see Chapter 3), but also recognized the occurrence of fatigue as an illness in the absence of disease. This was the condition labelled 'neurasthenia' by George Beard in 1869[60]. This diagnosis was frequently made during the latter years of the last century but subsequently declined in usage. During the ensuing decades chronic fatigue continued to trouble patients and physicians alike, and to be attributed to a range of diagnoses (see Chapter 5).

In more recent years chronic fatigue has again returned to prominence. The various diagnoses have coalesced into the concept of a chronic fatigue syndrome (CFS). This was first defined in 1988[61] in terms of a symptom of fatigue (amongst others) that was chronic and associated with a reduction in the patient's functional capacity. This syndrome has subsequently been the focus of much research and debate. Unfortunately, this has often been conducted in ignorance of the rich literature concerning both the phenomenon of fatigue and other clinical fatigue syndromes. The nature, aetiology, and management of CFS is the subject of much of the remainder of this book.

1.4 Measurement of fatigue

One of the tasks of the British Industrial Fatigue Board was to develop a measure of fatigue. This enterprise failed. In a report to the Board in 1921 Muscio argued that a test for fatigue was neither available, nor likely to be possible[1]. Muscio was concerned with the measurement of fatigue as mechanism or process and the continuing absence of evidence for a single physiological or psychological process appears to confirm his pessimism. Nonetheless, the conceptual analysis we have completed makes it clear that the individual components of the broad concept are amenable to measurement, and consequently to valid scientific investigation. We will end this chapter by briefly reviewing some of these measures.

Measurement of fatigue as behaviour

Function can be affected by fatigue in a number of ways. The measurement of alterations in function has been categorized into impairment, disability, and handicap by the WHO[62]. Impairment refers to a reduction in physical or mental capabilities; disability to the inability to perform a human function such as walking; and handicap to the social disadvantage that results from the disability. Disability and handicap are particularly important in persons with chronic fatigue where we are concerned with interference with living and are generally measured by self-report. Many of the self-report scales actually measure a combination of impairment, disability, and handicap.

Impairment of physical function

Impairment in physical function can be assessed by self-report – for example 'ability to sustain physical functioning' is an item on a self-report fatigue scale[63]. Perhaps the most direct way to measure impairment due to fatigue is to ask a person to exert themselves until they can go on no longer[64]. For isolated muscles, neurophysiological measures of muscle-force generation may be employed[65]. The power of specific muscle groups can be assessed by machines such as the dynamometer to measure grip strength[66]. Whole body power output can be measured using a cycle ergometer (a fixed cycle with a device that allows the resistance encountered when the pedals are rotated to be varied) or a treadmill[46,64]. Measures of physical performance are listed in Table 1.5.

Table 1.5 Measures of fatigue behaviour

Impairment	
Physical	e.g. ergometer
Mental	e.g. CANTAB
Disability	e.g. physical function scale of SF-36
Handicap	e.g. employment status

Impairment of mental function

As with physical impairment, this may be measured either by self-report or by direct assessment. One self-assessment scale is the cognitive failures questionnaire[67] which comprises items such as 'do you find you forget people's names?' Direct tests of cognitive performance include simple reaction time, attention span, memory, reasoning, vigilance tasks, and decision-making. An example of a test of cognitive function would be the Cambridge automated neuropsychological test battery (CANTAB) test battery which runs on a personal computer[68].

Disability

The effect of physical and mental impairment on daily function can be assessed either by self-report[69] or by an observer[70]. A variety of generic scales are available, some of which combine disability subsales with others assessing symptoms and well-being to provide a measure of 'quality of life'[71,72] A widely used example of self-rated scales are the physical and role-function subscales of the Medical Outcomes Survey: 36-item short form or SF-36.[72] A popular observer-rated measure is the 100 point scale devised by Karnofsky[70]. A scale has also been devised specifically to assess fatigue-related disability[73]

Handicap

This reflects social consequences of disability, and may be measured in terms of lost earnings or employment status. It is worth noting that some individuals such as athletes may be handicapped by chronic fatigue of modest severity, whereas those in other occupations are not.

Measurement of fatigue as a feeling

The acceptance of feeling states in general, and the feeling of fatigue in particular, as valid and measurable phenomena has been important in enabling systematic research[74]. Measures may be classified according to content (e.g. physical or mental fatigue), format (questionnaire or interview), number of items (single question or multiple), scoring method, and the time period they cover.

Questionnaires

Self-rated questionnaires are easy to administer and can yield summary scores for correlation with other measures. A variety of rating scales are available.[74] In some of these fatigue is simply one component of a more general enquiry, in others the measurement of fatigue is the principal purpose of the scale.

Single-item scales

These have the benefit of simplicity. Unfortunately, because they invite a rating of a single word (often 'fatigue') they are prone to idiosyncratic responses and may not adequately tap the overall concept. Existing scales designed to measure emotional disturbance often include items that address fatigue. For example, the Beck Depression Inventory (BDI) includes the item 'get tired', the Zung Depression Scale 'get tired for no reason', and the Centre for Epidemiological Studies Depression Scale (CES-D) 'everything an effort'. These items are usually scored in only a crude categorical way.

More sensitive methods of scoring single-item questions allow a greater range of responses. One such method is the visual analogue scale (VAS)[75]. In its most common form the VAS is a 100 mm horizontal line with descriptive phrases or anchors placed at each end. For example 'not at all fatigued' on the far left and 'extremely fatigued' on the far right. The subject is asked to make a mark on a line to indicate their level of fatigue. Likert-type scales are similar to the VAS but has instead of a simple line a number of categories (up to seven) for the subject to choose from[75]. Because each point is anchored, changes on a Likert scale may be more readily interpreted than changes on a VAS. A simple VAS and a Likert scale for measuring fatigue are shown in Table 1.6

Table 1.6 Single-item visual analogue and Likert-type scale measure of fatigue

A.	10 cm VAS				
	Not at all fatigued	_____		Completely fatigued	
B.	Likert scale				
	I am fatigued:				
	Not at all	A little	Moderately	A great deal	Extremely

Multi-item scales

As we have seen, a number of words and concepts describe the feeling state of fatigue. Using a larger number of words and synonyms in the measures produces a better sampling of the concept. An example is the scale of Lee *et al.*[76], which includes 18

descriptors of the feeling of fatigue, and the scale of Piper *et al.* which attempts to measure affective and evaluative as well as sensory dimensions. A widely used scale is that
of Chader *et al.* which comprises separate physical and mental subscales[77]. It is shown in Table 1.7.

Table 1.7 The fatigue scale of Chalder *et al.*[77]

Physical symptoms
1.	Do you have problems with tiredness?
2.	Do you need to rest more?
3.	Do you feel sleepy or drowsy?
4.	Do you have problems starting things?
5.	Do you start things without difficulty but get weak as you go on?
6.	Are you lacking in energy?
7.	Do you have less strength in your muscles?
8.	Do you feel weak?

Mental symptoms
9.	Do you have difficulty concentrating?
10.	Do you have problems thinking clearly?
11.	Do you make slips of the tongue when speaking?
12.	Do you find it more difficult to find the correct word?
13.	How is your memory?
14.	Have you lost interest in the things you used to do?

The scale is scored by offering the four response categories of 'better than usual', 'no more than usual', 'worse than usual', 'much worse than usual'.

As with single-item scales a variety of scoring methods have been used in multi-item scales. The Profile of Mood States (POMS) uses Likert scales and has been widely used. Others have used both categorical and VAS scoring formats[77]. An alternative method is to use an adjective checklist. Subjects indicate on the checklist whether they feel 'better than', 'the same as', or 'worse than' each of the ten feeling levels described[78]. A range of questionnaires purporting to measure the feeling of fatigue are listed in Table 1.8; they sample the aspects of the feeling listed in Table 1.4 with varying degrees of adequacy; none is ideal.

Interviews

Interviews have been less widely used to measure fatigue. As with questionnaires it is worth noting that most standard psychiatric interviews such as the PSE[79] include items that assess fatigue, usually as part of the assessment of depression. Although attempts have been made to construct observer-rated fatigue scales (one such 20-item scale requires the observer to rate items such as 'spiritless eyes' and 'pale face'[80]) these are of questionable validity as measures of a private subjective state.

Table 1.8 Questionnaires measuring the feeling of fatigue

Reference	Name	Content (no. of items)	Scoring	Time frame	Comment
Brunier and Graydon[101]	VAS	Fatigue (1)	VAS	Past week	Simplest scale
Borg[102]	Borg scale	Effort (1)	Scale 6–20	Right now	Perceived exertion or effort
Chalder et al.[77]	Fatigue scale	Fatigue; physical (7) mental (4)	Each item 0–3	Last week	Widely used
Lee et al.[76]	Visual analogue scale:fatigue	General fatigue (13)	VAS	Right now	List of synonyms for fatigue
McNair and Lorr[88]	Profile of mood states	General fatigue (6)	Each item 0–4	Last week	Measures 'mood' states also
Pearson[78]	Fatigue feeling checklist	Fatigue (energy) (10)	Each item 0–3	Right now	Adjective checklist scoring
Krupp et al.[103]	Fatigue severity scale	General fatigue (9)	Each item 1–7	Right now	Scale is confounded with disability
Schwartz et al.[63]	Fatigue assessment instrument	Fatigue (11); associations (11)	Each item 1–7	Last 2 weeks	Expanded version of Krupp et al. scale
Ray et al.[104]	Profile of fatigue related symptoms	Fatigue (12) and associations (42)	Each item 0–6	Past week	Measures range of aspects of illness
Bentall et al.[105]	Mental fatigue scale	Mental fatigue (9)	Each item 0–4	Last month	Report of cognitive difficulties
Smets et al.[106]	Multidimensional fatigue inventory	Multidimensional (20)	Each item 0–7	Previous days	Measures symptoms and behaviour
Piper et al.[107]	Piper fatigue scale	Multidimensional (7)	VAS	Variable	Assesses other dimensions of fatigue

Measurement of fatigue as mechanism

A large range of measures have been used in attempts to investigate the process or internal mechanism hypothesized to underlie fatigue. The choice of measure is wide and depends on the theoretical thrust of the investigation. Only a small sample will be mentioned here (see Table 1.9).

Table 1.9 Measures of the mechanism of fatigue

Field of investigation	Example of measure
Biochemistry	Plasma cortisol
Physiology	Muscle work output
Psychology	Arousal by flicker fusion frequency

Physiological and biochemical processes

For the exploration of physiological mechanisms of fatigue a variety of techniques have been used. Prominent amongst these are neurophysiological studies of muscle stimulation[81] and polysomnographic measures of sleep[82]. Biochemical and hormonal assays have sought to capture key abnormalities[83,84], and challenge tests to uncover specific neuroendocrine dysfunction[85]. More recently, imaging methods have been used to examine possible CNS abnormalities[86].

Psychological processes

Similarly, a variety of psychological measures have been used. These include interview techniques to assess beliefs[87], and questionnaires to measures of mood[88], attribution[89], somatic focus[90], and coping behaviour[91].

Measurement of fatigue in context

Aspects of the context of the fatigued person and possible measures are listed in Table 1.10. The cultural influence is hard to measure. Insights must therefore be drawn from analysis of cross-cultural studies[92,93], historical records[94], in-depth interviews of persons with fatigue[95], and from reports in the current popular literature[96]. The person's immediate social environment is a little easier to measure; standard and reliable measures of social support and life stresses or events[97,98] are available. More subtle interpersonal influences are more difficult to capture. Finally, some aspects of the physical environment such as temperature and noise are relatively easy to measure although others such as traces of allergens[99] and the essence of 'sick buildings'[100] can be more elusive.

Table 1.10 Measure of context of fatigue

Cultural	Cross-cultural comparisons
Social	Recent life event interview
Physical	Ambient temperature measurement
Task	Measurement of work incentive

Clinical assessment

In clinical practice fatigue presents as a general problem but must be analysed into specific components. This requires a multidimensional approach in which specific measures of the range of fatigue phenomena are used together. This approach to assessment of the patient with chronic fatigue is described further in Chapter 16.

1.5 Conclusion

We have seen that the term 'fatigue' is at once meaningful and imprecise. We have argued that our understanding of what it means can be enhanced by 'deconstructing' it into components, each of which may be measured. In the laboratory, individual components of fatigue may be studied, whereas in the clinical situation the many aspects of fatigue commonly coexist and require a multidimensional approach. This comprehensive approach to the problem of fatigue is a major theme of this book and is developed further in the chapters that follow.

References

1 Muscio B. Is a fatigue test possible? *Br. J. Clin. Psychol.* 1921; **12**: 31–46.
2 Rabinbach A. *The Human Motor – Energy, Fatigue and the Origins of Modernity.* Berkeley, Universty of California Press, 1992.
3 Mosso A. *Fatigue.* London: Swan Sonnenschein and Co., 1904.
4 Bartley SH, Chute E. *Fatigue and Impairment in Man.* New York, McGraw-Hill, 1947.
5 Ioteyko J. *La Fatigue.* Paris, 1920.
6 Cameron C. A Theory of Fatigue. *Ergonomics* 1973; **16**: 633–548.
7 Lehmann M, Foster C, Keul J. Overtraining in endurance athletes: a brief review. *Med. Sci. Sports Exerc.* 1993; **25**: 854–862.
8 MacDougall R. Fatigue. *Psychol. Rev.* 1899; **6**: 203–208.
9 Broadbent DE. Neglect of the surroundings in relation to fatigue decrements in output. In Floyd WF, Welford AT (ed.) *Fatigue.* London, H. K. Lewis, 1953: 173–178.
10 Davis RD. The disorganization of behaviour in fatigue. *J. Neurol. Psychiat.* 1947; **9**: 1–23.
11 Davis RD. Satiation and frustration as determinants of fatigue. In Floyd WF, Welford AT (ed.) *Fatigue.* London, H. K. Lewis 1953: 179–182.
12 Neville KJ, Bisson RU, French J, Boll PA, Storm WF. Subjective fatigue of C-141 aircrews during Operation Desert Storm. *Human Factors* 1994; **36**: 339–349.
13 Bonnet MH, Arand DL. We are chronically sleep deprived. *Sleep* 1995; **18**: 908–911.
14 Berrios GE. Feelings of fatigue and psychopathology: a conceptual history. *Compr. Psychiatry* 1990; **31**: 140–151.
15 Steege JF, Stout AL, Somkuti SG. Chronic pelvic pain in women: toward an integrative model. *Obstet. Gynecol. Surv.* 1993; **48**: 95–110.
16 Fowler HW, Fowler FG. *The Concise Oxford Dictionary of Current English.* Oxford University Press, 1964.
17 Bartley SH, Chute E. A preliminary clarification of the concept of fatigue. *Psychol. Rev.* 1945; **53**: 169–174.
18 Ream E, Richardson A. Fatigue: a concept analysis. *Int. J. Nurs. Stud.* 1996; **33**: 519–529.
19 Waller AD. The sense of effort: an objective study. *Brain* 1891; **14**: 179–249.

20 Nixon PG. The grey area of effort syndrome and hyperventilation: from Thomas Lewis to today. *J. R. Coll. Physicians Lond.* 1993; **27**: 377–383.
21 Guilleminault C. Disorders of excessive sleepiness. *Annals. of Clinical Research* 1985; **17**: 209–219.
22 Bartley SH. Conflict, frustration and fatigue. *Psychosom. Med.* 1943; **5**: 160–162.
23 Smythe HA. Fibrositis syndrome: a historical perspective. *J. Rheumatol.* 1989; **19(suppl):** **2–6.**
24 McFarland RA. Understanding fatigue in modern life. *Ergonomics* 1971; **14**: 1–10.
25 Barmack JE. The length of the work period and the work curve. *J. Exp. Psychol. 1939;* **25**: 109–115.
26 Muncie W. Chronic fatigue. *Psychosom. Med.* 1941; **3**: 277–285.
27 Snaith RP. The concept of mild depression. *Br. J. Psychiatry* 1987; **150**: 387–393.
28 Petrie KJ, Moss-Morris R, Weinman J. The impact of catastrophic beliefs on functioning in chronic fatigue syndrome. *J. Psychosom. Res.* 1995; **39**: 31–38.
29 Surawy C. Hackmann A. Hawton KE, Sharpe M. Chronic fatigue syndrome: a cognitive approach. *Behav. Res. Ther.* 1995; **33**: 535–544.
30 Holding DH. Fatigue. In Hockey GJR (ed.) *Stress and Fatigue in Human Performance.* London, Wiley, 1983: 145–167.
31 Poteliakhoff A, Adrenocortical activity and some clinical findings in acute and chronic fatigue. *J. Psychosom. Res.* 1981; **25**: 91–95.
32 Meeusen R, De Meirleir K. Exercise and brain neurotransmission. *Sports Med.* 1995; **20**: 160–188.
33 Newsholme EA, Blomstrand E. Hassmen P, Ekblom B. Physical and mental fatigue: do changes in plasma amino acids play a role? *Biochem. Soc. Trans.* 1991; **19**: 358–362.
34 Chao CC, DeLaHunt M, Hu SX, Close K, Peterson PK. Immunologically mediated fatigue: a murine model. *Clin. Immunol. Immunopathol.* 1992; **64**: 161–165.
35 Edwards RHT. Human muscle function and fatigue. In Edwards R (ed.) *Human Muscle Fatigue: Physiological Mechanisms.* London, Pitman Medical, 1971: 1–18.
36 Zorbas YG, Matveyev IO. Man's desirability in performing physical exercises under hypokinesia. *Int. J. Rehabil. Res.* 1986; **9**: 170–174.
37 Kottke FJ. The effect of limitation of activity upon the human body. *J. Am. Med. Assoc.* 1966; **196**: 825–830.
38 Horne J. *Why We sleep.* Oxford University Press, 1988.
39 Reite M. Buysse D. Reynolds C. Mendelson WB. The use of polysomnography in the evaluation of insomnia. *Sleep* 1995; **18**: 58–70.
40 Eysenck M. *Attention and Arousal.* Berlin, Springer, 1982.
41 Weber A. Jermini C. Grandjean EP. relationship between objective and subjective assessment of experimentaly induced fatigue. *Ergonomics* 1975; **18**: 151–156.
42 Johnson SK, DeLuca J, Fiedler N, Natelson BH. Cognitive functioning of patients with chronic fatigue syndrome. *Clin. Infect. Dis.* 1994; **18(suppl. 1)**: S84–S85.
43 Snyder M, Schulz R, Jones EE. Expectancy and apparent duration as determinants of fatigue. *J. Pers. Soc. Psychol.* 1974; **29**: 426–434.
44 Barsky AJ. Amplification, somatization, and the somatoform disorders. *Psychosom.* 1992; **33**: 28–34.
45 Pennebaker JW, Lightner JM. Competition of internal and external information in an exercise setting. *J. Pers. Soc. Psychol.* 1980; **39**: 165–174.
46 Jones M, Mellersh V. A comparison of the exercise response in anxiety states and normal controls. *Psychosom. Med.* 1946; **8**: 180–187.
47 Cohen RM, Weingartner H, Smallberg SA, Pickar D, Murphy DL. Effort and cognition in depression. *Arch. Gen. Psychiatry* 1982; **39**: 593–597.

48 Shands H, Finesinger JE. A note on the significance of fatigue. *Psychosom. Med.* 1952; **14**: 309–314.

49 McCranie EJ. Neurasthenic neurosis: psychogenic weakness and fatigue. *Psychosom.* 1980; **21**: 19–24.

50 Bartley SH. *Fatigue: Mechanism and Management.* Springfield, Illinois, Charles C Thomas, 1947.

51 Vernon HM. *Industrial Fatigue and Efficiency.* London, Routledge, 1921.

52 Edholm OG. Tropical fatigue. In Floyd WF, Welford AT (ed.) *Fatigue,* London, H. K. Lewis, 1953.

53 Cameron C. Fatigue problems in modern industry. *Ergonomics* 1971; **14**: 713–720.

54 Grandjean E. Fatigue in industry. *Br. J. Ind. Med.* 1979; **36**: 175–186.

55 Schwab RS. Motivation in measurements of fatigue. In Floyd WF, Welford AT (ed.) *Fatigue* London, H. K. Lewis, 1953; 143–148.

56 Finkelman JM. A large database study of the factors associated with work-induced fatigue. *Human Factors* 1994; **36**: 232–243.

57 Lydeard S, Jones R. Factors affecting the decision to consult with dyspepsia: comparison of consultants and non-consulters. *J. R. Coll. Gen. Pract.* 1989; **39**: 495–498.

58 Verbrugge LM, Ascione FJ. Exploring the iceberg. Common symptoms and how people care for them. *Med. Care.* 1987; **25**: 539–569.

59 Wessely S. Old wine in new bottles; neurasthenia and "M.E.". *Psychol. Med.* 1990; **20**: 35–53.

60 Beard G. Neurasthenia or nervous exhaustion. *Boston Med. Surg. J.* 1869; **3**: 217–221.

61 Holmes GP, Kaplan JE, Gantz NM, *et al.* Chronic fatigue syndrome: a working case definition. *Ann. Intern. Med.* 1988; **108**: 387–389.

62 World Health Organization. *International Clasification of Impairments, Disabilities and Handicaps. A Manual of Classification Relating to the Consequences of Disease.* Geneva, WHO, 1980.

63 Schwartz JE, Jandorf L, Krupp LB. The measurement of fatigue: a new instrument. *J. Psychosom. Res.* 1993; **37**: 753–762.

64 Riley MS, O'Brien CJ, McCluskey DR, Bell NP, Nicholls DP. Aerobic work capacity in patients with chronic fatigue syndrome. *Br. Med. J.* 1990; **301**: 953–956.

65 Goodgold J, Eberstein A. Clinical neurophysiology in the evaluation of "weakness". *Med. Clin. North Am.* 1969; **53**: 625–632.

66 Pugh LC. Childbirth and the measurement of fatigue. *J. Nurs. Meas.* 1993; **1**: 57–66.

67 Broadbent DE, Cooper DF, Fitzgerald P, Parkers KR. The cognitive failures questionnaire (CFQ) and its correlates. *Br. J. Clin. Psychol.* 1982; **21**: 1–16.

68 Sahakian BJ, Owen AM. Computerized assessment in neuropsychiatry using CANTAB: discussion paper. *J. R. Soc. Med.* 1992; **85**: 399–402.

69 Tait RC, Pollard A, Margolis RB, Duckro PN. The pain disability index: psychometric and disability data. *Arch. Phys. Med. Rehabil.* 1987; **68**: 438–441.

70 Karnofsky DA, Abelmann WH, Craver LF, Burchenal JH. The use of the nitrogen mustards in the palliative treatment of carcinoma. *Cancer* 1948; **1**: 634–656.

71 Bergner M, Bobbitt RA, Carter WB, Gilson BS. The sickness Impact Profile: Development and final revision of a health status measure. *Med. Care.* 1981; **19**: 787–805.

72 Ware JE. Sherbourne CD. The MOS 36-item short-form health survey. *Med. Care* 1992; **30**: 473–481.

73 Fisk JD, Ritvo PG, Ross L, Haase DA, Marrie TJ, Schlech WF. Measuring the functional impact of fatigue: initial validation of the fatigue impact scale. *Clin. Infect. Dis.* 1994; **18(suppl. 1)**: S79–S83.

74 Barofsky I, Legro MW. Definition and measurement of fatigue. *Rev. Infect. Dis.* 1991; **13(suppl. 1)**: S94–S97.

75 Guyatt GH. Townsend M, Berman LB, Keller JL. A comparison of Likert and visual analogue scales for measuring change in function. *J. Chron. Dis.* 1987; **40**: 1129–1133.

76 Lee KA, Hicks G. Nino-Murcia G. Validity and reliability of a scale to assess fatigue. *Psychiatry Res.* 1991; **36**: 291–298.

77 Chalder T. Berelowitz G. Pawlikowska T, *et al.* Development of a fatigue scale. *J. Psychosom. Res.* 1993; **37**: 147–153.

78 Pearson RG. Scale analysis of a fatigue checklist. *J. Applied Psychol.* 1957; **41**: 186–191.

79 World Health Organization. *Schedules for Clinical Assessment in Neuropsychiatry* (SCAN). Geneva, WHO, 1992.

80 Kashinwagi S. Psychological rating of human fatigue. *Ergonomics* 1971; **14**: 17–21.

81 Connolly S, Smith DG, Doyle D, Fowler CJ. Chronic fatigue: electromyographic and neuropathological evaluation. *J. Neurol.* 1993; **240**: 435–438.

82 Morriss RK, Sharpe M, Sharpley A, Cowen PJ, Hawton KE, Morris JA. Abnormalities of sleep in patients with chronic fatigue syndrome. *Br. Med. J.* 1993; **306**: 1161–1164.

83 Jacobson W, Saich T. Borysiewicz LK, Behan WM, Behan PO, Wreghitt TG. Serum folate and chronic fatigue syndrome. *Neurol* 1993; **43**: 2645–2647.

84 Demitrack MA, Dale JK, Straus SE, *et al.* Evidence for impaired activation of the hypothalamic–piturity–adrenal axis in patients with chronic fatigue syndrome. *J. Clin. Endocrinol Metab.* 1991; **73**: 1224–1234.

85 Sharpe M, Clements A, Hawton KE, Young AH, Sargent P, Cowen PJ. Increased prolactin response to busiprone in chronic fatigue syndrome. *J. Affect. Disord.* 1996; **41**: 71–76.

86 Cope H, David AS. Neuroimaging in chronic fatigue syndrome. *J. Neurol Neurosurg. Psychiatry* 1996; **60**: 471–473.

87 Clements A, Sharpe M, Borrill J, Hawton K. Chronic fatigue syndrome: a qualitative investigation of patients' beliefs about the illness. *J. Psychosom. Res.* 1997; **42:** 615–624.

88 McNair DM, Lorr M. An analysis of mood in neurotics. *J. Ab. Soc. Psychol.* 1964; **69**: 620–627.

89 Wessely S, Powell R. Fatigue syndromes: a comparison of chronic "postviral" fatigue with neuromuscular and affective disorder. *J. Neurol. Neurosurg. Psychiatry* 1989; **52**: 940–948.

90 Barsky AJ, Goodson JD, Lane RS, Cleary PD. The amplification of somatic symptoms. *Psychosom. Med.* 1988; **50**; 510–519.

91 Ray C, Jefferies S, Weir W. Coping with chronic fatigue syndrome: illness responses and their relationship with fatigue, functional impairment and emotional status. *Psychol. Med.* 1995; **25**: 937–945.

92 Kleinman A. Neurasthenia and depression: a study of somatization and culture in China. *Cult. Med. Psychiatry* 1982; **6**: 117–190.

93 Starcevic V. Neurasthenia: a paradigm of social psychopathology in a transitional society. *Am. J. Psychother.* 1991; **45**: 544–553.

94 Wessely S. The history of chronic fatigue syndrome. In Straus SE (ed.) *Chronic Fatigue Syndrome* New York, Marcel Dekker, 1994: 3–44.

95 Ware NC. An anthropological to understanding chronic fatigue syndrome. In Straus SE (ed.) *Chronic Fatigue Syndrome* New York: Marcel Dekker, 1994: 85–100.

96 MacLean G, Wessely S. Professional and popular views of chronic fatigue syndrome. *Br. Med. J.* 1994; **308**: 776–777.

97 Paykel E. Life events, social support and depression. *Acta Psychiat. Scand.* 1994; **377(suppl):** 50–58.

98 Ray C, Jefferies S, Weir WR. Life-events and the course of chronic fatigue syndrome. *Br. J. Med. Psychol.* 1995; **68**: 323–331.

99 Simon GE, Katon WJ, Sparks PJ. Allergic to life: psychological factors in environmental illness. *Am. J. Psychiatry* 1990; **147**: 901–906.

100 Bauer RM, Greve KW, Besch EL, Schramke CJ. The role of psychological factors in the report of building-related symptoms in sick building syndrome. *J. Consult. Clin. Psychol.* 1992; **60**: 213–219.

101 Bruner G, Graydon J. A comparison of two methods of measuring fatigue in patients on chronic haemodialysis: visual analogue vs Likert scale. *Int. J. Nurs. Stud.* 1996; **33**: 338–348.

102 Borg GAV. Perceived exertion as an indicator of somatic distress. *Scand. J. Rehabil. Med.* 1970; **2**: 92–98.

103 Krupp LB, LaRocca NG, Muir-Nash J, Steinberg AD. The fatigue severity scale. *Arch. Neurol.* 1989; **46**: 1121–1123.

104 Ray C, Weir WR, Phillips S, Cullen S. Development of a measure of symptoms in chronic fatigue syndrome: The Profile of Fatigue-Related Symptons (PFRS). *Psychol. Health.* 1992; **7**: 27–43.

105 Bentall RP, Wood GC, Marrinan T, Deans C Edwards RHT. A brief mental fatigue questionnaire. *Br. J. Clin. Psychol.* 1993; **32**: 375–379.

106 Smets EM, Garssen B, Bonke B, De Haes JC. The Multidimensional Fatigue Inventory (MFI) psychometric qualities of an instrument to assess fatigue. *J. Psychosom. Res.* 1995; **39**: 315–325.

107 Piper BF, Lindsey AM, Dodd MJ, Ferketich S, Paul SM, Weller S. The development of an instrument to measure the subjective dimension of fatigue in Funk SG, Tornquist EM, Champagne MT, Archer Cop L, Wiese RA (ed.) *Key Aspects of Comfort Management of Pain, Fatigue and Nausea*, New York, Springer, 1989: 187–198.

2. Epidemiology of fatigue

2.1 Epidemiology and its application to fatigue

Epidemiology is the population-based, quantitative study of the distribution, determinants, and outcome of disease. The epidemiological approach offers a methodology for the acquisition and evaluation of new information about the cause of disease. There are several reasons why the study of chronic fatigue is suited to this approach; these include the ubiquity of the symptom of fatigue, the lack of a definitive fatigue test, and the number of possible causes. We hope to show that the application of epidemiological principles can shed light on the nature of fatigue as both symptom and syndrome.

This chapter will focus on the following questions:

1. What is the relationship between normal fatigue and pathological fatigue?
2. How much fatigue is there in the population?
3. What does research on patient samples tell us about fatigue in the population?
4. What does epidemiological research tell us about associations of fatigue?

2.2 The problem of the definition of fatigue for epidemiological surveys

In order to examine the prevalence of a symptom or illness we first need a definition. The definition and measurement of fatigue was addressed in Chapter 1 where we argued that fatigue was best considered as a multidimensional concept. We also noted the many and varied synonyms that have been used to describe that elusive sensation. Despite the limitations of subjective report we concluded that there is no objective fatigue test to come to our rescue. Instead, we can only judge fatigue second hand – it is present when a person says it is. Validity will always be elusive – we must instead aim for reliability.

Which symptom should we measure?

Most epidemiological studies that give information on fatigue have relied on a single question. Given the difficulties in definition it is not surprising that the findings of such studies are substantially different. For example, in the National Ambulatory

Medical Care Survey (NAMCS) fatigue was defined as feelings of weakness, being run down, tired, or worn out. After 1977 the definition was changed to include only the feelings of 'tiredness and exhaustion'. 'General weakness' was considered as a separate symptom. As a consequence fatigue appeared to decrease in prevalence between the two surveys.[1] Those unaware of this change may have wasted effort considering why the complaint of fatigue was decreasing in the population of the USA[2].

The importance of the precise linguistic definition of fatigue can be seen in the differing prevalence of symptoms which may be considered as synonyms for fatigue. For example, fatigue is up to ten times commoner than weakness (Table 2.1). Similarly, general fatigue appears to be twice as common as exhaustion[3], or nearly ten times commoner that feeling 'generally run down'[4]. Terminology is not just a problem between professionals and patients, but also between different professional groups. Given the close relationship between fatigue and depression (see below), the finding that of 16 adjectives used by psychiatrists to signify sadness, six were applied by patients to states of fatigue[5], is of particular interest. Even small differences in terminology can therefore result in considerable differences in research findings.

Table 2.1 Fatigue or weakness?

Author(s)	Fatigue (%)	Weakness (%)
David *et al.* (1990)[6] (males)	40	24
David *et al.* (1990)[6] (females)	54	26
Epidemiologic Catchment Area Program	24	11
Hannay (1978)[7]	23	2
Kellner and Sheffield (1973)[8]	45	12
Reidenberg and Lowenthal (1968)[9]	37	3

Dimension or category?

There are two ways of approaching the measurement of fatigue. One is to assume that fatigue is something one either has, or does not have. This dichotomous approach is an essential prerequisite for determining conventional epidemiological measures such as incidence and prevalence. It is in line with conventional medical practice – one either has cancer, or one does not, or one has had a heart attack, or not. Researchers seeking to find the cause of a condition need to know who has the condition, and who is free from it for the purposes of comparison.

This is a conceptually simple approach, and is the basis of such activities as service planning, but how much does it reflect reality? A simple division between health and disease is not even true for such apparently well-defined conditions as cancer – in cervical cancer, for example, there are degrees of malignancy. What is the situation as regards fatigue? Is there a qualitative difference between 'normal' fatigue and 'abnormal' fatigue? Is there a clear division between those with, and those without, fatigue? We suggest not.

There is considerable evidence to support a dimensional, rather than a categorical, view of fatigue. To quote the late Geoffrey Rose – 'the real question in population studies is not "Has he got it?", but "How much of it has he got?" '[10]. Considering symptoms in the community Goldberg and Huxley wrote – 'it would be tedious to enumerate the surveys which have shown that symptoms are continuously distributed in the population: rather than attempt to do this, we will observe that we are unaware of a single survey that shows anything else'[11]. The evidence concerning the severity of fatigue in the community confirms that it is indeed continuously distributed. A survey of general practice attenders in South London[6] used a nine-item scale to measure fatigue severity, based on the assumption that the greater the number of synonyms for fatigue endorsed, the greater the fatigue problem. They reported that the number of fatigue items followed a continuous distribution. A UK population study using a fatigue scale that incorporated a range of fatigue symptoms, and allowed for a measure of severity also showed a continuous distribution of risk (Fig. 2.1).

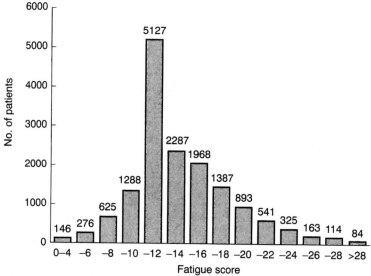

Fig. 2.1 Dimensions of fatigue in a population sample (from Pawlikowska *et al.*[12]).

A larger study from the USA included ten items on tiredness, weakness, slow recovery from viral infections, and need to rest, grouped together under the heading of 'asthenia'[13]. Once again, plotting the number of items endorsed against the number of persons with each score yielded a continuous distribution[14] (Fig. 2.2.). Fatigue is not, however, normally distributed, but in all these studies shows a positive skew, although changing the scoring system ('Likert scoring') does normalize the distribution[12].

No obvious cut-off exists between the normal and abnormal, and no 'point of rarity' can be found by statistical methods. Hence, if we are to use only severity to define when fatigue becomes abnormal the precise point must be arbitrary. This observation is not new. Back in 1908 Wells advocated 'shifting the viewpoint from the measurement of discrete states of fatigue to continuous determinants of susceptibility'[15]. How can a dimensional model of fatigue be reconciled with fatigue as illness? It may be helpful to consider the example of blood pressure and the definition of hypertension; during the 1960s there was a famous debate between Platt and Pickering on the nature of high blood pressure, with the former maintaining that a discrete disease ('hypertension') existed, the latter that there was a continuous distribution of blood pressure across the community, and no discrete entity. It is now concluded that the evidence supports the dimensional view, and that no discrete disease called 'high blood pressure' exists.

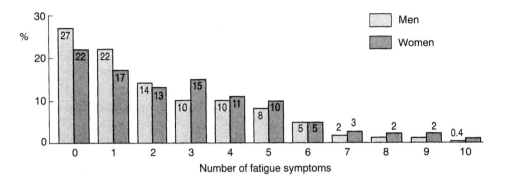

Fig. 2.2 'Fatigue and asthenic symptoms: U.S. population' (from Cloninger[13] and Lewis and Wessely[14]).

Thus epidemiology favours, as it usually does, a dimensional rather than a categorical view of fatigue. Whether or not increasing severity of fatigue is also associated with an increased risk of a defined disease, currently called chronic fatigue syndrome, remains a moot point, to which we will return in Chapter 7.

Fatigue: normal or abnormal?

As will be seen when we review community surveys, 'feeling tired' is so common as to be considered normal. The late Henry Miller once said 'the vague sense of being under the weather is what most people, if asked, will admit to most of the time'[16]. It is, said another, 'the normal chaff of living'[17]. If fatigue is so common as to affect up to half the population should we consider all these persons as ill? Clearly there is more to illness than the occurrence of a symptom. What possible differences are there between this seemingly benign symptom that affects all of us on occasion, and fatigue as illness?

Before addressing this issue we need to consider the differences between illness and disease. Medical anthropologists such as Arthur Kleinman have helped us to understand the difference between these two concepts. Kleinman has argued that illness refers to the patient's perception, expression, and pattern of coping with symptoms, whilst disease is a medical interpretation of pathology[18].

Using this framework, fatigue becomes an illness when the sufferer regards it as a sufficient problem to seek help, but becomes a disease only when it is the result of a definable medical pathology. The reasons for and against fatigue as a disease make up the middle section of this book. In this section we will consider the differences between normal and abnormal fatigue in terms not of possible aetiology, but instead via the concepts of help-seeking behaviour and functional impairment.

Fatigue and illness behaviour

One way of separating 'normal' and 'abnormal' fatigue is to assume that fatigue ceases to be part of normal experience and acquires the status of illness when a person starts to view it as a problem, and begins the process of requesting help.

There is a rich literature on the general topic of illness behaviour, seeking to explain which people consult doctors for symptoms, and when. Several factors are particularly important. First, the nature of the person. Introspection, and the general tendency to focus on symptoms, is a trait leading to more medical utilization, increased symptoms, and greater distress. Second, the character of the symptom. Highly visible symptoms, such as fever or a broken leg, and those which interfere with social functioning, such as fatigue, are more likely to cause concern than other symptoms which although lacking significant social impact, may none the less be medically significant.

Two other factors are important determinants of when fatigue crosses the threshold from a normal part of existence to a problem that may require medical attention. These are the duration of the symptom ('chronicity'), and the impact it has on people's lives ('intensity').

Duration

All of us have experienced transient fatigue, and it is thus tempting to extrapolate from this and assume that fatigue in the community is generally of a benign, short-term nature. Not so. In a British population study 38 per cent of respondents reported symptoms of fatigue, with 18 per cent reporting that this had existed for six months or longer[12]. Chronicity is also the rule in primary care. Studies in that setting have found that patients attending with a complaint of fatigue have already suffered it for a considerable length of time. The reported mean duration of fatigue varies from 16 months[19], and 17 months[20] to more than 3 years[21]. Looked at another way, two studies in UK primary care[22] found that at the time of presentation about one-third of those consulting the general practitioner with a primary complaint of fatigue had had their symptoms for longer than six months. Most studies from primary care report that fatigue is usually a chronic complaint, rather than a short term discomfort[20,23]. Not surprisingly, patients seen in secondary and tertiary care have even longer histories – one study of a specialist fatigue clinic reported a mean duration of 13 years[24] (see Chapter 7). All these studies are cross-sectional in design, and thus include an over-representation of those with chronic illness (known as prevalence bias). Nevertheless, long-lasting fatigue states can be identified in the community, primary, and secondary care settings.

In addition to long-lasting fatigue, it is reasonable to assume that a second group should also be identifiable. This is those with transient fatigue states, associated with minor psychiatric or physical morbidity (such as life events, minor viral illnesses, and so on), and those with fatigue of long duration. These will be harder to detect in cross-sectional studies, because of the previously mentioned problem of duration bias, and it is true that there are fewer studies with the power to detect short-term fatigue states. In a retrospective chart review of an Israeli general practice, asthenia was most likely to be an episodic problem, with only 10 per cent reported as 'chronic persistent asthenia'[25]. Simon Wessely and Geoff van der Linden, in an unpublished analysis of data from a three-wave study of the outcome of common viral infections, confirmed that there is also a large group of subjects in whom fatigue was transient. In the general population Angst has identified two neurasthenic syndromes, 'recurrent brief' and 'extended' neurasthenia that corresponds to these two populations[26], with the brief form outnumbering the extended version.

Overall, we suspect that the natural history of fatigue is similar to the natural history of neurotic disorders. In the community short-lived states outnumber more chronic conditions. In primary care the contribution of chronic and/or recurrent disorders increases. At any one time about one-quarter of those with minor psychiatric disorders have short-lived conditions of good prognosis, another quarter contributing to the burden of chronic illness, but the majority show a fluctuating course[27].

It will also be apparent that duration and severity may be correlated. A study in primary care[6] and a community survey[12] both found that the severity of fatigue increased with duration. Thus fatigue can well be a short-term complaint of little social importance, but fatigue presenting to the doctor is more severe[20], and perhaps has lasted longer. Nevertheless, the only study that directly compared fatigue in the community with fatigue in general practice did not confirm this plausible suggestion. In an interesting study Ingham and Miller compared those attending their general practitioner with various symptoms, including fatigue, with symptomatic people identified by a community survey who did not attend[23]. The emotional response to the symptom was important – those who presented rated the symptom as more unpleasant, and were more distressed by it. Severity also played a part, but mainly in those with more chronic symptoms. Perhaps surprisingly duration of symptoms was not a crucial factor – attenders did not consist solely of those whose symptoms had failed to resolve over time.

Functional impairment

Another basis for judging fatigue as abnormal is the extent to which it impairs functioning. For some authors functional impairment is part of the definition of fatigue itself. For example, one medical dictionary[28] defines fatigue as a 'state of increased discomfort and decreased efficiency resulting from prolonged or excessive exertion', thus combining subjective discomfort and functional impairment. However, as Armon and Kurland[28] point out in a brief but incisive review, how do we interpret *prolonged* or *excessive*?

Fatigue is by its nature a profoundly disabling state. Doctors often underestimate the impact of fatigue, perhaps because they are misled by how infrequently they are able to identify a discrete biomedical cause for the complaint. Doctors do not view fatigue with anything like the same degree of concern as patients, nor do they rate it with the same degree of importance[30]. Despite that, there is little question that fatigue can have a profound functional impact. Of the symptoms studied by Morrell in a population sample drawn from a single inner London general practice, fatigue had the strongest association with functional impairment. Of those who admitted tiredness, 26 per cent said it had forced them to restrict their normal activities, and 28 per cent reported needing to lie down in response to the symptom. The corresponding figures for toothache were 7 and 2 per cent[31]. Still in primary care, Nelson and colleagues wrote that 'about one-third of sufferers indicate that it seriously erodes their overall enjoyment of life and renders them unable to carry out their usual role activities'[20]. In the American primary care study already discussed[19], 28 per cent of patients had been completely bedridden as a result of fatigue at some stage of their illness.

In a UK systematic survey carried out in primary care chronically fatigued subjects had worse mental health, more bodily pain, worse perception of their health, and greater physical impairment than non-fatigued controls[32]. For comparison the data from the Medical Outcomes Study showed higher scores (indicating better functioning) for subjects with diabetes, hypertension, and arthritis. Only angina and advanced coronary artery disease scored less[33].

Summary

Fatigue is an important symptom in terms of its likely duration and associated functional impairment. There is no simple way of separating normal from abnormal fatigue. One approach is to leave that judgement to the person themself, and consider fatigue to be abnormal when a fatigued person starts to view him- or herself as ill. Many variables contribute to this decision. These include the duration of the fatigue, its severity and associated disability, and the presence of other symptoms. Fatigue that causes a person to visit a doctor is another measure of severity and importance, although this cannot be separated from other influences on illness behaviour. Normal and abnormal fatigue thus differ on a number of dimensions – drawing precise boundaries will also be an arbitrary decision.

2.3 Prevalence of fatigue

Community

We have already drawn attention to the fundamental problems in the measurement of fatigue, and hence determining its prevalence in the community, primary care, and hospital. Nevertheless, the conventional epidemiological measure of prevalence remains an important part of descriptive research, and has been addressed by numerous studies. The question 'how common is fatigue?' must be answered by the word 'very'. Most surveys find that of all somatic symptoms only headache is more common, and in some fatigue occupies the top place. The precise prevalence of fatigue as determined by a number of studies is shown in Table 2.1. The estimates are not surprising given differences in definition.

Having any symptom is so common as to be almost normal. In one early survey, only 14 per cent of a community sample reported having no symptoms at all[7]. An American study of healthy university students taking no medication found that no fewer than 81 per cent had experienced at least one somatic symptom during the last three days[9]. During a six-week period normal American women reported at least one somatic symptom on 43 per cent of days – the figure for men being only slightly less at 31 per cent[34]. Of these symptoms, fatigue was either the commonest[9], or was second only to headache in frequency[34].

Of the numerous studies that have attempted to determine the prevalence of symptoms in the population two are worth considering in more detail. The first is the OPCS survey of psychiatric morbidity in the United Kingdom – the first national population-based study to date. Twenty-seven per cent of all adults (33 per cent of women and 22 per cent of men) reported significant fatigue in the week before interview[35]. The second is the Health and Lifestyle Survey[36] which is the most comprehensive population-based health survey to be carried out in the United Kingdom to date (Table 2.2). The sampling frame for the survey was the entire adult population of England, Wales, and Scotland, aged 18 and over. A random sample of 12 254 addresses was obtained. From this number 9003 agreed to be interviewed and to complete the 30-item General Health Questionnaire[37]. This large sample was found to be representative of the general population.

Table 2.2 Prevalence of fatigue: Health and Lifestyle Survey

Age	Males ($n = 3905$)		Females ($n = 5098$)	
	%	95% confidence interval	%	95% confidence interval
18–24	21.7	18.9–24.5	34.6	30.9–38.3
25–34	19.1	16.3–21.9	33.0	33.0–35.9
35–49	18.7	15.9–21.5	30.8	28.4–33.2
50–64	18.8	15.9–21.6	26.3	23.8–28.8
65 +	17.6	14.7–20.3	26.1	23.3–28.9
Total	19.0	17.7–20.1	29.8	28.5–31.0

Fatigue was assessed by the response to a single item included as part of a comprehensive self-report questionnaire – 'Within the last month have you suffered from any problems with always feeling tired?' Tiredness was found to be the second-most common symptom after headache and was more common than bad back, indigestion, nerves, or painful joints. We shall return to this survey when we discuss the influence of risk factors such as social class, age, psychological and physical morbidity later in this chapter.

The picture is similar in other countries. Fatigue or fatigability was the commonest symptom in both French and Algerian housewives[38]. In Germany 26.2 per cent of a population survey in Mannheim reported experiencing 'states of fatigue and exhaustion' during a seven-day period[39]. In the USA 24 per cent of a population sample reported excessive fatigue[40]. Twenty-nine per cent of Mexican Americans reported that everything was an effort, with 14 per cent saying the symptom had persisted for at least a week[41]. Seventeen per cent of Taiwanese report fatigue[42]. Of a community sample in Finland 16 per cent reported excessive tiredness[43], as did 14 per cent of an Icelandic birth cohort, even after excluding patients with psychiatric disorders[44].

Primary care

Given the frequency with which fatigue is encountered in the community, one would not expect every feeling of tiredness to be reported to the doctor. Of those identified as either tired or feeling 'very run down all the time' during the previous 14 days, less than one-fifth had brought the symptoms to medical attention[45]. How common, therefore, is fatigue in primary care?

There are several ways of answering this question. First, the prevalence of tiredness among all general practice attenders. Second, the number consulting for a specific complaint of fatigue. Third, the number labelled by the doctor as cases of 'fatigue'.

There have been several systematic studies addressing prevalence of fatigue in primary care in both Britain and the United States. Kroenke and colleagues[21] surveyed 1159 consecutive attenders at a US Army medical centre providing general care for US servicemen and their families, a sample which the authors regard as similar to civilian practice. Of those surveyed 24 per cent felt that fatigue was a 'major problem' for more than one month, the mean duration being 3.3 years. Of those surveyed in Australian primary care 24 per cent also reported prolonged fatigue[46], whilst another American survey, this time from Boston[19], found a point prevalence of 21 per cent for fatigue of six months' duration, associated with other somatic symptoms such as sore throat, myalgia, and headache. Of those attending an Israeli general practice 32 per cent reported at least one asthenic symptom[25].

In the UK the first systematic study of psychiatric illness in general practice was carried out in 1966 under the supervision of the late Michael Shepherd at the Institute of Psychiatry[47]. They found that 16 per cent of males and 24 per cent of females admitted to rising in the morning feeling tired and exhausted. Researchers from the same department 24 years later narrowed their enquiries to the specific topic of tiredness[6,48]. In a single general practice in South London 10.2 per cent of men and 10.6 per cent of women complained of feeling tired all or most of the time throughout the previous month.

Tiredness is also a common reason for medical consultation beyond the developed world. In a study in Senegal 29 per cent of attenders to primary care services complained of being easily tired, and 25 per cent felt tired all the time[49]. Tiredness was the commonest somatic symptom in Kenya[50], whilst 10 per cent of primary care attenders in Guinea Bissau complained of weakness, making it the fifth commonest symptom encountered[51].

These studies record the prevalence of fatigue in all attenders. Only a few of those will have actually consulted their doctor with a specific complaint of fatigue. Studies of the reasons given for presentation give a different perspective. From the patient's perspective 13.6 per cent of patients presented with fatigue in a single practice in Canada[52], with 6.7 per cent having it as a major problem, similar to the figure of 7.6 per cent found in French primary care[53]. Both the US National Ambulatory Care and the UK National Morbidity Surveys record the doctor's view of why patients consult. The 1985 American survey reported that 0.9 per cent of visits to primary care physicians were for a specific complaint of fatigue, making it commoner than 'cold', rash, headache, or chest pain. The demographic pattern of fatigued attenders resembled that found in community surveys – i.e. patients attending complaining of fatigue were more likely to be female, whilst there was no particular age distribution except that fatigue was uncommon before adolescence. Of those attending Australian primary care 1.3 per cent were similarly given a specific label of chronic fatigue, lethargy, or chronic tiredness[46]. In a British survey, when the definition was slightly widened to include lethargy, fatigue, 'being knackered', 'needing a tonic', and so on, and both as presenting and supporting symptoms, the prevalence rose to 7.5 per cent, in keeping with the patient-reported data. Comparing these figures with the prevalence of fatigue among all primary care attenders confirms Morrell's findings that although fatigue was an extremely common symptom, it was an unusual reason for medical consultation[31].

For most fatigued patients attending the general practitioner diagnoses other than fatigue are made – since although around 10 to 30 per cent of those attending primary care have significant fatigue lasting more than a few weeks, it is recorded as a 'diagnosis' in only 1 to 2 per cent of primary care consultations[53, 55–59]. For example, the penultimate UK National Morbidity Survey[58] included a category of 'malaise, fatigue, debility, tiredness'. New presentations, a measure of incidence, were 12 per 1000, and the total annual consultation rates were 17.9 per 1000. The National Morbidity Survey revealed that approximately 1 per cent of consultations were listed as 'malaise, fatigue, debility, tiredness'. As there were innumerable other diagnostic categories available, it is reasonable to assume that the general practitioner reserved this category for those in whom he was either only able to make a very tentative alternative diagnosis, or none at all.

We will consider the range of diagnoses made in fatigued patients in primary care in a later section, but for now it is sufficient to conclude that the majority of fatigued patients receive a diagnosis, either of physical or psychological disorders. What do we make of those without an explanation – approximately one-quarter in those studies that systematically examine all fatigued attenders, or alternatively the 1 per cent of all attenders who, in naturalistic studies, simply receive a 'fatigue' diagnosis? One explanation is that these cases represent missed examples of the same conditions affecting the majority for whom a confident diagnosis was made. The authors of the National Morbidity Survey considered this when they wrote 'many consultations for such symptoms as [fatigue] may be more indicative of other concerns of the patient, perhaps emotional or stress related'. Such explanations are akin to the 'hidden' burden of psychiatric illness in general practice[60], partly explained by the difficulties many doctors have in detecting psychological illness. However, this is only a partial, albeit important, explanation, since studies utilizing standardized interviews and/or questionnaires, in which such information bias is minimized, show that a considerable proportion of fatigue in population samples is not accompanied by conventional signs of psychological illness.

What happens to this group of patients? At present we can only speculate. It is reasonable to assume that the general practitioner may refer at least a proportion to hospital for further investigations, and some of the answers can be provided by studies looking at fatigue in hospital practice.

Hospital care

Observant clinicians have long noted the prevalence of fatigue among those attending, or admitted to, hospital. One of the standard neurology textbooks states that 'more than half of all patients attending a general hospital register a direct complaint of fatiguability or admit it when questioned'[61]. However, as Kurt Kroenke points out: 'Fatigue, dizziness, insomnia, constipation and various pain syndromes are among the leading complaints in ambulatory care. Research regarding common symptoms, however, is meagre'[62]. This was elegantly expressed in the title of a recent editorial – ' "minor" illness symptoms: the magnitude of their burden and of our ignorance'[63].

In an early paper Ffrench studied 1170 medical outpatients by questionnaire. Nine per cent reported 'tiredness, lassitude or exhaustion' as principal complaints[64]. Nearly 30 years passed before another systematic enquiry. Kroenke and Mangelsdorff looked at the records of 1000 patients seen in one general medical outpatients in an American hospital[62] (Fig. 2.3). The results were striking. Fatigue was the presenting complaint in 8 per cent of clinic attendances, second only to chest pain. Looking at all symptoms experienced by hospital attenders, the same group found that 33 per cent reported fatigue, making it the commonest overall symptom[65].

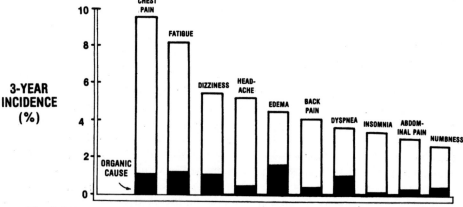

Fig. 2.3 'Symptoms in the general hospital' (from Kroenke and Mangelsdorff[62]).

No comprehensive surveys of medical practice have been conducted in the UK. British neurologists were asked to keep a log of all new patient consultations, and to record their diagnoses[66]. Five per cent were given the diagnosis of 'giddiness, fatigue', in addition to those felt to be suffering from either discrete neurological or psychological disorder. However, neurological diagnostic practice is variable – another survey found that the percentage of patients seen by neurologists whose illnesses were thought to lack organic basis varied from 0 to 80 per cent, with a median of 20 per cent, and the similar figures for illnesses thought to be psychological in origin varied from 1 to 90 per cent[67]. Despite the lack of systematic surveys, clinical impressions seem similar to those from the United States – a recent editorial considered that about half of those attending hospital clinics with a complaint of lassitude would be depressed or anxious, and that 'failure to diagnose depression is usually due to failure to seek it rather than to any confusion in diagnostic symptoms'[68].

What can be concluded from these surveys? Fatigue is common in hospital practice. A substantial minority will be readily diagnosed. The remainder are not so readily classifiable, but many will fulfil criteria for psychiatric disorders after detailed examination (although this will in practice be rarely performed in normal medical outpatient settings). This group may be considered as analogous to the 'hidden' psychiatric morbidity familiar from primary care studies. Finally, even after exhaustive examination, a minority remain without any satisfactory diagnosis. Cases of CFS are most likely to come from these last two categories.

2.4 Epidemiology and aetiology of fatigue

Sampling and bias

We have not drawn on the extensive literature concerning fatigue syndromes in this chapter for two reasons. First, because they are the subject of the middle section of this book. Second, because that literature does not contribute much in the way of epidemiologically sound observations. In the place of population-based studies which are the *sine qua non* of the epidemiological method are numerous, sophisticated, investigations of groups of patients encountered in hospital practice or specialist clinics. Unfortunately, there are several reasons why such samples cannot always yield reliable information about aetiology.

First, nearly all such samples contain an over-representation of severe, long-standing cases, who are more likely to be referred to hospital, or to join self-help organisations, the two principal sources of subjects for the majority of studies to date. Such cases will differ on a variety of factors, and any observed associations may explain not aetiology, but poor prognosis. The upper socio-economic groups are frequently over-represented, with a particular predominance of a few professions, such as teachers and doctors and an under-representation of ethnic minorities (see Chapter 7).

A different type of selection bias comes from studies of psychiatric morbidity. As the literature on irritable bowel syndrome shows, the presence of psychiatric morbidity is one reason for consultating a doctor and being referred to a specialist, and thus hospital samples might contain an excess of those with psychiatric problems, especially in those with more chronic or severe disorders

(Chapter 10). An opposite bias may result from a subject having a previous psychiatric history. In those with new-onset fatigue and a previous history of emotional disorders, the primary care doctor is more likely to diagnose a psychiatric condition, and to refer to a psychiatric, rather than a medical, specialist. In contrast, depressed patients with prominent fatigue and sleep difficulties are more likely to be referred to physicians than those with cognitive features such as guilt and suicidal ideation[69].

Third, hospital cases are usually long-standing. Recall of important events has been influenced by a variety of factors, such as memory, search after meaning, and, recently, the political climate surrounding the topic of CFS. All of these will lead to *recall* bias. Psychological state also influences recall – for example, depressed patients differentially recall unpleasant rather than pleasant events in their past.

Conventional epidemiological associations of fatigue

In the last section of this chapter we will consider the epidemiological associations of fatigue. We will restrict discussion at this stage to the conventional measures of gender, social class, and age. Other associations, in particular psychological or physical illness, as well as other variables such as exercise and sleep, will be considered in later chapters.

Epidemiological associations of fatigue: gender

A common finding in studies of fatigue is that women are more often affected than men. In the Health and Lifestyle Survey[36] 29.8 per cent of women reported feeling tired all the time for every day in the previous month, the equivalent figure for men was 18.9 per cent. Other studies are listed in Table 2.3. The absolute values listed in Table 2.3 are dependent upon the exact criteria used and the sample characteristics which differ markedly between studies, so the more meaningful comparisons are of the relative risks. Similar patterns are seen for symptoms such as inertia[70].

Not every study finds substantial gender differences. For example, the study by Tony David and colleagues[6] of a general practice in South London, failed to find a statistically significant sex difference in the overall rates of fatigue, although Morrell, in a nearby practice, had found a substantial over-representation of women[55]. Instead, David *et al.* did find that women were more likely to complain of tiring more easily and needing more rest. Similarly, a French-Canadian study also reported no significant gender excess for fatigue[52]. However, if one looks more closely the odds ratios for both studies (1.3) indicate a consistent female excess. Fuhrer and Wessely in their study of French primary care, were able to separate those presenting with fatigue from all fatigued subjects[53]. The odds ratios found for a principal complaint of fatigue, 1.2, were towards the lower end of the range, whilst those for any complaint of fatigue, 1.7, were towards the upper end of the literature.

Table 2.3 Gender differences in the prevalence of fatigue

Principal author(s)	Proportion fatigued: females (%)	Proportion fatigued: males (%)	Ratio female: male
Cathebras et al.[52]	15.2	11.2	1.4
Chen[71]	20.4	14.3	1.4
Hagnell et al[72]	31.0	21.0	1.5
Cox [et al.36]	29.8	18.9	1.6
David [et al.6]	12.0	9.0	1.3
Garcia and Marks[41]	29.6	29.3	1.0
Hammond[73]	45.7	33.0	1.4
Ingham and Miller (community)[23]	27.9	16.9	1.7
Ingham and Miller (primary care)[23]	44.6	28.5	1.6
Jenkins[74]	36.7	29.3	1.3
Kroenke [et al.21]	28.0	19	1.5
Montgomery[75]	10.9	6.9	1.6
Morrison[56]	16.8	6.9	2.4
Shepherd et al.[47]	18.0	10.7	1.7
Tarnopolsky et al.[76]	17.1	9.8	1.7

What are the possible explanations? First, is the gender difference the result of differences in illness behaviour? Women are greater users of medical services, especially for minor health problems[77]. However, this cannot explain the over-representation of females in population-based studies.

Second, all the studies listed in Table 2.3 are cross-sectional or prevalence studies, consisting of snapshots of the community taken at one time. We have already noted that the chances of any particular individual being included as a 'case' in such a cross-sectional survey increase with the length of time he or she has been fatigued ('prevalence bias'). Thus one possible explanation of these findings is that women do not become fatigued at any greater rate than men, but instead remain tired for longer. A brief communication from an American chronic fatigue clinic did indeed suggest this[78], whilst an Israeli study reported that the excess of women was most marked in those with chronic fatigue[25], although this was not confirmed by a better designed general practice survey[6].

Third, is the excess of fatigue in females explained by depression? One of the most robust findings in psychiatric epidemiology is that depressive disorders, however defined, are commoner in women than men. Depression is itself a strong association of fatigue (see Chapter 4). A secondary analysis of the National Health and Nutrition Examination Survey (NHANES 1) used logistic regression to model the effect of several different variables on the risk of fatigue in 2800 subjects[71]. The unadjusted data showed that women were 1.5 times more likely to be fatigued than men, but this disappeared when depression, anxiety, and emotional stress, were taken into account. Chen suggested that the higher rates of fatigue in women are actually due to their higher rates of other symptoms, largely psychological[71].

An alternative approach is to use the technique of stratification. If the higher rates of fatigue are due to the higher rates of psychological disorder in women, then stratifying (dividing) the sample into those with, and those without, psychological illness would result in an equal sex distribution for fatigue in both strata. In both the Health and Lifestyle Survey[36,79] and a community study in the south of England[12], stratification failed to account for the gender differences, and hence failed to confirm Chen's observations[72]. Likewise, even when fully adjusted for psychiatric disorder, being female was still associated with an increased risk of fatigue in the Epidemiologic Catchment Area data set[80].

Hence, simple explanations, such as illness behaviour, prevalence bias, and confounding by depressive illness are not complete explanations of the excess of women. What other reasons are possible? It is sometimes suggested that women have lower thresholds for reporting all symptoms, but this has not been confirmed[81]. Monica Briscoe found that women are more likely to express feelings, both positive and negative, than men[82]. Unlike women, men are more likely to express distress by a fall in positive feelings, rather than a rise in negative feelings, such as depression or fatigue. She concludes that the different degrees of affective response in females and males are underpinned by biological differences, but on which are superimposed additional social frustrations. It was noticeable than even in one of the few studies that failed to find substantial gender differences in fatigue[6], women were more likely than men to cite social explanations, such as family, as an explanation for their fatigue. In one of the classics of social psychiatry, Brown and Harris established that social circumstances, such as the lack of a confidante, lack of employment, and presence of young children, contributed to depression in women[83]. It seems very likely that similar relationships will be found for fatigue – for example, Jenny Popay found a relationship between fatigue symptoms in women and the presence of children under six[84]. At its simplest, women have many more reasons to feel fatigued than men[85].

In one of the best conducted studies in this area, Rachel Jenkins confined her study to a single grade of the British Civil Service, thus looking at samples of males and females that were closely comparable in terms of social class and work[74]. Sex differences in overall psychiatric morbidity disappeared. Jenkins argued that social factors affecting the role of women are a major determinant of gender differences in symptoms. Hence differences in the social environment and gender roles may play a part in explaining sex differences in fatigue – but even in Jenkins' study, in which social, employment, and family factors were carefully controlled for, women were still more fatigued than men.

Psychosocial factors are not the only explanations proposed in the literature, and both Briscoe and Jenkins consider the role of biological differences. Biological explanations have centred around the role of genes and hormones. Genetic explanations for depression have been most convincing for bipolar disorder (manic depression), yet bipolar disorder is the one category of affective disorder in which females do not appear to be at greater risk than males. The influence of hormones is more difficult to study – it is virtually impossible to make direct male–female comparisons, since such observations are totally confounded by other sex differences[86]. Nevertheless, in at least some disorders, such as post partum psychosis, the influence of hormonal changes on mood seem to be indisputable.

Epidemiological associations of fatigue: age

Overall, the prevalence of fatigue in the community shows little variation with age, with one exception. A striking feature is that fatigue is uncommon before adolescence (see Chapter 13). Once childhood has been successfully negotiated, nearly every study agrees that the prevalence of fatigue and related symptoms are relatively stable across adult life (see Table 2.2)[1,70]. However, there is more doubt about fatigue at the other extreme, old age. Two Swedish population studies reported a decline in the prevalence reporting general fatigue from middle age onwards, either in women only[3], or in men and women[87], but an American survey found the opposite, a steady increase from middle to old age[73]. In a US sample over half of a random sample of subjects over 65 had experienced tiredness during the previous month[88]. Just as in younger samples, many had not mentioned their symptoms to either families or doctors. One reason for the lack of consensus about the pattern of fatigue in old age, as opposed to childhood and adult life, is that the importance of physical illness as a cause of fatigue becomes more important.

Epidemiological associations of fatigue: social class

If one only considered fatigue syndromes, one might be forgiven for thinking that fatigue appears to be associated with higher social status, social class, or membership of the professional classes. Much of the current writings on chronic fatigue syndrome assume such a social class distribution, reflected in the term 'yuppie flu' (see Chapters 7, 15), although the idea that fatigue syndromes are commoner amongst the upper classes is nothing new (Chapter 5). However, population studies reveal a different story.

Data from the Health and Lifestyle Survey (Table 2.4) shows that fatigue is commoner in lower social classes, and thus displays a negative socio-economic gradient. This is confirmed by the results of the Epidemiologic Catchment Area Program in the USA[80]. Primary care studies in the United States and Scotland report that social class or education level, a customary marker for social class, were inversely correlated with fatigue[89,90]. In their study of fatigue in French general practice Fuhrer and Wessely[53] noted that fatigue as a symptom shows little variation by socio-economic status, and is no more common in upper social class groups – the highest group is again the least fatigued. Similarly, in Australian primary care fatigue is commonest in the lowest social class[46]. As we shall see later, it is only when considering fatigue as diagnosed by the doctor than an upper social class excess appears. Also, contrary to expectations, health workers appear no more fatigued than the rest of the population.[6,90].

Table 2.4 Prevalence of 'always feeling tired during previous month': Health and Lifestyle Survey[36]

Household socio-economic group	Males (%)	Females (%)
Professional, employers/managers	17.9	27.0
Other non-manual	17.8	29.1
Skilled manual	18.6	29.2
Semi- and unskilled manual	22.0	33.8

Part of the association with social class is because it acts as a proxy for social adversity. Being widowed, being unemployed, having young children at home, and living on a new housing estate were all associated with fatigue in primary care[88 – 91]. Other associations of chronic fatigue are equally predictable – in a community study it was commoner in those who were widowed, divorced, or separated.[45]

2.5 Conclusion

The experience of fatigue is extremely common, but all efforts to distinguish reliably between normal and abnormal tiredness are less than satisfactory. One way of separating 'normal' from 'abnormal' fatigue is to allow the individual to make that decision for him/herself, and regard it as abnormal only when the fatigued person becomes a patient. In that case abnormal fatigue also has certain characteristics. It is associated with more symptoms, particularly those of emotional distress, and with greater functional impairment. It is not, however, abnormal simply because it has been present for a longer period.

There is no simple solution to the measurement of fatigue in epidemiological studies. No objective 'fatigue test' will come to our rescue. Some of the problems can be partially overcome by using operational criteria, a necessary precursor to sound aetiological research. Operational criteria will not, however, completely overcome the problem of distinguishing between normal and abnormal tiredness.

However we chose to record it, fatigue is more common in women, and in lower socio-economic groups. It is relatively constant over the adult years. Finally, the literature also shows that fatigue is not just a frequent complaint in primary care, but is an important public health problem associated with disability comparable with that found in chronic medical patients[20,21,32].

References

1 US Dept of Health and Human Statistics. *National Ambulatory Medical Care Survey, USA: 1975–1981 and 1985 Trends.* Series 13, No 93. Hyattsville, Maryland, National Center for Health Statistics, 1988.

2 Barofsky I, Legros M. Definition and measurement of fatigue. *Rev. Infect. Dis.* 1991; **13 (suppl 1):** 94–97.

3 Tibblin G, Bengtsson C, Furunes B, Lapidus L. Symptoms by age and sex. *Scand. J. Prim. Care* 1990; **8:** 9–17.

4 Langer T. A twenty-two item screening score of psychiatric symptoms indicating impairment. *J. Health Human Behav.* 1962; **3:** 269–276.

5 Pinard G, Tetreault L. Concerning semantic problems in psychological examination. In Pichot P (ed.) *Psychological Measures in Psychopharmacology,* 1974: Vol.7 8–22.

6 David A, Pelosi A, McDonald E, *et al.* Tired, weak or in need of rest: fatigue among general practice attenders. *Br. Med. J.* 1990; **301:** 1199–1122.

7 Hannay D. Symptom prevalence in the community. *J. R. Coll. Gen. Pract.* 1978; **28:** 492–499.

8 Kellner R, Sheffield B. The one week prevalence of symptoms in neurotic patients and normals. *Am. J. Psych.* 1973; **130:** 102–105.

9 Reidenberg M, Lowenthal D. Adverse non-drug reactions. *N. Engl. J. Med.* 1968; **279:** 678–679.

10 Rose G, Barker D. What is a case? Dichotomy or continuum? *Br. Med. J.* 1978; **ii:** 873–874.

11 Goldberg D, Huxley P. *Common Mental Disorders: A Bio-social Model.* London, Tavistock, 1992.

12 Pawlikowska T, Chalder T, Hirsch S, Wallace P, Wright D, Wessely S. A population based study of fatigue and psychological distress. *Br. Med. J.* 1994; **308:** 743–746.

13 Cloninger, C.R. A systematic method for clinical description and classification of personality variants. *Arch. Gen. Psych.* 1987: **44:** 573–8.

14 Lewis G, Wessely S. The epidemiology of fatigue: more questions than answers. *J. Epidemiol. Commun. Health* 1992; **46:** 92–97.

15 Wells F. A neglected measure of fatigue. *Am. J. Psychol.* 1908; **19:** 345–358.

16 Dixon B. Scientifically Speaking. *Br. Med. J.* 1987; **294:** 317.

17 Ridsdale L. Chronic fatigue in family practice. *J. Fam. Pract.* 1989; **29:** 486–488.

18 Kleinman A. *Rethinking Psychiatry.* New York, Free Press, 1988.

19 Buchwald D, Sullivan J, Komaroff A. Frequency of 'chronic active Epstein Barr virus infection' in a general medical practice. *J. Am. Med. Assoc.* 1987; **257:** 2303–2307.

20 Nelson E, Kirk J, McHugo G, *et al.* Chief complaint fatigue; a longitudinal study from the patient's perspective. *Fam. Pract. Res.* 1987; **6:** 175–188.

21 Kroenke K, Wood D, Mangelsdorff D, Meier N, Powell J. Chronic fatigue in primary care: Prevalence, patient characteristics and outcome. *J. Am. Med. Assoc.* 1988; **260:** 929–934.

22 Ridsdale L, Evans A, Jerrett W, Mandalia S, Osler K, Vora H. Patients with fatigue in general practice: a prospective study. *Br. Med. J.* 1993; **307:** 103–106.

23 Ingham J, Miller P. Symptom prevalence and severity in a general practice population. *J. Epidemiol. Commun. Health* 1979; **33:** 191–198.

24 Manu P, Lane T, Matthews D. The frequency of chronic fatigue syndrome in patients with symptoms of persistent fatigue. *Ann. Int. Med.* 1988; **109:** 554–556.

25 Shahar E, Lederer J. Asthenic symptoms in a rural family practice: epidemiologic characteristics and a proposed classification. *J. Fam. Pract.* 1990; **31:** 257–262.

26 Angst J, Koch R. Neurasthenia in young adults. In Gastpar M, Kielholz P (ed.) *Problems of Psychiatry in General Practice.* Toronto, Hogrefe & Huber, 1991: 37–48.

27 Mann A, Jenkins R, Belsey E. The 12 month outcome of neurotic disorder in general practice. *Psychol. Med.* 1981; **11:** 535–550.

28 Anon. *Dorland's Illustrated Medical Dictionary,* 25th edn. Philadelphia, Saunders, 1974.

29 Armon C, Kurland L. Chronic fatigue syndrome: issues in the diagnosis and estimation of incidence. *Rev. Infect. Dis.* 1991; **13(suppl 1):** 68–72.

30 Dohrenwend B, Crandell D. Psychiatric symptoms in community, clinic and mental hospital groups. *Am. J. Psychol.* 1970; **126:** 1611–1621.

31 Morrell D, Wade C. Symptoms perceived and recorded by patients. *J. R. Coll. Gen. Pract.* 1976; **26:** 398–403.

32 Wessely S, Chalder T, Hirsch S, Wallace P, Wright D. The prevalence and morbidity of chronic fatigue and chronic fatigue syndrome: a prospective primary care study. *Am. J. Pub. Health* 1997; **87;** 1449–1455.

33 Wells K, Stewart A, Hays R, *et al.* The functioning and well-being of depressed patients: results from the Medical Outcomes Study. *J. Am. Med. Assoc.* 1989; **262:** 914–919.

34 Verbrugge L, Asione S. Exploring the iceberg: common symptoms and how people care for them. *Med. Care* 1987; **25:** 539–563.

35 Meltzer H, Gill D, Petticrew M, Hinds K. *The Prevalence of Psychiatric Morbidity amongst Adults Living in Private Households.* London, HMSO, 1995.

36 Cox B, Blaxter M, Buckle A, *et al. The Health and Lifestyle Survey.* London, Health Promotion Research Trust, 1987.

37 Goldberg D. *The Detection of Psychiatric Illness by Questionnaire.* Oxford University Press, 1972.

38 Brunetti P, Vincent P, Neves J, Benmami S. Epidemiological study of psychological status in French and Algerian samples. *L'encephale* 1982; **8:** 615–636.

39 Schepank H. *Epidemiology of Psychogenic Disorders; The Mannheim Study.* Berlin, Springer, 1987.

40 Kroenke K, Price R. Symptoms in the community: prevalence, classification and psychiatric comorbidity. *Arch. Intern. Med.* 1993; **153:** 2474–2480.

41 Garcia M, Marks G. Depressive symptomatology among Mexican-American adults: an examination with the CES-D scale. *Psychiatry Res.* 1989; **27:** 137–148.

42 Cheng TA. Symptomatology of minor psychiatric morbidity: a crosscultural comparison. *Psychol. Med.* 1989; **19:** 697–708.

43 Hyyppa M, Lindholm T, Lehtinen V, Puukka P. Self-perceived fatigue and cortisol secretion in a community sample. *J. Psychosom. Res.* 1993; **37:** 589–594.

44 Lindal E, Stefansson J. The frequency of depressive symptoms in a general population with reference to DSM-III. *Int. J. Soc. Psychol.* 1991; **37:** 233–241.

45 Wadsworth M, Butterfield W, Blaney R. *Health and Sickness: The Choice of Treatment.* London, Tavistock, 1971.

46 Hickie I, Koojer A, Hadzi-Pavlovic D, Bennett B, Wilson A, Lloyd A. Fatigue in selected primary care settings: socio-demographic and psychiatric correlates. *Med. J. Aust.* 1996; **164:** 585–588.

47 Shepherd M, Cooper B, Brown A, Kalton G. *Psychiatric Illness in General Practice,* 2nd edn. Oxford University Press, 1981.

48 McDonald E, David A, Pelosi A, Mann A. Chronic fatigue in general practice attenders. *Psychol. Med.* 1993; **23:** 987–998.

49 Diop B, Collignon R, Gueye M, Harding T. Diagnosis and symptoms of mental disorder in a rural area of Senegal. *African. J. Med. Sci.* 1982; **11:** 95–103.

50 Ndetei D, Muhangi J. The prevalence and clinical presentation of psychiatric illness in a rural setting in Kenya. *Br. J. Psychiat.* 1979; **135:** 269–272.

51 De Jong J, De Klein G, Horn S. A baseline study on mental disorders in Guinea-Bissau. *Br. J. Psychiat.* 1986; **148:** 27–32.

52 Cathebras P, Robbins J, Kirmayer L, Hayton B. Fatigue in primary care: prevalence, psychiatric comorbidity, illness behaviour and outcome. *J. Gen. Intern. Med.* 1992; **7:** 276–286.

53 Fuhrer R, Wessely S. Fatigue in French primary care. *Psychol. Med.* 1995; **25:** 895–905.

54 Jerrett W. Lethargy in general practice. *Practitioner* 1981; **225:** 731–737.

55 Morrell D. Symptom interpretation in general practice. *J. R. Coll. Gen. Pract.* 1972; **22:** 297–309.

56 Morrison J. Fatigue as a presenting complaint in family practice. *J. Fam. Pract.* 1980; **10:** 795–801.

57 Sugarman J, Berg A. Evaluation of fatigue in a family practise. *J. Fam. Pract.* 1984; **19:** 643–647.

58 OPCS. *Morbidity Statistics from General Practice; Third National Morbidity Survey,* 3rd edn. London, HMSO, 1985.

59 Wessely S, Chalder T, Hirsch S, Pawlikowska T, Wallace P, Wright D. Post infectious fatigue: a prospective study in primary care. *Lancet* 1995; **345:** 1333–1338.

60 Goldberg D, Williams P. *A User's Guide to the General Health Questionnaire.* Windsor, NFER-Nelson, 1988.

61 Adams R, Victor M. *Principles of Neurology*, 3rd edn. New York, McGraw Hill, 1985.
62 Kroenke K, Mangelsdorff D. Common symptoms in ambulatory care: incidence, evaluation, therapy and outcome. *Am. J. Med.* 1989; **86:** 262–266.
63 Komaroff A. 'Minor' illness symptoms; the magnitude of their burden and of our ignorance. *Arch. Intern. Med.* 1990; **150:** 1586–1587.
64 Ffrench G. The clinical significance of tiredness. *Can. Med. Assoc. J.* 1960; **82:** 665–671.
65 Kroenke K, Arrington M, Mangelsdorff D. The prevalence of symptoms in medical outpatients and the adequacy of therapy. *Arch. Intern. Med.* 1990; **150:** 1685–1689.
66 Hopkins A, Menken M, DeFriese G. A record of patient encounters in neurological practice in the United Kingdom. *J. Neurol. Neurosurg. Psychiat.* 1989; **52:** 436–438.
67 Mace CJ, Trimble MR. 'Hysteria', 'functional' or 'psychogenic'? A survey of British neurologists' preferences. *J. R. Soc. Med.* 1991; **84:** 471–475.
68 Havard C. Lassitude. *Br. Med. J.* 1985; **i:** 299.
69 Dew M, Dunn L, Bromet E, Schulberg H. Factors affecting help-seeking during depression in a community sample. *J. Affect. Disord.* 1988; **14:** 223–234
70 National Center for Health Statistics. *Selected Symptoms of Psychological Distress.* Hyattsville, Maryland, US Department of Health, Education and Welfare, 1970.
71 Chen M. The epidemiology of self-perceived fatigue among adults. *Prev. Med.* 1986; **15:** 74–81.
72 Hagnell O, Grasbeck A, Ojesjo L, Otterbeck L. Mental tiredness in the Lundby Study; incidence and course over 25 Years. *Acta Psychiat. Scand.* 1993; **88:** 316–321.
73 Hammond E. Some preliminary findings on physical complaints from a prospective study of 1,064,004 men and women. *Am. J. Pub. Health* 1964; **54:** 11–23.
74 Jenkins R. Sex differences in minor psychiatric morbidity. *Psychol. Med. Monogr.* 1985 **(supplement 7)**.
75 Montgomery G. Uncommon tiredness among college undergraduates. *J. Consult. Clin. Psychol.* 1983; **51:** 517–525.
76 Tarnopolsky A, Watkins G, Hand D. Aircraft noise and mental health: 1. Prevalence of individual symptoms. *Psychol. Med.* 1980; **10:** 683–698.
77 Verbrugge LM. Gender and health: an update on hypotheses and evidence. *J. Health Soc. Behav.* 1985; **26:** 156–182.
78 Matthews D, Lane T, Manu P. Gender differences among patients with chronic fatigue. *Clin. Res.* 1989; **37:** 320A.
79 Wessely S. The epidemiology of fatigue, MSc thesis, London School of Hygiene and Tropical Medicine, 1989.
80 Walker E, Katon W, Jemelka R. Psychiatric disorders and medical care utilisation among people who report fatigue in the general population. *J. Gen. Intern. Med.* 1993; **8:** 436–440.
81 Tousignant M, Brosseau R, Tremblay L. Sex biases in mental health scales: do women tend to report less serious symptoms and confide more than men? *Psychol. Med.* 1987; **17:** 203–15.
82 Briscoe M. *Sex Differences in Psychological Well-being.* Cambridge University Press, 1982.
83 Brown G, Harris T. *The Social Origins of Depression.* London, Tavistock, 1978.
84 Popay J. 'My health is all right, but I'm just tired all the time': women's experience of ill health. In Roberts H (ed.) *Women's Health Matters.* London, Routledge, 1992: 99–120.
85 Tierney D, Romito P, Messing K. She ate not the bread of idleness: exhaustion is related to domestic and salaried working conditions among 539 Quebec hospital workers. *Women's Health* 1990; **16:** 21–42.
86 Paykel ES. Depression in women. *Br. J. Psychiat.* 1991 **(suppl 10)** 22–29.
87 Essen-Moller E. Individual traits and morbidity in a Swedish Rural Population. *Acta Psychiat. Scand.* 1956 **(suppl 100)** 1–160.

88 Brody E, Klenban M. Physical and mental health symptoms of older people. Whom do they tell? *J. Am. Gerontol. Soc.* 1981; **24:** 442–449.

89 Valdini A, Steinhardt S, Jaffe A. Demographic correlates of fatigue in a university family health center. *Fam. Pract.* 1987; **4:** 103–107.

90 Lawrie S, Pelosi A. Chronic fatigue syndrome in the community: prevalence and associations. *Br. J. Psychiat.* 1995; **166:** 793–797.

91 Hare E, Shaw G. *Mental Health on a New Housing Estate.* Oxford University Press, 1965.

3. Physical mechanisms of fatigue

3.1 Introduction

This chapter is concerned with the mechanism of fatigue in health and disease. As we saw in Chapter 1, fatigue may be conceptualized as either a *decrement in performance* or as a *feeling*. This book is concerned with the latter definition of fatigue, and apart from a brief excursion into the physiology of muscle fatigue, the main focus of this chapter is on fatigue as a feeling.

As Chapter 1 emphasized, fatigue has many manifestations and may be apparent in many situations. Fatigue is familiar to everybody as a normal experience following physical exercise or after a sleepless night. Despite being troublesome, most people recognize the experience of fatigue in these situations as a passing nuisance – something essentially benign and self-limiting.

In other circumstances, fatigue becomes more pervasive, chronic, and disabling: from being a self-limiting irritant it becomes a symptom. To those with a medical training the most obvious causes for fatigue as a symptom are some of the physical and psychiatric disorders discussed in this and later chapters. However, we also emphasize the importance of less clearly defined states in causing fatigue, and examine the role of such states in the genesis of fatigue in physical and psychiatric disorders. For example, we will describe the role of sleep disorders and deconditioning as potential explanations for fatigue in physical disease. As the chapter unfolds we distinguish specific biomedical mechanisms from general factors common to many diseases, including sleep disturbance, pain, depression, and limitation of activities.

This chapter covers a wide range of topics, and it will become clear that fatigue is a non-specific symptom in the sense that it has many causes and associations. Furthermore, although it is nearly always possible to point to several potential mechanisms for fatigue in any one situation, it is very difficult to single out any one mechanism above all others. Our conclusion is that both as a symptom and as a decrement in performance, fatigue is multifactorial. Fatigue may perhaps be best understood as a final common neurobiological manifestation of physical or psychological stress.

From a clinical perspective, however, the main argument will relate to the relative importance of narrowly defined biological mechanisms versus a broader biopsychological conceptualization in the management of patients presenting with this common symptom.

3.2 Muscle fatigue

Muscle fatigue[1] refers to a *decrease in the force generated by muscles during a repeated neuromuscular task*. Unlike the sensation of fatigue, this phenomenon can be measured in animals as well as humans. Most of the studies reviewed here have defined and measured fatigue as a decrement in performance of a physical task over time. These studies do not (as we have seen in Chapter 1) tell us about the feeling of fatigue or about chronic fatigue states.

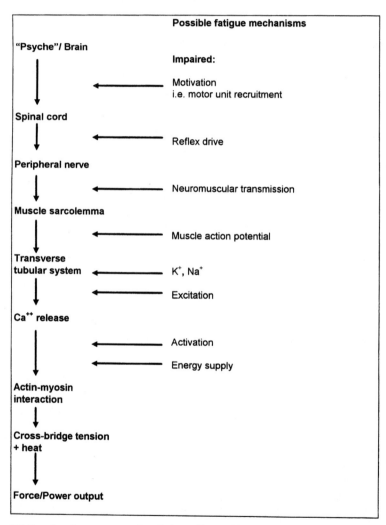

Fig. 3.1 Levels of neuromuscular fatigue (from Gibson, H.R. and Edwards, R.H.T. Muscular exercise and fatigue. *Sports Medicine* 1985; **2**: 120–132).

One key question to be repeated in this chapter is: 'where is the fatigue?' This has been perhaps the central question concerning neuro- and muscle-physiologists exploring fatigue. The generation of a voluntary muscular contraction involves a chain of processes (see Fig. 3.1). Starting at the level of the cerebral cortex, the nerve impulse is generated. This impulse travels down the upper motor neurone to the level of the relevant spinal segment and then passes through synaptic transmission to the lower motor neurone (LMN). The motor neurone then transmits to the muscle via the neuromuscular junction (NMJ) and the muscle is stimulated. Each LMN stimulates several muscle fibres, known collectively as a motor unit. The stimulation of the muscle fibre via the NMJ leads to the influx of calcium into the muscle and the generation of activated myosin. Activated myosin breaks down adenosine triphosphate (ATP) to adenosine diphosphate (ADP) and phosphate. It is this reaction which allows the formation of actomyosin and the contraction of muscle. In order for muscle to contract it requires an adequate supply of fuel: glycogen, glucose, and free fatty acids. Theoretically, fatigue may occur due to processes occurring at any level in this system. A recent important book on muscle fatigue[1] emphasizes this by grouping chapters according to the level of fatigue: from single muscle cells, to the brain. For example, fatigue may occur due to a failure of activation of the motor cortex, a failure of transmission of nerve impulses down the upper or lower motor neurone, failure of transmission at the level of the neuromuscular junction, or processes within the muscle itself. Fatigue may also be due to reduced energy supply to the muscle, or an inability of muscle to make use of available supply. Fatigue may be subdivided into central fatigue (which is fatigue demonstrated at the level of the upper motor neurone or above), and peripheral fatigue which involves fatigue in the LMN or below. Note that this definition of central fatigue is different to that frequently used in the clinical literature to describe certain symptoms such as difficulty concentrating, poor motivation, or slowed thinking.

Mechanisms for muscle fatigue

Even with fatigue used in this physiological sense, there are a variety of potential mechanisms within muscle. Decreased intracellular pH, changes in electrolytes such as potassium, and fuel alterations have all been proposed. Muscles use ATP to generate force. ATP is broken down to ADP and phosphate. ATP must then be regenerated and this require the oxidation of fuels. Muscle uses two main fuels: carbohydrates and lipids. The main source of carbohydrate is the glycogen stored within muscle. The main source of lipid is free fatty acid. Muscle may also use free plasma glucose and phosphocreatine, which is stored in muscle for short-term energy demands. The fuel used by muscle depends on several factors: oxygen supply, plasma free fatty acid concentrations, glycogen concentrations, and the duration and intensity of exercise. Light exercise (below 50 per cent of VO_{2max} – VO_{2max} refers to the maximum oxygen consumption of an organism and is a measure of energy intensity) is essentially aerobic and predominantly uses free fatty acids. In more intense exercise (60–90 per cent VO_{2max}), glycogen is used and energy supply is limited by pre-exercise glycogen levels. Athletes may improve performance, by exercising to exhaustion before an event, and then gorging on carbohydrates. This increases levels of stored glycogen and improves exercise endurance. At still higher levels of exercise (>100 per cent VO_{2max}) metabolism is anaerobic and there is an accumulation of lactic acid within muscle. Mechanisms of muscle fatigue are likely to vary according to the intensity of exercise. Newsholme et al.,[2] suggest, for example, that sprinting is limited by phosphocreatine depletion, middle-distance runners are affected by hydrogen ion accumulation (due to lactic acidosis), and long-distance running is limited by glycogen depletion.

High-intensity exercise is accompanied by hydrogen ion accumulation resulting in an intracellular fall in pH which has long been considered an important cause of fatigue. Much of the literature on intracellular pH and fatigue is contradictory. Allen et al.[3] have considered some of the reasons for this confusion. One problem is that whilst a fall in pH is seen in intense exercise and is therefore associated with fatigue, it is not a *necessary* cause of fatigue. For example, rare metabolic muscle diseases described in more detail below[4-6] involve rapid muscle fatigue in the absence of acidosis. Similarly, experimental preparations of single muscle fibres have demonstrated that fatigue occurs in the absence of acidosis, but is accelerated if acidosis is enhanced by blocking the lactic acid transportation system[7]. Other potential mechanisms of intracellular fatigue include levels of calcium and potassium ions[8].

Inborn errors of metabolism and muscle fatigue

Three inborn errors of metabolism have attracted attention because they are associated with muscle fatigue and the mechanisms – specific alterations in the use of fuel by muscle – are relatively well understood. They are of interest because of the specific pattern of the symptoms, summarized in Table 3.1. McArdle's syndrome is due to a lack of phosphorylase[5,9]. This enzyme is involved in the metabolism of glycogen. Affected individuals are unable to make use of muscle glycogen, but are able to metabolize glucose and free fatty acids. Sufferers are able to do low-intensity exercise, but the build up of ADP which results from higher intensity exercise (where they are unable to use glycogen to replenish ATP) leads to painful cramps. Since muscle can metabolize glucose in McArdle's syndrome, giving it to sufferers whilst they exercise improves their exercise endurance.

Table 3.1 Pattern of fatigue in three inborn errors of metabolism

Enzyme deficient	Fuel affected	Pattern of fatigue
Phosphorylase (McArdle's syndrome)	Glycogen	High-intensity exercise Improved with glucose
Phosphofructokinase	Glucose and glycogen	High-intensity exercise Worsened with glucose
Carnitine palimityltransferase	Free fatty acids	Low-intensity exercise Especially following fasting

Another rare inborn error is phosphofructokinase deficiency which prevents *all* carbohydrate use by muscle, including glucose. The pattern of exercise tolerated is similar to that seen in McArdle's syndrome except that giving glucose to people with phosphofructokinase deficiency makes their performance *worse*. This is because increased levels of glucose cannot be used by their muscles, and lead to decreases in plasma free fatty acids – the only fuel they can utilize[10].

The pattern of fatigue is completely different in a third rare metabolic disorder, carnitine palimityltransferase deficiency. This enzyme deficiency prevents use of long chain fatty acids. Individuals with this condition are able to exercise quite intensely, since they can make use of glycogen and glucose. Problems arise for them if they fast before exercise, or if they do prolonged low-intensity exercise which would normally depend on free fatty acid use. The final common pathway for all three syndromes is the build up of ADP in muscle and painful muscle cramps which may be associated with muscle damage. Note that the fatigue seen in these syndromes is closely associated with exercise and each syndrome has its own *specific* pattern of fatigue dependent on the type of exercise attempted. As we shall see this contrasts with other physical illnesses associated with fatigue where the relationship between fatigue and exercise is much less clear.

Fatigue at the neuromuscular junction and myasthenia gravis

The neuromuscular junction is not considered an important site of fatigue in normal individuals, but it is in a neuromuscular disease characterized by *painless* muscle fatigue called myasthenia gravis (MG). This usually has an autoimmune basis, the key abnormality being autoantibodies to the acetylcholine receptor on the motor end plate, which compete for the binding site with acetylcholine. This leads to a reduction of transmission at the neuromuscular junction. The most common symptom of MG is fatigue whose onset may be sudden or insidious. The muscle weakness is usually more severe in proximal muscles, and muscles enervated by cranial nerves are frequently severely affected. Fatigue in MG is usually more severe after exercise and at the end of the day. The course of symptoms is extremely variable, developing slowly over many years in some patients and rapidly in others. MG is an important differential diagnosis of chronic fatigue syndrome and misdiagnosis is common[11,12]. Important pointers to the diagnosis of MG are the involvement of cranial nerves, the absence of myalgia, physical signs such as ptosis, facial weakness, and reduced reflexes after exertion, and a reversal of symptoms and signs following the administration of anticholinesterases.

Central fatigue

There is no doubt that fatigue can be demonstrated in exercising muscle, although the exact mechanisms are not yet fully understood. Other potential sites are at levels above the neuromuscular junction. To demonstrate such fatigue (so-called central fatigue) one needs to show that stimulating the muscle leads to an improvement in performance. This implies one of two things: either the motor units are being stimulated submaximally or only a proportion of units in the muscle are being enervated.

To demonstrate central fatigue, volunteers are asked to contract a muscle, for example the quadriceps, for a fixed period of time and to maintain a fixed force in the muscle. Over time the force diminishes. If an electrical stimulus is applied to the nerve supplying the muscle at a level sufficient to cause tetany, any increase in the force generated would be seen as evidence of central fatigue[13]. Thus, any increase in force generation by the muscle is indicative of a failure of stimulation from levels above the neuromuscular junction. The implication of studies which demonstrate central fatigue is that the nerves supplying muscle are stimulating submaximally.

If central fatigue implies that the decrement in performance is not exclusively situated in the muscle, is it possible to locate its source elsewhere? In a series of recent experiments Gandevia and colleagues[14] have applied transcranial stimulation to the motor cortex during voluntary isometric contractions, and demonstrated that such stimulation is capable of overcoming force decrement. This implies that some of the loss of force in central fatigue is due to mechanisms at a level higher than the primary motor cortex. This finding begs the question whether this decrement in performance is due to reflex mechanisms – perhaps feedback from muscle mechanoreceptors operating at higher levels, or due to conscious processes. The 'volunteers' for these sorts of experiments tend to be highly motivated individuals, often working in the same laboratory as the investigators. Clearly motivation to maintain the muscular force is an important factor and one which will vary markedly between subjects. The next section deals with some of the findings regarding perception of effort during exercise.

Summary of muscle fatigue studies.

The clearest lesson this very brief review of fatigue in the neuromuscular system provides is that many levels and physical mechanisms may be involved. As Gandevia *et al.*[1] state:

. . . it is now widely accepted that sustained physical activity causes a reduction in the maximal force a muscle can exert due to the concurrent impairments of several (more of less) simultaneous processes which begin upstream of the motor cortex and go down to the myofibril.

In other words, the physiology of fatigue even in this narrow sense, is best understood as an integrated phenomenon: it is easy to find evidence that *one* part of the system is responsible for *some* aspects of fatigue in *some* experimental circumstances. However, there is no *single* underlying mechanism responsible for neuromuscular fatigue in all situations in healthy individuals.

3.3 Fatigue and exercise

The remainder of this chapter concerns fatigue as a sensation or symptom. The sensation of fatigue is closely associated with exercise. Recalling the first thought experiment in Chapter 1, imagine going on a five mile cross-country run. During the exercise you would experience a sensation of effort. This is likely to be under the influence of physical and psychological factors, for example, previous level of physical fitness, lactic acidosis, motivation, or the degree of pain suffered. Immediately after the run you would experience fatigue, which would increase over the next few hours. This sensation of fatigue, unlike that described elsewhere in this book, tends to be pleasant and passes after a good night's sleep. However, the next morning there may be considerable muscle pain and stiffness. These three phenomena – the sensation of effort during exercise, fatigue, and muscle pains afterwards are the subjects of this section. We shall also mention a rare fatigue syndrome affecting athletes: the 'overtraining syndrome'.

Perception of effort during exercise

Sports physicians frequently measure ratings of perception of effort (RPE) using the Borg scale[15], described in Chapter 1. There is an extensive body of literature on psychological, metabolic, and physiological factors which may affect RPE[16]. Metabolic factors include lactic acid production, hypoxia, and glycogen levels. Physiological factors include mechanoreceptor output from the exercising limb, heart rate, and respiratory effort. Psychological factors include aspects of personality and motivation as well as cognitive strategies used during exercise.

It is very difficult to interpret associations detected in research on perception of effort. During exercise a variety of different physiological and biochemical parameters change. These changes happen simultaneously, and as increasing levels of exercise are associated with increasing perceived effort, it is all too easy to correlate RPE with a physiological or biochemical marker of exercise intensity and then to propose a (spurious) casual relationship. One way around this is to study the same parameter in subjects with markedly different responses to exercise such as trained athletes and untrained controls.

An example of this sort of physiological experiment is a study by Demello *et al.*[17]. The level of training an individual has before performing exercise is likely to affect perception of effort. Trained athletes have higher exercise capacity indicated by higher VO_{2max} and lactate threshold (the point at which lactic acid reaches a certain concentration in the blood) indicating that they are capable of exercising harder. When subjects exercised it was found that for any per cent VO_{2max}, perceived effort was lower in trained subjects compared with those who were untrained. In other words, per cent VO_{2max} is unlikely to be a key determinant of RPE. However, lactate threshold was found to be closely correlated with RPE, with all subjects experiencing a similar level of exertion at the lactate threshold, despite the fact that the trained and untrained subjects were performing very different workloads at this point. Another study has indicated that increasing the buffering capacity of the blood by giving subjects sodium bicarbonate may reduce RPE for any level of exercise severity, again confirming the role of lactic acidosis in the sensation of effort[18].

There is no doubt that these sorts of metabolic factors play a role in determining the perception of effort in exercise. However, the nature of what is being measured (i.e. perception), would make it unlikely that metabolic factors were the sole mechanism. Perception is strongly influenced by context, and attentional style may play a role in determining RPE. This is well recognized by trainers in athletics who frequently work on focusing the athlete's mind rather than their body. There is some experimental evidence for the role of perceptual style in perception of effort. For example, distraction tends to increase RPE (the so-called 'dissociative style') and feedback information on performance may reduce it (so-called associative style; see Chapter 1)[19].

One theory of fatigue during exercise has been proposed by Newsholme and others[20]. This theory is of special interest as it may provide a link between central fatigue as described in the previous section and fatigue the symptom, described in future sections. The hypothesis is that exercise increases the brain's absorption of tryptophan. Tryptophan is an amino acid and precursor of the neurotransmitter serotonin. Increasing tryptophan levels should cause a rise in serotonin. Serotonin is involved in sleep regulation and there is some evidence to suggest it has a role to play in the pathogenesis of CFS and depression (see Chapter 11). Why should brain levels of tryptophan increase during exercise? First, there is competitive uptake of serotonin and aromatic amino acids into the brain. These amino acids are taken up by exercising muscle, so during exercise their levels fall[21], making the absorption of tryptophan easier. Second, tryptophan is transported in free and bound forms. During exercise the ratio of free to bound tryptophan increases due to increased free fatty acid levels which compete for albumin binding sites.

Evidence from the 1986 Stockholm marathon suggested that giving runners a drink rich in aromatic amino acids led to improved performance (at least for the so-called 'slow' runners, who completed in three to three and a half hours). Runners who were given the drink felt better during the race, and a subgroup of them showed some improvement in psychometric performance[22]. Further evidence for the role of serotonin in reducing performance and increasing sensations of fatigue comes from the finding that giving healthy subjects paroxetine (a serotonin-selective re-uptake inhibitor which increases central availability of serotonin), reduces their exercise capacity, without altering metabolic or cardiorespiratory responses[23]. There is also some evidence from the animal literature which supports a role for serotonin in the aetiology of fatigue[24,25]. These experiments show that whilst the organ involved in exercise is most obviously muscle, the sensation of fatigue involves central processes occurring in the brain.

Fatigue following exercise

Anyone who has done strenuous exercise will experience the sensation of fatigue a few hours after completing exercise. In contrast to fatigue as a symptom, this experience is often described as a pleasant sensation, and accompanied by sleepiness.

Exercise is associated with an increase in the stress hormones, adrenocorticotrophic hormone (ACTH) and cortisol[26]. These hormones change less in trained athletes than those who are untrained. This suggests that the hypothalamic–pituitary–adrenal axis (HPA) adapts to training, and it is possible that changes to these stress hormones are responsible for the sensation of fatigue following exercise. The decreased stress response associated with training might account for the reduced fatigue athletes feel compared to untrained individuals. Another possible mechanism is via the release of cytokines. The role of these hormones is discussed at the end of this chapter, and it is enough to say here that exercise is associated with an increase in blood levels of interleukin-1, interferons, tumour necrosis factor, and antitrypsin[27–29].

Delayed-onset muscle soreness

Anyone who attempts unaccustomed levels of exercise will experience muscle tenderness, which usually starts a matter of hours following the exercise and continues for several days following it, reaching a peak at 24–48 hours and subsiding over the next three to five days. This phenomenon is referred to as delayed-onset muscle soreness in the sports medicine literature. It is germane to chronic fatigue and CFS because myalgia following exercise is a prominent symptom of CFS, frequently seen as evidence of relapse. The acute effects of exercise have been reviewed elsewhere[30].

The exercise which most commonly leads to muscle pain is eccentric exercise. This occurs when a muscle is forcibly extended during activation, for example in the quadriceps when one walks downhill. It is for this reason that activities such as hill walking or skiing are associated with considerably more muscle soreness than cycling, which involved predominantly concentric contractions. A variety of structural and functional changes are seen following exercise and these are thought to reflect muscle damage. Muscle proteins such as creatine kinase, which may be used as markers of cell damage, are raised following exercise[31]. There is evidence from histological studies that exercise is associated with ultrastructural changes to muscle cells. Further, magnetic resonance imaging and spectroscopy studies have demonstrated changes indicative of cell damage. The delay associated with pain and tenderness following exercise and the associated swelling suggests that delayed-onset muscle soreness is due to an inflammatory response to cell damage.

One notable aspect of delayed-onset muscle soreness is that the same severity of exercise leads to less intense pain if it is repeated several times. Thus Newham *et al.*[31] found that healthy subjects who were asked to perform eccentric exercise on three occasions in a two-week period, had the worst pain after the first episode. Creatine kinase levels (which indicate muscle damage) were raised after the first, but not following subsequent bouts of exercise. Strength fell after each episode and did not recover to previous levels. This implies that training may protect against delayed-onset muscle soreness and that deconditioning associated with rest is likely to lead to the sensation at a lower intensity of exercise.

Another important aspect of delayed-onset muscle soreness is that the pain is not usually described as especially unpleasant. This is surprising since the pain may be intense and severe enough to render the sufferer incapable of climbing stairs for several days. MacIntyre *et al.*[30] used a visual analogue scale to assess both the intensity of soreness and the unpleasantness of pain in subjects who performed eccentric quadriceps exercises. Scores of unpleasantness were considerably lower than for the pain itself, a finding which is unusual: most pain is perceived – almost by definition – as something unpleasant. The conclusion these investigators made was that delayed-onset muscle soreness was perceived as less unpleasant than other pain because it was *expected*, and most people recognized it as something familiar and transitory. The implication of this is that any alteration of expectations – for example, that the pain was evidence of a sinister underlying disease process – would lead to it being perceived as considerably more distressing. This fits in with other models of symptom perception which demonstrate, for example, the importance of previous expectations on whether the physical symptoms of hyperventilation are experienced as pleasant or distressing[32]. This theme will be further explored in Chapter 12.

The overtraining syndrome

A well-recognized consequence of physical training in athletes is the overtraining syndrome[33–35]. The process of physical training involves a gradual incremental increase in exercise with scheduled periods of rest. This process is referred to as 'overload' as it is accompanied by acute fatigue, which in normal circumstances is self-limiting. Overtraining occurs when this fatigue becomes chronic and there is an objective fall in performance. It is seen as a consequence of failed adaptation to the stress of training. To make the diagnosis, performance has to have fallen over a two-week period in the absence of any physical ailments, apart from common infections[33].

Overtraining syndrome has a multitude of symptoms[35]. Many of these are non-specific and show considerable overlap with those of CFS. The cardinal features are fatigue with accompanying loss of performance. Other symptoms include headache, joint and muscle pains, loss of appetite, loss of co-ordination, gastrointestinal symptoms, depression, anxiety, low self-esteem, and poor concentration. It is widely claimed that the overtraining syndrome is associated with minor infections. More severe physical associations are recognized, such as ECG changes, and rhabdomyolysis (a severe form of muscle damage).

Finding a single pathophysiological pathway to explain the association between heavy physical training and this multitude of symptoms is not easy. This is partly because it is difficult to separate the physiological effects of proper training from those of over-training, and it is often difficult to establish a clear direction of causality. One theory suggests that overtraining syndrome is a hypothalamic disorder. Normal training is associated with changes to the hypothalamic–pituitary–adrenal axis consistent with mild hypercortisolism[26]. Overtraining syndrome is associated with a number of hormonal changes including attenuation of the stress response of growth hormone, and ACTH and cortisol to insulin[36] and this is reversed after rest. Other researchers have noted a reduction in plasma cortisol levels in overtraining[37]. In Chapter 11 we shall examine the possible role of the hypothalamic–pituitary–adrenocortical axis in the aetiology of CFS.

3.4 Fatigue, sleep, and sleep disorders

'I didn't get much sleep and I feel so tired!' Certainly sleep often relieves fatigue and fatigue and tiredness are commonly experienced as a result of disturbed or missed sleep. It is therefore reasonable to ask whether problems with sleep contribute as important causes of fatigue. The role of abnormalities of sleep in causing specific fatigue syndromes will be examined in Chapter 11.

The nature of sleep

First we must what ask: what is sleep? Of course we all know what it is in so far as we all do it. A more precise description, however, is of a rhythmic diurnal pattern of reduced activity and responsiveness, accompanied by physiological changes, especially in the brain[38]. We appear to require regular sleep in order to function, although the precise reasons for this remain unclear. As Horne has remarked, despite 50 years of sleep research many people feel that all we can conclude about the function of sleep is that it overcomes sleepiness. However, if there is a more optimistic conclusion it is that studies suggest that the organ most needy of sleep for its continuing function, and most affected by inadequate sleep, is the brain[38].

Measurement of sleep

By its nature sleep is relatively inaccessible to study. Studies of sleep must rely either on the report of the sleeper (with the obvious limitation that they will be unconscious most of that time) or on objective measures. The simplest objective measures are observable behaviour during sleep and sleep duration. Such observations indicate that sleep is not a homogeneous state, and that two main types of sleep are distinguishable. One type is associated with rapid movements of the eyes and loss of muscle tone (and is associated with reports of dreaming). This is called rapid eye movement (REM) sleep. The other type is not associated with these characteristics and is called (somewhat unimaginatively) non-REM (NREM) sleep[38].

In order to go beyond subjective reports, physiological measures are required. The principal investigatory tool of the sleep researcher is the electroencephalogram (EEG). This measures the gross electrical activity of the brain by amplifying electrical signals recorded from the scalp. In sleep research it is usual to also include measures of muscle tone and eye movements – the complete record being referred to as a polysomnograph[39]. Polysomnographic records reveal that the EEG of REM sleep is characterized by relatively fast EEG waves, whereas the other part of sleep (NREM sleep) is characterized by slower waves.

Sleep researchers have used the combination of wave frequency, muscle tone, and eye movement to create a convention for describing sleep. This scheme divides sleep first into REM and NREM, and then subdivides NREM into four types or stages depending on the wave frequency of the EEG. The stages with the lowest-frequency waves (3 and 4) are conventionally termed slow-wave sleep (SWS) or delta sleep.

Sleep not only has different components but also has a structure. The sleep stages described normally occur in orderly sequence in a cyclical pattern approximately every 90 minutes punctuated by periods of REM sleep. The proportion of sleep occupied by the REM phase increases and SWS decreases as the night progresses. The stages of sleep are shown in Table 3.2. These stages of sleep can also be graphically portrayed on a chart or hypnogram. An example of a normal hypnogram is shown in Fig. 3.2.

Table 3.2 Stages of sleep, EEG changes, and relative time spent in each

Type	EEG	Proportion of sleep (%)
REM (rapid eye movement)	Similar to stage 1	20–25
NREM (non-REM)		
Stage 1	Transition from wake to sleep	5
Stage 2	Sleep spindle and K complexes	50
Stages 3 and 4	Slow waves	10–20

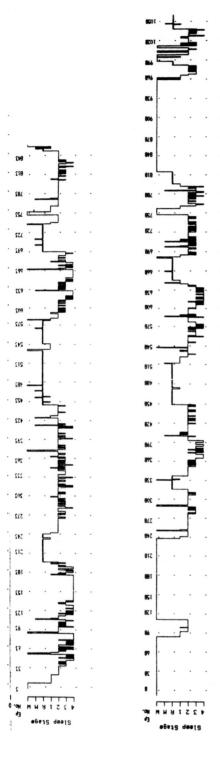

Fig. 3.2 Sleep hypnograms. The time elapsed from when the person signalled his/her intention to go to sleep in along the top. Sleep stages 1–4, rapid eye movement sleep (R), awake (W), and movements (M) are indicated on the left of the trace. The top trace is the hypnogram of a healthy person and the bottom trace the hypnogram of a patient with CFS.

Fatigue and sleepiness

Before considering the association of sleep and fatigue it is important to be precise about what we mean by fatigue. Fatigue is a complex phenomenon (see also Chapter 1). When reviewing the research literature concerning sleep and fatigue we must first distinguish between fatigue as impaired performance and fatigue as a subjective feeling. Then within subjective fatigue we must differentiate 'lack of energy' from the desire to go to sleep, usually called 'sleepiness'[40]. When assessing subjective fatigue it is particularly important to clarify whether the complaint is predominantly one of lack of energy or one of sleepiness as we will see below.

Sleep disorder and sleep abnormality

Sleep then has a duration, distinguishable components, a structure, and a place in the person's circadian rhythm. We are therefore interested not only in the total amount of sleep but also in the effect of disruption of sleep, selective loss of the components of sleep, and changes in its timing. In order to address these questions we will first consider the association of fatigue with each of the most relevant clinically defined sleep disorders. We will first review the association of fatigue with recognized clinical sleep disorders and second, review studies in which the effect of experimental manipulation of sleep on fatigue has been examined.

Types of sleep disorder

There are two principal classifications of sleep disorders; the International Classification of Sleep Disorders[41], and DSM-IV[42]. These use a combination of the patient, complaints and the (presumed) cause as the basis for classification. The main types of complaint and the categories of causes used in DSM-IV[42] are shown in Table 3.3. In order to consider the effect of sleep on fatigue we will focus on those sleep disorders that are uncomplicated by other conditions. These so-called primary disorders are listed in Table 3.4.

Table 3.3 DSM-IV classification of sleep disorders

A. By presumed aetiology

Primary	None of aetiologies below apply
Related to mental disorder	Often depression or anxiety-related
Related to medical condition	Direct physiological effect of medical condition
Substance-induced	Associated with current or recent substance use

B. By sleep complaint

Dyssomnia type: disturbance in amount, quality, or timing of sleep

Insomnia	Difficulty falling asleep, staying asleep, or feeling unrefreshed next day
Hypersomnia	Excessive duration of nocturnal sleep or sleepiness during the day

Parasomnia type: abnormal behavioural events in relation to sleep

Table 3.4 Primary dyssomnias

Primary insomnia
Primary hypersomnia (including narcolepsy)
Breathing-related sleep disorders (including obstructive sleep apnoea)
Circadian rhythm sleep disorder (including jet lag)
Others (including periodic limb movement disorders and restless legs syndrome)

Insomnia

People with insomnia complain of daytime fatigue that they attribute to inadequate sleep. The sleep complaints are typically difficulty in getting to sleep or staying asleep. An episode of insomnia is reported by as many as half of all adults in a one-year period[43]. A typical polysomnographic record may be normal, or may show disturbance of sleep continuity. Insomnia may be of unknown cause and is then referred to as primary. It is, however, very frequently associated with depression and anxiety[44,45] or with other medical conditions, particularly those associated with pain[46]. Certain substances such as excess coffee and alcohol intake can cause poor sleep.

It should, however, not be assumed that the sleep disturbance of patients with insomnia is the sole or even principal cause of fatigue. For example, the fatigue may be more closely related to the degree of 'trait' anxiety and to other somatic symptoms than to the sleep disturbance[47,48].

Hypersomnia

In hypersomnia, fatigue is associated with an excessive need for sleep (normal or long nocturnal sleep periods and daytime naps). The fatigue is predominantly a feeling of *sleepiness* and can be measured objectively in terms of the time to fall asleep in standard conditions[49]. The pattern of the sleep EEG may be normal or may show fragmented sleep. The population prevalence is about 3 per cent[50], and whilst some cases are primary, depression is a strong association. Hypersomnia is especially associated with depression in young persons[51], bipolar depression[52], and so-called atypical depression[53] In such cases fatigue is at least as likely to be caused by the depressive process as by the sleep abnormality[54].

Narcolepsy

The hallmark of this condition is irresistible daytime sleepiness resulting in napping. Other characteristic symptoms include cataplexy (sudden loss of muscle tone associated with emotion) and sleep paralysis (total muscular paralysis at sleep onset or awakening). The sleep EEG may show fragmented sleep and increased REM sleep. It has a prevalence of approximately 0.5 per cent in the general population. Narcolepsy is important to detect clinically because it is potentially treatable (but not curable) with stimulant drugs[55].

Obstructive sleep apnoea

This is the most important of the breathing-related sleep disorders. Patients with obstructive sleep apnoea may present with fatigue associated with insomnia (interrupted or unrefreshing sleep). Daytime sleepiness is prominent, however[55]. It occurs in up to 10 per cent of the adult population and is much more common in males, especially those who are overweight. Polysomnographic recording with continual measurement of arterial oxygen saturation shows that sleep is repeatedly interrupted ('fragmented') by obstruction of the upper airway and hypoxia. Associated features are loud snoring and morning headache. Treatment is by dieting or by maintaining the airway at night using continuous positive airway pressure (CPAP). This may relieve daytime sleepiness but is often poorly tolerated[56].

Circadian rhythm sleep disorder

These disorders are characterized by feeling of fatigue and insomnia in circumstances where there is a mismatch between the individual's endogenous sleep–wake cycle and actual sleep–wake pattern[42]. It may also be caused by time zone travel, shift working, or simply chaotic sleeping habits. Polysomnographs of such individuals may be normal or show disturbance sleep continuity[57]. The fatigue generally improves when the sleep pattern is normalized. There is also some evidence that the sleep and fatigue can be improved by light therapy in circumstances where such sleep disruption is inevitable – such as persons working on NASA space shuttle missions[58].

Restless legs and periodic limb movements

These conditions are associated with disturbance of sleep and daytime fatigue. Patients with restless legs suffer from an unpleasant feeling in their legs at night relieved by moving them. Such symptoms occur to a mild degree in as many as 5 per cent of the population – severe symptoms are less common[59].

Periodic limb movements are episodic repeated involuntary brief movements of the legs that can disrupt sleep[60]. The disorder can be primary or can be associated with a variety of medications and conditions. In both cases sleep EEG may be fragmented. Restless legs may be diagnosed by the patient's complaints but periodic limb movements may require nocturnal EMG recording.

What do experiments tell us about sleep and fatigue?

In clinically defined sleep disorders it is difficult to know whether daytime fatigue is due to the abnormality of sleep itself or to the cause of the sleep disturbance. Furthermore several parameters of sleep may be disrupted simultaneously – for example in insomnia, reduced sleep duration is often confounded with disrupted sleep. We therefore need to perform experimental manipulations of sleep to determine the effect on fatigue of specific changes in sleep. The main types of experiment are listed in Table 3.5.

Table 3.5 Experimental manipulations of sleep

Deprive of sleep
Allow prolonged sleep
Alter timing of sleep in circadian rhythm
Disrupt sleep

Reduction in sleep duration

It is a common experience that going to bed late or getting up very early leads one to feel more tired the next day, and it has long been noticed that fatigue states are similar to those induced by sleep deprivation[61]. Junior hospital doctors provide a natural experiment in the effects of sleep deprivation (let us ignore any cries of 'never did me any harm!'). Studies certainly confirm that junior doctors feel fatigued and sleepy after long periods 'on call'[62], but do sleepless nights affect performance the next day? The answer is 'yes and no'. Assessments of performance of junior doctors and earlier experiments in aircraft pilots show that motivated individuals can go on for incredibly long periods without sleep and yet still make physical efforts and solve complex problems. Any deficit in performance appears in routine, prolonged, and repetitive tasks[62].

Laboratory experiments in which subjects are deprived of sleep under controlled conditions reveal similar findings. Some of these experiments have been truly heroic; an experiment conducted in the late 1960s in Los Angeles required that volunteers stayed awake for over a week. To ensure that they did so they were paid on a sliding scale – the amount increasing with time spent without sleep. This and other studies show that sleep-deprived subjects feel fatigued and sleepy! In addition, tests of cognitive and motor function find that the subjects report increased subjective effort but relatively small objective deficits in cognitive and physical performance[63–66].

Increase in sleep duration

The finding that a reduction in sleep duration causes fatigue is perhaps not surprising. What about an increase in sleep duration? Observational studies of longer sleepers find that they often report more fatigue on those occasions when they sleep in. In a much cited study, Globus[67] gave questionnaires to nurses and found that they often slept in for several hours in the morning! On these occasions they rated themselves as more fatigued, less alert, and having impaired concentration for several hours after waking. He termed this the 'worn-out syndrome' (see also CFS fibromyalgia, and sleep in Chapter 11). This observation has been extended by experimental alterations of sleep duration in which volunteers are encouraged to sleep as long as they wish, and report an increase rather than a decease in fatigue[51,68].

Abnormal sleep–wake cycle

We all know that a disturbance in our normal sleeping pattern can make us feel sleepy and fatigued, and many of us have suffered the consequences of so-called jet lag[69]. A systematic study of healthy university students found that those with irregular sleep habits experienced more daytime fatigue[70]. In experimental studies Taub found that manipulations of the timing of sleep in the 24-hour cycle caused a feeling of fatigue and sleepiness and also impaired performance on vigilance tasks. These findings were independent of the total amount of sleep[71] and were therefore attributed to the timing of sleep. He also found that such changes in the pattern of sleep caused discontinuity and fragmentation of sleep on the sleep EEG[57].

Disrupted sleep

There is an association between the amount of disruption and fragmentation of the sleep EEG pattern and daytime fatigue and sleepiness[72]. Experimental studies have investigated this association by deliberately disrupting sleep[73]. One night of experimentally induced brief awakenings of healthy subjects using a noise tone every two minutes, not only makes subjects fatigued and sleepy the next day, but also has an effect on their performance in tasks requiring sustained attention[73]. A much cited experiment examined the effect of selective disruption of either NREM (stage 4) or REM sleep using a similar technique but also co-ordinating the noise with the appropriate sleep stage on the sleep EEG. Both groups reported fatigue but those who had stage 4 sleep disrupted were more symptomatic – experiencing more aches and being more profoundly fatigued.[74]

Sleep and fatigue: conclusion

It seems obvious that if we miss sleep we feel generally tired and lethargic, have less inclination toward activity, and difficulty with concentration. On the whole, the research literature confirms that conclusion. It also tells us that too much sleep, sleep at the wrong time, and broken or fragmented sleep can also make us feel tired. In fact it seems that any disturbance of sleep can result in fatigue. There is some evidence that slow-wave sleep is the most important for cerebral recovery and perhaps for relieving fatigue.

The fatigue produced by sleep disturbance is usually strongly coloured by a feeling of sleepiness rather than simply lack of energy. Subjective effort is increased and performance is subtly reduced in both mental and physical tasks. In most clinically encountered fatigue states, sleep has a part to play – but is rarely the whole story.

3.5 Fatigue and inactivity

Bedrest was an important treatment for many diseases in the first half of this century, but its harmful effects have been appreciated for at least 50 years[75–77]. Medically ill patients confined to bed were noted to be especially at risk of bedsores, chest infections, deep venous thrombosis and pulmonary embolus, muscle contractions and stiffness, urinary retention and calculi, constipation, retention of faeces, demoralization, and 'dismal lethargy'. Since then a combination of human and animal experiments have been able to demonstrate the specific effects of inactivity. Reduced activity, whether secondary to injury, immobilization, or simple disuse, results in profound alterations in most bodily systems, and appears to be a potent cause of fatigue. For current purposes it will be sufficient to focus on the effects of rest to muscles, heart, and mind (see Table 3.6).

Table 3.6 Effects of deconditioning

---

1. Muscular effects:
   Reduced muscle bulk
   Reduced turnover of proteins
   Atrophy of type I fibres
   Reduced muscle strength

2. Cardiac effects:
   Reduced blood volume
   Increased heart rate and decreased stroke volume
   Reduced VO_{2max}

3. Psychological effects:
   Reduced desire to perform activity
   Increased sensations of fatigue on exercise
   Sleep disturbance
   Depression

Muscle changes

Immobilization leads to structural changes in muscle. Animal experiments can show reduced muscle bulk following hind leg suspension in rats[78]. Reduced muscle protein turnover has been shown in humans after prolonged quadriceps immobilization and some reduction is detectable within six hours of immobilization[79]. Muscle histology alters, too, with atrophy especially affecting type I (slow twitch) muscle fibres[80] which are involved in maintenance of posture. Muscle function studies reflect these structural changes. Young healthy males may lose as much as 20 per cent of muscle strength after immobilization[81].

Cardiovascular changes

Effects of immobilization on cardiac function are also profound. An early experiment[82] submitted five young physically healthy men to three weeks' bedrest and found that blood volume decreased by 9 per cent and performance on a bicycle ergometer was reduced with increased heart rates. Saltin *et al.*[83] restricted five young fit males subjects to 20 days' strict bedrest. Two of the subjects were trained athletes whereas the remainder led sedentary lifestyles as students. Whilst most conventional measures of respiratory function were unchanged, there were important changes in cardiac function. Resting cardiac output remained the same, but when the subjects attempted exercise, stroke volume was reduced, heart rate increased, and overall cardiac output fell. These changes were accompanied by a reduction in plasma volume, and total oxygen consumption (a measure of exercise capacity) fell by approximately 25 per cent during this time. Subsequent work has replicated these results: one study[84] described the effects of ten days' bedrest. Bedrest was accompanied by a fall in VO_{2max} and anaerobic threshold, (the highest work rate achieved without lactic acidosis). These effects may take several weeks to reverse[85].

Psychological changes

These physiological effects of bedrest are mirrored by psychological ones: Zorbas and Matveyev[86] reported the effects of 120 days' hypokinesia on four physically healthy men. This led to a reduced desire to perform physical activity. Following the experiment, they all reported increased fatiguability of muscles, and a sensation of heaviness, clumsiness, and muscle pain. It is easy to appreciated how a vicious cycle could become established in inactive subjects, by which the symptoms caused by inactivity lead to further avoidance of exercise (Fig. 3.3). Another study demonstrated that normal volunteers who remain immobile for one week develop impaired neuropsychological function and EEG changes[87]. Sleep is also affected in prolonged bedrest: with alterations in sleep architecture and alterations in the balance of light as opposed to heavy sleep stages[85].

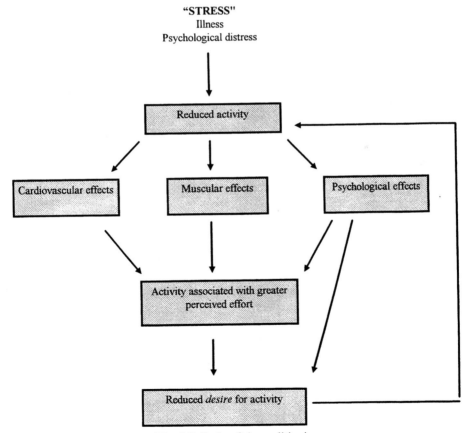

Fig. 3.3 Cycle of deconditioning.

These observations have led to physical activity being evaluated as a possible treatment for depression. In an overview of 10 randomized controlled studies of physical activity in depression, Martinsen[88] concluded that it was as effective as control interventions such as relaxation or brief psychotherapies. These studies are all small and suffer from not being able to determine the 'active ingredient' – if any – in exercise. The effect may be more to do with improved mastery than any physiological mechanism. Aerobic training, for example, does not appear to be a prerequisite: any exercise seems beneficial.

Inactivity is of course a consequence of many illnesses. It may also be a risk factor for future symptoms and disability. In an important study Stewart *et al.*[89] assessed levels of activity in a number of illnesses, including hypertension, heart failure, myocardial infarction, diabetes, and depression. They noted the degree to which low levels of physical activity at baseline predict problems two years later. They found that low levels of physical activity predicted poor outcome in terms of physical functioning, emotional problems, social activity, fatigue, pain, and sleep disorder. The results were not statistically significant for all outcomes and diseases, but the overall pattern was very clear: low levels of physical activity in these conditions predict future disability and symptoms.

In summary, lack of exercise is associated with changes in muscle and cardio-vascular physiology shown in Table 3.6. These changes are accompanied by a reduced drive to exercise, subjective fatigue, and other changes in mood. We speculate that lack of exercise is associated with depression, and exercise may be used as a treatment for depression. Lack of exercise is also associated with a poor outcome in patients with specific physical and psychiatric disorders. The remainder of this chapter is devoted to exploring this relationship between physical illness and fatigue in more depth.

3.6 Fatigue and physical illness: introduction

We will see elsewhere in this book that there is an important disparity between patients' and their doctors' perceptions of the importance of fatigue as a symptom. This is reflected in the sparse literature on physical diseases and fatigue. Many of the papers on this subject comment on how common and disabling fatigue is as a symptom is, and bemoan the small output of medical research on the subject. For example, one review of the cancer literature[90] performed a MEDLINE search from 1980 to 1991 and found only nine papers with fatigue and cancer together in the title. All but one of these papers were in the nursing literature. The same paper noted that fatigue is one of the most common and universal symptoms of cancer. Another paper illustrates the same phenomenon in multiple sclerosis (MS)[91]. The symptom is common, disabling, and yet is frequently ignored in the literature on symptoms in MS. There are probably several reasons for this; the most obvious being that fatigue is universal, and therefore non-specific, and of little diagnostic interest. A related reason is that due to its very ubiquity it becomes an expected consequence and therefore there is little interest in understanding the mechanisms of this symptom.

Table 3.7 Physical illness and fatigue: potential mechanisms

1. Specific biological mechanisms: disease activity and treatment
2. General mechanisms:
   Effects of deconditioning
   Effects of psychiatric disorder and psychological symptoms
   Effects on sleep
   Effects of pain

There are no shortage of candidate mechanisms for fatigue in physical illness (see Table 3.7). First there are general factors which are non-specific and apply to most diseases: these factors include sleep disturbance, pain, depression, and inactivity. Then there are more specific factors related in a more narrow biological sense to the pathophysiology of the disease itself, or its treatment. For our purposes these narrow factors will be referred to as 'disease activity', and include direct measures of nutritional state, endocrine, or inflammatory changes. To make matters worse such factors are all interrelated. Thus depression is common in physical illness, leads to sleep disturbance, and is likely to reduce activities. It may therefore lead to deconditioning. Furthermore, depression is associated with increased perception of pain. Disease activity in, for example, a rheumatological condition, may be associated with pain which in turn leads to sleep disturbance and depression. In other words there are endless possible interrelated mechanisms (Fig. 3.4).

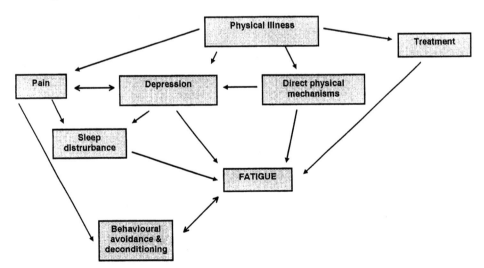

Fig. 3.4 Integrated scheme of potential mechanisms between physical illness and fatigue.

Methodology

One difficulty researchers have is determining which of these associations is causal. This difficulty is made worse by the fact that most of the literature reviewed here is cross-sectional. Cross-sectional studies, which measure potential risk factors and symptoms simultaneously, may be able to detect associations, but cannot comment on the direction of causality. To do this, cohort or intervention studies are required. These would follow subjects with a disease over time and examine which factors at baseline are associated with increased risk of fatigue at follow-up. Another methodological problem is that many constructs such as fatigue, disability, pain, sleep disturbance, and depression are so closely linked that it may be impossible to detect meaningful causal pathways between them.

Despite these misgivings, one meaningful thing these studies can do is to determine the extent to which variation in fatigue is accounted for by differences in disease activity measured by objective laboratory criteria. This is a very important point for clinicians. If fatigue is closely correlated to markers of physical disease, this implies that vigorous treatment aimed at the underlying physical disease should reverse the fatigue. On the other hand, if fatigue does not correlate with any marker of physical disease activity, it implies that the clinician should look for alternative associations. As we shall see, in most circumstances fatigue is *not* closely related to markers of disease activity. We shall now review physical illness and fatigue according to medical specialities.

3.7 Fatigue and cardiology: the case of chronic heart failure

Fatigue is an almost universal experience to patients with chronic heart failure (CHF) and physiological mechanisms for fatigue (in both meanings of the word) have been more thoroughly studied in this condition than in any other. If the *sine qua non* of CHF is the failure of the heart to pump blood efficiently, one obvious candidate mechanism for fatigue is restricted blood flow to skeletal muscle. There is certainly evidence that exercise intolerance correlates with measures of reduced cardiac function. Thus one study[92] found those with lowest VO_{2max} (indicating poor exercise tolerance) had increased pulmonary wedge pressure at rest and reduced cardiac output during exercise. Furthermore, exercise intolerance was associated with a considerably increased death rate. Poor exercise tolerance in CHF is therefore related to cardiac functioning.

Blood flow

A series of studies have assessed local blood flow to skeletal muscle during exercise. Exercise intolerance was associated with reduced cardiac output during exercise and reduced blood flow and oxygen consumption by the exercising limb[93]. If reduced cardiac output during exercise was responsible for this finding one would anticipate that the use of a positive inotrope (a drug, such as dobutamine, which increases cardiac output) would reverse this change. Whilst dobutamine does improve limb blood flow and cardiac output, this does not necessarily lead to improvements in exercise duration and biochemical markers of nutritive flow[94]. Thus it seems that a modest reversal of pump failure does not improve muscle function, indicating the possibility that there are secondary changes within muscles in CHF. Another study found that in about a quarter of CHF patients limb blood flow is normal but exercise tolerance in the limb is reduced[95]. Finally, there is evidence that although reduced blood flow may be a cause of fatigue in large muscle groups like the quadriceps; fatigue in small muscles (such as adductor pollicis) cannot be explained by this mechanism[96]. Taken together, these results suggest that blood flow and cardiac output are important indicators of severity of CHF, and therefore correlate with exercise intolerance. However, they do not necessarily explain muscle fatigue in these patients.

Muscle function

What other mechanisms might exist for the fatigue in CHF? Minotti *et al.*[97] compared neurophysiological properties of skeletal muscle in CHF in patients and controls. CHF patients had similar muscle strength, but poorer endurance. In other words their strength was not impaired but they fatigued quicker. External tetanic stimulation (see above) applied to the peroneal nerve did not increase muscle force, indicating the fatigue was not of central origin. Nor was there any evidence for neuromuscular junction dysfunction. This suggested that the fatigue in CHF was situated in the muscles themselves.

There is certainly evidence for a myopathy in CHF. The histology of skeletal muscle shows a shift from type I to type II fibres[98,99]. There is clear evidence of reduced oxidative capacity with changes to mitochondrial volume and surface density[99] and reduced oxidative enzymes[98]. Patients with CHF show reduced levels of phosphocreatine in skeletal muscle and greater depletion of phosphocreatine and increased levels of lactic acid even with modest levels of exercise[100,101]. These changes do not closely correlate with blood flow[101]. The exact cause of these changes are unclear. An obvious candidate is deconditioning, although the not all the changes are identical to those seen in the experiments reviewed in Section 3.5.

Symptoms of fatigue in CHF

Relatively few studies have compared objective markers of fatigue in CHF with the subjective complaints of patients. In an important (and unusually large) study, Wilson *et al.*[102] did just this. They took 52 ambulatory patients with CHF and assessed symptoms such as fatigue and dyspnoea using questionnaires. These were compared with the results of physiological measures, such as blood lactate and pulmonary wedge pressures. When the patients were subdivided into three groups on the basis of cardiac function, they complained of very similar severity of symptoms at the same workload. The implication of this paper is that *perception* of symptoms is not a function of more direct measures of disease activity. This is an extremely important point, both clinically and theoretically. To the clinician it implies that simply treating the underlying disease may not improve the symptom, and alternative explanations and interventions may be more fruitful. In theoretical terms it suggests that although the *association* between physical diseases such as CHF and fatigue are not in question, it implies that the narrow disease-specific factors may not provide the full picture: to fully understand fatigue in physical illness we need to examine general non-specific factors as well. This theme will be reviewed later in this chapter.

At present it may not be entirely possible to synthesize these findings into a coherent explanation of fatigue in CHF; however, we can be confident that skeletal muscle changes in CHF appear to play an important role. Once again these changes are unlikely to be due to a single cause: reduced nutritive flow, deconditioning, and endocrine changes[103] may all play a part. The myopathy may also be accompanied by alterations in feedback mechanisms which affect the sympathetic response to exercise, and could theoretically be important in the subjective experience of fatigue.

Exercise and CHF

These findings are based on cross-sectional designs which, as we have already seen, cannot determine direction of causality. One way of overcoming this limitation is to use an intervention study and see what, if anything reduces the experience of fatigue in CHF patients. Exercise was once considered to be contraindicated in chronic heart failure. However, an elegant blinded cross-over trial demonstrated this was erroneous[104,105]. A brief programme of exercise was associated with no harmful effects and patients reported improvements of symptoms. In particular, sensations of tiredness and breathlessness improved, and patients reported improved general well-being. Exercise tolerance also improved as did peak oxygen consumption.

Despite the modest size of this trial the results are important. First, they suggest that whilst the abnormalities of skeletal muscle described in the previous section are still causes of fatigue, they are potentially reversible. Second, they suggest that fatigue in heart failure may, to a large extent, be due to deconditioning, i.e. the effects of prolonged periods of rest. Third, this has implications for clinicians managing patients with this common condition. Modern medicine with its emphasis on technological advances is inclined to overlook this simple, cheap, and effective intervention. We shall see elsewhere in this and later chapters how beneficial exercise is in reducing fatigue associated with many chronic diseases.

From this overview it seems likely that the fatigue of CHF is in part reversible with exercise and this would suggest that deconditioning is an important mechanism for the changes seen. The most obvious conclusion is that fatigue in heart failure does not have a single cause, but deconditioning is one reversible one.

3.8 Fatigue and neurological disorders

We have already seen that fatigue is a feature of disorders such as myasthenia gravis and inborn errors of metabolism affecting muscle metabolism. The following describes fatigue in two other neurological disorders: multiple sclerosis and Parkinson's disease.

Multiple sclerosis

Multiple sclerosis (MS), dominates the literature on fatigue in neurological disorders. That fatigue is common in MS there can be no doubt. Approximately 80 per cent of patients complain of fatigue and for many it is their most disabling symptom[91]. Most of those who suffer from fatigue experience it daily or nearly every day, and crucially the most common strategy patients use to overcome fatigue is to reduce their levels of activity[91]. These results have been replicated other studies[105,107]. Those with the chronic progressive variant of the disease appear most at risk. Some neurological symptoms and signs may be more closely associated than others[107].

There are plausible physical mechanisms for the fatigue in MS. For example, nerve conduction studies show increased conduction times[108], and the well-recognized feature of fatigue in MS, namely that it is made worse by warm conditions, implies that the fatigue may be due to slowing of neurotransmitter release. Other studies have attempted to relate the fatigue of MS to pineal calcification (which implies low levels of melatonin)[109], or alterations in other monoaminergic neurotransmitters[110]. Psychological factors are also associated. Thus Vercoulen *et al.*[111] found that whilst fatigue in MS was not associated with depression, it was related to focusing on bodily symptoms, and low sense of control.

Treatments for the fatigue associated with MS have been assessed. The antiviral amantadine (which also has anti-parkinsonian effects) has been found to be useful for patients with debilitating fatigue and MS[112–114]. There is rather less evidence for the central stimulant pemoline[112,115]. The pharmacological basis of any treatment effect these drugs may have in alleviating the fatigue associated with MS is unknown, despite confident claims that their action (and that of electromagnetic fields, which have also been used to treat fatigue in MS) is on central monoamines[110]. Exercise has also been assessed as a treatment for the symptoms of MS[116]. It was found that aerobic training was associated with improvements in mood and fatigue on one measure but curiously not on another. Most other measures of quality of life were improved with exercise.

Parkinson's disease

Parkinson's disease is also associated with fatigue and sleep disturbance[117]. Friedman and Friedman[118] compared patients with Parkinson's with matched controls. The patients were more depressed and fatigued than controls as we would expect. Using a factor analytic technique they identified nine fatigue factors of which six correlated significantly with depression, but only one correlated to disease activity as measured by physician rating. This item was related to the disability caused by fatigue. These findings suggest that depression is an important predictor of fatigue in Parkinson's disease, and that disease severity may be less important. However, the choice of a tertiary care sample may have biased the study towards a more homogeneously disabled sample of patients, thus disguising a genuine effect of disease severity.

The literature on fatigue in MS has not examined the competing roles of specific versus general pathways in enough depth to allow a clear conclusion. Nonetheless, there it is clear that the general factors play an important role in the fatigue of Parkinson's disease which may be more important than the specific.

3.9 Fatigue and rheumatological disorders

The most widely researched association between a rheumatological disorder and fatigue is fibromyalgia, which is discussed in Chapter 14. Of the rheumatological diseases with established disease pathology two predominate in this literature: rheumatoid arthritis (RA) and systemic lupus erythematosus (SLE).

Rheumatoid arthritis

Fatigue is common in RA. Belza *et al.*[119] assessed correlates of fatigue in 133 elderly sufferers. They assessed the role of three groups of factors: sociodemographics, those related to disease activity, and psychosocial ones. These variables were then entered into a hierarchical multiple regression model, which took sociodemographic details at the top of the hierarchy, then disease activity, and finally psychosocial variables. The key finding was that measures of disease activity were the most important predictors of fatigue. They accounted for approximately 42 per cent of variance in fatigue whereas demographics accounted for 14 per cent and psychosocial factors only 5 per cent. The paper concludes that fatigue is largely a consequence of these measures of disease activity, and psychosocial factors have less importance. This is an important finding, and one which would have clinical implications in terms of finding strategies to treat fatigue in RA.

However, we believe the conclusion they drew from these data was flawed. The measures of disease activity they used were all essentially subjective (pain, level of functioning, and sleep disturbance). These symptoms are all strongly correlated to depression, and the imposition of the hierarchy creates a false distinction between these symptoms and depression. If the model supposed that depression was a key determinant of sleep and pain in RA and placed it on the second rung of the hierarchy, we suspect the results would have been very different.

This problem is reflected in another paper from the same group[120]. In this they assessed self-reported fatigue in patients with RA and age and sex matched controls. All participants completed a questionnaire on fatigue and mood states at six to eight week intervals. As one would expect, fatigue scores were worse in the RA sample, and the symptom did not alter much over time. There was a strong association between poor sleep, functional disability, depressive symptoms, and low haematocrit, and similar associations were found in the healthy controls. Apart from haematocrit, other markers of disease activity like C reactive protein only had a minor relationship with fatigue.

A recent paper[121] assessed fatigue in a mixed population of 1488 consecutive rheumatological patients. Patients with rheumatoid arthritis, osteoarthritis (OA), and fibromyalgia were all included. The key findings were that whilst fatigue was common in all three conditions, being present in 88–98 per cent of patients, it was more likely to be disabling in fibromyalgia than in RA and OA. Approximately 90 per cent of the variance in fatigue scores was explained by pain, sleep disturbance, and depression. When patients with RA were assessed alone, it was found that only a weak correlation existed between measures of disease activity such as erythrocyte sedimentation rate (ESR), and the number of joints affected, although grip strength had a somewhat stronger relationship. The relationship between these variables and fatigue was abolished by controlling for depression, pain, and sleep. This important study indicates that whereas pain, disability, and depression are determinants of fatigue in patients with RA they are also determinants of fatigue in rheumatological disorders such as OA and fibromyalgia where there is less evidence for an inflammatory process. This again emphasizes the multifactorial basis of fatigue in medical patients, and the relative dissociation between fatigue and disease activity when measured on a marker of systemic inflammatory processes.

Sleep has also been assessed in RA. Whilst there is no evidence that duration of sleep is reduced there are important alterations of sleep architecture in many patients. In one study of 15 subjects[122] two had sleep apnoea, and most had frequent arousal awakenings and excessive limb movements, suggesting that sleep in RA is fragmented. A further study compared objective and subjective measures of sleep in patients and controls[123]. Again RA patients showed evidence of sleep fragmentation. Patients perceived their sleep to be very much altered, probably more so than the objective evidence suggested. As we saw in the section on sleep disorders, sleep fragmentation and sleep apnoea are associated with fatigue, and may play a causal role.

Systemic lupus erythematosus (SLE)

Over 80 per cent of patients with SLE see fatigue as a problem[124] and it is associated with impairments in physical, social, and emotional functioning in the majority of patients. The majority of SLE patients rate fatigue as their most disabling symptom[125]. Fatigue correlates with ratings of depression, the doctor's assessment of disease activity but not laboratory tests of disease activity (including the erythrocyte sedimentation rate, complement, and anti-DNA antibodies). McKinley et al.[126] assessed the role of sleep disorders, disease activity, and depression in causing fatigue in SLE. They devised a model based on depression ratings and sleep disturbance which could explain 50 per cent of the variance of fatigue in their sample. Thus fatigue in SLE is associated with sleep disturbance and depression.

In summary fatigue is common in all rheumatological disorders studied, and has been consistently related to general factors, such as pain, sleep disturbance, depression, and inactivity. There is some evidence for it to be related to specific markers of disease activity, although this is less compelling and may not be independent of disability, pain, and depression.

3.10 Fatigue and cancer

Fatigue is a particular problem for those with cancer since chemotherapy and radiotherapy are known to cause severe and disabling fatigue. Reviews of cancer and fatigue[90,127] tend to emphasize the multifactorial nature of the problem: malnutrition, anaemia, drugs, depression, and immobilization have all been implicated. The small literature available emphasizes many of these factors. Thus Smith Blesch et al.[128] suggested that fatigue was a universal experience in cancer patients, and correlated with depression, pain, and duration of illness. Another paper showed the powerful, but reversible, effects of radiation on fatigue[129]. In a study over five weeks of radiotherapy there was a strong relationship between peaks of fatigue and timing of radiation.

There is some literature on treatments for fatigue related to cancer. Questad[130] studied the effects of a rehabilitation programme consisting of exercise and stress management. This was compared with a less intensive intervention. The chief finding was that although there was not much change in overall levels of activities achieved in either group, symptomatic fatigue improved in the treated group. A trial of a structured psychiatric intervention consisting of supportive, educative, and problem solving group work in malignant melanoma sufferers[131] found that patients given the intervention had a better outcome in terms of depressive symptoms, lack of vigour, and fatigue. Another finding was that the coping strategies used appeared to be a predictor of adverse mood states including lack of vigour. For example, patients who had an active–cognitive or active–behavioural coping strategy did better than those who used avoidance. Another tiny study[132] found that aerobic training was beneficial in terms of functional ability for women with breast cancer.

3.11 Fatigue and HIV

Darko *et al.*[133] compared patients with HIV and controls. The HIV positive men were in stage 3 or 4 (the latter of which includes full-blown AIDS). This paper related fatigue to markers of disease activity, for example CD4 cell count. There was a general pattern of worsening fatigue with worsening medical illness. Medical parameters appeared to predict fatigue in subjects of the same severity of clinical illness as well as between stages of illness. However, the paper did not assess psychosocial measures, thus they cannot be discounted. An important though rare mechanism of fatigue in HIV is through a myasthenic syndrome which open trials suggest may respond to pyridostigmine[134]. Another mechanism is via low cortisol levels: an addisonian syndrome is not uncommon in the latter stages of HIV, and an association with fatigue has been reported in an uncontrolled study[135], although this has not been replicated in a controlled study[136]. Finally, a small proportion of HIV sufferers go on to develop a syndrome of glucocorticoid resistance – akin to an extremely rare familial illness characterized by end organ insensitivity to cortisol – which is also associated with extreme fatigue[137].

Fatigue associated with HIV does, therefore, appear to have a stronger relationship with the disease process than in many other defined organic diagnoses, and in rare cases important biological mechanisms may be demonstrated. We suspect that the same associations between fatigue, depression, pain, and deconditioning will be found in HIV as in other medical illnesses, if they are sought.

3.12 Fatigue and renal failure

Fatigue is prominent symptom in renal failure with well over one-half of dialysis patients reporting moderate to severe fatigue[138]. This study suggested that patients with renal failure secondary to SLE are at greater risk than those with other diagnoses, suggesting that the systemic nature of this illness adds to the effect of renal disease. Interestingly, there was no correlation between fatigue and any of the markers of renal disease activity measured, including creatinine and haematocrit, a finding which has been replicated elsewhere[139]. Fatigue was related to use of haemo-dialysis as opposed to peritoneal dialysis. Interestingly, patients who had been dialysed for many years had lower levels of fatigue than recent cases, indicating that fatigue may relate to the difficulties of adjusting to dialysis. Fatigue related to employment status, but the majority of patients with mild or no fatigue were unemployed. Once again depression was common and strongly related to fatigue. Another study[139] indicates a strong relationship between fatigue and reduced levels of physical activity: implying that fatigue could either lead to reduced activity or be caused by it.

3.13 Post-operative fatigue

The phenomenon of post-operative fatigue is well recognized[140]. It is most apparent in patients who have undergone abdominal or thoracic surgery. Symptoms are usually worst in the first week following surgery, but one-third of patients have. disabling fatigue at one month. As ever, a number of potential risk factors have been advocated including the type and duration of surgery or anaesthesia, pre-operative anxiety, anthropometric measures, and so on. Studies of post-surgical fatigue have the important advantage of being able to assess possible risk factors prospectively with relative ease.

Post-operative fatigue gets better with time. Indeed for some conditions pre-operative fatigue may be reversed. For example a study by Kjerulff *et al.*[141] assessed fatigue by questionnaire in 1205 patients undergoing hysterectomy who were fol-lowed up for two years. A high proportion (over two-thirds) of women reported significant fatigue before surgery and this proportion to fell to just over one-quarter by six months after surgery. Post-operative fatigue was correlated with the now familiar general factors: pain, activity limitation, and psychological dysfunction. The women with significant fatigue at six months had used more services and were less satisfied by the surgery.

Nutrition and post-operative fatigue

Nutrition and anthropometric parameters have been assessed in the development of post-operative fatigue. Christensen and Kehlet[142] assessed the nutritional status of patients undergoing abdominal surgery. The age and gender of the patients and duration of surgery did not predict fatigue one month later, and it was difficult to identify any pre-operative predictor of fatigue apart from transferrin levels. Fatigue was accompanied by a fall in nutritive status: patients who became fatigued also lost more weight and skinfold thickness, indicating that post-operative fatigue correlated with catabolic changes, which could be due to neuroendocrine mechanisms. Other studies by the same group[143,144] have confirmed the importance of weight loss and pre-operative thinness as predictors of post-operative fatigue.

Muscle function and surgery

Another question is whether muscle function is altered in surgery. Although increased cardiorespiratory effort is required to undertake low-intensity exercise early post-operatively there is less evidence of physiological muscle fatigue[145]. Other studies have assessed changed in muscle enzymes[146] and muscle amino acids[144] according to patients' subjective complaints of fatigue. Whilst alterations in both enzymes and amino acids were common, these did not correlate with subjective fatigue.

Cardiovascular function and post-operative fatigue

Cardiovascular function is affected following surgery. Increased levels of fatigue post-surgery correlate with increases in heart rate for a given amount of work[147,148] and there are similar correlations between subjective fatigue and blood lactate concentrations and catecholamines for the same level of work[148]. These findings may be due to the non-specific effects of deconditioning and the authors concluded that this suggested that exercise might be a useful treatment for post-operative fatigue.

Stress, catecholamines, and anxiety

Surgery is accompanied by changes in catecholamine levels which may be determined by pre-surgical anxiety, although these changes are not consistent and are dissimilar to the classic stress response[149]. Pick *et al.*[150] assessed both psychological and physical aspects of post-operative fatigue following coronary artery bypass surgery. One month after surgery fatigue was predicted by high levels of noradrenaline perioperatively and to depression and anxiety. The suggestion was that both pre-operative anxiety and high levels of noradrenaline were signs of an exaggerated stress response which was responsible for fatigue. Another smaller study[151] suggested that whilst there was a strong cross-sectional correlation between fatigue and anxiety, pre-operative anxiety was not a predictor of post-operative fatigue. In contrast a larger study showed that post-operative fatigue correlates with negative mood states pre-operatively as well as pre-operative levels of fatigue[152].

Post-operative fatigue: conclusions

This review of post-operative fatigue emphasizes it is multifactorial. This lends support to the view that fatigue is a non-specific reaction to stress – caused either by the surgery itself, unrelated psychological factors, pain, or limitations of activity. There are probably important physical associations: for example reduced cardiovascular fitness and catabolic changes. Some of the changes seen in post-operative fatigue appear similar to those seen in deconditioning, and it is through early mobilization and exercise that patients are likely to avoid fatigue. Psychological symptoms such as low mood is also associated both cross-sectionally and prospectively. Different factors may be responsible for fatigue at different stages post-operatively. Thus psychological factors including anxiety may not be major factors in determining who is fatigued at one month, although we suspect they may be more powerful predictors of fatigue at six months or one year.

3.14 Mechanisms of fatigue in physical illness: conclusions

This review of fatigue in physical illnesses has covered many diseases and treatments. Are there any unifying themes which may allow clinicians to approach fatigue in their physically ill patients? Firstly, it is clear that fatigue is a common experience in physical illness, and that physical illness is a risk factor for fatigue. None the less many studies suggest that direct and specific biochemical or physiological measures of disease activity are not important predictors of fatigue. Does this mean that fatigue is due purely to these general factors? We doubt this is the case. Many of the samples selected homogeneous groups of patients (e.g. ambulant patients in outpatient clinics) and these will probably restrict the variation in disease activity such that it will be a less powerful predictor of fatigue. Were studies to include the range of all patients with a condition from those who are asymptomatic in community settings to those admitted to general medical wards, we anticipate disease activity would be a more important predictor.

However, there is no doubt that general factors such as pain, depression, inactivity, and sleep disturbance are strongly associated with fatigue in physical illness. We are faced with a philosophical problem here: fatigue, depression, and pain are all *symptoms*. Can one symptom lead to another? We do not believe this is a sufficient explanation. We suspect that the relationship between fatigue and depression in physical illness reflects a single underlying process: these symptoms may be viewed as the final, common, neurobiological effects of illness on the individual.

Pathophysiological pathways connecting symptoms should also be explored in further research. For example, the pain and fatigue may be connected because pain leads to behavioural changes such as avoidance, and avoidance (if it is exercise which is avoided) may lead to deconditioning.

There is, however, an important *clinical* point in emphasizing this interaction between symptoms. If a doctor views fatigue in a patient with physical illness solely as evidence of disease progression (i.e. assumes a specific aetiology to do with disease pathophysiology) he or she may miss treatable general associations of disease. Thus the doctor may alter drug treatment but overlook other aspects of rehabilitation. The patient may have depression, which worsens their perception of pain, leads to restriction in activity, and thereby to deconditioning. Rehabilitation might aim to treat depression, but also to improve mobility and pain management. We shall further explore this multifactorial view of fatigue in subsequent chapters of this book.

Another implication of these studies, also to be explored in more detail elsewhere, is that the *original* cause of fatigue in a disease may differ from factors which *perpetuate* it. Thus in patients with chronic systemic diseases, it may very well be that fatigue is first experienced as a direct result of the disease process. When the disease becomes more chronic it is likely that secondary factors, such as inactivity, other symptoms, and disability come into play perpetuating fatigue. Thus a vicious circle may be established since fatigue leads to reduced activity (see Fig. 3.3).

As we have previously stated, fatigue may ultimately be best understood as a non-specific reaction to stress. This view sees fatigue as evidence for a final common neurobiological pathway for many different stressors, whose distal mechanisms may be varied, but whose central effects are similar. The next section explores one possible unifying explanation for fatigue.

3.15 Cytokines, cortisol, and fatigue

Cytokines are trophic hormones which are involved in the regulation of the immune system. They act on a wide variety of tissues. The number of recognized cytokines has rapidly grown over the last decade, although the function of many remains poorly understood. In Chapter 9 we will examine the role (if any) of cytokines in the pathogenesis of chronic fatigue and CFS. Their role as possible agents of fatigue comes from several observations.

First, animal and human experiments show that some cytokines lead to a range of behavioural and subjective changes which are germane to fatigue. Animals given interleukin-1 (IL-1) show drowsiness, decreased activity, and changes to operant performance. For example mice given IL-1 exhibit less social exploratory behaviour, an effect which may work through prostaglandins[153]. Healthy human subjects given interferon show specific changes related to reasoning speed which are said to mimic those of acute influenza infections[154,155]. Interferon also makes people feel ill: it is associated with pyrexia (fever), fatigue, and sleepiness. Uncontrolled studies of those treated with interferons for cancer or hepatitis indicate that they almost universally experience severe systemic side effects such as lethargy, pyrexia, anorexia, poor concentration, and psychomotor slowing[156,157]. On formal psychological testing they are not associated with any specific cognitive impairment, and with strong motivation subjects on interferon are capable of performing most tasks. However, the poor concentration and slowing caused by interferons leads to poor performance on psychometric testing[157]. This pattern of psychological symptoms has been likened to a frontal lobe syndrome. Patients on a controlled trial of interferon for hepatitis demonstrated increased levels of psychiatric disorders. These included a neurasthenic syndrome as well as depression, anxiety states, phobias, and rarely delusions[158] in those given the active treatment. These mental state changes are usually reversible but may remain chronic in a minority of patients[159]. Thus interferons are associated with mental state changes which include prominent symptoms of fatigue and a syndrome akin to CFS.

The second strand of evidence that cytokines may play a key role in fatigue comes from their role in sleep. IL-1[22,160], the interferons, and tumour necrosis factor (TNF)[160] all have effects on sleep. IL-1 and TNF have been shown to increase slow-wave sleep, an effect which has been likened to the 'sleep rebound' phenomenon seen after sleep deprivation. There is evidence to suggest some of these effects are mediated through hypothalamic releasing hormones such as growth hormone releasing hormone and corticotrophin releasing factor[22,161]. The role of cytokines in the regulation of normal sleep is uncertain, but circulating levels of the cytokines IL-1 and TNF fall after periods of sleep[162]. Animal studies also suggest that these cytokines accumulate during periods of wakefulness and promote fatigue and sleep.

Third, cytokines are released following exercise. We have seen above how exercise is associated with an immune response. There is evidence for a transitory increase in IL-1, tumour necrosis factor, and interferon levels following exercise[27-29]. These changes are produced by relatively modest exercise which may not necessarily be associated with an inflammatory response in the muscles. Exercise leads to an increase in levels of interferon lasting approximately one hour. For IL-1 the effect may be longer, and there is evidence that muscle levels are elevated for several days following exercise[163].

Fourth, cytokines are involved in inflammatory disease. Apart from being a part of the acute phase response to infections, they are active in chronic inflammatory diseases such as rheumatoid arthritis. There is some evidence to suggest that IL-1 is associated with many of the symptoms of RA such as pain and malaise[164].

The mechanism by which cytokines cause fatigue is poorly understood. IL-1 is known to bind to the gamma-aminobutyric acid (GABA) receptor[165]. GABA is the main inhibitory neurotransmitter in the brain and it may be that the somnogenic and motor-depressant effects of IL-1 are related to this[165]. Cytokines have effects upon several levels of the hypothalamic–pituitary–adrenal axis, for example stimulating cortisol secretion (an effect which may be mediated via peripheral prostaglandins[166]), stimulating ACTH release[167] and corticotrophin releasing hormone (CRH) release[161]. Any or all these mechanisms may be involved.

These strands of evidence suggest that cytokines might be part of a common pathway to the experience of fatigue. A case could be made for their involvement in most of the physical causes of symptomatic fatigue we have reviewed in this chapter, but there are some problems which should be overcome. There is some contradictory evidence. For example, a study of a gruelling military exercise, which involved subjecting previously healthy cadets to a programme of strenuous exercise, sleep deprivation, and hunger, did not lead to any overall increase in IL-1, -2, or -4, although there was decrease in IL-6 and an increase in granulocyte macrophage colony stimulating factor[168]. This result shows how difficult it is sometimes to translate laboratory findings to real-life situations. A further study suggested that exhausting exercise was associated with a *fall* in tumour necrosis gene expression[169]. Another problem is that the specific central effects of cytokines are properly understood. Finally there is the difficulty that whilst cytokines may very well be important in the genesis of acute symptoms of fatigue familiar to anyone who has had influenza, they may be less relevant in the genesis of chronic fatigue and CFS. This is reviewed in Chapter 9.

Many cytokines interact with the hypothalamic–pituitary–adrenal axis leading to secretion of CRH, ACTH, and cortisol. A case can be made for the stress hormones acting as a final common pathway for fatigue. Addison's disease (primary hypocortisolaemia) is almost always accompanied by profound fatigue. The rare familial syndrome of glucocorticoid resistance in which end organs may be insensitive to cortisol is also associated with profound fatigue[170].

Many of the disease and non-disease states described above are associated with a stress response with the release of cortisol. Because cortisol is so sensitive to stress, it is easy to demonstrate links between stressors and alterations in cortisol levels. Unfortunately, the correlation between the severity and chronicity of fatigue and cortisol is less compelling: so for example in a study of post-operative fatigue no correlation was detected between changes in fatigue and changes in cortisol levels[148]. We do not believe this is sufficient evidence to propose cortisol as a 'final common pathway' for fatigue. Indeed there is epidemiological evidence that cortisol levels do not correlate with complaints of fatigue in population-based samples[171]. Low cortisol, like high interferon, is clearly a potent cause of fatigue. It is unlikely to be able to explain all causes of fatigue.

3.16 Conclusion

This chapter has reviewed many causes of several manifestations of fatigue. Whilst the literature has sometimes been bewilderingly varied, a few recurring themes are worth emphasizing (summarized in Table 3.8). First, symptoms of fatigue are strongly associated with psychological symptoms even when there is a very clear-cut physical cause of fatigue. This association between fatigue and psychological symptoms is certainly not proof that fatigue has no physical basis. None the less, it reiterates our view that complaints of fatigue in patients with chronic physical illnesses should not be viewed solely as evidence of disease progression. Second, apart from the over-training syndrome and a few rare neuromuscular disorders, regular exercise is nearly always associated with improvements in fatigue, even in the presence of a clear-cut physical illness. Third, the corollary of this – that prolonged inactivity is associated with fatigue – is also true. Finally, whilst there are undoubtedly a number of neurochemical and physiological mechanisms for acute fatigue, such as cytokines and fluctuations in cortisol or central serotonin levels, these mechanisms remain poorly understood. We do not believe any one of these mechanisms is likely to appear as a sufficient explanation for fatigue across the board.

Table 3.8 Physical illness and fatigue: conclusions

Most physical illnesses are associated with fatigue
Fatigue in physical illness is a multifactorial phenomenon
Disease activity does not correlate closely with fatigue
Psychological symptoms (especially depression) correlate strongly with fatigue
Regular exercise is well tolerated in most physical illnesses
Exercise is associated with a reduction in fatigue in physical illnesses
Prolonged inactivity causes fatigue

From a clinical perspective what this means is that when a patient with a physical illness complains of fatigue the most likely factors to be responsible are mood disorder and deconditioning. Whilst it is naturally reasonable to briefly review disease progression and instigate new physical therapies if thought appropriate, this course of action is only occasionally likely to have much impact on the patient's symptoms. The symptom of fatigue should lead to an assessment of the patient's mood and level of activities, treatment of any mood disorder, and examination of strategies to increase activity levels.

References

1 Gandevia SC, Enoka RM, McComas AJ, Stuart DG, Thomas CK. *Fatigue: neural and muscular mechanisms*. New York, Plenum Press, 1996.

2 Newsholme EA, Blomstrad E, Ekblom B. Physical and mental fatigue: metabolic mechanisms and importance of plasma amino acids. *Br. Med. Bull.* 1992; **48:** 477–495.

3 Allen DG, Westerblad H, Lannergren J. The role of intracellular acidosis in muscle fatigue. In Gandevia SC, Enoka RM, McComas AJ, Stuart DG, Thomas CK (ed.) *Fatigue: Neural and Muscular Mechanisms*. New York, Plenum Press, 1996; 577–68.

4 Anon. Fatigue. *Lancet* 1988; **2:** 546–548.

5 Layzer RB. How muscles use fuel. *New Engl. J. Med.* 1991; **324:** 411–412.

6 Cady EB, Elshove H, Jones DA, Moll A. The metabolic causes of slow relaxation in fatigued human muscle. *J. Physiol.* 1989; **418:** 327–337.

7 Westerblad H, Allen DG. Changes in intracellular pH during repeated tetani in single mouse skeletal muscle fibres. *J. Physiol.* 1992; **449:** 49–71.

8 Sjogaard G, McComas AJ. Role of interstitial potassium. In Gandevia SC, Enoka RM, McComas AJ, Stuart DG, Thomas CK (ed.) *Fatigue: Neural and Muscular Mechanisms*. New York, Plenum Press, 1996; 69–80.

9 Layzer RB. Muscle metabolism during fatigue and work. *Ballière's Clinical Endocrinology and Metabolism* 1990; **4:** 441–459.

10 Friedland JS, Paterson DJ. Exertional fatigue in disorders of muscle. *New Engl. J. Med.* 1991; **324:** 1896–1897.

11 Lishman WA. *Organic Psychiatry*. Oxford, Blackwell, 1987.

12 Nicholson C, Wilby J, Tennant C. Myasthenia gravis: the problem of 'psychiatric' misdiagnosis. *Med. J. Aust.* 1986; **144:** 632–638.

13 Bigland-Ritchie B, Jones DA, Hosking GP, Edwards RHT. Central and peripheral fatigue in sustained maximum voluntary contractions of human quadriceps muscle. *Clin. Sci. Molec. Med.* 1978; **54:** 609–614.

14 Gandevia SC, Allen GM, Butler JE, Taylor JL. Supraspinal factors in human muscle fatigue: evidence for suboptimal output from the motor cortex. *J. Physiol.* 1996; **490:** 529–536.

15 Borg G. Perceived exertion as an indicator of somatic stress. *Scand. J. Rehabil. Med.* 1970; **2:** 92–98.

16 Pandolf KB. Differentiated ratings of perceived exertion during physical exercise. *Med. Sci. Sports Exerc.* 1982; **14:** 397–405.

17 Demello JJ, Cureton KJ, Boineau RE, Singh MM. Ratings of perceived exertion at the lactate threshold in trained and untrained men and women. *Med. Sci. Sports Exerc.* 1987; **19:** 354–362.

18 Robertson RJ, Falkel JE, Drash AL, *et al.* Effect of blood pH on peripheral and central signals of perceived exertion. *Med. Sci. Sports Exerc.* 1986; **18:** 114–122.

19 Russell WD, Weeks DL. Attentional style in ratings of perceived exertion during physical exercise. *Percept. Motor Skills* 1994; **78:** 779–783.

20 Newsholme EA, Blomstrad E. Tryptophan, 5-hydroxytryptamine and a possible explanation for central fatigue. In Gandevia SC, Enoka RM, McComas AJ, Stuart DG, Thomas CK (ed.) *Fatigue: Neural and Muscular Mechanisms*. New York, Plenum Press, 1996; 315–320.

21 Blomstrand E, Celsing F, Newsholme EA. Changes in plasma concentrations of aromatic and branched chain amino acids during sustained exercise in man and their possible role in fatigue. *Acta Physiol. Scand.* 1988; **133:** 115–121.

22 Krueger JM, Majde JA. Cytokines and sleep. *Int. Arch. Allergy Immunol.* 1995; **106:** 97–100.

23 Bailey SP, Davis JM, Ahlborn EN. Neuroendocrine and substrate responses to altered brain 5-HT activity during prolonged exercise to fatigue. *J. Appl. Physiol.* 1993; **74:** 3006–3012.

24 Blomstrand E, Perrett D, Parry-Billings M, Newsholme EA. Effect of sustained exercise on plasma amino acid concentrations and on 5-hydroxytryptamine metabolism in six different brain regions in the rat. *Acta Physiol. Scand.* 1989; **136:** 473–481.

25 Wilson WM, Maughan RJ. Evidence for a possible role of 5-hydroxytryptamine in the genesis of fatigue in man: administration of paroxetine, a 5-HT re-uptake inhibitor, reduces the capacity to perform prolonged exercise. *Exp. Physiol.* 1992; **77:** 921–924.

26 Luger A, Deuster PA, Kyle SB, *et al.* Acute hypothalmic-pituitary-adrenal responses to the stress of treadmill exercise. *New Engl. J. Med.* 1987; **316:** 1309–1315.

27 Dufaux B, Order U. Plasma elastase-alpha 1-antitrypsin, neopterin, tumour necrosis factor, and soluble interleukin-2 receptor after prolonged exercise. *Int. J. Sports Med.* 1989; **10:** 434–438.

28 Cannon JG, Kluger MJ. Endogenous pyrogen activity in human plasma after exercise. *Science* 1983; **220:** 617–619.

29 Viti A, Muscettola M, Paulesu L, Bocci V, Almi A. Effect of exercise on plasma interferon levels. *J. Appl. Physiol.* 1985; **59:** 426–428.

30 MacIntyre DL, Reid WD, McKenzie DC. Delayed muscle soreness: the inflammatory response to muscle injury and its clinical implications. *Sports Med.* 1995; **20:** 24–40.

31 Newham DJ, Jones DA, Clarkson PM. Repeated high-force eccentric exercise: effects on muscle pain and damage. *J. Appl. Physiol.* 1987; **63:** 1381–1386.

32 Salkovskis PM, Clark DM. Affective responses to hyperventilation: a test of the cognitive model of panic. *Behav. Res. Ther.* 1990; **28:** 51–61.

33 Budgett R. Overtraining syndrome. *Br. J. Sports Med.* 1990; **24:** 231–236.

34 Lehmann M, Foster C, Keul J. Overtraining in endurance athletes: a brief review. *Med. Sci. Sports Exerc.* 1993; **25:** 854–862.

35 Fry RW, Morton AR, Keast D. Overtraining in athletes: an update. *Sports Med.* 1991; **12:** 32–65.

36 Barron JL, Noakes TD, Levy W, Smith C, Millar RP. Hypothalamic dysfunction in overtrained athletes. *J. Clin. Endocrinol. Metabol.* 1985; **60:** 803–806.

37 Lehmann M, Gaustmann U, Petersen KG, *et al.* Training – overtraining: performance, and hormone levels, after a defined increase in training volume versus intensity in experienced middle- and long-distance runners. *Br. J. Sports Med.* 1992; **26:** 233–242.

38 Horne J. *Why we Sleep.,* Oxford University Press, 1988.

39 Standards of Practice Committee of the American Sleep disorders Association. Practice parameters for the use of polysomnography in the evaluation of insomnia. *Sleep* 1995; **18:** 55–57.

40 Guilleminault C. Disorders of excessive sleepiness. *Ann. Clin. Res.* 1985; **17:** 209–219.

41 American Sleep Disorders Association. *International Classification of Sleep Disorders: ICSD Diagnostic and Coding Manual.* Rochester, MN, American Sleep Disorders Association, 1990.

42 American Psychiatric Association. *Diagnostic and Statistical Manual of Mental Disorders: DSM-IV.* Washington DC, APA, 1994.

43 Mellinger GD, Balter MB, Uhlenhuth EH. Insomnia and its treatment. Prevalence and correlates. *Arch. Gen. Psychiatry* 1985; **42:** 225–232.

44 Reynolds CF, Shaw DH, Newton TF, Coble PA, Kupfer DJ. EEG sleep in outpatients with generalized anxiety: a preliminary comparison with depressed outpatients. *Psychiatry Res.* 1983; **8:** 81–89.

45 Arriaga F, Rosado P, Paiva T. the sleep of dysthymic patients: a comparison with normal controls. *Biol. Psychiatry* 1990; **74**: 649–657.

46 Hirsch M, Carlander B, Verge M, *et al.* Objective and subjective sleep disturbances in patients with rheumatoid arthritis. A reappraisal. *Arthritis Rheum.* 1994; **37**: 41–49.

47 Chambers MJ, Alexander SD. Assessment and prediction of outcome for a brief behavioral insomnia treatment program. *J. Behav. Ther. Exp. Psychiatry* 1992; **23**: 289–297.

48 Chambers MJ, Kim JY. The role of state-trait anxiety in insomnia and daytime restedness. *Behav. Med.* 1993; **19**: 42–46.

49 Carskadon MA, Dement WC. The multiple sleep sleep latency test: what does it measure? *Sleep* 1982; **5**: 67–72.

50 Ford DE, Kamerow DB. Epidemiologic study of sleep disturbances and psychiatric disorders. An opportunity for prevention? *J. Am. Med. Assoc.* 1989; **262**: 1479–1484.

51 Hawkins DR, Taub JM, Van de Castle RL. Extended sleep (hypersomnia) in young depressed adults. *Am. J. Psychiatry* 1985; **142**: 905–910.

52 Nofzinger EA, Thase ME, Reynolds CF, *et al.* Hypersomnia in bipolar depression: a comparison with narcolepsy using the multiple sleep latency test. *Am. J. Psychiatry* 1991; **148**: 1177–1181.

53 Davidson JRT, Miller RD, Turnbull CD, Sullivan JL. Atypical depression. *Arch. Gen. Psychiatry* 1982; **39**: 527–534.

54 Van Moffaert MM. Sleep disorders and depression: the 'chicken and egg' situation. *J. Psychosom. Res.* 1994; **38(suppl 1)**: 9–13.

55 Kales A, Vela Bueno A, Kales JD. Sleep disorders: sleep apnoea and narcolepsy. *Ann. Int. Med.* 1987; **106**: 434–443.

56 De Backer WA. Central sleep apnoea, pathogenesis and treatment: an overview and perspective. *Eur. Respir. J.* 1995; **8**: 1372–1383.

57 Taub JM. Nocturnal electrographic features of frequently changing-irregular sleep-wakefulness rhythms. *Int. J. Neurosci.* 1981; **14**: 227–237.

58 Stewart KT, Hayes BC, Eastman CI. Light treatment for NASA shiftworkers. *Chronobiol. Int.* 1995; **12**: 141–151.

59 O'Keeffe ST. Restless legs syndrome. A review. *Arch. Int. Med.* 1996; **156**: 243–248.

60 Saskin P, Moldofsky H, Lue FA. Periodic movements in sleep and sleep-wake complaint. *Sleep* 1985; **8**: 319–324.

61 Cameron C. A theory of fatigue. *Ergonomics* 1973; **16**: 633–648.

62 Samkoff JS, Jacques CH. A review of studies concerning effects of sleep deprivation and fatigue on residents' performance. *Acad. Med.* 1991; **66**: 687–693.

63 Herscovitch J, Stuss D, Broughton R. Changes in cognitive processing following short-term cumulative partial sleep deprivation and recovery oversleeping. *J. Clin. Neuropsychol.* 1980; **2**: 301–319.

64 Myles WS. Sleep deprivation, physical fatigue, and the perception of exercise intensity. *Med. Sci. Sports Exerc.* 1985; **17**: 580–584.

65 VanHelder T, Radomski MW. Sleep deprivation and the effect on exercise performance. *Sports Med.* 1989; **7**: 235–247.

66 Reilly T, Piercy M. The effect of partial sleep deprivation on weight-lifting performance. *Ergonomics* 1994; **37**: 107–115.

67 Globus GG. Sleep duration and feeling state. *Int. Psychiatry Clin.* 1970; **7**: 78–84.

68 Taub JM. Individual variations in awakening times, daytime alertness and somnograms as a function of ad libitum extended sleep. *Int. J. Neurosci.* 1983; **21**: 237–250.

69 Arendt J, Marks V. Physiological changes underlying jet lag. *Br. Med. J. Clin. Res. Ed.* 1982; **284**: 144–146.

70 Taub JM. Behavioral and psychophysiological correlates of irregularity in chronic sleep routines. *Biol. Psychol.* 1978; **7**: 37–53.

71 Taub JM, Berger RJ. The effects of changing the phase and duration of sleep. *J. Exp. Psychol. Hum. Percept.* 1976; **2**: 30–41.

72 Stepanski E, Lamphere J, Badia P, Zorick F, Roth T. Sleep fragmentation and daytime sleepiness. *Sleep* 1984; **7**: 18–26.

73 Martin SE, Engleman HM, Deary IJ, Douglas NJ. The effect of sleep fragmentation on daytime function. *Am. J. Respir. Crit. Care Med.* 1996; **153**: 1328–1332.

74 Moldofsky H, Scarisbrick P. Induction of neurasthenic musculoskeletal pain syndrome by selective sleep stage deprivation. *Psychosom. Med.* 1976; **38**: 35–44.

75 Menninger K. The abuse of rest in psychiatry. *J. Am. Med. Assoc.* 1944; **125**: 1087–1090.

76 Dock W. The evil sequelae of complete bed rest. *J. Am. Med. Assoc.* 1944; **125**: 1083–1085.

77 Asher RAJ. The dangers of going to bed. *Br. Med. J.* 1947; **2**: 967–968.

78 Winiarski AM, Roy RR, Alford EK, Chiang PC, Edgerton VR. Mechanical properties of rat skeletal muscle after hind limb suspension. *Exp. Neurol.* 1987; **96**: 650–660.

79 Booth F. Physiologic and biochemical effects of immobilization on muscle. *Clin. Orthopaedics* 1987; **10**: 15–20.

80 Jaffe D, Terry R, Spiro A. Disuse atrophy of skeletal muscle. *J. Neurol. Sci.* 1978; **35**: 189–200.

81 Muller E. Influence of training and of inactivity on muscle strength. *Arch. Phys. Med. Rehab.* 1970; **51**: 449–452.

82 Taylor HL, Erickson L, Henschel A, Keys A. The effect of bed rest on the blood volume of normal young men. *Am. J. Physiol.* 1945; **144**: 227–232.

83 Saltin B, Blomquist G, Mitchell J, Johnson R, Wildenthal K, Chapman C. Response to exercise after bed rest and training: a longitudinal study of adaptive changes in oxygen transport and body composition. *Circulation* 1968; **38(suppl 7)**: 1–55.

84 Convertino VA, Karst GM, Kirby CR, Goldwater DJ. Effect of simulated weightlessness on exercise-induced anaerobic threshold. *Aviation Space Environ. Med.* 1986; **57**: 325–331.

85 Ryback RS, Lewis OF. Effects of prolonged bed rest on EEG sleep patterns in young, healthy volunteers. *Electroencephalogr. Clin. Neurophysiol.* 1971; **31**: 395–399.

86 Zorbas YG, Matveyev IO. Man's desirability in performing physical exercises under hypokinesia. *Int. J. Rehab. Res.* 1986; **9**: 170–174.

87 Zuber J, Wilgosh L. Prolonged immobilization of the body: changes in performance and the electroencephalogram. *Science* 1963; **140**: 306–308.

88 Martinsen EW. Physical activity and depression: clinical experience. *Acta Psychiatr. Scand.* 1994 **(suppl 377)**: 23–27.

89 Stewart AL, Hays RD, Wells KB, Rogers WH, Spritzer KL, Greenfield S. Long-term functioning and well-being outcomes associated with physical activity and exercise in patients with chronic conditions in the medical outcomes study. *J. Clin. Epidemiol.* 1994; **47**: 719–730.

90 Smets EMA, Garssen B, Shuster-Uitterhoeve ALJ, de Haes JCJM. Fatigue in cancer patients. *Br. J. Cancer* 1993; **68**: 220–224.

91 Freal JE, Kraft GH, Coryell JK. Symptomatic fatigue in multiple sclerosis. *Arch. Phys. Med. Rehab.* 1984; **65**: 135–138.

92 Szlachcic J, Massie BM, Kramer BL, Topic N, Tubau J. Correlates and prognostic implications of exercise capacity in chronic congestive heart failure. *Am. J. Cardiol.* 1985; **55**: 1037–1042.

93 Wilson JR, Martin JL, Schwartz D, Ferraro N. Exercise intolerance in patients with chronic heart failure: role of impaired nutritive flow in skeletal muscle. *Circulation* 1984; **69**: 1079–1087.

94 Wilson JR, Martin JL, Ferraro N. Impaired skeletal muscle nutritive flow during exercise in patients with congestive heart failure: role of cardiac pump dysfunction as determined by the effect of dobutamine. *Am. J. Cardiol.* 1994; **53**: 1308–1315.

95 Wilson JR, Mancini DM, Dunkman WB. Exertional fatigue due to skeletal muscle dysfunction in patients with heart failure. *Circulation* 1993; **87**: 470–475.

96 Buller NP, Jones D, Poole-Wilson PA. Direct measurement of skeletal muscle fatigue in patients with chronic heart failure. *Br. Heart J.* 1991; **65**: 20–24.

97 Minotti JR, Pillay P, Chang L, Wells L, Massie BM. Neurophysiological assessment of skeletal muscle fatigue in patients with congestive heart failure. *Circulation* 1992; **86**: 903–908.

98 Sullivan MJ, Green HJ, Cobb FR. Skeletal muscle biochemistry and histology in ambulatory patients with long-term heart failure. *Circulation* 1990; **81**: 518–527.

99 Drexler H, Riede U, Munzel T, Konig H, Funke E, Just H. Alterations in skeletal muscle in chronic heart failure. *Circulation* 1992; **85**: 1751–1759.

100 Massie BM, Conway M, Yonge R, *et al.* Skeletal muscle metabolism in patients with congestive heart failure: relation to clinical severity and blood flow. *Circulation* 1987; **76**: 1009–1019.

101 Wiener DH, Fink LI, Maris J, Jones RA, Chance B, Wilson JR. Abnormal skeletal muscle bioenergetics during exercise in patients with heart failure: role of the reduced muscle blood flow. *Circulation* 1986; **73**: 1127–1136.

102 Wilson JR, Rayos G, Gothard P, Bak K. Dissociation between exertional symptoms and circulatory function in patients with heart failure. *Circulation* 1995; **92**: 47–53.

103 Francis GS, Goldsmith SR, Levine BT, Olivari MT, Cohn JN. The neurohumoral axis in congestive heart failure. *Ann. Int. Med.* 1984; **101**: 370–377.

104 Coats AJS, Adamopoulos A, Meyer TE, Conway J, Sleight P. Effects of physical training in chronic heart failure. *Lancet* 1990; **335**: 63–66.

105 Coats AJS, Adamopoulos A, Radaelli A, *et al.* Controlled trial of physical training in chronic heart failure. *Circulation* 1992; **85**: 2119–2131.

106 Fisk JD, Pontefract A, Ritvo PG, Archibald CJ, Murray TJ. The impact of fatigue on patients with multiple sclerosis. *Can. J. Neurol. Sci.* 1994; **21**: 9–14.

107 Colosimo C, Millefiorini E, Grasso MG, *et al.* Fatigue in MS is associated with specific clinical features. *Acta Neurol. Scand.* 1995; **92**: 353–355.

108 Hess CW, Mills KR, Murray NMF, Schreifer TN. Magnetic brain stimulation: central motor conduction studies in multiple sclerosis. *Ann. Neurol.* 1987; **22**: 744–752.

109 Sandyk R, Awerbuch GI. Pineal calcification and its relationship to the fatigue of multiple sclerosis. *Int. J. Neurosci.* 1994; **74**: 95–103.

110 Sandyk R. Treatment with weak electromagnetic fields improves fatigue associated with multiple sclerosis. *Int. J. Neurosci.* 1996; **84**: 177–186.

111 Vercoulen JHMM, Hommes OR, Swanink CMA, *et al.* The measurement of fatigue in patients with multiple sclerosis. *Arch. Neurol.* 1996; **53**: 642–649.

112 Krupp LB, Coyle PK, Doscher C, *et al.* Fatigue therapy in multiple sclerosis: results of a double-blind, randomized, parallel trial of amantadine, pemoline and placebo. *Neurology* 1995; **45**: 1956–1961.

113 Rosenberg GA, Appenzeller O. Amantadine, fatigue, and multiple sclerosis. *Arch. Neurol.* 1988; **45**: 1104–1106.

114 The Canadian MS Research Group. A randomized controlled trial of amantadine in fatigue associated with multiple sclerosis. *Can. J. Neurol. Sci.* 1987; **14**: 273–278.

115 Weinshenker BG, Penman M, Bass B, Ebers GC, Rice GPA. A double-blind, randomized, crossover trial of pemoline in fatigue associated with multiple sclerosis. *Neurology* 1992; **42**: 1468–1471.

116 Petajan JH, Gappmaier E, White AT, Spencer MK, Mino L, Hicks RW. Impact of aerobic training on fitness and quality of life in multiple sclerosis. *Ann. Neurol.* 1996; **39**: 432–441.

117 van Hilten JJ, Weggeman M, van der Velde EA, Kerkhof GA, van Dijk JG, Roos RAC. Sleep, excessive daytime sleepiness and fatigue in Parkinson's disease. *J. Neural Transmission* 1993; **5**: 235–244.

118 Friedman J, Friedman H. Fatigue in Parkinson's disease. *Neurology* 1993; **43**: 2016–2019.

119 Belza BL, Henke CJ, Yelin EH, Epstein WV, Gilliss CL. Correlates of fatigue in older adults with rheumatoid arthritis. *Nursing Res.* 1993; **42**: 93–99.

120 Belza BL. Comparison of self report fatigue in rheumatoid arthritis and controls. *J. Rheumatol.* 1995; **22**: 639–643.

121 Wolfe F, Hawley DJ, Wilson K. The prevalence and meaning of fatigue in rheumatic disease. *J. Rheumatol.* 1996; **23**: 1407–1417.

122 Mahowald MW, Mahowald ML, Bundlie SR, Ytterberg SR. Sleep fragmentation in rheumatoid arthritis. *Arthritis Rheum.* 1989; **32**: 974–983.

123 Hirsch M, Carlander B, Verge M, *et al.* Objective and subjective sleep disturbances in patients with rheumatoid arthritis. *Arthritis Rheum.* 1994; **37**: 41–49.

124 Hastings C, Joyce K, Yarboro C, Berkebile C, Yocum D. Factors affecting fatigue in systemic lupus erythematosus. *Arthritis Rheum.* 1986; **29(suppl)**: 176.

125 Krupp LB, LaRocca NG, Muir J, Steinberg AD. A study of fatigue in systemic lupus erythematosus. *J. Rheumatol.* 1990; **17**: 1450–1452.

126 McKinley PS, Ouellette SC, Winkel GH. The contributions of disease activity, sleep patterns, and depression to fatigue in systemic lupus erythematosus. *Arthritis Rheum.* 1995; **38**: 826–834.

127 Aistars J. Fatigue in the cancer patient: a conceptual approach to a clinical problem. *Oncol. Nursing Forum* 1987; **14**: 25–30.

128 Smith Blesch K, Paice JA, Wickham R, *et al.* Correlates of fatigue in people with breast or lung cancer. *Oncol. Nursing Forum* 1991; **18**: 81–87.

129 Haylock PJ, Hart LK. Fatigue in patients receiving localized radiation. *Cancer Nursing* 1979; December: 461–467.

130 Questad KA. An empirical study of a rehabilitation program for fatigue related to cancer. *Dissertation Abstracts Int.* 1983; **44**.

131 Fawzy FI, Cousins N, Fawzy NW, Kemeny ME, Elashoff R, Morton D. A structured psychiatric intervention for cancer patients: I. Changes over time in methods of coping and affective disturbance. *Arch. Gen. Psychiatry* 1990; **47**: 720–725.

132 MacVicar M, Winnighar M. Effect of aerobic training on functional status of women with breast cancer. *Oncol. Nursing Forum* 1991 **(suppl)**: 62.

133 Darko DF, McCutchan JA, Kripke DF, Gillin JC, Golshan S. Fatigue, sleep disturbance, disability, and indices of progression of HIV infection. *Am. J. Psychiatry* 1992; **149**: 514–520.

134 Cupler EJ, Otero C, Hench K, Luciano C, Dalakas MC. Acetylcholine receptor antibodies as a marker of treatable fatigue in HIV-1 infected individuals. *Muscle Nerve* 1996; **19**: 1186–1188.

135 Piedrola G, Casado JL, Lopez E, Moreno A, Perez-Elias MJ, Garcia-Robles R. Clinical features of adrenal insufficiency in patients with acquired immunodeficiency syndrome. *Clin. Endocrinol. Oxf.* 1996; **45**: 97–101.

136 Abbott M, Khoo SH, Hammer MR, Wilkins EG. Prevalence of cortisol deficiency in late HIV disease. *J. Infection* 1995; **31**: 1–4.

137 Norbiato G, Galli M, Righini V, Moroni M. The syndrome of acquired glucocorticoid resistance in HIV infection. *Ballière's Clin. Endocrinol. Metabol.* 1994; **8**: 777–787.

138 Cardenas DD, Kutner NG. The problem of fatigue in dialysis patients. *Nephron* 1982; **30**: 336–340.

139 Brunier GM, Graydon J. The influence of physical activity on fatigue in patients with ESRD on hemodialysis. *ANNA J.* 1993; **20**: 457–461.

140 Christensen T. Postoperative fatigue *Danish Med. Bull.* 1995; **42**: 314–322.

141 Kjerulff KH, Langenberg PW. A comparison of alternative ways of measuring fatigue among patients having hysterectomy. *Med. Care* 1995; **33(suppl)**: 5156–5163.

142 Christensen T, Kehlet H. Postoperative fatigue and changes in nutritional status. *Br. J. Surg.* 1984; **71**: 473–476.

143 Christensen T, Hougard F, Kehlet H. Influence of pre- and intra- operative factors on the occurrence of postoperative fatigue. *Br. J. Surg.* 1985; **73**: 63–65.

144 Christensen T, Kehlet H, Vesterberg K, Vinnars E. Fatigue and muscle amino acids during surgical convalescence. *Acta Chir. Scand.* 1987; **153**: 567–570.

145 Zeiderman MR, Welchew EA, Clark RG. Changes in cardiorespiratory and muscle function associated with the development of postoperative fatigue. *Br. J. Surg.* 1990; **77**: 576–580.

146 Christensen T, Nygaard E, Stage JG, Kehlet H. Skeletal muscle enzyme activities and metabolic substrates during exercise in patients with postoperative fatigue. *Br. J. Surg.* 1990; **27**: 312–315.

147 Christensen T, Bendix T, Kehlet H. Fatigue and cardiovascular function following abdominal surgery. *Br. J. Surg.* 1982; **69**: 417–419.

148 Christensen T, Stage JG, Galbo H, Christensen NJ, Kehlet H. Fatigue and cardiac and endocrine metabolic response to exercise after abdominal surgery. *Surgery* 1989; **105**: 46–50.

149 Salmon P, Pearce S, Smith CCT, *et al.* Anxiety, type A personality and endocrine responses to surgery. *Br. J. Clin. Psychol.* 1989; **28**: 279–280.

150 Pick B, Molloy A, Hinds C, Pearce S, Salmon P. Post-operative fatigue following coronary artery bypass surgery: relationship to emotional state and to the catecholamine response to surgery. *J. Psychosom. Res.* 1994; **38**: 599–607.

151 Christensen T, Hjortso NC, Mortensen E, Riis-Hansen M, Kehlet H. Fatigue and anxiety in surgical patients. *Acta Psychiatr. Scand.* 1986; **73**: 76–79.

152 Aarons H, Forester A, Hall G, Salmon P. Fatigue after major joint arthroplasty: relationship to preoperative fatigue and postoperative emotional state. *J. Psychosom. Res.* 1996; **41**: 225–233.

153 Crestani F, Seguy F, Dantzer R. Behavioural effects of peripherally injected interleukin-1: role of prostaglandins. *Brain Res.* 1991; **542**: 330–335.

154 Smith AP, Tyrrell DAJ, Coyle K, Willman JS. Selective effects of minor illnesses on human performance. *Br. J. Psychol.* 1987; **78**: 183–188.

155 Smith A, Tyrrell D, Coyle K, Higgins P. Effects of interferon alpha on performance in man: a preliminary report. *Psychopharmacology* 1988; **96**: 414–416.

156 Smedley H, Katrak M, Sikora K, Wheeler T. Neurological effects of recombinant human interferon. *Br. Med. J.* 1983; **286**: 262–264.

157 Adams F, Quesada JR, Gutterman JU. Neuropsychiatric manifestations of human leukocyte interferon therapy in patients with cancer. *J. Am. Med. Assoc.* 1984; **252**: 938–941.

158 McDonald EM, Mann AH, Thomas HC. Interferons as mediators of psychiatric morbidity. *Lancet* 1987; **ii**: 1175–1178.

159 Meyers CA, Scheibel RS, Forman AD. Persistent neurotoxicity of systemically administered interferon-alpha. *Neurology* 1991; **41**: 672–676.

160 Shoman S, Davenne D, Cady AB, Dinarello CA, Krueger JM. Recombinant tumor necrosis factor and interleukin 1 enhance slow-wave sleep. *Am. J. Physiol.* 1987; **253**: R142–R149.

161 Payne LC, Obal F, Krueger JM. Hypothalamic releasing hormones mediating the effects of interleukin-1 on sleep. *J. Cellular Biochem.* 1993; **53:** 309–313.

162 Uthgenannt D, Schcolmann D, Pietrowsky R, Horst-Lorenz F, Born J. Effects of sleep on the production of cytokines in humans. *Psychosom. Med.* 1995; **57:** 97–104.

163 Cannon JG, Fielding RA, Fiatorone MA, Orenocole SF, Dinarello CA, Evans WJ. Increased interleukin-1 beta in human skeletal muscle after exercise. *Am. J. Physiol.* 1989; **257:** 451–r455.

164 Eastgate J, Wood NC, di Giovane FS, Symons JA, Grinlinton FM, Duff GW. Correlations of plasma interleukin 1 levels with disease activity in rheumatoid arthritis. *Lancet* 1988; **2:** 706–709.

165 Miller LG, Galperin WR, Dunlap K, Dinarello CA, Turner TJ. Interleukin-1 augments gamma aminobutyric acid A receptor function in brain. *Mol. Pharmacol.* 1991; **39:** 105–108.

166 Winter JSD, Gow KW, Perry YS, Greenberg AH. A stimulatory effect of interleukin-1 on adrenocortical cortisol secretion mediated by prostaglandins. *Endocrinology* 1990; **127:** 1904–1909.

167 O'Grady MP, Hall NRS, Menzies RA. Interleukin-lbeta stimulates adrenocorticotropin and corticosterone release in 10-day-old rat pups. *Psychoneuroendocrinology* 1993; **18:** 241–247.

168 Boyum A, Wiik P, Gustavsson E, *et al.* The effects of strenuous exercise, calorie deficiency and sleep deprivation on white blood cells, plasma immunoglobulins and cytokines. *Scand. J. Immunol.* 1996; **43:** 228–235.

169 Natelson BH, Zhou X, Ottenweller JE, *et al.* Effect of acute exhausting exercise on cytokine gene expression in men. *Int. J. Sports Med.* 1996; **17:** 299–203.

170 Lambert SWJ, Koper JW, Biemond P. Cortisol receptor resistance: the variability of its clinical presentaions and response to treatment. *J. Clin. Epidemiol. Metabol.* 1992; **74:** 313–321.

171 Hyppa MT, Lindholm T, Lehtinen V, Puukka P. Self-perceived fatigue and cortisol secretion in a community sample. *J. Psychosom. Res.* 1993; **37:** 589–594.

4. Fatigue and emotional disorders

4.1 Introduction

In this chapter we consider fatigue and psychiatric disorders. Psychiatric disorder is a term not without problems of concept and definition (see Sharpe[1] and Chapter 10). For this chapter we shall consider psychiatric disorders from a pragmatic rather than a philosophical perspective. Psychiatric disorders are what the international classifications of diseases say they are – operationally defined concepts based on particular constellations of symptoms. In practice although the number of psychiatric disorders is so vast that it is covered by a separate volume of the *International Classification of Diseases* (ICD-10), and a large and indigestible manual produced by the American Psychiatric Association (DSM-IV), most of this chapter will be devoted to the two most common disorders, depression and anxiety[2].

4.2 Fatigue and depression

Depression is both a symptom and a syndrome. As a symptom it means a lowering of mood – the feeling of being unhappy. As a syndrome it is defined by the presence of certain symptoms. There are numerous criteria and concepts for the syndrome, but, as the introduction to the *International Classification of Diseases* states, in all the patient suffers from lowering of mood, reduction of energy, and decrease in activity. The criteria for depressive episodes (F 32) continue:

In typical depressive episodes the individual usually suffers from depressed mood, loss of interest and enjoyment, and reduced energy leading to increased fatiguability and diminished activity. Capacity for enjoyment, interest and concentration is reduced, and marked tiredness after even minimum effort is common.

From the beginning, modern investigations of depressed patients emphasized the importance of fatigue. 'The earliest complaint is of a general slowing of activity, accompanied by a sense of effort and a subjective sense of fatigue'[3]. Others noted that 'the fatigue was often overwhelming, and made daily activity difficult'[4]. The investigators remarked on the phenomenology of depressive fatigue – 'the tiredness after muscular exertion is a pleasant feeling. Depressive fatigue, on the other hand, is unpleasant, and not relieved by relaxation'. Fatigue has long been considered as an integral part of our concept of depression. It is not therefore surprising that numerous epidemiological studies have confirmed the association of fatigue and lowered mood. In the next sections we will consider this evidence grouped, as before (Chapter 2), by the setting in which the study was performed.

Community samples

Wherever one looks depressive disorder and fatigue go together. For example, a survey of college students found that over 80 per cent of those scoring over a predetermined cut-off on the Center for Epidemiological Studies Depression Scale (CES-D) also felt that everything is an effort[5]. In another unselected sample of American college students there were associations between fatigue and self-reports of both depression and anxiety[6]. Walker *et al.*[7], using the Epidemiologic Catchment Area (ECA) data, showed a tenfold difference in the rates of both current and lifetime major depression between those with and without a history of fatigue, even if fatigue was excluded from the criteria used to diagnosis depression. In Switzerland Jules Angst and colleagues found that exhaustion was three times as common in those with depression than those without[8]. A similar relationship exists for both major depression and dysthymia[9]. The association between depression and fatigue is found throughout adult life, persisting into old age[10].

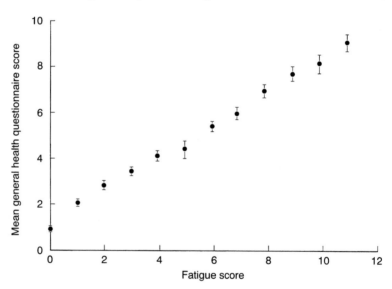

Fig. 4.1 Fatigue and psychological morbidity[11].

These studies use arbitrary cut-offs to define cases of both fatigue and depression or anxiety. An alternative way of exploring the relationship is to consider both fatigue and emotional disorder as dimensional measures, an approach we favour (see Chapter 2). This approach was used in a large population sample[11]. The results (Fig. 4.1) showed a close correlation between the score on the 12-item General Health

Questionnaire (GHQ-12) and that on a fatigue questionnaire[12]. The GHQ-12 does not contain an item directly measuring fatigue, although it does measure concentration difficulties. A high score is associated with a high probability of depressive or anxiety disorder. The relationship between feeling tired and the probability of having an emotional disorder is clear – the more of one, the more of the other ('a dose response'). These results were confirmed by the relationship between fatigue and feeling tired all the time found in the Health and Lifestyle Survey (Table 4.1).

Table 4.1 Feeling tired all the time and GHQ score: Health and Lifestyle Survey[13]

GHQ Score	Males		Females	
	(%)	No.	(%)	No.
0–4	10.3	78	11.6	84
5–9	14.2	129	21.1	214
10–14	23.6	157	36.1	357
15–19	34.9	125	46.2	269
20–24	35.8	29	54.9	83
25–29	64.3	18	71.9	41

Primary care

In Chapter 2 we considered the prevalence of fatigue in primary care. Some of the studies we quoted also looked at the links between fatigue, psychological symptoms, and psychiatric disorder. Kroenke and colleagues noted that 56 per cent of those with fatigue in a primary survey scored above a predefined cut-off on the Beck Depression Scale.[14] Of those with a fatigue syndrome attending a Boston ambulatory care clinic 70 per cent were depressed[15]. An Australian primary care study found that those with chronic fatigue were six times more likely to have probable psychiatric disorder (measured by the GHQ) than those without chronic fatigue[16]. The relationship between fatigue and depression holds in other cultures, such as South East Asian refugees[17] and in Israel[18]. It was the commonest symptom of depression in a Japanese primary care sample[18].

Most credence should be given to studies that involved direct interviews. A Canadian study of patients with chronic fatigue found increased rates of both current and lifetime psychiatric disorder, especially depression[19]. Patients with fatigue had higher levels of distress and worry than those without. Nevertheless, the majority of fatigued patients received no formal psychiatric diagnosis. In contrast, when psychiatrists interviewed those with substantial fatigue attending a London general practice[20] the majority fulfilled criteria for or more psychiatric disorders. The psychiatrist made an ICD-9 diagnosis in 72 per cent of cases, of which 43 per cent were depression[21]. The same group carried out a further study in a wider sample of general practices. Those with chronic fatigue were eight times more likely to meet criteria for depressive disorder, and nearly ten times more likely to have any psychiatric disorder, than a non-fatigued comparison[22]. Another prospective study carried out in UK primary care similarly found that those with chronic fatigue or CFS were between five and six times more likely to fulfil criteria for psychiatric disorder on both questionnaire and interview[23]. Both groups were also considerably more likely to have previous episodes of psychiatric disorder or to have previously been prescribed psychotropic drugs[23]. As in the general population, fatigue and emotional distress are closely correlated[24].

Many of the epidemiological features of the common psychiatric disorders resemble those of fatigue – the over-representation of women, the particular risk for younger adults, and the negative socio-economic gradient, and the associations with demographic factors such as divorce, unemployment, and having young children at home (see Chapter 2 and Goldberg and Huxley[25]).

Secondary care

Study after study shows that fatigue is one of the most prominent symptoms of depression found in secondary or tertiary care samples. Typical findings are that 93 per cent of outpatients with major depression complained of loss of energy[26], as did 97 per cent of another sample[27]. We are unaware of any exceptions.

Conversely, depression is commonly seen in association with chronic fatigue in medical outpatients. Komaroff, a Boston general physician with extensive experience of chronic fatigue, puts it thus: 'Depression, with or without associated anxiety disorder or somatization, is by far the most common cause of fatigue among all patients who seek medical care for fatigue'[28].

4.3 Fatigue and anxiety

Psychiatrists classify the symptoms of anxiety under two headings. The first are the 'psychological' symptoms of anxiety – dread, nervousness, fear, anguish, agitation, and worry. The second are called the 'somatic' symptoms of anxiety. These result from the overactivity of the sympathetic and parasympathetic nervous systems, and include such well recognized symptoms as tremor, palpitations, stomach pain, headache, chest pain, dry mouth, irritable bowel, and many others. They provide a classic example of how emotional disorders may result in physical symptoms via well recognized physiological processes.

Anxiety can be free-floating, in which case it is called 'generalized anxiety disorder' (GAD), or episodic, in which case it is called panic disorder, as the subject experiences panic attacks. Panic attacks can either arise in no particular situation ('free-floating') or in specific places, such as trains, supermarkets, or any crowded setting. If the latter, the sufferer will usually tend to avoid similar situations in the future, for fear of provoking a similar distressing attack. In that case the person is said to have developed a phobia.

Like depression, fatigue is part and parcel of our concepts of anxiety[3]. The major classification systems all include fatigue amongst the criteria for several of the anxiety disorders. Fatigue is listed as a symptom of GAD, and hence fatigue, myalgia, and sleep disorders are found in the majority of those with GAD[23]. Fatigue is also listed as a symptom of episodic anxiety ('panic disorder').

In the ECA sample the presence of fatigue was associated with a considerable increase in the lifetime prevalence of panic disorder, although the actual proportions were relatively modest. Eighty-four per cent of a clinical sample of patients with anxiety disorders complained of chronic fatigue[30]. Angst *et al.* showed that exhaustion was the second commonest symptom of anxiety disorder[31]. Individual symptoms including weakness, exhaustion, poor concentration, hypersensitivity, and fatigue were all between five and ten times commoner in cases than normal controls[31]. In US primary care 58 per cent of those with substantial fatigue were cases of anxiety according to a standard questionnaire[14]. A similar number of those with chronic fatigue in another US primary care clinic rated themselves as anxious[15].

4.4 Fatigue and somatization

'Somatization' is a term frequently encountered in the CFS literature, but opinions differ on its importance, not the least because of the many different usages of the term. We prefer the concept of somatization as a process by which patients experience physical symptoms, which are most probably the result of psychological distress, but which are attributed by the patient to a physical cause[32].

Defined thus, somatization is a very common process by which patients present with psychological disorders to their doctors. Patients with psychiatric disorders are nearly four times more likely to present to their general practitioner with physical rather than psychological symptoms[32]. Somatization is indeed the commonest way for psychiatric disorder to present[33]. Contrary to popular prejudice, somatization is a ubiquitous phenomenon, not restricted to any particular class, gender, ethnic group, or level of intelligence. Instead, comparing somatic with psychological presentations, somatizers were less depressed, had less social dysfunction, but had more unsympathetic attitudes to mental disorder. In common with other investigations, it was reported that those who presented with physical rather than psychological symptoms were more likely to have received previous medical care both as adults and as children[34].

When somatic symptoms are severe and numerous, some subjects will fulfil criteria for somatization disorder, also known as Briquet's syndrome. This diagnosis, first proposed by researchers in St Louis, refers to a chronic condition, usually beginning during adolescence (and certainly no later than 30), characterized by the experience of multiple unexplained medical symptoms affecting multiple organ systems. It is approximately ten times more common in women than men[35]. It is associated with considerable suffering, morbidity, and use of medical resources, but no increase in mortality[36].

Chronic fatigue as a symptom is associated with an increased number of other unexplained physical symptoms, both with and without the inclusion of symptoms that overlap with the concept of CFS[7]. In somatization disorder itself fatigue and weakness are invariably prominent complaints among the many other somatic symptoms encountered[37,38].

4.5 Fatigue – depression or anxiety?

Fatigue is part of the experience of many psychiatric disorders. Are the links closer for any particular disorder than others? Many have suggested that fatigue is characteristic of depression. Low energy successfully classified 93 per cent of another series as depressed or non-depressed, a more accurate marker than psychosocial variables[39] – It was the most efficient symptom for correctly classifying depression[26]. In 1042 primary care patients fatigue significantly discriminated between depressed and non-depressed patients, with a positive predictive value of 61 per cent[40].

However, many studies do not confirm such a simple picture. Depression is certainly not the only psychological symptom associated with fatigue. In one community study 92 per cent of depressives scored highly on a factor representing decreased energy, but so did 46 per cent of agoraphobics, 45 per cent of those with a diagnosis of generalized anxiety, and 29 per cent of those with other phobias[41]. A survey of 2299 adults in Chicago showed that feeling low in energy or slowed down loaded on a factor for depression – but also on the three other factors, labelled anxiety, anger, and cognitive disturbance[42]. The ECA data[7] also showed strong associations for lifetime and current histories of somatization disorder, panic disorder, dysthymia, and so on. In one series of over 2000 consecutive GP attenders, fatigue occurred in the majority of depressed patients, but was also found, albeit with less frequency, in those with either other psychiatric disorders or physical illness. The presence of fatigue was not helpful in discriminating between depressed and non-depressed cases[43]. Depressed mood and anhedonia were both characteristic and discriminating. A study of French primary care[44] found that although the risk of fatigue increases at least seven-fold between the least and most depressed, the absolute figures revealed that fatigue is not characteristic of depression, except in the most severely depressed cases, or those of longer duration[44]. Similar conclusions were reached in Swiss and Icelandic studies[8,9].

In the French study Fuhrer and Wessely[44] also concluded that there exists a similar association between fatigue and non-psychiatric diagnoses; hence fatigue is not a discriminating symptom for depression. A similar result was found in medical patients in the general hospital – fatigue was twice as common in depressed medical cases compared with non-depressed medical cases, but low mood, diurnal variation, and hopelessness were more discriminating[45]. The conclusion is that fatigue and/or weakness is more closely associated with depressive disorder than any other psychiatric diagnosis[46], but is certainly not specific.

4.6 Stress and personality

Personal experience convinces most people that stress and fatigue go together. Fatigued patients in primary care reported greater perceived stress in the previous three months than non-fatigued controls[19]. Emotional strain was associated with fatigue in a large population sample[47]. 'Stress' is a notoriously unreliable term, however; difficult to define, subjective in nature, and prone to recall bias. Social researchers prefer to assess the role of specific events, known as life events, which are easier to record, particularly if using some of the rigorous methodologies that have been developed for the purpose. Major life events are associated with onset of psychiatric disorders such as depression or anxiety, but there is a suggestion that fatigue may be associated with less severe events. One study reports a hierarchy of life events. Severe events such as loss or threat were associated with severer symptoms such as depression or anxiety, but milder events involving choice or uncertainty were associated with fatigue[48]. In another study, however, there was no association between self-reported life events and fatigue[19].

The literature on stress is dominated by the influence of the workplace. Work stress influences the development of neurasthenic symptoms[49], and is related to both fatigue and poor psychological health[50]. Another study reported that job stress was associated with fatigue and multiple symptoms[51]. The links between workplace stress, physical load, musculoskeletal symptoms and fatigue are complex, in particular determining cause and effect is not straightforward. The general conclusion appears to be that short-term workload does contribute to transient feeling of fatigue and muscle discomfort – which of us have not returned from work tired at the end of a hard day? On the other hand, more persistent symptoms are linked to psychosocial distress at the workplace. A recent systematic review found 76 relevant references, and concluded that monotonous work and feeling under pressure were closely associated with musculoskeletal symptoms and fatigue[52]. In general, the risk of developing symptoms such as muscle pain and fatigue is about twice as high in an office with a bad psychosocial environment as in an office with a good one.

4.7 The nature of the association between fatigue and psychiatric disorders

There can be no doubt that fatigue is closely associated with a range of psychiatric disorders. There are many plausible explanations for this association. The first is that the fatigue is the cause of subsequent psychiatric disorder. People become depressed because they are tired. The second is that psychiatric disorder leads to fatigue; for example, a person becomes inactive because they are depressed, and in turn becomes fatigued. Finally, both fatigue and psychiatric disorder may have a common origin.

That fatigue and psychiatric disorder may arise from a common pathology is certainly true and has been discussed in the previous chapter. Cushing's disease or Parkinson's disease provide examples. We will therefore not repeat those arguments, and instead address the question of fatigue and psychiatric disorder which cannot be simply explained by a comorbid medical diagnosis.

One way of addressing these issues is to consider which comes first, the fatigue or the psychiatric disorder? Most of the evidence to answer this question comes from the study of depression, where, in general, the answer appears to be the fatigue. It has long been observed that depressed subjects recall a period of generalized fatigue, myalgia, and malaise before the onset of more typical mood disorder[3,53]. In a study of primary care, somatic complaints, amongst which fatigue was second only to insomnia in importance, preceded the development of the typical affective changes of depression[54,55]. The incidence of fatigue was increased fourfold prior to the diagnosis of depression in primary care[56]. The most convincing evidence comes from the Epidemiologic Catchment Area Program, in which a large sample of community subjects in the United States were given two psychiatric interviews separated by one year[57]. Looking back at those who, free from depression at the first interview, had developed major depression at the one year follow-up, Dryman and Eaton[57] showed that women with fatigue were three times, and males with fatigue seven times, more likely to develop depression over the next year. A 30-month follow-up study in New Zealand gave very similar results[58]. The only exception comes from a longitudinal study[59] in which depressed affect preceded the development of somatic symptoms such as fatigue, the effect being most apparent after several months. This seems to be an isolated finding.

In general there is little doubt that the symptom of fatigue is a significant precursor of later depression. Nevertheless, that does not necessarily imply that fatigue is the cause of subsequent depression. Instead, we prefer to view fatigue as a prodrome of depression – in other words the temporal sequence in which fatigue precedes depression does not imply causality, but is an intrinsic part of the natural history of mood disorder. We feel this is the most likely explanation, although this is not to downplay the significant effect that the experience of fatigue can have on mood. We will return to the question of the direction of causality when we consider the literature on CFS, depression, and physical illness (Chapter 10).

Issues of causality also arise when considering the nature and origin of disability in chronic fatigue. In Chapter 2 we drew attention to the considerable impact of chronic fatigue on various measures of functional impairment, and will do so again when we turn to CFS. This impairment is closely related to the presence of emotional disorder[60]. A similar link was noted in the multinational WHO study of psychiatric disorder in primary care[61] using the ICD-10 diagnosis of neurasthenia (see Chapter 5). Second, the presence of emotional disorder has a significant and deleterious effect on the prognosis of chronic fatigue (see Chapter 7).

Once again, these observations do not tell us the direction of causality. It is not possible to infer that emotional disorder causes functional impairment in chronic fatigue, it might be the other way around. What is important is to note that the two go together. From the clinical perspective this observation does imply that when assessing someone with substantial fatigue that interferes with many aspects of life, and does not speedily resolve, then a careful assessment of mental state is always indicated.

4.8 Fatigue – neither depression nor anxiety?

Given the intimate association between fatigue, depression, and anxiety, is there a fatigue syndrome that exists independently of the two commonest psychiatric disorders? This is a matter of some dispute. For example, Sir David Goldberg argues that the common symptoms found in the community and primary care can largely be accounted for by the twin concepts of depression and anxiety, pointing to the high correlations that exist between somatic symptoms in general, and fatigue in particular, and both depression and anxiety. Neurasthenia is always closely associated with mood disorder[62,63].

On the other hand, others suggest that there is a place for a third factor, labelled neurasthenia[63] or chronic fatigue[22]. In one of Goldberg's own studies[64] a third dimension representing neurasthenic symptoms existed in between depression and anxiety. Cope and colleagues[22] showed that chronic fatigue could be separated from general psychosocial morbidity, but not the tendency to have somatic symptoms.

The nature of psychiatric diagnoses almost mandates the existence of a separate fatigue syndrome. Symptoms are always commoner than diagnoses – the OPCS study of psychiatric disorder in Great Britain found that fatigue was reported by 27 per cent of the population (see Chapter 2), whilst the commonest psychiatric diagnosis, mixed anxiety depression, was only found in 8 per cent[2]. Fatigue is most unlikely to be fully congruent with any particular categorical diagnosis. On the one hand, if you have no psychological symptoms, then you are unlikely to complain of fatigue, and at the other extreme if you are depressed you almost certainly will also experience fatigue. In between these two extremes comes a large area in which fatigue exists in combination with other symptoms, but falls short of fulfilling criteria for recognized diagnostic categories. Some call this neurasthenia, and view it is as a separate diagnostic category in its own right. Others see it as a statistical artefact of the manner in which diagnoses are constructed, lying somewhere in between depression and anxiety without exactly fulfilling criteria for each. The issue may be more semantic than real, since it is accepted by all that neurasthenia is always closely associated with depressive and anxiety disorders, but is never totally congruent. Hence we conclude that there is an independent fatigue syndrome in the community. It is usually, but by no means always, comorbid with the common psychiatric disorders. Whether or not it is called a fatigue syndrome or neurasthenia is a matter of taste[65]. Whether or not it is a separate nosological entity (in terms of aetiology, epidemiology, outcome, and treatment) is a matter of dispute, and will be discussed in succeeding chapters.

4.9 Myalgia and psychiatric disorder

The experience of muscle pain (myalgia) is closely related to that of fatigue. Many patients find it hard to distinguish between the two sensations, and are often unable to be certain whether they are limited by one or the other. The term 'myalgia' is incorporated into the title of one of the most popular current chronic fatigue syndromes, myalgic encephalomyelitis (ME).

Given the overlap between pain and fatigue, it is not surprising that many of the same psychiatric disorders that are associated with fatigue are also associated with self-report of pain. This is confirmed by population studies. For example, in a well conducted study of a Health Maintenance Organisation in Seattle[66] self-reported measures of somatization using the SCL-90 (although one may argue that is more a measure of somatic distress than somatization), were significantly associated with self-reported somatic pain complaints, even when adjusted for sociodemographic variables and depression.

In a population sample of 1254 adults in the USA an association was found between muscle pain and self-reported stress[67]. Of the low-stress sample, 45 per cent reported some degree of muscle pain within the previous 12 months, compared with

62 per cent in the medium-stress, and 63 per cent in the high-stress group. A more linear relationship was observed for 'daily hassles', a measure of chronic stressors. A population based study in the north of England also found that chronic widespread pain was closely associated with feelings of depresion, anxiety, and fatigue[68].

Further understanding of the links between psychiatric disorder and musculoskeletal symptoms comes from studies of the workplace. A Finnish survey[69] found a close association between a questionnaire measure of stress (which recorded a variety of somatic symptoms, including fatigue), and the number of rheumatic symptoms, such as muscle pain and tenderness. A dose-response curve was observed in both men and women – the higher the number of somatic 'stress' symptoms, the higher the rheumatic morbidity. A similar association was observed with the results of a physiotherapist assessment of functional limitation.

The same study also helped to resolve the difficult question of which came first, the psychological or the pain symptoms. A follow-up was performed five years after the initial survey. Symptoms of stress five years previously significantly predicted rheumatic symptoms and musculoskeletal functional impairment. The author suggests that stress produces changes in the physical state of the musculoskeletal system, although an alternative explanation is that psychiatric morbidity predicted functional musculoskeletal impairment[69]. The same authors then performed a similar study, this time over a ten-year period, and looking at neck and shoulder pain. The presence of depression predicted the onset of musculoskeletal pain ten years later[70].

4.10 The causes of fatigue in the community

This chapter and the previous one confirm that fatigue can be a symptom of ill health. The list of possible causes reads like a combined edition of the Oxford Textbooks of both Medicine and Psychiatry. However, in practice the range of options is considerably less.

Some idea of the relative contributions made by the different categories comes from studies that look at the frequencies with which particular diagnoses are made in particular settings. As expected, general practitioners most often attribute tiredness to psychological causes. Of the 58 patient visits for fatigue in Morrell's study of a British primary care practice[71], the doctor diagnosed psychiatric disorders in 30. Other surveys of diagnostic practice in the United Kingdom[72] or the United States[73,74] found that the majority (albeit a slim one) of those presenting with fatigue states received a psychiatric diagnosis. Depression was the largest single diagnostic category, accounting for a quarter of all new presentations[75]. However, psychiatric disorders are certainly not the only diagnoses made. Still in American primary care, Nelson and colleagues reported that 43 per cent of attenders with a chief complaint of fatigue received mixed physical and psychiatric diagnoses[76].

Epidemiological measures can also shed some light on the same issue. If you are depressed, you are between three and eight times more likely to be complaining of chronic fatigue than if you are not depressed. This is labelled 'relative risk'. However, in population terms, what contribution does depression make to the overall levels of fatigue? This is called the 'attributable risk'. How much less tired would the population be if depression did not exist, or if glandular fever disappeared, and so on? Fuhrer and Wessely[44] calculated the population attributable risk of psychiatric disorder and fatigue to be 40 per cent. In other words, if psychiatric disorders could be totally prevented the number of fatigued patients presenting to general practitioners would decrease by that amount. When we consider practical assessment, investigation, and management (Chapter 16), and in particular consider the practical yield of various investigative strategies, we will revisit these figures.

A third and final way of assessing the relative contributions of different factors is to use a statistical technique called logistic regression. This enables the calculation of the odds of being a case (of fatigue), whilst adjusting simultaneously for a number of confounders. As with all multivariate techniques, it requires a large data set (Table 4.2). This gives what we consider to be a reasonable picture of the contribution made by various factors to the experience of fatigue in the community. It will be seen that psychiatric illness ('GHQ case') is a strong association, closely followed by physical illness (as detailed in Chapter 3), but with lifestyle factors such as low exercise also contributing. How these diagnoses are made in practice, and what to do about them, will be the subject of the final section of this book.

Table 4.2 Risk factors for tiredness : Health and Lifestyle Survey. Adjusted odds ratios (logistic regression)

	Odds ratios	95% confidence limits	Probability
Social class 3[1]	1.1	(1.0–1.3)	.057
Social class 4/5	1.2	(1.0–1.5)	.026
Being female	1.5	(1.3–1.7)	<.001
GHQ case	2.5	(2.2–2.8)	<.001
Physical illness	1.5	(1.3–1.7)	
Prescribed drug use	1.2	(1.0–1.4)	
Average exercise[2]	0.9	(0.8–1.1)	.22
High exercise	0.8	(0.7–1.0)	.01

[1] Compared with social class 1.
[2] Compared with low exercise category.

4.11 The story so far

Chronic fatigue is common. It is associated with a wide spectrum of illnesses. Given the central role that fatigue plays in our concepts of common psychiatric disorders, most particularly depression and anxiety, it is not surprising, but noteworthy, that in both the community and primary care the strong associations are between depression, anxiety, and chronic fatigue. However, physical illnesses and behavioural/lifestyle factors also make substantial contributions to the overall burden of fatigue.

What surveys also reveal, whether of the population, primary, or secondary care, is that there is also a category in which clear-cut physical or psychiatric diagnoses cannot be made. If symptoms of depression and/or anxiety are found, they are insufficient to justify a diagnosis of psychiatric disorder. No clear-cut physical abnormality accounts for the fatigue either. It is from this area, the borderlands between medicine and psychiatry, that the concept of syndromes characterized by fatigue *per se* has arisen. It is here that we find the historical syndrome of neurasthenia, and latterly the modern chronic fatigue syndrome.

The nature of these syndromes form the middle section of the this book. We will consider them from a variety of physical and psychological perspectives, but before that we wish to trace their historical origins.

References

1 Sharpe M. Chronic Fatigue Syndrome. *Psych. Clin. North. Am.* 1996; **19:** 549–573.
2 Meltzer H, Gill D, Petticrew M, Hinds K. *The Prevalence of Psychiatric Morbidity Amongst Adults Living in Private Households.* London, HMSO, 1995.
3 Hemphill R, Hall K, Crookes T. A preliminary report on fatigue and pain tolerance in depressive and psychoneurotic patients. *J. Ment. Sci.* 1952: 433–440.
4 Stoeckle J, Davidson G. Bodily complaints and other symptoms of depressive reaction. *J. Am. Med. Assoc.* 1962; **180:** 134–139.
5 Wells VE, Klerman GL, Deykin EY. The prevalence of depressive symptoms in college students. *Soc. Psychiatry* 1987; **22:** 20–28.
6 Montgomery G. Uncommon tiredness among college undergraduates. *J. Consult. Clin. Psychol.* 1983; **51:** 517–525.
7 Walker E, Katon W, Jemelka R. Psychiatric disorders and medical care utilisation among people who report fatigue in the general population. *J. Gen. Intern. Med.* 1993; **8:** 436–440.
8 Angst J, Dobler Mikola A, Binder J. The Zurich study – a prospective epidemiological study of depressive, neurotic and psychosomatic syndromes: I. Problem, methodology. *Eur. Arch. Psychiatry Neurol. Sci.* 1984; **234:** 13–20.
9 Lindal E, Stefansson J. The frequency of depressive symptoms in a general population with reference to DSM-III. *Int. J. Soc. Psychiat.* 1991; **37:** 233–241.
10 Brody E, Klenban M. Physical and mental health symptoms of older people. Whom do they tell? *J. Am. Ger. Soc.* 1981; **24:** 442–449.
11 Pawlikowska T, Chalder T, Hirsch S, Wallace P, Wright D, Wessely S. A population based study of fatigue and psychological distress. *Br. Med. J.* 1994; **308:** 743–746.
12 Chalder T, Berelowitz G, Pawlikowska T, *et al.* Development of a fatigue scale. *J. Psychosom. Res.* 1993; **37:** 147–153.
13 Wessely S. The epidemiology of fatigue. MSc Thesis. London School of Hygiene and Tropical Medicine, 1989.
14 Kroenke K, Wood D, Mangelsdorff D, Meier N, Powell J. Chronic fatigue in primary care: Prevalence, patient characteristics and outcome. *J. Am. Med. Assoc.* 1988; **260:** 929–934.
15 Buchwald D, Sullivan J, Komaroff A. Frequency of 'chronic active Epstein – Barr virus infection' in a general medical practice. *J. Am. Med. Assoc.* 1987; **257:** 2303–2307.
16 Hickie I, Koojer A, Hadzi-Pavlovic D, Bennett B, Wilson A, Lloyd A. Fatigue in selected primary care settings: socio-demographic and psychiatric correlates. *Med. J. Aust.* 1996; **164:** 585–588.
17 Beiser M, Cargo M, Woodbury M. A comparison of psychiatric disorder in different cultures: depressive typologies in southeast Asian refugees and resident Canadians. *Int. J. Method Psychiat. Res.* 1994; **4:** 157–172.
18 Froom J, Aoyama H, Hermoni D, Mino Y, Galambos N. Depressive disorders in three primary care populations: United States, Israel, Japan. *Fam. Pract.* 1995; **12:** 274–278.

19 Cathebras P, Robbins J, Kirmayer L, Hayton B. Fatigue in primary care: prevalence, psychiatric comorbidity, illness behaviour and outcome. *J. Gen. Intern. Med.* 1992; **7:** 276–28.

20 David A, Pelosi A, McDonald E, *et al.* Tired, weak or in need of rest: fatigue among general practice attenders. *Br. Med. J.* 1990; **301:** 1199–1122.

21 McDonald E, David A, Pelosi A, Mann A. Chronic fatigue in general practice attenders. *Psychol. Med.* 1993; **23:** 987–998.

22 Cope H, Mann A, Pelosi A, David A. Psychosocial risk factors for chronic fatigue and chronic fatigue syndrome following presumed viral infection: a case control study. *Psychol. Med.* 1996; **26:** 1197–1209.

23 Wessely S, Chalder T, Hirsch S, Wallace P, Wright D. Psychological symptoms, somatic symptoms and psychiatric disorder in chronic fatigue and chronic fatigue syndrome: a prospective study in primary care. *Am. J. Psychiat.* 1996; **153:** 1050–1059.

24 Ridsdale L, Evans A, Jerrett W, Mandalia S, Osler K, Vora H. Patients who consult with tiredness: frequency of consultation, perceived causes of tiredness and its association with psychological distress. *Br. J. Gen. Practice* 1994; **44:** 413–416.

25 Goldberg D, Huxley P. *Common Mental Disorders: A Bio-social Model.* London, Tavistock, 1992.

26 Buchwald A, Rudick-Davis D. The symptoms of major depression. *J. Abnorm. Psychol.* 1993; **102:** 197–205.

27 Baker M, Dorzab J, Winokur G, Cadoret R. Depressive disorder: classification and clinical characteristics. *Comprehensive Psychiatry* 1971; **12:** 354–365.

28 Komaroff A. Clinical presentation of chronic fatigue syndrome. In Straus S, Kleinman A (ed.) *Chronic Fatigue Syndrome.* Chichester, Wiley, 1993: 43–61.

29 Brawman-Mintzer O, Bruce Lydiard R, Crawford M, *et al.* Somatic symptoms in generalised anxiety disorder with and without comorbid psychiatric disorders. *Am. J. Psychiat.* 1994; **151:** 930–932.

30 Winokur G, Holeman E. Chronic anxiety neurosis: clinical and sexual aspects. *Acta Psychiat. Scand.* 1963; **39:** 384–391.

31 Angst J, Dobler Mikola A. The Zurich Study. V. Anxiety and phobia in young adults. *Eur. Arch. Psychiatry Neurol. Sci.* 1985; **235:** 171–8.

32 Goldberg D, Bridges K. Somatic presentations of psychiatric illness in primary care. *J. Psychosom. Res.* 1988; **17:** 461–470.

33 Murphy M. Somatisation: embodying the problem. *Br. Med. J.* 1989; **298:** 1331–1332.

34 Bridges K, Goldberg D, Evans B, Sharpe T. Determinants of somatisation in primary care. *Psychol. Med.* 1991; **21:** 473–481.

35 Golding J, Smith R, Kashner M. Does somatization disorder exist in men? *Arch. Gen. Psychol.* 1991; **48:** 231–235.

36 Smith G. The course of somatization and its effects on utilization of health care resources. *Psychosomatics* 1994; **35:** 263–267.

37 Smith G, Monson R, Ray D. Patients with multiple unexplained symptoms. *Arch. Intern. Med.* 1986; **146:** 69–72.

38 Fink P. Physical complaints and symptoms of somatizing patients. *J. Psychosom. Res.* 1992; **36:** 125–136.

39 Christensen L, Duncan K. Distinguishing depressed from nondepressed individuals using energy and psychosocial variables. *J. Consult. Clin. Psychol.* 1995; **63:** 495–498.

40 Gerber P, Barrett J, Barrett J, *et al.* The relationship of presenting physical complaints to depressive symptoms in primary care patients. *J. Gen. Intern. Med.* 1992; **7:** 170–173.

41 Uhlenhuth H, Balter M, Mellinger G, Cisin I, Clinthorne J. Symptom checklist syndromes in the general population. *Arch. Gen. Psychiat.* 1983; **40:** 1167–1173.

42 Illfield F. Psychologic status of community residents along major demographic dimensions. *Arch. Gen. Psychiat.* 1978; **35**: 716–724.

43 Blacker R. Depression in primary care. MD. University of London, 1989.

44 Fuhrer R, Wessely S. Fatigue in French primary care. *Psychiat. Med.* 1995; **25**: 895–905.

45 Hawton K, Mayou R, Feldman E. Significance of psychiatric symptoms in general medical patients with mood disorders. *Gen. Hosp. Psychiat.* 1990; **12**: 296–302.

46 Mumford D. Can 'functional' somatic symptoms associated with anxiety and depression be differentiated? *Int. J. Method Psychol. Res.* 1994; **4**: 133–141.

47 Chen M. The epidemiology of self-perceived fatigue among adults. *Prev. Med.* 1986; **15**: 74–81.

48 Miller PM, Ingham JG. Dimensions of experience and symptomatology. *J. Psychosom. Res.* 1985; **29**: 475–88.

49 van Vliet C, Swaen GM, Meijers JM, Slangen J, de Boorder T, Sturmans F. Prenarcotic and neuraesthenic symptoms among Dutch workers exposed to organic solvents. *Br. J. Indust. Med.* 1989; **46**: 586–90.

50 Estryn Behar M, Kaminski M, Peigne E, *et al.* Stress at work and mental health status among female hospital workers. *Br. J. Indust. Med.* 1990; **47**: 20–8.

51 Bromet EJ, Dew MA, Parkinson DK, Cohen S, Schwartz JE. Effects of occupational stress on the physical and psychological health of women in a microelectronics plant. *Soc. Sci. Med.* 1992; **34**: 1377–83.

52 Bongers PM, de Winter CR, Kompier MA, Hildebrandt VH. Psychosocial factors at work and musculoskeletal disease. *Scand. J. Work Environ. Health* 1993; **19**: 297–312.

53 Lindberg B. Somatic complaints in the depressive symptomatology. *Acta Psychiat. Scand.* 1965; **41**: 419.

54 Cadoret R, Wilmer R, Troughton E. Somatic complaints; harbinger of depression in primary care. *J. Affect. Disord.* 1980; **2**: 61–70.

55 Wilson D, Widmer R, Cadoret R, Judiesch K Somatic symptoms: a mojr feature of depression in a family practice. *J. Affect. Disord.* 1983; **5**: 199–207.

56 Widmer R, Cadoret R. Depression in primary care-changes in pattern of patient visits and complaints during a developing depression. *J. Fam. Pract.* 1978; **7**: 293–302.

57 Dryman A, Eaton W. Affective symptoms associated with the onset of major depression in the community; findings from the US National Institute of Mental Health Epidemiologic Catchment Area Program. *Acta Psychol. Scand.* 1991; **84**: 1–5.

58 Romans S, Walton V, McNoe B, Herbison G, Mullen P. Otago Women's Health Survey 30-month follow-up: 1. Onset patterns of non-psychotic psychiatric disorder. *Br. J. Psychiatry* 1993; **163**: 733–738.

59 Brenner B. Depressed affect as a cause of associated somatic problems. *Psychol. Med.* 1979; **9**: 737–746.

60 Wessely S, Chalder T, Hirsch S, Wallace P, Wright D. The prevalence and morbidity of chronic fatigue and chronic fatigue syndrome: a prospective primary care study. *Am. J. Pub. Health* 1997; **87**, 1449–1455.

61 Ormel J, VonKorff M, Ustun B, Pini S, Korten A, Oldehinkel T. Common mental disorders and disabilities across cultures: results from the WHO Collaborative Study on Psychological Problems in General Health Care. *J. Am. Med. Assoc.* 1994; **272**: 1741–1748.

62 Persson L, Sjoberg L. Mood and somatic symptoms. *J. Psychosom. Res.* 1987; **31**: 499–511.

63 Angst J, Koch R. Neurasthenia in young adults. In Gastpar M, Kielholz P (ed.) *Problems of Psychiatry in General Practice.* Toronto, Hogrefe & Huber, 1991: 37–48.

64 Goldberg D, Bridges K, Duncan Jones P, Grayson D. Dimensions of neuroses seen in primary-care settings. *Psychol. Med.* 1987; **17**: 461–70.

65 Farmer A, Jones I, Hillier J, Llewelyn M, Borysiewicz L, Smith A. Neuraesthenia revisited: ICD-10 and DSM-III-R psychiatric syndromes in chronic fatigue patients and comparison subjects. *Br. J. Psychiatry* 1995; **167:** 503–506.

66 Von Korff M, Dworkin S, Le Resche L, Kruger A. An epidemiologic comparison of pain complaints. *Pain* 1988; **32:** 173–183.

67 Sternbach R. Pain and 'hassles' in the United States: findings of the Nuprin pain report. *Pain* 1986; **27:** 69–80.

68 Croft P, Schollum J, Silman A. Population study of tender point counts and pain as evidence of fibromyalgia. *Br. Med. J.* 1994; **309:** 696–699.

69 Leino P. Symptoms of stress predict musculoskeletal disorders. *J. Epidemiol. Community Health* 1989; **43:** 293–300.

70 Leino P, Magni G. Depressive and distress symptoms as predictors of low back pain, neck-shoulder pain, and other musculoskeletal morbidity: a 10-year follow-up of metal industry employees. *Pain* 1993; **53:** 89–94.

71 Morrell D. Symptom interpretation in general practice. *J. R. Coll. Gen. Pract.* 1972; **22:** 297–309.

72 Jerrett W. Lethargy in general practice. *Practitioner* 1981; **225:** 731–737.

73 Morrison J. Fatigue as a presenting complaint in family practice. *J. Fam. Pract.* 1980; **10:** 795–801.

74 Sugarman J, Berg A. Evaluation of fatigue in a family practice. *J. Fam. Pract.* 1984; **19:** 643–647.

75 Elnicki D, Shockcor W, Brick J, Beynon D. Evaluating the complaint of fatigue in primary care: diagnoses and outcomes. *Am. J. Med.* 1992; **93:** 303–307.

76 Nelson E, Kirk J, McHugo G, *et al.* Chief complaint fatigue: a longitudinal study from the patient's perspective. *Fam. Pract. Res.* 1987; **6:** 175–188.

Section II:

The history of chronic fatigue

5. Neurasthenia

So far we have considered the question of fatigue, or more specifically chronic fatigue, as an isolated symptom. However, fatigue can be more than just a symptom. Recently the popular imagination has been caught by the concept of fatigue as specific illness, encapsulated in the term 'chronic fatigue syndrome' (CFS), or, as it is better known in the vernacular, ME. It is frequently stated that these illnesses are either new, or at least on the increase, and the popular and professional literature contains numerous possible explanations for this phenomenon.

But just how new are these syndromes? In this chapter we will argue that these syndromes, and the claims made about them, are not new to medicine or popular thinking. This chapter considers the original fatigue syndrome, neurasthenia. The story of neurasthenia is fascinating in its own right, but we hope to show that an historical analysis remains relevant to the discussion of the modern fatigue syndromes that follow.

5.1 What was neurasthenia?

Neurasthenia was 'a disease of the nervous system, without organic lesion, which may attack any or all parts of the system, and characterized by enfeeblement of the nervous force, which may have all degrees of severity, from slight loosening of these forces down to profound and general prostration' (Bouveret, cited by Deale and Adams[1]). 'Neurasthenia is a condition of nervous exhaustion, characterised by undue fatigue on [the] slightest exertion, both physical and mental . . . the chief symptoms are headache, gastrointestinal disturbances, and subjective sensations of all kinds'[2]. According to Ballet, neurasthenia consisted of 'weakening of the motor energy . . . subjects cannot complete the simplest act in one effort, however short, without feeling immediate and insurmountable lassitude. To stand, to walk or to talk, each causes fatigue'. These definitions outline the core concepts of neurasthenia – that it was the disease of excessive fatigability, and that fatigability could affect physical and mental (which meant the processes of thought, speech, and memory) functioning equally. There was a consensus that although the symptoms of neurasthenia could vary, essential to the diagnosis was that the patient be 'incapacitated for all forms of mental and physical exertion'[1].

Beyond that core concept, neurasthenia was an exceptionally broad church. Several strands can be discerned[3]. First, neurasthenia was chronic fatigue[4,5]. In neurasthenia chronic fatigue was always the 'primary or essential' symptom[6], its 'cardinal characteristics being an inordinate sense of physical or mental fatigue'[7]. The commonest manifestation of fatigue was either a 'neuromuscular weakness – by all writers this is accounted for as the most frequently observed objective sign of disease'[8] or 'unusually rapid exhaustion mainly affects the mental activities; the power of attention becomes quickly exhausted and the capacity for perception is paralysed'[9]. Whether mental or physical, fatigue had certain characteristics – it 'comes early, is extreme and lasts long'[10], and is 'the first, and most important symptom'[11] – hence neurasthenics had 'abnormally quick fatigability and slow recuperation'[12], their fatigue not being relieved by rest. Neurasthenics, with 'every appearance of normal values of power, are speedily exhausted in the process of moderate exercise', and that 'prolonged or severe mental effort' was equally impaired[13]. These and many other quotations give little doubt that what was being described is directly comparable to modern descriptions of CFS or ME.

Second, neurasthenia was depression. This could mean depression of 'cortical activity'[14] or latterly depression in a more psychological sense. Déjerine and Gauckler[15] felt that melancholia and neurasthenia could only be distinguished on the basis of history, previous episodes of depression or mania favouring the former diagnosis. Many authors equated neurasthenia with a mild melancholia[8,16].

Third, neurasthenia was a masculine form of hysteria – women developed hysteria whilst men developed neurasthenia[17]. Freud felt that the 'male nervous system has as preponderant a disposition to neurasthenia as the female to hysteria'[18]. (It is important to note that hysteria did not have its modern meaning of non-organic, almost the opposite was true.)

Fourth, Beard himself viewed neurasthenia as the prototype of many diseases, both physical and mental. Others agreed that neurasthenia was the soil from which all mental illnesses spring[19,20]. These intermediate stages were, according to Durkheim, 'the various anomalies usually combined under the common name of neurasthenia'[21].

Regardless of the classification of neurasthenia adopted, most noted the discrepancy between physical disability and physical examination. Neurasthenia was also 'destitute of the objective signs which experimental medicine of our times more particularly affects'[22]. Sufferers looked normal, and were typically 'well nourished, muscularly well developed'[23], despite often profound functional disability. It also had no significant mortality (indeed, George Beard claimed the opposite[24]).

5.2 The arrival of neurasthenia

The New York neurologist George Beard (Fig. 5.1) is widely credited with introducing the term 'neurasthenia' in a brief paper presented in the *Boston Medical and Surgical Journal* in 1869[25]. However, the psychiatrist Van Deusen has an equal claim to the authorship of neurasthenia, as he introduced the term in the *American Journal of Insanity* in the same year[26]. The rival claims of Van Deusen, an alienist treating farmers in unfashionable Kalamazoo, and Beard, an East Coast neurologist with clients drawn from the Social Register, mirrored the wider confrontation between neurology and psychiatry at that time[27]. As with the larger professional conflict, it was Beard who triumphed and the neurologist who became most credited with the 'discovery' of neurasthenia.

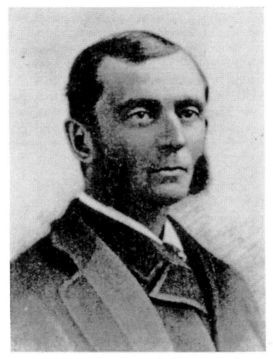

Fig. 5.1 George Beard.

The concept of nervous exhaustion was not new, and a few contemporaries took care to elaborate the history of the disease before Beard, tracing its origins to nervosisme, neurospasm, spinal irritability, and so on[19,28]. Later historians have pointed out the debt Beard owed to hypochondria, spinal irritation, and the Brownian doctrine of asthenia and esthenia[17,29].

Whatever the provenance of neurasthenia, it spread rapidly, especially to France and Germany. By the turn of the century a French doctor wrote that 'the name of neurasthenia was on everybody's lips, the fashionable disease'[30], the 'maladie à la mode'[31], even 'La Maladie du Beard'[32,33]. Many of Charcot's pupils wrote texts on the illness; the most popular was probably that by Adrien Proust, ironically, the father of the most famous neurasthenic of the age, Marcel Proust. Bumke later wrote that there was no instance in the history of medicine of a label having the impact of neurasthenia[34]. Beard's success was because he articulated his ideas to a receptive audience. He was able to incorporate many of the exciting new discoveries in medicine, physiology, and physics, and hence his new illness assisted medical thought in moving away from the outdated doctrines of sentiments and passions no longer suitable for a society preoccupied with 'La Vie Moderne'[35].

5.3 The aetiologies of neurasthenia

Peripheral

During the early years of interest in neurasthenia the prevailing neurological para-digm was the reflex hypothesis. Excessive irritation of the nervous system led to exhaustion of the peripheral nerves, which could spread to any tissue (see Shorter[3] and Lopez-Pinero[29]). One cause of this was over-stimulation, which fitted easily into Beard's theory. However, the remarkable flourishing of neurophysiology soon discredited the reflex hypothesis. Many of the early advocates of neurasthenia in England were emphatic in their condemnation of reflex theory, and in particular of the practice of 'local treatment' of the female genital organs. In ridiculing the reflex theory Allbutt explained that neither muscles nor reflex arc were in a state of exhaustion, nor were the neurasthenic cells too excitable – 'to be excitable is their business'[36]. All these authorities espoused the new central paradigm of nervous disease, which soon replaced reflex theories.

The central paradigm

As views of the nervous system changed, especially under the impact of the new laws of thermodynamics and conservation of energy, so did the nature of neurasthenia. Before the arrival of neurasthenia doctors were beginning to discuss not only the body, but also the mind in terms of heat and energy: George Johnson, the Chair of Medicine at King's College Hospital, wrote about the mind as a 'set of complex psychological energies'[37], and it was only a short step to see neurasthenia as an exhaustion of that supply of energy within the central nervous system. The con-sequence was 'cortical weakness'[38] or 'cortical irritability'[39]. Irritable weakness of the brain permitted some remnants of reflex theory to survive, but many other causes of cerebral exhaustion were identified. These could be directly involving the brain – a failure of cerebral blood supply was a popular explanation[40]. The brain could also be exhausted by either a deficiency in local energy sources or as a result of the effect of toxins and infections elsewhere in the body. Hence the increased demands on the system could result from overwork, or be the result of toxic, metabolic, or infective insults. All of the above were acquired in adult life, but individuals could also be predisposed to react to each or all of these factors by heredity, or could inherit neurasthenia itself.

The social paradigm

The doctrine of overwork and nervous exhaustion linked neurasthenia with a variety of contemporary changes in society. Medical authorities viewed overwork, the agent by which the nervous system became exhausted (which could be purely physical, mental, or a mixture of both), as the inevitable consequence of a host of new social ills. Even before the introduction of neurasthenia, a variety of medical authorities were writing about the dangers of overwork[37,41,42]. It was Beard, with his facility for similes, who joined together a number of discontents into an explanatory model for his disease[24,43]. His particular skill was to mix scientific advances with social theory and moral exhortation, and constructing out of these sources a single disease, designed to appeal to the social concerns of the age, but couched in what seemed to many (but by no means all) acceptable scientific terminology. We will encounter similar skills in modern popular writings on CFS and other twentieth-century illnesses (see Chapter 15). For example, Beard, and many others, ascribed neurasthenia to the new, acquisitive nature of society summed up as 'modern civilisation'[43]. Much of this was conveyed by metaphors drawn from business life, the exhausted businessman overdrawn on his nervous capital, overspent nervous resources, and so on (see Oppenheim[44] and Lutz[45]). Another social preoccupation was of the possible untoward consequences of the new educational reforms and the changing status of women. Beard, Mitchell, and their contemporaries were thus able to translate what were essentially social and cultural fears into a quasi scientific idiom – the female nervous system, inheritantly weaker than the male, giving way as a result of excessive occupational demands, or the children made vulnerable to neurasthenia by similar excessive educational demands.

The psychogenic paradigm

Unfortunately for the organic view of neurasthenia, the central paradigm could not be sustained. Fatigue could only be measured with the greatest of difficulty[46], if at all[47], nor could any discrete neuropathological lesion be located. Adolf Meyer[48] wrote that the 'remarkable changes in the nerve cells' which others had found, were 'highly fashionable and a matter of pride to both patient and diagnostician . . . but could not be replicated. Fatigue exhaustion is no longer tenable'. The consequence was a loss of faith in simple neurological explanations. In the first issue of the prestigious *Journal of Abnormal Psychology* Donley criticized the previous 'mechanical symbolism' of descriptions of neurasthenia, with the false belief that 'for every pathological manifestation there must be an underlying, definite "disease process" ', and the 'futility of the purely anatomical concept' expressing itself in 'apologetic reproductions of nerve cells in a state of fatigue'[49]. Two years later neurasthenia could be described as 'a state of habitual valetudinarianism with no corresponding characteristic organic lesion'[50].

Social aetiologies were also changing. It was doubted if neurasthenia really was a disease of modern life[51], except that 'we had become more tender in our ills'[30]. Neurasthenia was more likely to result from idleness than overwork[52,53], reflected in the increased emphasis on activity and exercise in place of the classic rest cure.

These last quotes suggest a further change, that of class. Neurasthenia had been sustained by the belief that it was a condition of the most successful people in society. 'It is a disease of bright intellects, its victims are leaders and masters of men, each one a captain of industry'[54], a view shared by many, including both Freud and Kraepelin[55]. Many noted the large number of doctors afflicted[22,56], which included some of those most closely identified with the condition, such as Beard, Dowse, and Mitchell.

However, the preponderance of the male professional classes amongst sufferers began to alter. Charcot was among the first to point this out[57], and by 1906 a series of papers were produced describing the illness in the working class[58–61]. The records of the Vanderbilt Clinic in New York[62] shows that neurasthenia was now mainly a disease of the lower social classes, and, as many of these comprised Jewish immigrants, it could no longer even be called the 'American Disease'. The illness had become the commonest cause of absenteeism among the garment workers of New York[63]. In 1906 Stedman pleaded in his presidential address to the American Neurological Association[64] for more attention to the need for facilities for the neurasthenic poor. Cobb noted sardonically that those who continued to believe the disease was restricted to the upper social echelons were those whose commitment was entirely to private practice[2].

These two factors – the failure of the organic paradigm and the social class changes – prepared the way for the psychological model. Initially, neurasthenia was retained, but viewed as a psychological, rather than a physical illness. The pendulum shifted; rather than psychological symptoms being a consequence of neurasthenia, they first became linked in a vicious circle, with neither having supremacy[65,66]. Next, psychological processes caused neurasthenia: thus Déjerine writes that 'many manifestations [of neurasthenia] are by nature purely phobic in origin'[15]. Finally, the category itself was dismembered, and replaced by new psychiatric diagnoses. It is well known that by 1893 Freud considered sexual exhaustion to be the sole cause of neurasthenia, either directly or indirectly. The following year saw his famous removal of anxiety neurosis from neurasthenia[67]. Just as important was the work of Pierre Janet. He also regarded fatigue as the key to psychological disorder, and, like his contemporaries blamed modern life for fatigue neurosis[68], However, like William James he derided the conventional economic metaphor of the neurasthenic overdrawing on a limited capital of physical energy, but emphasized instead the emotional demands on the psychic economy[68]. Janet replaced neurasthenia with psychasthenia, containing what we now recognize as the obsessional and phobic neuroses[69], but even this category did not last long.

Freud, Bernheim, and others continued to believe in a physical neurasthenia, not amenable to psychotherapy, but thought it was rare. Freud retained an interest in neurasthenia – of the seven book reviews he is known to have written four are concerned with neurasthenia, but their tone became increasingly sceptical[70]. Freud's biographer Ernest Jones later wrote that fewer than 1 per cent of neurasthenics were correctly diagnosed[71]. Janet also believed in a physical neurasthenia for a brief period, but then abandoned this altogether.

The organicists countered such observations in two ways. First, the present methods of investigation were too crude to detect the organic changes[9]. Second, psychological symptoms, if present, were part of the physical neurasthenic state[72,73], or were an understandable reaction to the illness. In a speech to the American Neurological Association, Weir Mitchell referred to his own early neurasthenia, and pointed out how depression could not be an explanation for his condition, since he had 'no depression that was abnormal or unreasonable'[11]. His own illness, and that of other distinguished contemporary medical men, made it inconceivable that neurasthenia could be 'a malady of the mind alone'.

Nevertheless, these became increasingly minority views. Charles Dana, Professor of Neurology at Cornell, read an influential paper to the Boston Society of Psychiatry and Neurology[74], expounding the 'renaissance' in psychiatric thinking, in contrast to the previous antagonism between neurology and psychiatry, and urging adoption of the new classifications. Only two years later the new President of the Neurological Association described an eminent patient as suffering from 'neurasthenia or mild melancholia'[64], the 'or' being unlikely a decade earlier. When the London Medical Society debated neurasthenia in 1913, Kinnier-Wilson wrote that 'it was clear . . . from the discussion that Beard's original description of "American Nervousness" as a physical and not a mental state was evidently not accepted by several of the speakers'[75]. Thomas Horder at St Bartholomew's remarked that in his experience the mental element in neurasthenia overshadowed any physical contribution[76]. The successive editions of one important English psychiatric text show how neurasthenia moved from the neuroses (still an organic neurological diagnosis) to the psychoneuroses[77]. Neurologists at the Massachusetts General Hospital had already done the same[78], as did both Dutil and Déjerine, pupils of Charcot – 'Beard's illness must now be seen as of mental origin'[79]. In a reminiscence of George Beard published in 1926 fellow neurologist Charles Dana casually referred to neurasthenia as 'what we now call psychoneurosis'[80].

Neurasthenia was replaced mainly by the new psychiatric diagnoses. Fatigue on the slightest exertion was now a symptom of anxiety[81], but the greatest beneficiary was the new concept of depression. A book which in 1901 had been entitled 'Les grands symptômes neurasthéniques', twenty years later had changed to 'Les états depressifs et la neurasthénie'. With the support of such figures as Jaspers and Bleuler ('What usually produces the so-called neurasthenia are affective disturbances'[82]) the view became widespread that 'all neurasthenic states are in reality depression – perhaps minor, attenuated, atypical, masked, but always forms of anxious melancholia'[83].

5.4 Changes in the treatment of neurasthenia

The change in the nosology of neurasthenia was also influenced by changing views of treatment. Victorian neurasthenics were treated with a bewildering variety of pharmacological and electrical treatments, mixing drugs to either stimulate a failing nervous system or sedate an overexcitable one[84]. For many, this treatment also involved a visit to a spa. By the 1880s neurasthenics made up most of the clientele of the great spas of Europe[85]. Here they would receive a variety of treatments, usually beginning with some form of hydrotherapy or 'cold bath' cure, a treatment recently resurrected for the management of CFS. Most popular of all was the rest cure. This consisted of five elements: rest, seclusion, massage, electricity, and diet. Weir Mitchell, the doyen of American neurology, first described the cure in 1875, and then popularized it in a series of best-sellers (although not initially concerned with neurasthenia), summed up in the contemporary catch phrase 'Doctor Diet and Doctor Quiet'. Nevertheless, it is often forgotten that Mitchell originally suggested the cure for the treatment of hysteria. In 1888 Freud was recommending a combination of Weir Mitchell's and Breuer's cathartic treatment for hysteria, but added that 'in the case of the other neuroses, for instance neurasthenia, the success of the treatment is far less certain'[18].

It was only as the distinctions between hysteria and neurasthenia became blurred, and perhaps as the financial advantages from treating neurasthenia became clearer, that rest cure became popular for neurasthenia. By 1881 the 'cure' was being used in England, largely due to William Playfair, Professor of Obstetrics at King's College Hospital and noted society doctor[86], who proclaimed it 'the greatest advance of which practical medicine can boast in the last quarter of the century'.

It was in Germany and the USA that the rest cure found its most ready acceptance. Mitchell's own hospital became the 'Mecca'[87] for neurasthenics. Playfair's book was available in German in 1883, only a year after its publication in English, and a German edition of Weir Mitchell was available by 1886, reviewed by Freud in the following year. Large numbers of 'retreats', private clinics, and rest homes appeared across Europe between 1880 and 1900[88-90]. It was financially vital to the neurologist, since, as one wrote in 1894, the neurologist should not '*undertake a thoroughgoing course of this sort of treatment unless in a private institution*'[91] (italics in original). The rest cure became the most used treatment for nervous disorder across Central Europe and America and the principal justification for the private clinic, since neither isolation, nor rest or the expensive apparatus of electrotherapy could be provided at home. As Shorter points out, 'physicians in these competitive, profit making clinics were happy to comply with the patients' desire for face saving [organic] diagnoses, and made great use of such expressions as . . . chronic fatigue and neurasthenia'[90].

The rest cure has attracted many criticisms over the years. The writings of famous patients treated by the cure, such as Virginia Woolf and Charlotte Perkins Gilman, have been important in highlighting the influence of male stereotypes of women, especially their moral and physical weaknesses (see Wood[92] and Cayleff[93]). Contemporaries, however, noted other failings. Principal among these was the failure of the somatic model. If there was no cellular basis to exhaustion, then what was the purpose of rest? The growing awareness that all the business of the cure, the diet, massage, electricity, etc., were just props for the physician to exhort and encourage the patient, meant that they could be dispensed with (see Dutil[79], Drummond[94], and Waterman[95]). It became increasingly difficult to deny the role of suggestion, of the doctor–patient relationship[15], and ultimately of the newer psychotherapies (see Shorter[85] and Hale[27]). Gradually authorities began to suspect that the rest cure might actually make the patient worse. For example, less than ten years separates two contributions on neurasthenia made by Dutil, another pupil of Charcot. In the first[33] he espouses a standard Weir Mitchell approach, but in the second[79] Mitchell's regime was seen as condemning the patient to a life of disability and hypochondriasis. 'It is quite evident that what a patient needs is not rest, but *exercise* . . . *a carefully graduated physical culture*'[96] (italics in original).

The decline of the rest cure and the corresponding rise of the new occupational and psychotherapies is a fundamental passage in the history of psychiatry. The eclipse of the rest cure further weakened the organic models of neurasthenia, and conversely increased the status of the new psychological school of thought. Inevitably, the management of the neurasthenic patient passed from the neurologist to the psychiatrist. By 1944 Karl Menninger's[97] disdainful account of the rest cure sealed this transfer, at least for a time.

5.5 The reaction against neurasthenia

What were the consequences of the failures of the simple organic models of both aetiology and treatment, and the rise of the psychological models? Physicians could either abandon the concept or concede that the patients were best cared for by the psychiatric profession. Many neurologists were soon persuaded that neurasthenia should be abandoned – in 1911 Browning[98] wrote that neurasthenics were rare in his neurological service (although not, he admitted, in his private practice), because 'Many of our best neurologists do not now recognise such as disease'. Particularly in the United Kingdom, neurology was establishing itself as a scientific speciality and many soon turned their backs on the now discredited neurasthenia. Although pleas were made for the same process in the USA[74], the concept was more deeply entrenched there. As late as 1927 one-third of patients seen by American neurologists were still either neurasthenic or psychasthenic[99]. Many physicians retained the diagnosis (and therefore the patients), but began gradually to incorporate the new psychological insights into their treatments – the 'rational psychotherapy' of Paul Dubois being particularly influential, perhaps because it repudiated notions of the unconscious that were often unpalatable to many neurologists. By the end of the 1920s the journals were full of articles and reviews questioning the diagnosis of neurasthenia; such critiques, always present, had now become a chorus[45]. A 1929 review concluded that 'neurasthenic disorders are a bit out of fashion'[100].

British neurologists were happy to drop neurasthenia, partly because they had always been sceptical about the illness anyway. Beard himself had a dismal reception when he visited England in 1880 and 1881. He committed his first social gaffe before he had even set foot in England, an incident that resulted in a letter of criticism in the *British Medical Journal*[101]. He failed to impress the British Medical Association, and finally upset no less a person than Crichton Browne[102]. Beard's own account of his visit made no mention of these troubles. However, when describing what we would now call a 'study tour' of the asylums of Europe he mentioned that his preferred method was to arrive without any letters of instructions or prior notice, nor to tell his hosts of the purpose of his visit[103].

After Beard's departure, Sir Andrew Clark, an eminent physician at the London Hospital, launched a blistering attack in *The Lancet*[104], and, although Playfair made a spirited defence[105], he was forced to concede that he had been unable to persuade the Collective Investigation Committee of the BMA to take an interest. Neurasthenia was never accepted by the neurological establishment. The giants of the profession, such as Gowers, Gordon Holmes, Ferrier, Buzzard, and Kinnier-Wilson based at the National Hospital for Nervous Diseases, declared themselves in various ways against an organic view of neurasthenia, and in favour of psychological interpretations. Gower devoted only one page of his two-volume 1888 text to the subject[106], and in the next edition was even briefer – neurasthenia 'occurs especially in those of a neurotic disposition'[107].

Whether or not this academic disdain was translated into clinical practice is an interesting question. When Simon Wessely was fortunate enough to be conducting outpatient clinics in a room at the National Hospital lined with the original case records of the period, reading them during gaps in the clinic showed that, despite their declarations, all the giants of neurology made the diagnosis with varying degrees of frequency. Contemporary accounts noted the same[76]. Nevertheless, unlike the United States, France, and Germany, in the United Kingdom the neurasthenic flag was flown in public by only a few – the most prominent being Clifford Allbutt in Cambridge. Even he had to admit that acceptance was at best grudging; in his eight-volume textbook he criticized those 'medical men who reject neurasthenia as in part a sham, and in part a figment of complacent physicians'[36]. Despite such efforts a reviewer conceded that neurasthenia had 'not taken deep root in Britain'[108]. British neurologists were, wrote one, far more concerned with organic than functional nervous disease[109]. The *British Medical Journal* did not 'take quite so serious a view of the prevalence of neurasthenia in modern life'[110], and by 1913 neurasthenia's 'servicableness as coin of the realm' was doubtful[111].

5.6 Neurasthenia, stigma, and prejudice

Issues of class and gender were intimately related to those of aetiology and treatment. The more 'organic' the account, the more likely was the author to insist on the predominance of upper social classes, the distinction from hysteria, and the over-representation of men and 'civilized' races. Physicians were more likely to view sympathetically those whose illnesses had been acquired by praiseworthy rather than contemptible means (as indeed they still do); neurasthenia, the disease of overwork, came into the former, hysteria the latter[112]. Groups allegedly not subject to such overwork, such as women, lower classes, degenerates, American Negroes, and all uncivilized races, thus were spared neurasthenia[43,113–115]. One writer considered that manual labourers were spared neurasthenia because 'their muscular development holds down their emotional centres to a safe level'[116].

We have already noted how the classic views of neurasthenia were sustained by the belief that it was a disease of the rich and succesful, but that by 1900 it had become increasingly hard to ignore the evidence that not only were women and the lower classes also susceptible to the condition, they were starting to make up the majority of cases. Writings on neurasthenia underwent a shift to explain this – women were more susceptible to the condition because of their smaller brains, frail constitution, and lower moral constitution. Women were unsuited for the stressors to which they were now being exposed, namely increased participation in the workforce and increased access to education[92,93,117]. Likewise Jews had a special predisposition for neurasthenia because of their excitable, emotional, and unstable temperaments[3].

We can detect these prejudices most clearly in the contrasts made between neurasthenia and hysteria. Those who supported the organic views of neurasthenia were the most likely to emphasize the differences the two conditions (see Chapter 6). Playfair, writing in Tuke's dictionary, stated that the difference between neurasthenics and hysterics was that the former 'give all they possess to be well, and heartily long for good health, if only they knew how to obtain it'[118]. Neurasthenics cooperated with the doctor, unlike hysterics[119]. The bluntest was Ernest Reynolds, Professor of Medicine in Manchester, who wrote that whereas hysteria was 'purely a mental condition, whose basis is a morbid craving for sympathy and notoriety', neurasthenia was 'entirely different . . . a functional disorder of chronic overuse of neurones' due to 'gross overwork and worry'[120].

Even within the sexes, such moral judgements were frequent – thus Sir Frederick Mott[121] wrote that 'neurasthenia . . . was more likely to be acquired in *officers of a sound mental constitution than men of the ranks*', because in the former the prolonged stress of responsibility which, in the officer worn out by the prolonged stress of war and want of sleep, causes anxiety less he should fail in his critical duties'[6] (italics in the original). Officers had greater moral fibre than the common soldier.

The consequence was the decline of the diagnosis. This was partially intended, as doctors dismantled the now overstretched concept, that 'mob of incoherent symptoms borrowed from the most diverse disorders'[104]. However, as the reception accorded Beard in the journals showed ('Dr Beard's book is not worth the ink with which it is printed, much less the paper on which this was done'[122] was a mild example), academic disdain was not new. It now vanished for more practical reasons. Neurasthenia had survived academic dissatisfaction because it was 'useful to the doctor'[111] as a code for non-psychotic illnesses for which the only effective treatments were psychologically based. The diagnosis was made 'for the comfort of the relatives and peace of mind of the patient'[123] since it avoided the stigma of psychiatric illness and the necessity to seek treatment in an asylum, where the neurasthenic would 'soon be subject to the usual stigma attached to the abode of mental patients . . . only in a general hospital could the psychic problem be solved under the happiest auspices'[124]. Others commented that even if the symptoms were psychological, it was better to talk about nervous diseases and neurasthenia since 'the patients and the patient's friends usually have a horror of mental disease'[20]. Several anecdotes attest to the consequences of not keeping to these codes. Drummond[94], the senior physician at the Royal Victoria Infirmary in Newcastle, describes a scene which many may still recognize today when he witnessed a 'kindly physician' let slip the word 'melancholia' during a consultation with a neurasthenic patient. 'The outcome of that visit was disastrous, involving serious trouble all round, in which even Sir Andrew himself shared, for he was pestered for weeks with letters to know whether in using the term "melancholia" he had the idea of insanity in his mind'.

As more doctors accepted the new psychological models, it became harder to maintain the obscurity of the codes. Statements such as 'functional illness means pooh poohed illness'[125] and 'neurotic, neurasthenic, hysterical and hypochondriacal are, on the lips of the majority of clinical teachers, terms of opprobrium'[94] show that the codes were being broken, and the demise of the category a matter of time. In 1868 patients were only too willing to confess to 'weakness of the nerves'[126], but 30 years later the *Spectator* observed that neurasthenia was no longer 'interesting' but 'discredited and disgraceful . . . shameful to confess'[127]. The changes in social class, and the rise of the psychogenic school, meant that aetiologies had also changed. Infection remained (see below), but in place of overwork came laziness, fecklessness, degeneration, and poor hygiene. Bad housing was now blamed[128], and even poor dental hygiene, due to the 'fashion of eating ice cream . . . prevalent among the children of the lower classes'[58].

Neurasthenia had once been a badge of honour[129] – 'It is certain that it is chiefly the people who have a neurasthenic constitution who are the most brilliant, original, energetic and influential. It is they who do the intellectual work of the world'[130]. In *The Guermantes way*, Proust has Dr du Boulbon, the 'alienist and brain doctor', who has 'special competence in cerebral and nervous matters' explain that only neurasthenics could create great art. 'The world will never realise how much it owes to them, and what they have suffered in order to bestow their gifts on it'[131]. However, neurasthenia was rapidly losing its distinction. In place of the hard-pressed businessman came the stereotype of the work-shy labourer, the Jewish garment worker, or the pampered hypochondriacal upper class female invalid[132]. Now doctors who had used the rise of neurasthenia as evidence of the advance of both civilization and medicine made the same observations on its decline – 'the gradual "passing of neurasthenia" is a sign of the times and of the advancement of medical science'[133]. It had 'outlived its usefulness'[134].

Successive editions of the *Surgeon General's Index* catalogue the decline of the diagnosis. Beard had always argued that neurasthenia was the precursor of a variety of conditions, both mental and physical. As the symptoms were so protean, this was not surprising, but physicians began to see little point in diagnosing neurasthenia in those with conditions adequately covered by other labels[134]. The space devoted to it in the classic neurological texts dwindled, and finally disappeared, or received a brief psychiatric coverage. In the first edition of Cecil's prestigious textbook of medicine neurasthenia has its own chapter[99]. In 1934 in the third edition it is listed under 'The neuroses or psychoneuroses', is reduced to a single sentence in the 1947 seventh edition, and disappears from the eighth.

In conclusion there were a number of reasons for the decline in neurasthenia. First, the neuropathological basis of the illness was discredited. Second, rest cure was seen either to be unsuccessful, or to be efficacious principally for psychological reasons. Third, the social class distribution of the illness altered. Finally, the interest and optimism shown by the neurologists was transferred to the new profession of psychiatry.

5.7 The disease that did not disappear

The rise of psychogenic explanations of neurasthenia had one unexpected side effect, it paradoxically prolonged the survival of neurasthenia. Sir Farquahar Buzzard had warned that although the advances in both neurology and psychiatry had illuminated the plight of the neurasthenic, the same could not be said of the exclusively psychogenic theories, which would lead to a polarization among doctors. 'On the contrary, Freudian doctrines have produced a reaction in the minds of medical men which has taken the form of a desire to ascribe all mental disorders, including neurasthenia, to some physical or chemical agent the result of disturbed glandular secretions, of septic tonsils or teeth, of intestinal stasis or infection, or of a blood pressure which is too high or too low'[135].

Before the acceptance of the psychogenic paradigm, neurasthenia served a purpose. It flourished when physicians felt comfortable only with clearly organic disorders; hence a diagnosis of neurasthenia permitted them to address clinical issues and to provide an essentially psychological therapy without loss of face to doctor or patient[89]. For a time the good physician now 'wanted to study all sides of the question'[48], which meant attention to emotional issues, but 'without overlooking the possibilities of infective and organic factors'. Conversely, the informed psychiatrist also accepted the possible role of organic factors; hence in 1911 Tredgold doubts the existence of a structural basis to neurasthenia, but accepts the probable role of a cerebral 'bio-chemical' abnormality[136]. This balanced approach did not last long, and, as Buzzard warned, was finally doomed by the success of the exclusively psychogenic view of neurasthenia.

The introduction of psychoanalysis, with its exclusive emphasis on mental origins, ended this for once appropriately labelled 'holistic' approach[137]. Narrow somaticism had failed, but in its place came 'belligerent Freudianism', as illustrated by statements such as 'there is only one certain cure for neurasthenia – viz psychoanalysis'[77] Ironically, this treatment attracted criticisms reminiscent of those of the rest cure, namely questionable efficacy, but unquestionable expense[27,111,135]. Others disliked the new approach because it appeared to encourage introspection, a quality which the neurasthenic apparently possessed to excess[99].

Paradoxically, it was the solely psychological explanations in the new 'official' consensus on neurasthenia that ensured the survival of a contradictory view familiar to Beard and Mitchell. One reason was financial. Beard had made a virtue out of the predominance of upper classes among his patients, claiming that 'the miseries of the rich, the comfortable and intelligent have been unstudied and unrelieved'[43]. Neurasthenia's 'habitat is in Fifth Avenue'[116]. Mitchell himself may have earned $70 000 in private practice per year[89,138]. In the 1920s the creator of *Dr Finlay's Casebook*, A. J. Cronin, was still making a decent living in fashionable London by treating society ladies for the illness[139], his use of magnesium injections being once again topical (see Chapter 17). American physicians and neurologists were particularly reluctant to abandon it; as late as 1927 Adolf Meyer wrote to Abraham Flexner complaining that neurologists continued to see neurasthenics in their clinics, although it was psychiatrists who had the necessary training[140]. Some physicians sympathetic to neurasthenia rejected what they perceived as the implications of the now ascendant psychological views. Such physicians often endorsed a division between organic and psychological, usually synonymous with a division between real and unreal illnesses. The argument would thus revolve around the status to be accorded neurasthenia. Those continuing to diagnose the condition would thus energetically refute 'the idea, now strongly held that neurasthenia is basically psychiatric, almost imaginary in nature'[73]. Only by continuing to affirm the organicity of neurasthenia could many doctors continue in their dealings with chronically fatigued patients. Such attitudes prolonged the survival of neurasthenia, and prepared the way for its modern re-emergence.

The result was that despite the obituaries, and the consignment of the condition to the 'dump heap'[98], 'garbage can'[119], 'rubbish heap'[141] or 'waste basket'[75,142], neurasthenia survived. 'Everywhere we meet with the statements that it is rare . . . yet no name is more often on the lips of both our profession and the laity'[143]. Buzzard, now the Regius Professor at Oxford, noted with regret that although he felt that most of the patients referred to him were depressed, nearly all came with a label of neurasthenia[135]. Abraham Brill commented 'in spite of all that was said and done about the inadequacy of the name, as well as the concept itself, neurasthenia is still very popular with the medical profession'[119].

5.8 Modern neurasthenia

Neurasthenia did gradually disappear. In the United States and United Kingdom formal interest had disappeared by 1960[141], and it was dropped from the influential DSM-III, the bible of the American psychiatric profession. The term does survive in other parts of the world, and is retained in the *International Classification of Diseases* (ICD-9 and ICD-10):

Two main types occur, with substantial overlap. In one type the main feature is a complaint of increased fatigue after mental effort, often associated with some decrease in occupational performance or coping efficiency in daily tasks. . . . In the other type the emphasis is on feelings of bodily or physical weakness or exhaustion after only minimal effort, accompanied by a feeling of muscular aches and pains and inability to relax. In both types a variety of other unpleasant physical feelings is common, such as dizziness, tension headaches and feelings of general instability. Worry about decreasing mental and bodily well being, irritability, anhedonia and varying minor degrees of depression and anxiety are all common. Sleep is often disturbed in its initial and middle phrases, but hypersomnia may also be prominent.

It is a common diagnosis in the Netherlands, Germany, Eastern Europe, and the former Soviet Union[145]. In Germany a systematic community survey gave a point prevalence of ICD-9 neurasthenia of 0.3 per cent[146]. It also flourished in parts of Asia, especially China, where it was seen as a physical illness, without stigma. During the 1950s and 1960s as many as 80 per cent of medical and psychiatric outpatients were labelled as neurasthenic[147]. Arthur Kleinman showed that many of these fulfilled criteria for depressive disorders[148]. Since the end of the Cultural Revolution the changing political and economic climate has, however, led to a decline in the use of neurasthenia. Something similar can be observed in Japan, where neurasthenia was, until recently, extremely popular, and was largely applied to patients who would be diagnosed as having anxiety disorders or hypochondriasis[149]. Another usage in Japan is as a euphemism for schizophrenia[150], since Japanese society has a particular abhorrence of serious mental illness.

Academic interest on neurasthenia in the West has started to return, perhaps stimulated by the rise of CFS, and reflected in a series of recent publications from transcultural psychiatry. The diagnosis has reappeared in modern epidemiological studies[151,152]. In the recent WHO study of primary care the prevalence of neurasthenia was 5.4 per cent, with a range across the centres of 1.1 to 10.5 per cent[153]. Of Chinese Americans living in Los Angeles 6.5 per cent were neurasthenic[154].

5.9 Conclusion

One of the striking features of both neurasthenia and CFS is their capacity to cause dissent. Non-believers consistently attacked the gullibility of those who willingly accepted neurasthenia *in toto* – many of the reviews that greeted Beard's books between 1880 and 1882 were extraordinarily vituperative. In return believers were hardly less tolerant – Weir Mitchell once reacted to a copy of Freud by saying 'Throw that nonsense on the fire'[155]. The accounts of the 'Congrès des Médicin Aliénists et Neurologists de France' in 1907 and 1908, the American Neurological Association on numerous occasions between 1880 and 1914, the American Medical Association in 1944[156], and many others, including many modern meetings on CFS, were characterized by arguments of varying degrees of intensity. Disputes also split the two camps; on the one hand Dubois and Déjerine devote much space to criticizing Bernheim and Freud (and vice versa), whilst on the organic side the arguments between Althaus and Arndt, and between Beard and Hammond, were even more ill tempered. Doctors have always found it easy to disagree about chronic fatigue.

After dissent came dismissal, as the personal scorn about which Beard and Mitchell so often complained became transferred to the patients themselves. Sir Andrew Clark[104] called neurasthenics 'always ailing, seldom ill', whilst the 'wealthy neurasthenic will be a useless, frivolous, noxious element of society'[157]. Charles Beevor joined Clifford Allbutt in reminding doctors that 'on no account should the patient's symptoms be laughed at'[158], but to little avail. At the Johns Hopkins Hospital 'the neurasthenic patient is treated by physicians . . . with ridicule or a contemptuous summing up of his case in the phrase "there is nothing the matter, he is only nervous" '[159], views echoed in the popular press – 'The majority of sufferers have better reason to complain of the weakening of their moral fibres than of either their mental or physical ones'[127]. All of these charges and counter charges will reappear in the modern era (see Chapter 15).

Even those sympathetic to neurasthenics could not avoid a note of irritation and condescension. Patients were 'the terror of the busy physician'[160] 'occupied by their symptoms beyond reason'[22], going from physician to physician where they 'write down their sensations in long memoranda which they hasten to read and to explain'[22]. Nowadays, such patients would be called 'high users' in the journals, and 'heartsink' in doctors' conversations.

This dissent revolves around differing interpretations of the physical and psychological. The supporters of neurasthenia argued that these must be physical illnesses, not because of the evidence, which remains inconclusive, but because psychological illnesses are unreal, malingered, or imaginary. This tendency of those committed to an exclusively organic view of such illnesses to juxtapose psychiatric and imaginary was criticised by contemporaries such as Dutil[79] and Tinel[83] both of whom denied that neurasthenia was a 'maladie imaginaire'. Drummond attacked with equal vigour those who viewed neurasthenia as a solely physical illness, and those who regarded it as a thinly veiled excuse for malingering[94]. Neurasthenia provided a haven for those uncomfortable with the psychological aspects of illness, who either insisted on its solely organic basis, or saw it as a refuge for the mentally infirm. Both extremes have resurfaced in the debate on CFS. The passions that these arguments created and continue to create was because what was at stake is the issue of legitimacy, namely what constitutes an acceptable disease, and what is legitimate suffering, deserving of support and sympathy?

The Victorians never provided satisfactory answers to these dilemmas. Hence when the latest fatigue syndromes, ME and CFS, made their appearance in the 1980s, it was inevitable that both doctors and patients would experience an almost identical sequence of claim and counter claim over the legitimacy or otherwise of the next syndromes. We will discuss these newest developments in the story of fatigue in the next chapter and in our review of the concepts of twentieth century illness (Chapter 15).

References

1 Deale H, Adams S. Neurasthenia in young women. *Am. J. Obstet.* 1894; **29:** 190–195.

2 Cobb I. *A Manual of Neurasthenia (Nervous Exhaustion).* London, Ballière, Tindall and Cox, 1920.

3 Shorter E. *From Paralysis to Fatigue: a History of Psychosomatic Illness in the Modern Era.* New York, Free Press, 1992.

4 Knapp P. The nature of neurasthenia. *J. Nerv. Ment. Dis.* 1896; **21:** 688–689.

5 Weiss E. A consideration of neurasthenia in its relation to pelvic symptoms in women. *Am. J. Obstet.* 1908; **57:** 230–235.

6 Dercum F. *Rest, Suggestion and Other Therapeutic Measures in Nervous and Mental Disease.* Philadelphia, Blakiston's Son & Co, 1917.

7 Neu C. Treatment and management of the neurasthenic individual. *Med. Record* 1920; **97:** 341.

8 Berkley H. *A Treatise on the Mental Diseases.* London, Henry Klimpton, 1901.

9 Oppenheim H. *Text-book of Nervous Diseases for Physicians and Students*, 5th edn. London, Foulis, 1908.

10 Mitchell S. *Fat and Blood*, 3rd edn. Philadelphia, J Lippincott, 1883.

11 Mitchell SW. The treatment by rest, seclusion etc., in relation to psychotherapy. *J. Am. Med. Assoc.* 1908; **25:** 2033–2037.

12 Jaspers K. *General Psychopathology.* Manchester University Press, 1963.

13 Jewell J. Nervous exhaustion or neurasthenia in its bodily and mental relations. *J. Nerv. Ment. Dis.* 1879; **6:** 45–55.

14 Hartenberg P. La psychothérapie chez les neurasthéniques. *Encephale* 1907; **7:** 266–267.

15 Déjerine J, Gauckler E. *Les Manifestations Functionelles des Psychonervoses; Leur Traitement par la Psychothérapie.* Paris: Masson, 1911.

16 Clouston T. *Clinical Lectures on Mental Diseases*, 3rd edn. London, Churchill, 1892.

17 Fischer-Homberger E. *'Hypochondrie'. Melancholie der Neurose, Krankenheiten und Zustandbilder.* Bern, Hans Huber, 1970.

18 Freud S. Hysteria. In Villaret A (ed.) *Handwörterbuch der gesamten Medizin*, Vol. 3. London, Hogarth Press, 1996: 39–57.

19 Arndt R. Neurasthenia. In Tuke D (ed.) *Dictionary of Psychological Medicine.* London, J Churchill, 1892: 840–850.

20 Barker L, Byrnes C. Neurasthenia and psychasthenic states, including the new phobias. In Forcheimer F (ed.) *Therapeutics of Internal Medicine.* New York; Appleton, 1913: 516–581.

21 Durkheim E. *Suicide: A Study in Sociology.* Glencoe, IL, Free Press, 1951.

22 Blocq P. Neurasthenia. *Brain* 1894; **14:** 306–314.

23 Ferrier D. Neurasthenia and drugs. *Practitioner* 1911; **86:** 11–15.

24 Beard G. *A Practical Treatise on Nervous Exhaustion (Neurasthenia): its Symptoms, Nature, Sequences, Treatment.* New York, William Wood, 1880.

25 Beard G. Neurasthenia, or nervous exhaustion. *Bost. Med. Sur. J.* 1869; **3:** 217–221.

26 Van Deusen E. Observations of a form of nervous prostration, (neurasthenia), culminating in insanity. *Am. J. Insanity* 1869: 445–461.

27 Hale H. *Freud and the Americans: the Beginnings of Psychoanalysis in the United States, 1876–1917.* New York, Oxford University Press, 1971.

28 Huchard H. Neurasthénie. In Axenfeld A, Huchard H (ed.) *Traite des Nevroses.* Paris, Germer Baillière, 1883: 873–907.

29 Lopez-Pinero J. *Historical Origins of the Concept of Neurosis.* Cambridge University Press, 1983.

30 Dubois P. *The Psychic Treatment of Nervous Diseases,* 6th edn. New York, Funk and Wagnalls, 1909.

31 Certhoux J. De la neurasthénie aux neuroses: le traitment des neuroses dans le passe. *Ann. Med. Psychol.* 1961; **119**: 913–930.

32 Levillain F. *La Neurasthenia, Maladie de Beard (Methodes de Weir-Mitchell et Playfair, Traitment de Vigoroux).* Paris, A Malvine, 1891.

33 Dutil A. Neurasthénie, or La Maladie de Beard. In Charcot J, Bouchard E, Brissaud E (ed.) *Traite de Médicine.* Paris, G Masson, 1894: 1281–1301.

34 Bumke O. Die Revision der Neurosenfrage. *Münch. Med. Wochenschr.* 1925; **72**: 1815–1819.

35 Zeldin T. *Intellect and Pride.* Oxford, Oxford University Press, 1980.

36 Allbutt T. Neurasthenia. In Allbutt T (ed.) *A System of Medicine.* London, Macmillan, 1899: 134–164.

37 Johnson G. Lectures on some nervous diseases that result from overwork and anxiety. *Lancet* 1875; **ii**: 85–87.

38 Foster G. Common features in neurasthenia and insanity: their common basis and common treatment. *Am. J.Insanity* 1900; **56**: 395–418.

39 Pershing H. The treatment of neurasthenia. *Med. News* 1904; **84**: 637–640.

40 Lowenfeld L. *Die moderne Behandlung der Nervenschwäche (Neurasthenie). Hysteria und verwandte Leiden.* Wiesbaden, Bergman, 1887.

41 Poore G. On fatigue. *Lancet* 1875; **i**: 163–164.

42 Savage G. Overwork as a cause of insanity. *Lancet* 1875; **ii**: 127.

43 Beard G. *American Nervousness.* New York, G.P Putnam's, 1881.

44 Oppenheim J. *'Shattered Nerves': Doctors, Patients and Depression in Victorian England.* Oxford University Press, 1991.

45 Lutz T. *American Nervousness: 1903.* Ithaca, Cornell University Press, 1991.

46 White W. *The Principles of Mental Hygiene.* New York, Macmillan, 1917.

47 Muscio B. Is a fatigue test possible? *Br. J. Psychol.* 1921; **12**: 31–46.

48 Meyer A. Discontent—a psychbiological problem of hygiene. In Winters E (ed.) *The Collected Papers of Adolf Meyer.* Baltimore, MD, Johns Hopkins Press, 1962: 383–400.

49 Donley J. On neurasthenia as a disintegration of personality. *J. Abnorm. Psychol.* 1906; **1**: 55–68.

50 Tanzi E. *A Textbook of Mental Diseases.* London, Rebman, 1909.

51 Schofield A. The psychology of neurasthenia and hysteria. *Lancet* 1908; **ii**: 400–401.

52 Brock A. 'Ergotherapy' in neurasthenia. *Edin. Med. J.* 1911: 430–434.

53 White W. *Neurasthenia. Outlines of Psychiatry.* Washington, Nervous and Mental Disease Publishing Company, 1921: 265–267.

54 Pritchard W. The American Disease: an interpretation. *Can. J. Med. Surg.* 1905; **18**: 10–22.

55 Kraepelin E. *Clinical Psychiatry.* London, Macmillan, 1902.

56 Jewell J. Influence of our present civilization in the production of nervous and mental disease. *J. Nerv. Ment. Dis.* 1881; **8**: 1–24.

57 Charcot J. *Leçons du Mardi a la Salpêtrière.* Paris, Lecrosniew & Babe, 1889.

58 Savill T. *Clinical Lectures on Neurasthenia*. London, Henry J Glaisher, 1906.
59 Leubuscher P, Bibrowicz W. Die Neurasthenie in Arbeitkreisen. *Deutsch. Med. Wochenscr.* 1905; **31:** 820–824.
60 Iscoueco. De la neurasthénie des pauvrès. *Bull. Med.* 1905; **19:** 359.
61 Cleghorn C. Notes on six thousand cases of neurasthenia. *Med. Rec.* 1907; **71:** 681–684.
62 Jelliffe S, Clark L. The work of a neurological dispensary clinic. *J. Nerv. Ment. Dis.* 1903; **30:** 482–488.
63 Schwab S. Neurasthenia among the garment workers. *Bull. Am. Econ. Assoc.* 1911; **4th Series, No. 2:** 265–270.
64 Stedman H. The public obligations of the neurologist. *J. Nerv. Ment. Dis.* 1906; **33:** 489–499.
65 Tuckey C. Treatment of neurasthenia by hypnotism and suggestion. *Practitioner* 1911: 185–192.
66 Hurry J. *The Vicious Circles of Neurasthenia and their Treatment*. London, Churchill, 1914.
67 Freud S. On the grounds for detaching a particular syndrome from neurasthenia under the description 'anxiety neurosis'. In Strachey J (ed.) *Standard Edition*. London, Hogarth Press, 1895: 87–115.
68 Rabinbach A. *The Human Motor: Energy, Fatigue and the Origins of Modernity*. New York, Basic Books, 1990.
69 Blumer G. The coming of psychasthenia. *J. Nerv. Ment. Dis.* 1906; **33:** 336–353.
70 Solms M. Three previously untranslated reviews by Freud from the Neue Freie Presse. *Int. J. Psychoanal.* 1989; **70:** 397.
71 Jones E. *The Life and Work of Sigmund Freud*. London, Penguin, 1961.
72 Starr M. The toxic origin of neurasthenia and melancholia. *Bost. Med. Surg. J.* 1901; **144:** 563.
73 De Fleury M. *Les Grands Symptômes Neurasthénique (Pathogénie et Traitement)*. Paris, Germer Baillière, 1901.
74 Dana C. The partial passing of neurasthenia. *Bost. Med. Surg. J.* 1904; **60:** 339–344.
75 Kinnier-Wilson S. Medical Society of London: discussion of neurasthenia. *Lancet* 1913; **ii:** 1542–1544.
76 Horder T. Neurasthenia: a critical inquiry. *St Bartholomew's Hosp. J.* 1903; February: 67–73.
77 Stoddart W. *The Psychoneuroses. Mind and Its Disorders*, 5th edn. London, HK Lewis, 1926: 224–243.
78 Walton O. Proceedings of the Boston Neurological Society. *J. Nerv. Ment. Dis. 1906;* **33:** 279.
79 Dutil A. Neurasthénie. In Ballet G (ed.) *Traite de Pathologie Mentale*. Paris, Octave Dion, 1903: 842–850.
80 Dana C. Dr George M Beard: a sketch of his life and character with some personal reminiscences. *Arch. Neuro. Psychol.* 1926; **10:** 427–435.
81 Ross T. *The Common Neuroses*, 2nd edn. London, Edward Arnold, 1937.
82 Bleuler E. *Textbook of Psychiatry*. New York, Macmillan, 1924.
83 Tinel J. *Conceptions et Traitment des États Neurasthéniques*. Paris, J B Ballière et fils, 1941.
84 Stea J, Fried W. Remedies for a society's debilities: medicines for neurasthenia in Victorian America. *N.Y. State Med. J.* 1993; **93:** 120–127.
85 Shorter E. *A History of Psychiatry*. New York, Wiley, 1996.
86 Playfair W. Notes on the systematic treatment of nerve prostration and hysteria connected with uterine disease. *Lancet* 1881; **i:** 857–859, 949–950, 991–992, 1029–1030.
87 Weisenburg T. The Weir Mitchell rest cure forty years ago and today. *Arch. Neurol. Psychol.* 1925; **14:** 384–389.

88 Haller J. Neurasthenia: the medical profession and urban 'blahs'. *N.Y. State Med. J.* 1970; **70:** 2489–2497.

89 Sicherman B. The uses of a diagnosis: doctors, patients and neurasthenia. *J. Hist. Med.* 1977; **32:** 33–54.

90 Shorter E. Private clinics in central Europe 1850–1933. *Soc. Hist. Med.* 1990; **3:** 159–195.

91 Ziemssen H. *Neurasthenia and Its Treatment. Clinical Lectures on Subjects Connected With Medicine and Surgery.* London, New Sydenham Society, 1894: 53–86.

92 Wood A. 'The fashionable diseases'; women's complaints and their treatment in nineteenth century American. *J. Interdiscip. Hist.* 1973; **4:** 25–52.

93 Cayleff SE. 'Prisoners of their own feebleness': women, nerves and Western medicine – a historical overview. *Soc. Sci. Med.* 1988; **26:** 1199–208.

94 Drummond D. The mental origin of neurasthenia, and its bearing on treatment. *Br. Med. J.* 1907; **ii:** 1813–1816.

95 Waterman G. The treatment of fatigue states. *J. Abnorm. Psychol.* 1909; **4:** 128–139.

96 McGrew, F. Neurasthenia and the rest cure. *J. Am. Med. Assoc.* 1900: **34:** 1466–8.

97 Menninger K. The abuse of rest in psychiatry. *J. Am. Med. Assoc.* 1944; **125:** 1087–1090.

98 Browning W. Is there such a disease as neurasthenia? A discussion and classification of the many conditions that appear to be grouped under that head. *N.Y. State Med. J.* 1911; **11:** 7–17.

99 Peterson F. Neurasthenia. In Cecil R (ed.) *A Textbook of Medicine*, Philadelphia, WB Saunders, 1927: 1419–1426.

100 Anon. Review of Prengowski, 'Les Maladies Neurasthenique'. *J. Nerv. Ment. Dis.* 1929; **69:** 353.

101 Fourness-Brice J. Medical etiquette on board ship. *Br. Med. J.* 1880; **i:** 238.

102 Crichton Browne J. Dr Beard's experiments in hypnosis. *Br. Med. J.* 1881; **ii:** 378–379.

103 Beard G. The asylums of Europe. *Bost. Med. Surg. J.* 1880; **53:** 605–608.

104 Clark A. Some observations concerning what is called neurasthenia *Br. Med. J.* 1886; **ii:** 853–855.

105 Playfair W. Some observations concerning what is called neurasthenia. *Br. Med. J.* 1886; **ii:** 843–845.

106 Gowers W. *A Manual of Diseases of the Nervous System*, 2nd ed. London, Churchill, 1888.

107 Gowers W. *A Manual of Diseases of the Nervous System*, 3rd ed. London, Churchill, 1899.

108 Ireland W. Review of 'The Treatment of Neurasthenia; Proust and Ballet'. *J. Ment. Sci.* 1907; **48:** 548–549.

109 Wilson S. Some modern French concepts of hysteria. *Brain* 1910; **33:** 293–338.

110 Anon. Neurasthenia and modern life. *Br. Med. J.* 1909; **ii:** 97–98.

111 Anon. The definition and treatment of neurasthenia. *Lancet* 1913; **ii:** 1557–1558.

112 Gosling F, Ray J. The right to be sick. *J. Soc. Hist.* 1986; **20:** 251–267.

113 Althaus J. *On Failure of Brain Power (Encephalasthenia); Its Nature and Treatment*, 5th edn. London, Longmans, Green and Co., 1898.

114 Mitchell Clarke J. *Hysteria and Neurasthenia.* London, Bodley Head, 1905.

115 Burr C. Neurasthenia. In Osler W, McCrae T (ed.) *A System of Medicine.* London, Henry Frowde 1910: 725.

116 Love I. Neurasthenia. *J. Am. Med. Assoc.* 1900; **22:** 539–544.

117 Dembe A. *Occupation and Disease: How Social Factors Affect the Conception of Work-Related Disorders.* New Haven, CT, Yale University Press, 1996.

118 Playfair W. The systematic treatment of functional neuroses. In Tuke D (ed.) *Dictionary of Psychological Medicine.* London, Churchill, 1892: 850–857.

119 Brill A. Diagnostic errors in neurasthenia. *Med. Rev.* 1930; **36:** 122–129.

120 Reynolds E. Hysteria and neurasthenia. *Med. Rev.* 1923; **ii:** 1193–1195.

121 Mott F. *War Neuroses and Shell Shock*. London, Hodder & Stoughton, 1919.

122 Spitzka E. Review of 'A Practical Treatise on Nervous Exhaustion (Neurasthenia)'. *St Louis Clin. Rec.* 1880; **7**: 92–94.

123 Risien Russell J. The treatment of neurasthenia. *Lancet* 1913; **ii**: 1453–1456.

124 Hallock F. The sanatorium treatment of neurasthenia and the need of a colony sanatorium for the nervous poor. *Bost. Med. Surg. J.* 1911; **44**: 73–77.

125 Anon. Review of Otto Binswanger; The Pathology and Treatment of Neurasthenia. *Br. Med. J.* 1897; **i**: 920–921.

126 Madden H. On nervousness. *Mon. Homeopath. Rev.* 1868; **12**: 211–221.

127 Anon. Nerves and nervousness. *The Spectator* 1894; **72**: 11–12.

128 Glorieaux. Neurasthenia among the working classes. *J. Nerv. Ment. Dis.* 1906; **33**: 607.

129 Haller J. Neurasthenia: the medical profession and the 'new woman' of the late nineteenth century. *N.Y. State Med. J. 1971;* **71**: 473–482.

130 Robertson W. The infective factors in some types of neurasthenia. *J. Ment. Sci.* 1919; **65**: 16–24.

131 Proust M. *Remembrance of Things Past*. London, Penguin Modern Classics, 1983.

132 Edes R. The New England invalid. *Bost. Med. Surg. J.* 1895; **133**: 53–57.

133 Ramsay Hunt J. Neurasthenia. *The Medical Annual*. Bristol, John Wright & Co., 1920: 416–417.

134 Clayton M. When is the diagnosis of neurasthenia justified? *US Veterans Bureau Med. Bull.* 1926; **2**: 61–64.

135 Buzzard F. The dumping ground of neurasthenia. *Lancet* 1930; **i**: 1–4.

136 Tredgold A. Neurasthenia and insanity. *Practitioner* 1911; **86**: 84–95.

137 Gosling F. *Before Freud: Neurasthenia and the American Medical Community: 1970–1910*. Springfield, IL, University of Illinois Press, 1987.

138 Olson M. The Weir Mitchell rest cure. *Pharos* 1988; **51**: 30–2.

139 Cronin AJ. *Adventures in Two Worlds*. London, Victor Gollancz, 1952.

140 Grob G. *The Inner World of American Psychiatry: 1890–1940*. New York, Rutgers University Press, 1985.

141 Culpin M. *Recent Advances in the Study of the Psychoneuroses*. London, Churchill, 1931.

142 Bassoe P. The origin, rise and decline of the neurasthenia concept. *Wisconsin Med. J.* 1928; **27**: 11–14.

143 Dicks H. Neurasthenia: toxic and traumatic. *Lancet* 1933; **ii**: 683–686.

144 Chatel J, Peele R. A centennial review of neurasthenia. *Am. J. Psychol.* 1970; **126**: 48–57.

145 Starevic V. Neurasthenia in European psychiatric literature. *Transcult. Psychiatric Res. Rev.* 1994; **31**.

146 Schepank H. *Epidemiology of Psychogenic Disorders; The Mannheim Study*. Berlin, Springer, 1987.

147 Lin T. Neurasthenia revisited: its place in modern psychiatry. *Cult. Med. Psychol.* 1989; **13**: 105–129.

148 Kleinman A. Neurasthenia and depression: a study of somatization and culture in China. *Cult. Med. Psychol.* 1982; **6**: 117–190.

149 Kitanishi K, Kondo K. The rise and fall of neurasthenia in Japanese psychiatry. *Transcult. Psychiatric Res. Rev.* 1994; **31**.

150 Munakata T. The socio-cultural significance of the diagnostic label 'neurasthenia' in Japan's mental health care system. *Cult. Med. Psychiatry* 1989; **13**: 203–13.

151 Merikangas K, Angst J. Neurasthenia in a longitidunal cohort study of young adults. *Psychol. Med.* 1994; **24**: 1013–1024.

152 Ormel J, Von Korff M, Ustun B, Pini S, Korten A, Oldehinkel T. Common mental disorders and disabilities across cultures: results from the WHO Collaborative Study on Psychological Problems in General Health Care. *J. Am. Med. Assoc.* 1994; **272:** 1741–1748.

153 Ustun T, Sartorius N (ed). *Mental Illness in General Health Care: an International Study.* Chichester, World Health Organization/Wiley, 1995.

154 Zheng Y, Lin K, Takeuchi D, Kurasaki K, Wang Y, Cheung F. A epidemiological study of neurasthenia in Chinese Americans in Los Angeles. *Comprehen. Psych.* 1997: **38:** 249–59.

155 Earnest E. *S Weir Mitchell: Novelist and Physician.* Philadelphia, University of Pennsylvania Press, 1950.

156 Allan F. The differential diagnosis of weakness and fatigue. *New Engl. J. Med.* 1944; **231:** 414–418.

157 Urquhart A. Austrian retrospect: review of the writings of Professor Benedikt of Vienna. *J. Ment. Sci.* 1889; **34:** 276–281.

158 Beevor C. *Diseases of the Nervous System: A Handbook for Students and Practitioners.* London, HK Lewis, 1898.

159 Mitchell J. Diagnosis and treatment of neurasthenia. *Johns Hopkins Hosp. Bull.* 1908; **19:** 41–43.

160 Rankin G. Neurasthenia; the wear and tear of life. *Br. Med. J.* 1903; **i:** 1017–1020.

6. From neurasthenia to CFS

6.1 Introduction

Much of the early part of this book concerned fatigue as a symptom. With the introduction of neurasthenia came the concept of fatigue as the principal symptom of a diagnostic entity. This chapter describes the origins of the latest disease of abnormal fatigue and fatigability, chronic fatigue syndrome, and its variants.

We have charted the rise and fall of neurasthenia, concluding that, in Western countries at least, it had to all intents and purposes vanished by the Second World War, partly because of the widespread acceptance of psychogenic explanations of the condition.

Between the demise of neurasthenia and the last 15 years, fatigue syndromes were not a major issue for doctors or the professional or lay journals. By the 1950s US psychiatrists had neither interest in, nor knowledge of, neurasthenia[1], nor, it is fair to say, did any other group of doctors. Certainly, fatigued patients did not disappear. After the demise of neurasthenia, general physicians continued to encounter the patient with chronic fatigue, often arising after a variety of insults, including infection. Perhaps mindful of the neurasthenia experience, physicians avoided specific nosological entities in preference to descriptive labels, such as 'tired, weak and toxic'[2] 'chronic nervous exhaustion'[3], 'fatigue and weakness'[4], or 'fatigue and nervousness'[5]. All had a psychological emphasis. Women whose profound fatigue caused them to be confined to a single room were usually regarded as hysterical[6].

The rise of the psychogenic school was only part of the story, albeit the closest to an official consensus. What happened to the physical paradigm of Beard, Mitchell, and so many others? There was a second line of descent from neurasthenia, traced in a series of illnesses embodying the concept of physical fatigue, due to external factors, allegedly easily and unfairly confused with psychological disorders, and usually regarded with some degree of academic scepticism. Thus, we encounter chronic brucellosis in the 1940s and 1950s, reactive hypoglycaemia in the 1960s, total allergy syndrome, and chronic candidiasis in the 1970s. There are several links between these conditions and CFS which we will consider as part of the social history of fatigue syndromes. There are also differences between all these conditions and neurasthenia, principally in the degree of professional acceptance. None achieved the same degree of professional support required to permit the spread of the condition. Many doctors remained unaware of such conditions as chronic brucellosis or neurocirculatory asthenia, and the professional discourse, such as it was, was often sceptical. Norma Ware has appropriately noted that throughout this period 'chronic fatigue had become invisible', with 'no name, no known etiology, no case illustrations or clinical accounts in the medical textbook, no ongoing research activity – nothing to relate it to current medical knowledge'[7].

These conditions only represent part of the neurasthenia heritage, and the true successor to neurasthenia only appeared in the 1980s, with the spread of myalgic encephalomyelitis (ME) and the arrival of chronic fatigue syndrome.

6.2 The beginnings of ME: from Los Angeles to the Royal Free Hospital, London

In the United Kingdom the first mention of the term 'myalgic encephalomyelitis' was in a leading article in 1956[8]. It was proposed as an explanation for a series of outbreaks of a contagious condition, causing symptoms referable to the central nervous system, which had occurred in various parts of the world in the preceding three decades. Some of these had been named by their place of origin (hence Iceland disease), others by the neuromuscular weakness that was a frequent feature (hence neuromyasthenia), and others by the presumed relation to poliomyelitis (hence atypical poliomyelitis). An exhaustive bibliography of these outbreaks is provided elsewhere[9].

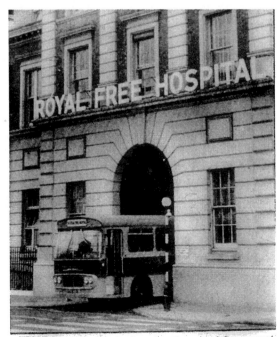

Start of it all . . . the old Royal Free where the outbreak first occurred

Fig. 6.1. The Royal Free Hospital – the beginning of ME.

Two episodes have attracted most attention. These took place at the Los Angeles County Hospital (LAC) in 1934, and the Royal Free Hospital (RFH) in London in 1955. Both concerned the nursing and medical staff of these hospitals, and not patients. The symptoms of these epidemics remain unclear, but at the core were mixtures of unusual motor and sensory symptoms, accompanied by myalgia and signs of emotional distress and lability. On the whole, the laboratory tests available to the clinicians of the day were unhelpful.

Some of the contemporary professional concerns about these epidemics centred around possible links to poliomyelitis, a theme that remains relevant today. Aronowitz elegantly demonstrates how these links began[10]. He shows that before the LAC epidemic in 1934 the incidence of polio in California had been declining for several years, and that, by the prevailing opinion of the time, this heralded a new severe episode. The cases were thus viewed with polio very much in mind, and described as 'atypical poliomyelitis'. McEvedy and Beard make similar points about the Middlesex Hospital outbreak in 1952, and although doctors at the Royal Free Hospital three years later were less taken with the similarity to polio, this was not the case among the non-medical personnel[11].

Despite the label, the nature of the outbreaks was unlike polio. Most of the cases in the LAC epidemic had unusually mild symptoms, and doctors experienced considerable diagnostic difficulties. The fatality rate was remarkably low, the spinal fluid normal, paralysis was usually absent, and muscular atrophy rare[12]. The public health report was unable to contain a calculation of the ratio of paralytic to non-paralytic cases, a conventional statistic of polio epidemics, because of the scarcity of paralytic cases – instead what was often recorded as paralytic polio was in fact minor neurological impairment detected by over vigorous testing[10]. Overall, the head of the Infectious Diseases Unit reported that 'it was the scarcity of the usual and the large volume of the unusual which gave the epidemic its bizarre aspects'[13]. Similar arguments soon convinced the RFH doctors that the illness was not poliomyelitis. Now that polio has virtually disappeared from our society, it is perhaps hard for us to understand just how frightening was the spectre of paralytic poliomyelitis, particularly amongst staff whose professional obligations required them to treat patients who might have the acute illness.

Having raised the possibility of infection, many of the original observers were reluctant to abandon it. Despite the lack of objective evidence of infection, and the observation that emotional disturbance was an integral part of nearly all of these outbreaks, the initial authors were keen to reinforce the organic aetiology of the syndromes, and in introducing names such as neuromyasthenia or myalgic encephalomyelitis, effectively ruled out any alternative explanation. For some years this position remained publicly unchallenged (although this might be a consequence of the fact that many professionals remained either unaware of, or indifferent to, neuromyasthenia, ME, and so on during this period).

The most influential critique of the organic position came from McEvedy and Beard[14,15]. They suggested that certain epidemics, including those at the RFH, were due to transmitted emotional distress ('mass hysteria'), whilst others were not epidemics at all, but clustering of small numbers of cases of heterogeneous illnesses combined with altered medical perception. This was not the first time such a suggestion had been made – similar accounts had been in circulation during the Royal Free outbreak itself[16], whilst two epidemiologists had made the same suggestion in print[17]. Paul, the historian of polio, came to a similar conclusion[18]. However, McEvedy and Beard's was the most public statement. Their evidence against an infective origin was strong; the disease almost invariably affected female staff, and never patients. It was a similar observation, of an illness that affected patients and never staff, that led to Goldberger's classic work refuting the alleged infectious origins of pellagra.

Both epidemics, at the Los Angeles County Hospital in 1934 and the London Royal Free Hospital in 1955, were associated with a climate of anxiety, partly linked to publicity concerning the possible threat of polio. At the Royal Free 'the anxiety of the lay population on this score was not at first appreciated'[11]. In Los Angeles, the chief of the California Department of Public Health stated that 'There is a well founded fear of this disease, and there is also an unfortunate terror that is wholly unnecessary' (quoted in Aronowitz[10]). Aronowitz details the alarmist media coverage, often at the instigation of the authorities to enforce hygiene regulations. The fear of disease was not restricted to non-professionals – staff at the LAC, running the risk of exposure, were not well supported by their colleagues. Aronowitz notes how the attending physicians preferred not to visit the contagion wards, instead carrying out consultations on the telephone[10]. Staff on the ward were required to have their temperature taken every day. The severe stress to which the professional staff were subjected was commented upon in an early account of the outbreak[19].

Against that background, the evidence for an emotional origin to symptoms was suggestive, albeit not conclusive. There was little doubt that emotional factors were responsible for a proportion of the cases in the best documented outbreaks. One case in Los Angeles developed 'psychic blindness', as well as psychosis[13], yet was still included as an epidemic case of atypical poliomyelitis. Observers constantly used terms such as 'bizarre' or 'remarkable' to describe the nature of the symptoms and signs, involving 'frank hysterical manifestations'[20]. Many suggested that the illness represented the 'functional end of a disorder with an organic beginning'[8]. Ramsay himself noted that the Royal Free disease resembled both polio and hysteria[21], and others felt the illnesses 'displayed features remarkably akin to hysteria'[22]. It was thus not far-fetched to suggest that the episodes actually were mass hysteria.

What did happen? We will never know. An infective agent cannot be dismissed, and has been cogently argued by Acheson[12] and subsequently Jenkins[23]. It is possible that cases were admitted of an infective disease with some similarities to polio, but the epidemiology of the episodes suggests this is not the sole or even main explanation. On the other hand, there are several arguments in favour of an emotional nature to the contagion[14,15]. Perhaps the initial infective cases served as a focus for natural anxiety, and in turn triggered others whose illnesses cannot be explained by an infective agent, but it is only in an occasional case that the diagnosis of factitious illness can be sustained[24,25]. The social pressures common to both hospitals, and the subsequent history of the condition, must be at least one factor in the sad tale of the future fate of those afflicted. Jenkin's conclusion seems the most reasonable: 'the majority of cases were a hysterical reaction to a small number of poliomyelitis cases among the staff'[23]. It is clear that the outbreaks grouped together under the label of

ME/neuromyasthenia, and so on are more heterogeneous than implied by a single label[26]. Finally, McEvedy and Beard's second proposition, that some episodes did not involve any clustering of new illness but altered medical perception of expected levels of morbidity, was certainly true in some 'epidemics'[27].

It was reasonable for McEvedy, Beard, and others to suggest that these epidemics were not satisfactorily explained by infection, but their psychogenic exposition had an unexpected and untoward consequence. As with neurasthenia[28], the arrival of the psychogenic hypothesis had the paradoxical effect of reinforcing the organic alle-giances of the supporters of the new illness. The mass hysteria hypothesis led to a retrenchment of the organic school of thought, and a polarized, bitter, and acrimo-nious debate which continues to this day. As with neurasthenia, many of the most active advocates of the organic camp remain afflicted physicians. Again, as the available evidence failed to determine the aetiology of the outbreaks, prejudice was called upon to affirm their organic nature. Poskanzer[29] suggested that rather than ME being a psychoneurosis, all cases of psychoneurosis were sporadic ME. In so doing he acknowledged that both conditions lay claim to the same clinical territory, hence non-clinical factors were needed to assert the organic aetiology. Neurasthenia and ME were both claimed to affect professionals of impeccable moral stature, 'level headed'[30], 'extravert types of stable personality'[31] and so on, were evidence against a psychiatric origin. A variation on this theme is that the staff at the Royal Free Hospital, and not the patients, were affected by the outbreak because the former were vulnerable because of the amount of exercise involved in their jobs, unlike the patients, rendered immune by resting in bed[32]. The idea that sufferers have a particular personality rendering them vulnerable to CFS/ME but immune to psy-chiatric disorder will reappear (see Chapter 10).

6.3 The origins of post-viral fatigue syndrome

Even the first descriptions of neurasthenia included a link with febrile illness. In 1869 Van Deusen highlighted malaria, since he worked in an area in which the disease was endemic[33], whilst Beard drew attention to wasting fevers. The link with infection persisted in the earliest accounts in France[34], whilst one of the first cases to be treated in this country by the Weir Mitchell regime was a woman with a 14-year history of neurasthenia, confined to bed in a darkened room, whose illness had begun with a persistent cold[35].

By 1914 the observation that neurasthenia and/or effort syndrome frequently followed an infection was widely acknowledged. For most, including Osler, Oppen-heim, and Kraepelin the principle candidate was influenza, but claims were also made for many others, especially typhoid, and latterly the effects of vaccination[36]. As the microbiological revolution spread, each organism was linked with neurasthenia. Everybody had a favourite culprit, until it was conceded that any infective agent could produce the state of chronic exhaustion[37–39], especially in combination with depression[40] or worry[41]. To a generation schooled on Virchow and Koch this was a major hurdle.

Such efforts did not cease after the decline of neurasthenia, since, starting with Reiter's disease, attempts to link infective organisms with previously mysterious clinical conditions had reaped dividends, and the list of *bona fide* post-infective conditions was growing. Specific post-infective syndromes identical with neurasthenia continued to be describe as each new infection was discovered, although some continued to be noticeable for their psychological flavour.

The story of chronic brucellosis is another link between neurasthenia and CFS. Although by 1930 the diagnosis of acute brucellosis was well established, there was less certainty about chronic brucellosis. One of its chief supporters was the public health specialist Alice Evans, who noted the similarities between neurasthenia and chronic brucellosis, but only in order to highlight the plight of the large numbers of those afflicted who suffered the indignity of receiving the erroneous, 'dishonourable' diagnosis of neurasthenia[42]. Thirteen years later she was still championing the disease, which remained 'extremely difficult to diagnose . . . however, an unrecognised mild form of brucellosis is a common ailment in this country'[43].

The end of the syndrome encapsulates on a smaller scale the eclipse of neurasthenia. Spink[44] studied a series of patients with acute brucella infection, and noted that a proportion failed to recover – the chronic brucellosis group. However, he found no objective evidence of disease, and instead noted high rates of psychological disorder. Spink linked it with worker's compensation claims and neurasthenia. Researchers from Johns Hopkins Hospital, in the first of a series of papers on the relationship between infection and psychological vulnerability, studied subjects with the label of chronic brucellosis in greater detail. They found no evidence of chronic infection[45] but high levels of psychiatric morbidity, coupled with reluctance to discuss psychological issues and a strong attachment to the 'organic' diagnosis[46]. Once this evidence became widely disseminated, chronic brucellosis largely disappeared.

The eclipse of chronic brucellosis seemed not to be associated with particular controversy, perhaps because the patients tended to be more isolated rural areas, or, as Shorter[47] suggests, medical authority was stronger. Whatever the explanation, chronic brucellosis vanished, only reappearing in an editorial on the social construction of mental illness[48].

6.4 ME: from epidemic to sporadic cases

After the Royal Free epidemic the story of ME is one of two shifts. The first is the change from epidemic to sporadic cases. The second is the merging of ME with the tradition of post-infectious fatigue syndromes outlined in the previous section.

Epidemics of ME or neuromyasthenia, whatever their provenance, gradually disappeared from the literature during the 1960s and 1970s, to be replaced by the wider problem of sporadic cases of chronic fatigue. As epidemic ME gave way to sporadic CFS, the nature of the illness itself was changing. In 1976 a group of doctors, including both sufferers and those involved in the Royal Free outbreak, formed a study group[49], and were instrumental in organizing a symposium at the Royal Society of Medicine. The content of the meeting showed that epidemic ME was still the dominant concern, but few new outbreaks were appearing for further study.

Attention shifted to the problem of sporadic cases. These had been considered before – some had been noted in the community surrounding the Royal Free Hospital, and others had also described sporadic cases elsewhere[50], but these were not the predominant concern until the early 1980s.

The result of this shift, largely unnoticed, was a gradual, but profound, change in the character of the illness. In the index episodes neurological signs, of whatever aetiology, were recorded in the majority, and were divided into cerebral, brainstem, and spinal[11] (just as in the first series of neurasthenic texts). An early report[51] of two cases of sporadic ME had neurological signs (and both required assisted ventilation). On the other hand persistent severe fatigability was either not mentioned, or given little prominence, in the reports of epidemics but gradually increased in importance until it became the hallmark of the disease. Neurological signs disappeared[26]. Unfortunately, whereas most epidemic cases recovered[52,53], this was no longer the case for sporadic CFS (see Chapter 7). Contagion, the key feature of the index episodes, all but disappeared.

It must be emphasized that the link between these epidemics and modern CFS is largely historical. The two conditions were very different. Epidemic ME was contagious, acute, and accompanied by paralysis and neurological signs (albeit of disputed origin). Sporadic CFS or ME, as seen today, is non-contagious, chronic, fatiguing, and has no neurological signs – we doubt whether any modern observers would consider a diagnosis of CFS in a patient requiring assisted ventilation. Hysteria is also a peripheral issue in most clinical encounters (see Chapter 10). Most of those affected by outbreaks of epidemic neuromyasthenia, Iceland disease, myalgic encephalomyelitis, and related conditions do not fulfil criteria for CFS[54]. Despite these differences, many advocates of the condition continue to lay claim to either the Los Angeles or Royal Free episodes as the origin of the disease. Because the same name, ME, has been attached to both sporadic and epidemic processes, supporters of ME continue to affirm the organicity of the original episodes with a vehemence at variance with the quality of the evidence available. Alternatively, much media coverage of the condition revolves around the accusation of hysteria.

The shift from epidemic to sporadic occurred in both the United Kingdom and United States, but transatlantic differences remained. Although there are no reliable methods of distinguishing between ME and CFS, and the professional literature treats them as largely synonymous, some cultural differences can be discerned. British texts on ME frequently assume a neuromuscular pathogenesis, and emphasize neurological symptoms and signs. American writings on CFS are less concerned with muscle symptoms and pathology, but instead emphasize central ('cognitive' or 'neuropsychiatric') symptoms. Similar differences exist in aetiological theories. In the United Kingdom more attention is given to viral causes, with the principal culprit the enterovirus family. In the United States immunological theories have achieved greater prominence. Viral aetiologies are by no means absent, but the chief culprit has been the Epstein–Barr virus (EBV).

In the United Kingdom the link between enterovirus and ME started with the controversial association between poliovirus and some outbreaks of epidemic ME. The next stage was when two eminent Glasgow virologists, Norman Grist and Eleanor Bell, who had already played a major role in linking the coxsackievirus to the pathogenesis of a number of diseases, joined forces with Glasgow neuroim-munologist Peter Behan, who was interested in ME. Together they studied new outbreaks of what appeared to be acute epidemic ME in the west of Scotland, and reported finding an association with high neutralizing antibody titres to coxsackie virus, to be succeeded by similar findings in sporadic cases. They were also instrumental in reintroducing the term 'post-viral fatigue' to replace ME[55]. Although the serological tests used are no longer seen as reliable it served as a spur to further work (reviewed in Chapter 9).

Particularly important to the rapid rise of interest in CFS/ME in the United Kingdom was the work carried out in the mid 1980s at St Mary's Hospital, London on enteroviral involvement in CFS (see Chapter 9). This was greeted with immense enthusiasm – 'all ME sufferers must have been elated by the news in January 1988 that a specific blood test for ME had been perfected'[56], and a doctor congratulated those responsible for 'the magnificent work with the VP-1 estimations'[57]. We will review the scientific findings later, and will conclude that, like the mononucleosis story in the USA, early claims were exaggerated. However, the significance of the early work on enteroviruses in the United Kingdom, coming as it did from prestigious institutions, was to confer the same degree of professional legitimacy on CFS in the United Kingdom as did the papers from Denver and the National Institutes of Health in the United States (see above).

6.5 From chronic Epstein–Barr virus to the CFS

The reconstruction of chronic fatigue began in the mid 1980s, with the emergence of 'chronic Epstein–Barr virus syndrome'. This began with a *Lancet* paper from Israeli researchers[58], followed by two papers in high-impact American journals[59,60]. These papers sought to link evidence of infection by the Epstein–Barr virus to chronic fatigue, leading to a consensus conference organized in 1985 by the National Institute of Allergic and Infectious Diseases[61]. As we will show when we discuss the evidence linking mononucleosis and chronic fatigue, it is now clear that the role of persistent EBV in the new condition was also exaggerated (Chapter 9). The same authors who had presented the original data themselves concluded that 'chronic mononucleosis' was a misnomer, and should be abandoned.

This did not happen. Concurrent with the Israeli and American research, others were beginning to recognize and lobby on behalf of patients with 'chronic active Epstein–Barr virus'. The crucial year appears to have been 1984 in which there was 'an unprecedented increase in sporadic and epidemic cases across North America', culminating in an impassioned testimony before a US Senate subcommitee in 1984[62]. The combination of this grass roots activism and the publication of prestigious papers triggered a surge of public media attention, for which the original proposers of chronic mononucleosis later declared themselves unprepared. One of the most striking features of chronic fatigue in the 1980s and 1990s is the extent of media interest in the subject. We will consider the background to the upsurge of media interest in Chapter 15, but for the narrative it is sufficient to document the size of the response. The immediate triggers appeared to be the ill-defined epidemic at Lake

Tahoe, together with the chronic mononucleosis papers already cited. Feiden[63] notes the 'key events' in the story of CFS in the USA as the Lake Tahoe epidemic, which coincided with 'two path-breaking articles in the *Annals of Internal Medicine*'[59,60]. The confluence of these two events made an extraordinary impact, described by one medical journalist as a 'proliferation of support groups, research foundations dominated by patients with the syndrome, and fund raising and lobbying groups'[64]. Between 1984 and 1987 a journalist/sufferer noted that support groups rose 'out of practically nothing to more than 200'[65]. Simultaneously 'Physicians throughout the United States were inundated with requests to evaluate chronic fatigue'[66] By 1990 a hotline at the Centers for Disease Control (CDC) was attracting over 2000 calls a month[67], a figure now nearer 4000. Only AIDS attracts more calls to the National Institutes of Health[68]. When the CDC published the latest case definition in the *Annals of Internal Medicine* in 1994 they received an unprecedented 250 000 reprint requests. As a final statistic on the public impact of CFS, a recent paper looked at the use of 'on-line' support groups for various diseases via the Internet. Looking at 'America Online', a commercial server, over a two-week period more 'posts' were made by the CFS support groups that for all the other support groups (arthritis, breast cancer, diabetes, heart disease, and prostate cancer) combined[69]. The length of the average communication was also longest for CFS[69].

In the United Kingdom a broadcast in 1980 on *Woman's Hour* led to 1000 letters[70], but many credit the article by Sue Finlay[71] in *The Observer* of 1 June 1986 ('An illness doctors don't recognise'), relating her own experiences as a sufferer, as playing a pivotal role in the surge of interest in ME in the UK and the founding of the ME Action Campaign[56]. The first medical adviser to the ME Association noted how the dramatic rise in membership of the other patients' organization in the United Kingdom, the ME Association, was also assisted by media coverage[72].

Did this coverage, itself labelled a 'media epidemic'[67], actually create the demand? Stewart's finding of the overlap between CFS, environmental illness, and candida may owe something to media publicity[73], but perhaps what is being influenced is the choice of label, rather than the development of illness. Interest must have preceded the media attention – Sue Finlay's article provoked an immediate response. Fourteen thousand fact sheets were requested in the following weeks[56], suggesting that the demand was already there, and was not created by the article.

The remarkable acceptance of CFS/ME in the late 1980s left the research community with a dilemma. Although little convincing evidence had been provided for the existence of a discrete syndrome, researchers were faced with a *fait accompli*. Chronic mononucleosis had captured the public imagination. The professional disillusionment with the role of EBV in the syndrome did nothing to diminish or delegitimize this – the new syndrome appeared to be here to stay. The medical reaction was therefore to change the label. Opportunity was therefore taken during a meeting of infectious diseases specialists in 1987 to arrive at a case definition and find a new name[74]. The authors were more successful in their second that their first objective. The name chosen, chronic fatigue syndrome (CFS), proved acceptable to most (but not all) parties, and appears to be durable. Researchers in Australia had reached the same conclusion and proposed the identical title[75]. Two years later the United Kingdom followed suit[76].

6.6 Fibromyalgia

This book is devoted to the topic of chronic fatigue, but we have already made reference to a closely related symptom, muscle pain (myalgia). The concepts of fatigue and pain have a considerable overlap, and many patients are often unable to determine whether they are limited by one or the other. Painful exhaustion can be difficult to separate from muscle pain. Just as severe fatigue has become the core feature of a specific syndrome (CFS), so, in recent years, has myalgia become the defining feature of an illness called fibromyalgia. This is a syndrome characterized by chronic pain and stiffness in skeletal muscle, associated with painful 'tender points' on palpation.

We have traced the historical origins of CFS to the Victorian illness of neurasthenia. Likewise, fibromyalgia can be traced to the concept of 'fibrositis'. Gowers described both muscle tenderness and increased pain sensitivity as characteristic of fibrositis[77,78]. Beard himself remarked on the overlap between neurasthenia and rheumatism[79]. Shorter notes how the diagnosis was used in a similar fashion to that of neurasthenia[47]. He also outlines how the lack of any objective evidence of inflammation gradually led to a disillusionment with the concept among orthodox rheumatologists.

The renaissance of fibromyalgia preceded that of CFS, albeit only by a decade. Commentators are agreed that it was studies by the Canadian physicians Hugh Smythe and Harvey Moldofsky, the former delineating specific sites of muscle tenderness, later to be called 'tender points', and the latter describing what was claimed to be a specific abnormality of sleep[80]. This research gathered pace during the 1980s, accompanied by the increasing enthusiasm of a fairly small group of active researchers, culminating in the publication by the American College of Rheumatology of a case definition and classification of fibromyalgia[81].

There are many similarities between fibromyalgia and CFS, although the two are not synonymous[82]. Whereas the research into CFS has been dominated by virological and immunological investigations, this has not been so in fibromyalgia. On the other hand, important studies of neuromuscular and neuroendocrinological function have been carried out in both conditions, with, as we shall note, rather similar findings. Although fibromyalgia is associated with some dispute and controversy within professional circles, usually related to the same objections raised concerning CFS[47,83], this has been generally conducted in a restrained atmosphere largely restricted to the normal forums of academic debate. The degree of professional and popular controversy and political action that is so striking in CFS is largely absent from fibromyalgia.

In the remainder of this book we will concentrate on chronic fatigue and chronic fatigue syndrome, but will draw attention to the literature on fibromyalgia where it informs our discussion of chronic fatigue (see also Chapter 14). This will be particularly evident in the sections on epidemiology, neurology, and treatment. On the other hand, fibromyalgia will figure very little in our discussions of the virological and immunological basis of CFS or in our account of the social history of CFS.

References

1 Chatel J, Peele R. A centennial review of neurasthenia. *Am. J. Psychiat.* 1970; **126:** 48–57.
2 Alvarez W. What is wrong with the patient who feels tired, weak and toxic? *New Engl. J. Med.* 1935; **212:** 96–104.
3 Macy J, Allen E. Justification of the diagnosis of chronic nervous exhaustion. *Ann. Int. Med.* 1934; **7:** 861–867.
4 Allan F. The clinical management of weakness and fatigue. *J. Am. Med. Assoc.* 1945; **127:** 957–960.
5 Wilbur D. Clinical management of the patient with fatigue and nervousness. *J. Am. Med. Assoc.* 1949; **141:** 1199–1204.
6 Shands H, Finesinger J. A note on the significance of fatigue. *Psychosom. Med.* 1952; **14:** 309–314.
7 Ware N. Suffering and the social construction of illness: the delegitimisation of illness experience in chronic fatigue syndrome. *Med. Anthropol. Q.* 1992; **6:** 347–361.
8 Anon. A new clinical entity? *Lancet* 1956; **i:** 789–790.
9 Parish J. Early outbreaks of 'epidemic neuromyasthenia'. *Postgrad. Med. J.* 1978; **54:** 711–717.
10 Aronowitz R. From myalgic encephalitis to yuppie flu: a history of chronic fatigue syndrome. In Rosenberg C, Golden J (ed.) *Framing Disease.* New Brunswick, Rutgers University Press, 1992: 155–181.
11 Crowley N, Nelson M, Stovin S. Epidemiological aspects of an outbreak of encephalomyelitis at the Royal Free Hospital. *J. Hygiene* 1957; **58:** 102–122.
12 Acheson D. The clinical syndrome variously called benign myalgic encephalomyelitis, Iceland Disease and epidemic neuromyasthenia. *Am. J. Med.* 1959; **26:** 569–595.
13 Bigler M, Nielsen J. Poliomyelitis in Los Angeles in 1934: neurologic characteristics of the disease in adults. *Bull. Los Angeles Neurol. Soc.* 1937; **2:** 47–58.
14 McEvedy C, Beard A. Royal Free Epidemic of 1955; a reconsideration. *Br. Med. J.* 1970; **i:** 7–11.
15 McEvedy C, Beard A. Concept of benign myalgic encephalomyelitis. *Br. Med. J.* 1970; **i:** 11–15.
16 Hare M. Epidemic malaise. *Br. Med. J.* 1970; **i:** 299.
17 Mausner J, Gezon H. Report on a phantom epidemic of gonorrhoea. *Am. J. Epidemiol.* 1967; **85:** 320–331.
18 Paul J. *A History of Poliomyelitis.* New Haven, CT, Yale University Press, 1971.
19 Stevens G. The 1934 epidemic of poliomyelitis in Southern California. *Am. J. Pub. Health* 1934; **12:** 1213–1214.
20 Daikos G, Garzonis S, Paleologue A, Bousvaros G, Papadoyannakis N. Benign myalgic encephalomyelitis: an outbreak in a nurses' school in Athens. *Lancet* 1959; **i:** 693–696.
21 Ramsay A. Encephalomyelitis in northwest London. An endemic infectious simulating poliomyelitis and hysteria. *Lancet* 1957; **ii:** 1196–2000.
22 Hill R, Cheetham R, Wallace H. Epidemic myalgic encephalomyelopathy. The Durban outbreak. *Lancet* 1959; **i:** 689–693.
23 Jenkins R. Introduction. In Jenkins R, Mowbray J (ed.) *Postviral Fatigue Syndrome.* Chichester, Wiley, 1991: 1–39.
24 Hope-Pool J, Walton J, Brewis E, Uldall P, Wright A, Gardner P. Benign myalgic encephalomyelitis in Newcastle-upon-Tyne. *Lancet* 1961; **i:** 733–737.
25 McEvedy C, Beard A. A controlled study follow up of cases involved in an epidemic of 'benign myalgic encephalomyelitis'. *Br. J. Psychiatry* 1973; **122:** 141–150.

26 Briggs N, Levine P. A comparative review of systemic and neurological symptomatology in 12 outbreaks collectively described as chronic fatigue syndrome, epidemic neuromyasthenia and myalgic encephalomyelitis. *Clin. Infect. Dis.* 1994; **18(suppl 1):** 32–42.

27 May P, Donnan S, Ashton J, Ogilvie M, Rolles C. Personality and medical perception in benign myalgic encephalomyelitis. *Lancet* 1980; **ii:** 1122–1124.

28 Buzzard F. The dumping ground of neurasthenia. *Lancet* 1930; **i:** 1–4.

29 Poskanzer D. Epidemic malaise. *Br. Med. J.* 1970; **ii:** 420–21.

30 Howell B. Epidemic malaise. *Br. Med. J.* 1970; **i:** 300.

31 Ramsay A. Benign myalgic encephalomyelitis. *Br. J. Psychiatry* 1973; **122:** 618–619.

32 Shepherd C. Fatigue that's viral, not hysterical. *MIMS,* Oct 15th 1987.

33 Van Deusen E. Observations of a form of nervous prostration, (neurasthenia), culminating in insanity. *Am. J. Insanity* 1869: 445–461.

34 Huchard H. Neurasthénie. In Axenfeld A, Huchard H (ed.) *Traite des Nevroses.* Paris, Germer Baillière, 1883: 873–907.

35 Young P. Two cases of neurasthenia of long standing successfully treated by the Weir Mitchell method. *Edin. Clin. Path. J.* 1884; **47:** 905–909.

36 Craig M. *Nerve Exhaustion.* London, Churchill, 1922.

37 Oppenheim H. *Text-book of Nervous Diseases for Physicians and Students,* 5th edn. London, Foulis, 1908.

38 Dubois P. *The Psychic Treatment of Nervous Diseases,* 6th edn. New York, Funk and Wagnalls, 1909.

39 Dicks H. Neurasthenia: toxic and traumatic. *Lancet* 1933; **ii:** 683–686.

40 Lane C. The mental element in the etiology of neurasthenia. *J. Nerv. Ment. Dis.* 1906; **33:** 463–466.

41 Ash E. Nervous breakdown: the disease of our age. *Med. Times* 1909; **37:** 35–54.

42 Evans C. Chronic brucellosis. *J. Am. Med. Assoc.* 1934; **103:** 665.

43 Evans C. Brucellosis in the United States. *Am. J. Pub. Health* 1947; **37:** 139–151.

44 Spink W. What is chronic brucellosis? *Ann. Int. Med.* 1951; **35:** 358–374.

45 Cluff L, Trever R, Imboden J, Canter A. Brucellosis: II. Medical aspects of delayed convalescence. *Arch. Intern. Med.* 1959; **103:** 398–405.

46 Imboden J, Canter A, Cluff L. Brucellosis: III. Psychologic aspects of delayed convalescence. *Arch. Intern. Med.* 1959; **103:** 406–414.

47 Shorter E. *From Paralysis to Fatigue: a History of Psychosomatic Illness in the Modern Era.* New York, Free Press, 1992.

48 Eisenberg L. The social construction of mental illness. *Psychol. Med.* 1988; **18:** 1–9.

49 Ramsay A. 'Epidemic neuromyasthenia' 1955–1978. *Postgrad. Med. J.* 1978; **54:** 718–721.

50 Holt G. Epidemic neuromyasthenia: the sporadic form. *Am. J. Med. Sci.* 1965: 124–138.

51 Price J. Myalgic encephalomyelitis. *Lancet* 1961; *i:* 737–738.

52 Compston N. An outbreak of encephalomyelitis in the Royal Free Hospital Group, London, 1955. *Postgrad. Med. J.* 1978; **554:** 722–724.

53 Levine P, Jacobson S, Pocinki A, *et al.* Clinical, epidemiologic, and virologic studies in four clusters of the chronic fatigue syndrome. *Arch. Intern. Med.* 1992; **152:** 1611–1616.

54 Levine P. Summary and perspective: epidemiology of chronic fatigue syndrome. *Clin. Infect. Dis.* 1994; **18(suppl 1):** S47–S60.

55 Behan P, Behan P, Bell E. The postviral fatigue syndrome: an analysis of the findings in 50 cases. *J. Infect.* 1985; **10:** 211–222.

56 Franklin M, Sullivan J. *The New Mystery Epidemic. M.E. What is it? Have you got it? How to get Better.* London, Century, 1989.

57 Merry P. Management of symptoms of myalgic encephalomyelitis. In Jenkins R, Mowbray J (ed.) *Postviral Fatigue Syndrome.* Chichester, Wiley, 1991: 281–296.

58 Tobi M, Morag A, Ravid Z, *et al*. Prolonged illness associated with serological evidence of persistent Epstein – Barr virus infection. *Lancet* 1982; **i:** 61–64.

59 Jones J, Ray G, Minnich L, Hicks M, Kibler R, Lucas D. Evidence for active Epstein – Barr virus infection in patients with persistent, unexplained illnesses; elevated anti-early antigen antibodies. *Ann. Int. Med.* 1985; **102:** 1–7.

60 Straus S, Tosato G, Armstrong G, *et al*. Persisting illness and fatigue in adults with evidence of Epstein – Barr virus infection. *Ann. Int. Med.* 1985; **102:** 7–16.

61 Tobi M, Straus SE. Chronic Epstein – Barr virus disease: a workshop held by the National Institute of Allergy and Infectious Diseases. *Ann. Intern. Med.* 1985; **103:** 951–3.

62 Coulter P. Chronic fatigue syndrome; an old virus with a new diagnosis. *J. Commun. Health Nursing* 1988; **5:** 87–95.

63 Feiden K. *Hope and Help for Chronic Fatigue Syndrome: The Official Guide of the CFS/ CFIDS Network*. New York, Prentice Hall, 1990.

64 Charatan F. Chronic fatigue in the US. *Br. Med. J.* 1990; **301:** 1236.

65 Johnson H. Journey into fear. *Rolling Stone* 3 August 1987; 42–57.

66 Jones J, Straus S. Chronic Epstein – Barr virus infection. *Ann. Rev. Med.* 1987; **38:** 195–209.

67 Anon. Chronic fatigue: all in the mind? *Consumer Rep.* 1990: 671–674.

68 Anon. In search of a cause. *Awake* 22 August 1992.

69 Davison K, Pennebaker J. Virtual narratives: illness representations in online support groups. In Petrie K, Weinman J (ed.) *Perceptions of Health and Illness: Current Research and Applications*. London, Harwood Academic Press, 1997, 463–486.

70 Wookey C. *Myalgic Encephalomyelitis: Post-viral Fatigue Syndrome and How to Cope With it*. London, Croom Helm, 1986.

71 Finlay S. Don't listen if your GP says it's 'just nerves'. *Scotsman* 18 August 1986.

72 Smith D. *Understanding ME*. London, Robinson Publishing, 1989.

73 Stewart D. The changing face of somatisation. *Psychosomatics* 1990; **31:** 153–158.

74 Holmes G, Kaplan J, Gantz N, *et al*. Chronic fatigue syndrome: a working case definition. *Ann. Int. Med.* 1988; **108:** 387–389.

75 Lloyd A, Wakefield D, Boughton C, Dwyer J. What is myalgic encephalomyelitis? *Lancet* 1988; **i:** 1286–1287.

76 Sharpe M, Archard L, Banatvala J, *et al*. Chronic fatigue syndrome: guidelines for research. *J. R. Soc. Med.* 1991; **84:** 118–121.

77 Gowers W. Lumbago, its lessons and analogues. *Br. Med. J.* 1904; **i:** 117–121.

78 Smythe H. Fibrositis syndrome: a historical perspective. *J. Rheumatol.* 1989; **16(suppl 19):** 2–6.

79 Beard G. Neurasthenia, or nervous exhaustion. *Bost. Med. Surg. J.* 1869; **3:** 217–221.

80 Smythe H, Moldofsky H. Two contributions to understanding of the 'fibrositis' syndrome. *Bull. Rheum. Dis.* 1977; **28:** 928–931.

81 Wolfe F, Smythe H, Yunus M, *et al*. The American College of Rheumatology 1990 criteria for the classification of fibromyalgia: report of the multicenter criteria committee. *Arth. Rheumat.* 1990; **33:** 160–173.

82 Buchwald D. Fibromyalgia and chronic fatigue syndrome: similarities and differences. *Rheumat. Dis. Clin. N. Am.* 1996; **22:** 219–243.

83 Bohr T. Fibromyalgia syndrome and myofascial pain syndrome. Do they exist? *Neurol. Clin.* 1995; **13:** 365–384.

Section III:

Chronic fatigue syndrome

7. CFS: definitions, epidemiology, presentation, prognosis

By the mid 1980s chronic fatigue syndrome had arrived. The story of the next ten years is the story of the professional community attempting to catch up on the dramatic entry of CFS into the public arena, and to bring the traditional methods of scientific inquiry to bear on the problem. As in all such endeavours, the appropriate starting point was to establish a case definition of the new syndrome. This was recognized with the publication in 1988 of what became known as the CDC or Holmes' criteria[1]. This was a milestone in the acceptance of the syndrome and the beginning of a new generation of scientific studies[2].

7.1 Definitions of CFS

Naturally, the first hurried attempts at establishing a definition encountered problems. The criteria require that the clinician routinely enquire about and exclude a large number of disorders, both physical and psychiatric[1]. If a diagnosis of major depression or other psychiatric conditions is made, then the subject cannot be considered a case of CFS. There are several objections to this strategy. First, it is clear from systematic studies (see below) that at least half of the reported series of CFS patients also fulfil criteria for psychiatric disorder. Thus clinicians are either not enquiring after such disorders, which is confirmed by the general evidence of the poor detection of psychiatric disorders by physicians, or are using their own judgement to decide retrospectively whether or not psychiatric disorder is responsible for CFS-like symptoms, or a consequence of CFS. For example, in one series the authors concluded that *all* of the observed psychiatric morbidity was secondary to CFS, and thus classified as an adjustment disorder[3]. This judgement is a very difficult one indeed, given the degree of overlap between depression and CFS, and is likely to be unreliable, especially in the absence of standardized interviews.

The strategy itself was based on a false premise, that CFS and psychiatric disorder are mutually exclusive (see Chapter 10). The authors who were largely responsible for the original Centers for Disease Control (CDC) criteria came to the same conclusion[4], and advised modification to remove at least part of the psychiatric exclusion criteria, the requirement to exclude anyone with a previous psychiatric history. Nevertheless, others continue to insist upon a 'normal' premorbid personality as a prerequisite before a making a diagnosis of CFS, without stating how this can be measured, or why those with premorbid psychological disorder should thus be immune from CFS.

Further problems were noted. First, if the CDC criteria are correctly applied, the condition seems extremely rare (see below). Second, the CDC criteria did not identify a distinct subgroup – for example, rates of psychiatric disorder were equally high when a large sample of chronically fatigued patients was divided into those who did, and those who did not, fulfil the criteria[5]. Immunological parameters also do not differ between the two groups[6]. Katon and Russo went one step further[7]. By using past psychiatric history data, they showed that the full CDC criteria did discriminate in favour of one group, namely those with a lifetime diagnosis of somatization disorder (see below).

New definitions were needed. Two of the current authors (Sharpe and Wessely), together with Peter White from St Bartholomew's Hospital, convened a consensus conference in Green College, Oxford in 1991. A new set of criteria were proposed which became known as the 'Oxford' criteria[8]. These retained some of the features of the CDC, namely a minimum duration of six months, a definite onset (i.e. not lifelong), and functional impairment. The defining characteristic of CFS was now physical and mental fatigability, with associated symptoms such as myalgia, mood, and sleep disturbance. Post-infectious fatigue was listed as a subcategory of CFS, with the same features but after a proven infective episode. The Oxford criteria also included suggestions for methodology, including the minimum information necessary to permit comparisons between studies, and research strategies that could prove fruitful. Finally, with the exception of substance abuse and psychosis, psychiatric illness was no longer an exclusion criterion, but instead should be recorded, permitting later stratification if desired.

The original CDC criteria were also modified following the 1991 Washington conference[9], and again following a further meeting in 1994 in Atlanta[10]. There are a number of similarities between the current US and UK criteria, such as the requirement for substantial functional impairment in addition to the complaint of fatigue (although all are vague on how this should be measured). Differences are also apparent. For example, the American criteria attach particular significance to certain somatic symptoms such as sore throats and painful muscles and lymph nodes, and, although the requirement for multiple symptoms has been modified in the latest revision, four somatic symptoms chosen from a list of eight are still required. The choice of symptoms reflects one school of thought that holds that an infective and/or immune process underlies CFS. In contrast, the British definition does not emphasize somatic symptoms, instead insisting on both physical and mental fatigue and fatigability (see Table 7.1).

One of the major unresolved problems, and hence criticisms, of the definitions of CFS lies in the role of somatic symptoms and the relationship with psychiatric disorder. As we shall see (Chapter 10) there is considerable overlap between the criteria for CFS and those for psychiatric disorders such as depression and anxiety. This is in part the inevitable consequence of the multiple symptom requirement in the CFS criteria. Katon and Russo showed that the greater the number of somatic symptoms in subjects with CFS, the greater the probability of all psychiatric disorders[7]. Our group has also confirmed this in a primary care sample[12]. These findings links CFS with the mainstream of psychiatric epidemiology, since it has been repeatedly demonstrated that a linear relationship exists between the number of somatic symptoms, and the risk of psychiatric disorder[13-16]. Jules Angst in a population survey in Zurich found that there was a consistent and linear relationship between the severity of depression and a number of somatic syndromes, identified at interview[17] – these included gastrointestinal, respiratory, circulatory, backache, headache, and, of course, exhaustion.

Table 7.1 Case definitions for chronic fatigue syndrome

	CDC-1988[1]	CDC-1994[10]	Australian[11]	UK[8]
Minimum duration (months)	6	6	6	6
Functional impairment	50% decrease in activity	Substantial	Substantial	Disabling
Cognitive or neuropsychiatric symptoms	May be present	May be present	Required	Mental fatigue required
Other symptoms	6 or 8 required	4 required	Not specified	Not specified
New onset	Required	Required	Not required	Required
Medical exclusions	Extensive list of known physical causes	Clinically important	Known physical causes	Known physical causes
Psychiatric exclusions	Psychosis, bipolar disorder, substance abuse	Melancholic depression, substance abuse, bipolar disorders, psychosis, eating disorder	Psychosis, bipolar, substance abuse, eating disorder	Psychosis, bipolar, eating disorder, organic brain disease

A similar relationship also exists for pain symptoms in general. Epidemiological studies have shown that there is no increased risk of depression in those with single acute pains, but this rises with both persistent and severity, until in those with multiple pains the risk of depression is greatly increased[18]. Thus insisting on criteria that include both duration and severity, and including pain symptoms (such as myalgia), CFS criteria again render inevitable an overlap with psychiatric disorder.

At its simplest, the more the number of symptoms required for the diagnosis of CFS, the greater the overlap with psychiatric disorder, and the greater the heterogeneity of the concept[19]. This has led both the Australian group and the current authors to argue that it would be more sensible to have a maximum rather than a minimum symptom criterion for CFS.

Most of the symptoms included in the definition of CFS are not specific to it, and thus cannot differentiate CFS from other causes of chronic fatigue, nor provide a satisfactory case definition. Myalgia, muscle weakness, and post-exertional fatigue did not differentiate CFS and severe depression[20,21], but did do so in another study[22]. That study[22] also suggested that infective symptoms (fevers and chills) differed between the groups. However, a number of other symptoms were also more common in CFS than depressed patients (cough, earache, nausea, puffy face, chest pain, and others), which raises the possibility that CFS patients report more somatic symptoms in general, an explanation in keeping with some other observations on symptom reporting in the illness (see Chapter 12) and epidemiological findings in chronic fatigue[23].

That myalgia may not be specific for CFS is not surprising, since it a common somatic symptom in its own right. In a population study 14 per cent of subjects aged between 18 and 45 complained of muscle pain at rest, and 22 per cent complained of muscle pain after exercise[24]. Myalgia was closely associated with fatigue. Those who reported muscle pain were more than three times more likely to experience substantial fatigue than those who did not. Many people find it difficult to distinguish between the two experiences, since the experience of painful muscles merges with the sense of painful weariness that is one expression of fatigue.

Definitions of CFS that involve various restricting criteria will have one obvious effect – they will reduce the prevalence of the condition. For example, in one UK population study[24] 18 per cent of the sample complained of excessive fatigue, but in only 1 per cent had this lasted for more than six months, been experienced all the time, and associated with myalgia. This minority group were distinguished from the rest by a female predominance, and a closer association with psychological distress.

We conclude that any specific diagnostic criterion for CFS risks imposing an arbitrary barrier where none exists in nature, and creating spurious associations, especially when the extreme end of the spectrum (CFS) is being compared with the other end of the spectrum (normal controls). Instead, it is more accurate to consider CFS as the morbid end of the dimension of fatigue.

7.2 CFS: dimension or category?

The difficulties of defining CFS, and hence estimating its prevalence, reflect the differences between categorical and dimensional approaches to classification, and the limitations of the former. A categorical approach assumes that there is an entity called 'chronic fatigue syndrome'. At some stage researchers will discover either a unique set of symptoms or a pathological marker which will enable the clinical boundaries of the syndrome to be delineated. This is the approach that underlies much of the current research effort in CFS. As we have seen and will see further, identifying either a unique symptom profile or validating a laboratory test continues to prove elusive.

The alternative is that there is no categorical condition called CFS. In Chapter 2 we showed that fatigue is dimensionally distributed in the community, and that no cut-off exists to separate normal from abnormal fatigue. We introduced an analogy with hypertension, which is similarly distributed in the community, with no single point at which blood pressure becomes abnormal, but instead a gradually increasing risk of adverse consequences. The nature of hypertension was famously debated by Platt, who proposed a categorical solution, and Pickering, who did not. It was Pickering's views that prevailed.

The two views are not totally incompatible. Continuing the analogy with hypertension, it can be argued that although the population studies do not find much evidence of a categorical syndrome of excessive fatigue, nor of a disease called hypertension, discrete causes do exist of both. In specialist practice cardiologists are always alert to the possibility of renal or endocrine causes of hypertension, such as renal artery stenosis or phaeochromocytoma, although their public health impact is slight. Likewise, severe hypertension is associated with a distinct constellation of pathology (e.g. damage to the kidneys, eyes, heart, and brain). Similarly, discrete diseases associated with severe fatigue also exist, some known, and no doubt others yet to be identified. Many of these conditions, both definite or more speculative, will be discussed in greater depth in other chapters. The role of epidemiology is to put them into a population perspective.

At present most thinking on CFS follows a 'Platt' model, but we favour a 'Pickering' view, and suggest that fatigue syndromes are often arbitrarily created syndromes that lie at the extreme end of the spectrum of polysymptomatic distress. The CDC criteria created a category known as 'idiopathic chronic fatigue'[10], which consisted of those with chronic fatigue who did not meet the full criteria for CFS. Little evidence has been shown of any fundamental differences between these two constructs – in one primary care study only post-exertional malaise, muscle weakness, and myalgia were more likely to be observed in CFS than idiopathic chronic fatigue, and not the other symptoms suggestive of immunological or infective processes[12]. On the basis of another set of comparisons Manu and colleagues conclude that CFS is a more severe subset of idiopathic chronic fatigue[21], a view we share. Definitive evidence to support or refute this view will come from primary care or community samples, not the study of specialist populations. A study that takes the extreme end of the spectrum, represented by selected samples of patients referred to CFS services, and compares them with non-fatigued controls, will produce a Platt categorical solution but for spurious reasons.

Researchers interested in the problem of fibromyalgia have drawn similar conclusions from a series of epidemiological studies confirming the dimensional nature of muscle pain and tender points in the community, and the similar difficulties of defining an arbitrary syndrome[25–28].

The example of hypertension has other lessons for those concerned with the study of fatigue. First, although fatigue is a dimensional variable that cannot be easily separated from the normal sensation and experience of tiredness, it can still be associated with specific disease processes, and requires understanding and treatment. Hypertension, even if labelled 'essential', is clearly not benign, and can be associated with both morbidity and mortality. No physician would hesitate to introduce vigorous treatment for high blood pressure. So it is with fatigue. Because one cannot detect a clear-cut division between 'normal' fatigue and the devastating illness so vividly detailed in the numerous first-person accounts of CFS sufferers, this no more invalidates the latter than the dimensional view of blood pressure invalidates the medical importance of severe hypertension.

7.3 Epidemiology of CFS

We have already shown in Chapter 2 that chronic fatigue is common, but what about CFS? The earliest estimates lacked both a population base and standardized criteria. Not surprisingly prevalence estimates varied widely. For example, one Scottish study reported 140 cases in six months in a general practice of 10 000, giving an annual rate of 2800 per 100 000[29], whilst, also in Scotland and using the same virologist, Behan and colleagues estimated the incidence to be between 3 and 5 per 100 000[30], a difference of approximately 600-fold. In between are Ho Yen, who on the basis of laboratory request forms, estimated the prevalence in the West of Scotland as 51 per 100 000[31], and Murdoch in New Zealand, who claimed a prevalence of 130 per 100 000[32].

The first attempt at a population-based study using an operational case definition came from Lloyd and colleagues in Australia[11]. Cases were identified using general practitioners as key informants. A point prevalence of 37 per 100 000 was recorded. However, only 25 per cent of those physicians approached agreed to participate. Ho Yen and McNamara[33] achieved a better response rate in their survey of Scottish general practitioners. They estimated a prevalence of 130 per 100 000, but recognition of CFS varied. The method chosen, known as a 'key informant' study, also has limitations. Case identification depended upon the patient attending the surgery, the doctor deciding to identify the problem as CFS, and then remembering the patient when approached by the researcher (the practices concerned did not have case registers). Thus the data tell us much about doctor's perceptions of CFS – that it is severe, and takes up a lot of medical time – but not how common it is. The substantial variations in prevalence are reminiscent of the variations in general practitioner use of the diagnosis of neurasthenia[34], and are likely to be influenced by similar factors. Geoff Clements also in Scotland, found that a diagnosis of CFS was made in between 1 in 60 and 1 in 10 000 general practice patients[35].

The Centers for Disease Control and Prevention (CDC) attempted to estimate the prevalence of CFS based on surveillance of selected physician's in four US cities[36]. The observed prevalence of CFS were lower than the Australian figures – between 2 and 7 per 100 000. The average duration of illness at presentation was seven years, suggesting this was very much a chronically ill sample. There was also considerable intrasite variation, as well as a marked female excess (four to one), and a high rate of psychiatric morbidity. All of these studies from Scotland, Australia, and the United States are examples of key informant/sentinel physician designs with all their drawbacks.

Price and colleagues used the Epidemiologic Catchment Area data (collected before the upsurge of interest in CFS) to develop loose approximations to the original CDC criteria[37]. Of the ECA sample, 23.6 per cent reported that they had ever experienced fatigue lasting two or more weeks. The authors then began to apply the CDC exclusion criteria. The figure of 23.6 per cent fell to 13.9 per cent when self-reported medical causes of fatigue were excluded. Excluding those who failed to meet the criteria for significant disability and interference with day-to-day functioning, left only 2.6 per cent. When psychiatric illness was also used as an exclusion criterion, no men, and only one woman out of the entire sample (13 538) fulfilled the approximation in the 1988 CDC criteria (7 per 100 000). Most of the possible cases were excluded because of the overzealous physical and psychological exclusion mandated by the 1988 CDC criteria.

Thus the first generation of quasi epidemiological studies all suggest that CFS is not a common problem in the population or primary care. Recent studies with systematic case ascertainment report a different picture.

Bates *et al.*[38] surveyed an American Ambulatory care clinic. In keeping with the literature, 27 per cent of those attending a primary care clinic had substantial fatigue lasting more than six months and interfering with daily life. The point prevalence of CFS according to the various definitions was 0.3 per cent (CDC 1988), 0.4 per cent (UK), and 1.0 per cent (Australia) respectively. Also in America a study[39] based on a Health Maintenance Organisation (HMO) found a point prevalence ranging between 0.08 per cent and 0.3 per cent, although this was using the over-restrictive 1988 criteria. In an occupational sample 0.9 per cent fulfilled CFS criteria[40].

Turning to the United Kingdom, a Scottish study reported a prevalence of 0.6 per cent, although the sample size was relatively small[41]. In a larger study of English primary care CFS had a prevalence ranging from 0.8 per cent (CDC 1988) to 2.6 per cent (CDC 1994), falling to 0.5 per cent if comorbid psychiatric disorders were excluded[42]. Only 0.1 per cent fulfilled the 1988 CDC criteria – similar to the American findings.

These primary care figures are an order of magnitude greater than those obtained in the first wave of primary care and community surveys. Why? The answer is that nearly all those who fulfilled operational criteria for CFS were not labelled as such by either themselves or their general practitioners, and thus would not be identified in a key informant survey, or a tertiary setting[42]. Among the vast numbers of subjects with excessive fatigue, only 1 per cent believed themselves to be suffering from CFS[24]. When we compared subjects who fulfilled the criteria for CFS identified in a systematic primary care survey with those attending a specialist clinic 12 per cent of the primary care, but 94 per cent of the hospital cases used the terms ME, PVFS or CFS to describe their illness[43].

This emphasises just how few of those who could be classified as CFS are labelled as CFS, or seek specialist help, and highlights the powerful role of selection bias in previous studies, which are almost all based on tertiary care samples of patients who have frequently made their own diagnosis before seeking specialist help, and are almost certainly an atypical and unrepresentative sample of CFS cases[15,44].

7.4 Social class and CFS

One of the most striking observations about CFS is its apparent social class and professional bias – too many studies to list show that the typical patient seen in a specialist clinic, or joining a self-help organization, comes from the upper social classes. Certain professions seem to be particularly over-represented. Forty per cent of the members of the main US patients' organization were associated with health care[45]. Several authors comment on the over representation of doctors amongst sufferers[46] – 'the number of doctors who are victims of the disease is quite out of proportion'[46]. Teachers are also considered a high risk group[47,48]. Similar observations have caused the headline writers to coin the term 'yuppie flu' to describe modern CFS. Although many including ourselves, dislike the flippancy of the word, few dispute the evidential basis of the soubriquet.

But how accurate are these observations? In Chapter 2 we noted that fatigue itself shows little in the way of social class variation, with, if anything, a tendency to be associated with lower socio-economic status. Surveys of CFS based in primary care and the population are also starting to confirm that the perception of the upper class CFS sufferer does not find empirical support[39,40,41,43,49], nor does the claimed susceptibility of the caring professions[41]. It is therefore very probable that the apparent social class distribution is another product of the selection bias introduced in the previous section.

It is therefore premature, and misleading, to invoke complex aetiological theories to explain alleged social class or professional biases, before considering more plausible explanations such as selection bias in referral, medical recognition, and symptom attribution. For example, reports that teachers are over-represented in hospital case series of 'ME'[47] is explained by assuming that teachers have greater exposure to certain infections, such as enteroviruses[47,48]. Such observations are more revealing of the social purpose of fatigue syndromes than the epidemiology of CFS.

7.5 Presentation

The hallmark of CFS is profound fatigue, made worse not only by physical effort, but also by mental effort. As we have noted (Chapter 2) patients use a variety of words to describe this elusive experience – encompassing the sense of tiredness, of effort, and of pain. Many will explain it is not a 'normal' tiredness, in order to convey both the intensity of the symptom, and also the fact that it occurs after activities which the patient does not expect to cause symptoms.

CFS is more, however, than just fatigue. We have already indicated that patients seen in specialist care frequently, if not invariably, complain of other discomforts as well, such as muscle pain, headache, sore throat, and so on. Much of the search for a satisfactory case definition of CFS has been the search for other symptoms to place alongside fatigue and fatigability. Whilst this search has not been entirely satisfactory, that it not to deny the important role that other symptoms play in the experience of CFS.

In Chapter 2 we noted that chronic fatigue can be associated with a range of disabilities, from the minor to the most serious. At the extreme end of the spectrum come patients who have many symptoms in addition to fatigue, and who show impairment in many aspects of their lives. This has been recognized in the current definitions of CFS, all of which include some requirement for functional disability. Patients with CFS seen in specialist clinics have greater disability and impairment in most aspects of their social, work, and domestic life, which is comparable to or often greater than those with a variety of other chronic medical conditions[50-53]. Even in primary care, the score on the MOS short form (SF-36) of 40 for physical functioning[42] is substantially worse than those recorded in the for a variety of chronic medical conditions[54]. Unemployment is common, and use of medical resources high[55]. The label 'benign' previously attached to one fatigue syndrome, 'benign myalgic ence-phalomyelitis', now seems particularly inappropriate.

To a certain extent the finding that functional impairment in CFS is profound is both unsurprising and tautologous, precisely because all the operational criteria for CFS include a requirement for the presence of substantial functional impairment. Nevertheless, this operational requirement itself reflects the clinical observation that CFS can be devastating in its impact to both sufferer and family. Both the popular literature and clinical experience confirm that those attending a CFS clinic are a very disabled group, often unable to manage even the basic tasks. The costs to the health service and society in terms of the use of health resources and the loss of income and productivity in a relatively young group of people is immense[55,56].

7.6 Physical signs and CFS

Early reports concerning ME often reported neurological signs, occasionally divided into cerebral, brainstem, and spinal varieties[57] (as in the first series of neurasthenia texts). Whatever their merit, which has been disputed, such signs were confined to epidemic outbreaks, and are no longer considered compatible with a diagnosis of CFS.

Other physical signs, such as lymphadenopathy, inflamed pharynx, mild fever, nystagmus, and so on, are claimed by enthusiasts to be 'usually present'[58]. The commonest physical sign reported in another series was tender points[59], which is not really a physical sign at all. The same authors do report low frequencies of signs such as hepatomegaly and splenomegaly, but this is not universally accepted. Most reports do not confirm objectively assessed physical abnormalities. Although nearly half of the patients in one series reported that at least one physical sign had been documented by physicians, the researchers could only substantiate this in 2 per cent[5]. Fever is a common symptom, but it too has proved difficult to define objectively[60]. A French study reported that in patients with unexplained fatigue and also fever, who had the usual constellation of physical and psychiatric symptoms typical of CFS, there was an unusual circadian rhythm to the fever[61]. Auscultation, standard ECGs, and 24-hour ambulatory monitoring have all been reported as normal[62,63].

The current consensus is that, like neurasthenia, 'abnormal physical signs are conspicuously absent'[64]. Clear-cut physical signs are not found, but there is still some dispute about the existence of 'softer' signs such as mildly enlarged lymph nodes. However, simply because alleged signs of CFS are 'soft' does not mean they should be discounted. The existence of 'soft' neurological signs in schizophrenia is one piece of the jigsaw suggesting a neurodevelopmental origin for that disease. Instead, if soft signs are proposed, it is essential that they be confirmed with rigorous methodology. To date that has not happened.

7.7 Prognosis

At first sight CFS appears to have a poor prognosis. By the time of presentation most studies report that the illness is already chronic, with *mean* length of illness ranging from 18 months to 13 years. Looking at the major papers on CFS published in the last five years, it is clear that what is being studied is a chronic disease.

Given the long duration of illnesses at presentation, it is not surprising that the prognosis of those in specialist care has long been considered gloomy. In 1934 researchers at the Mayo Clinic carried out a six-year follow-up of 235 patients with a diagnosis of chronic nervous exhaustion[65]. There was a surprising degree of diagnostic stability, with only 6 per cent receiving new diagnoses. The prognosis was not good, since most remained symptomatic, although precise figures are not given. A total of 173 cases of neurocirculatory asthenia seen by a single cardiologist were followed up for an average of 20 years[66]. Only 11 per cent were asymptomatic, whilst 38 per cent were mildly, and 15 per cent severely disabled.

Anecdotal impressions in the modern era are equally gloomy. The first wave of studies into CFS contained observations on prognosis. In one of the key early papers that launched chronic mononucleosis (see Chapter 6) the authors noted that all the subjects showed 'persistent or recurrent symptoms' up to four years later[67]. Behan and Behan write that 'most cases do not improve, give up their work and become permanent invalids, incapacitated by excessive fatigue and myalgia'[68].

Formal follow-up studies are only slightly less pessimistic[69]. Two American studies reported that half the patients referred had significantly improved after one year – but half had not, and only 6 per cent were symptom-free[70,71]. In a systematic follow-up of 177 cases referred to a single infectious disease clinic in Oxford short-term prognosis was poor, although two-thirds had shown some improvement by four years[72]. Only 13 per cent considered themselves 'fully recovered', a similar figure to that reported for neurocirculatory asthenia a generation earlier[66]. Similarly, although two-thirds of a series of Australian patients reported improvement three years later, only 5 per cent had completely recovered[73]. Only 3 per cent of a Dutch cohort had recovered 18 months after assessment[74].

The studies on the prognosis of fibromyalgia report a remarkably similar picture. Of those followed up in a Nottingham clinic, 97 per cent still had typical symptoms four years later and one-third remained 'heavily dependent'[75]. Other studies are equally discouraging[76–78].

Given that most patients who present to specialist clinics have already suffered from several years of illness, their relatively poor outcome may not be surprising, and may be another manifestation of selection bias, to which we have already drawn attention. It is therefore plausible that in primary care or the community the natural history is rather more optimistic. There have been a number of outcome studies of chronic fatigue in primary care, admittedly of relatively short duration[79–82]. When we merged comparable studies we found that even in primary care at one year only 32 per cent had improved or recovered[69]. This was better than the outcome of specialist studies, but not by much. A more favourable outcome has also been reported for a primary care sample of fibromyalgia, but again the majority remained symptomatic[83]. One explanation may be that even in primary care many of those presenting are already established cases (see Chapter 2).

Two unusual features of the natural history of CFS are its apparent tendency to relapse, and the absence of any effect on mortality. It is often anecdotally claimed that CFS has a peculiar pattern of relapse and remission. No formal studies have confirmed this, and even if confirmed, such a pattern would not be unique, as is sometimes claimed, since a similar pattern is found in affective disorder[84,85].

Another feature is that despite apparent persistent morbidity, no increase in mortality has ever been claimed[69]. The diagnosis seems remarkably stable over time. In a review of all the follow-up studies we found that even the most meticulous investigation found that only 5 per cent of CFS cases developed new diagnoses that might explain their symptoms over time – usually the figure was far lower[69]. The same applied to fibromyalgia. Hence CFS did not appear to increase the risk of developing other conditions, nor did it turn out to be the prodrome of another illness. There was also no evidence of any increase in mortality, with the possible exception of death by suicide.

The lack of association with mortality has been noted before. Indeed, both Wheeler[66] and even Beard himself, claimed that neurasthenia was associated with increased longevity (although this may have been due to the confounding effect of high social class). The absence of any increase in mortality is an important epidemiological feature, which should be borne in mind when considering the claims made concerning aetiology on behalf of either persistent viruses, or substantial immune defects.

One must not assume that the prognosis of CFS is always poor. We again emphasize that most of the cited studies are based on the unsystematic assessment of highly selected patients. All are cross-sectional studies of prevalent cases, and thus will always overestimate those with prolonged illness. Similarly, nearly all such patients will already have been fully investigated prior to joining any study, often on more than one occasion. The lack of any new diagnoses revealing themselves does not mean that patients with CFS do not require investigation – just that it does not need to repeated.

Most important of all, simply because such patients are not treated, should not imply that they are *untreatable* (see Chapter 17). Instead, the perception of ME and related illnesses as incurable can become a self-fulfilling prophecy. Table 7.2 gives a summary of the prognosis for CFS and Table 7.3 is concerned with predictors of outcome. It will be clear that both cultural and psychological factors play an important role in determining outcome. We will return to this in Chapter 12.

Table 7.2 Prognosis: summary points

1. Between 20% and 50% of CFS patients seen in specialist care improve in the medium term, but fewer than 10% return to premorbid functioning
2. The prognosis is better in children and in primary care
3. The principal predictors of poor outcome are intensity of illness beliefs and psychiatric morbidity
4. There is no increase in mortality (with the possible exception of suicide)

Table 7.3 Predictors of outcome

Study	Demography	Initial illness	Psychological	Physical
Bombardier et al.[86]	Older age did worse	Longer duration of symptoms and shorter duration of follow-up associated with worse outcome	Lifetime dysthymia associated with poor outcome	Raised oral temperature associated with better outcome
Calder et al.[29]	No report	Good outcome if presented with paraesthesiae, dyspnoea, or anorexia	No report	No association between recovery and viral titres, lymphocyte levels, or liver function
Clark et al.[87]	Older age and less schooling associated with poor outcome	Multiple physical symptoms, longer duration of fatigue associated with poor outcome	Lifelong dysthymia associated with poor outcome	No report
Hellinger et al.[70]	No report	No report	No report	EBV serology not associated with outcome
Hinds and McCluskey[88]	Patients under 20 years had better outcome	No report	No report	No report
Kroenke et al.[81]	Old age associated with poorer outcome but no association for education	More disability associated with poorer outcome; non-significant association with longer duration of fatigue and poorer outcome. No association with fatigue severity or somatic symptoms	BDI not associated	BMI not associated

Table 7.3 Predictors of outcome (*contd*)

Study	Demography	Initial illness	Psychological	Physical
Sharpe et al.[72]	Gender, age, or marital status *not* associated with outcome	Better outcome with increasing duration of follow-up. No association with duration of symptoms at start	Emotional disorder, and belief in viral aetiology associated with poor outcome	No report
Vercoulen et al.[74]	No associations found	Short duration of fatigue and lower fatigue scores associated with a good outcome	Positive self-efficacy, and not attributing to a physical cause associated with good outcome	
Wilson et al.[73]	Age at onset *not* associated	Duration of illness not associated	Strength in belief of a physical cause and psychiatric disorder developing during the illness associated with a poor outcome. No association for neuroticism and premorbid psychiatric disorder	No association with cell-mediated immunity

References

1 Holmes G, Kaplan J, Gantz N, *et al.* Chronic fatigue syndrome: a working case definition. *Ann. Int. Med.* 1988; **108:** 387–389.

2 David A, Wessely S, Pelosi A. Post-viral fatigue: time for a new approach. *Br. Med. J.* 1988; **296:** 696–699.

3 Petersen P, Schenck C, Sherman R. Chronic fatigue syndrome in Minnesota. *Minnesota Med.* 1991; **74:** 21–26.

4 Komaroff AL, Straus SE, Gantz NM, Jones JF. The chronic fatigue syndrome. *Ann. Int. Med.* 1989; **110:** 407–8.

5 Lane T, Manu P, Matthews D. Depression and somatization in the chronic fatigue syndrome. *Am. J. Med.* 1991; **91:** 335–344.

6 Swanink C, Vercoulen J, Galama J, *et al.* Lymphoctye subsets, apoptosis and cytokines in patients with chronic fatigue syndrome. *J. Infect. Dis.* 1996; **173:** 460–463.

7 Katon W, Russo J. Chronic fatigue syndrome criteria: a critique of the requirement for multiple physical complaints. *Arch. Intern. Med.* 1992; **152:** 1604–1609.

8 Sharpe M, Archard L, Banatvala J, *et al.* Chronic fatigue syndrome: guidelines for research. *J. R. Soc. Med.* 1991; **84:** 118–121.

9 Schluederberg A, Straus S, Peterson P, *et al.* Chronic fatigue syndrome research: definition and medical outcome assessment. *Ann. Int. Med.* 1992; **117:** 325–331.

10 Fukuda K, Straus S, Hickie I, Sharpe M, Dobbins J, Komaroff A. The chronic fatigue syndrome: a comprehensive approach to its definition and study. *Ann. Int. Med.* 1994; **121:** 953–959.

11 Lloyd A, Hickie I, Boughton R, Spencer O, Wakefield D. Prevalence of chronic fatigue syndrome in an Australian population. *Med. J. Aust.* 1990; **153:** 522–528.

12 Wessely S, Chalder T, Hirsch S, Wallace P, Wright D. Psychological symptoms, somatic symptoms and psychiatric disorder in chronic fatigue and chronic fatigue syndrome: a prospective study in primary care. *Am. J. Psych.* 1996; **153:** 1050–1059.

13 Goldberg D, Huxley P. *Common Mental Disorders: A Bio-social Model.* London, Tavistock, 1992.

14 Simon G, VonKorff M. Somatization and psychiatric disorder in the NIMH Epidemiologic Catchment Area Study. *Am. J. Psych.* 1991; **148:** 1494–1500.

15 Wessely S. The epidemiology of chronic fatigue syndrome. *Epidemiol. Rev.* 1995; **17:** 139–151.

16 Russo J, Katon W, Sullivan M, Clark M, Buchwald D. Severity of somatization and its relationship to psychiatric disorders and personality. *Psychosomatics* 1994; **35:** 546–556.

17 Angst J, Dobler Mikola A, Binder J. The Zurich study – a prospective epidemiological study of depressive, neurotic and psychosomatic syndromes: I. Problem, methodology. *Eur. Arch. Psychiatry Neurol. Sci.* 1984; **234:** 13–20.

18 Dworkin S, VonKorff M, LeResche L. Multiple pains and psychiatric disturbance: an epidemiological investigation. *Arch. Gen. Psychiat.* 1990; **47:** 239–244.

19 Hickie I, Lloyd A, Hadzi-Pavlovic D, Parker G, Bird K, Wakefield D. Can the chronic fatigue syndrome be defined by distinct clinical features? *Psychol. Med.* 1995; **25:** 925–935.

20 Wessely S, Powell R. Fatigue syndromes: a comparison of chronic 'postviral' fatigue with neuromuscular and affective disorder. *J. Neurol. Neurosurg. Psychiatry* 1989; **52:** 940–948.

21 Manu P, Lane T, Matthews D. Idiopathic chronic fatigue: depressive symptoms and functional somatic complaints. In Demitrack M, Abbey S (ed.) *Chronic Fatigue Syndrome: An Integrative Approach to Evaluation and Treatment.* New York, Guilford Press, 1996: 36–47.

22 Komaroff A. Fagioli L, Geiger A, *et al.* An examination of the working case definition of chronic fatigue syndrome. *Am. J. Med.* 1996; **100:** 56–64.

23 Walker E, Katon W, Jemelka R. Psychiatric disorders and medical care utilisation among people who report fatigue in the general population. *J. Gen. Intern. Med.* 1993; **8:** 436–440.

24 Pawlikowska T, Chalder T, Hirsch S, Wallace P, Wright D, Wessely S. A population based study of fatigue and psychological distress. *Br. Med. J.* 1994; **308:** 743–746.

25 Croft P, Schollum J, Silman A. Population study of tender point counts and pain as evidence of fibromyalgia. *Br. Med. J.* 1994; **309:** 696–699.

26 Wolfe F, Ross K, Anderson J, Russell IJ, Hebert L. The prevalence and characteristics of fibromyalgia in the general population. *Arth. Rheumat.* 1995; **38:** 19–28.

27 Wolfe F, Ross K, Anderson J, Russell I. Aspects of fibromyalgia in the general population: sex, pain threshold and fibromyalgia symptoms. *J. Rheumatol.* 1995; **22:** 151–156.

28 Croft P, Burt J, Schollum J, Thomas E, Macfarlane G, Silman A. More pain, more tender points: is fibromyalgia just one end of a continuous spectrum? *Ann. Rheum. Dis.* 1996; **55:** 482–485.

29 Calder B, Warnock P, McCartney R, Bell E. Coxsackie B viruses and the post-viral syndrome: a prospective study in general practice. *J. R. Coll. Gen. Pract.* 1987; **37:** 11–14.

30 Behan P, Behan W, Bell E. The postviral fatigue syndrome: an analysis of the findings in 50 cases. *J. Infect.* 1985; **10:** 211–222.

31 Ho-Yen D. The epidemiology of post viral fatigue syndrome. *Scot. Med. J.* 1988; **33:** 368–9.

32 Murdoch J. The myalgic encephalomyelitis syndrome. *Fam. Pract.* 1988; **5:** 302–306.

33 Ho-Yen D. General practitioners' experience of the chronic fatigue syndrome. *Br. J. Gen. Pract.* 1991; **41:** 324–326.

34 OPCS. *Morbidity Statistics from General Practice; Third National Morbidity Survey*, 3rd edn. London, HMSO, 1985.

35 Clements G. Survey of diagnosis of chronic fatigue. *Communicable Diseases and Environmental Health in Scotland: Weekly Report* 1991; **25:** 4.

36 Gunn W, Connell D, Randall B. Epidemiology of chronic fatigue syndrome: the Centers for Disease Control Study. In Kleinman A, Straus S (ed.) *Chronic Fatigue Syndrome.* Chichester, Wiley, 1993: 83–101.

37 Price R, North C, Fraser V, Wessely S. The prevalence estimates of chronic fatigue syndrome (CFS) and associated symptoms in the community. *Pub. Health Rep.* 1992; **107:** 514–522.

38 Bates D, Schmitt W, Lee J, Kornish R, Komaroff A. Prevalence of fatigue and chronic fatigue syndrome in a primary care practice. *Arch. Intern. Med.* 1993; **153:** 2759–2765.

39 Buchwald D, Umali P, Umali J, Kith P, Pearlman T, Komaroff A. Chronic fatigue and the chronic fatigue syndrome: prevalence in a Pacific Northwest Health Care System. *Ann. Int. Med.* 1995; **123:** 81–88.

40 Shefer A, Dobbins J, Fukuda K, *et al.* Fatiguing illness among employees in three large state office buildings, California, 1993: was there an outbreak? *J. Psych. Res.* 1997; **31:** 31–43.

41 Lawrie S, Pelosi A. Chronic fatigue syndrome in the community: prevalence and associations. *Br. J. Psychiatry* 1995; **166:** 793–797.

42 Wessely S, Chalder T, Hirsch S, Wallace P, Wright D. The prevalence and morbidity of chronic fatigue and chronic fatigue syndrome: a prospective primary care study. *Am. J. Pub. Health* 1997: **87:** 1449–55.

43 Euba R, Chalder T, Deale A, Wessely S. A comparison of the characteristics of chronic fatigue syndrome in primary and tertiary care. *Br. J. Psychiatry* 1996; **168:** 121–126.

44 Richman J, Flaherty J, Rospenda K. Chronic fatigue syndrome: have flawed assumptions been derived from treatment-based studies? *Am. J. Pub. Health* 1994; **84:** 282–284.

45 Coulter P. Chronic fatigue syndrome; an old virus with a new diagnosis. *J. Commun. Health Nursing* 1988; **5:** 87–95.

46 Ramsay M. *Postviral Fatigue Syndrome: The Saga of Royal Free Disease.* London, Gower Medical, 1986.

47 Dowsett E, Ramsay A, McCartney R, Bell E. Myalgic encephalomyelitis – a persistent enteroviral infection? *Postgrad. Med. J.* 1990; **66:** 526–530.

48 Colby J. The school child with ME. *Br. J. Special Ed.* 1994; **21:** 9–11.

49 Fukuda K, Dobbins J, Wilson L, Dunn R, Wilcox K, Smallwood D. An epidemiologic study of fatigue with relevance for the chronic fatigue syndrome. *J. Psychiat. Res.* 1997; **31:** 19–29.

50 Packer T, Sauriol A, Brouwer B. Fatigue secondary to chronic illness; postpolio syndrome, chronic fatigue syndrome, and multiple sclerosis. *Arch. Phys. Med. Rehab.* 1994; **75:** 1122–1126.

51 Schweitzer R, Kelly B, Foran A, Terry D, Whiting J. Quality of life in chronic fatigue syndrome. *Soc. Sci. Med.* 1995; **41:** 1367–1372.

52 Buchwald D, Pearlman T, Umali J, Schmaling K, Katon W. Functional status in patients with chronic fatigue syndrome, other fatiguing illnesses, and healthy controls. *Am. J. Med.* 1996; **171:** 364–370.

53 Komaroff A, Fagioli L, Doolittle T, *et al.* Health status in patients with chronic fatigue syndrome and in general population and disease comparison groups. *Am. J. Med.* 1996; **101:** 281–290.

54 Wells K, Stewart A, Hays R, *et al.* The functioning and well-being of depressed patients: results from the Medical Outcomes Study. *J. Am. Med. Assoc.* 1989; **262:** 914–919.

55 Bombardier CH, Buchwald D. Chronic fatigue, chronic fatigue syndrome, and fibromyalgia. Disability and health-care use. *Med. Care* 1996; **34:** 924–30.

56 Lloyd A, Pender H. The economic impact of chronic fatigue syndrome. *Med. J. Aust.* 1992; **157:** 599–601.

57 Crowley N, Nelson M, Stovin S. Epidemiological aspects of an outbreak of encephalomyelitis at the Royal Free Hospital. *J. Hygiene* 1957; **55:** 102–122.

58 Cheney P, Lapp C. The diagnosis of chronic fatigue syndrome: an assertive approach. *CFIDS Chronicle Physicians Forum*, 1992: 13–19.

59 Komaroff A, Buchwald D. Symptoms and signs in chronic fatigue syndrome. *Rev. Infect. Dis.* 1991; **13:** S8–S11.

60 Straus S, Dale J, Tobi M, *et al.* Acyclovir treatment of the chronic fatigue syndrome: lack of efficacy in a placebo-controlled trial. *New Engl. J. Med.* 1988; **319:** 1692–1698.

61 Camus F, Henzel D, Janowski M, Raguin G, Leport C, Vilde J. Unexplained fever and chronic fatigue: abnormal circadian temperature pattern. *Eur. J. Med.* 1992; **1:** 30–36.

62 Kannel W, Dawber T, Cohen M. The electrocardiogram in neurocirculatory asthenia (anxiety neurosis or neurasthenia): a study of 203 neurocirculatory asthenia patients and 757 healthy controls in the Framlingham study. *Ann. Int. Med.* 1958; **49:** 1351–1360.

63 Montague T, Marrie T, Klassen G, Bewick D, Horacek B. Cardiac function at rest and with exercise in the chronic fatigue syndrome. *Chest* 1989; **95:** 779–784.

64 Webb H, Parsons L. Chronic PVFS in the neurology clinic. In Jenkins R, Mowbray J (ed.) *Postviral Fatigue Syndrome.* Chichester, Wiley, 1991: 233–239.

65 Macy J, Allen E. Justification of the diagnosis of chronic nervous exhaustion. *Ann. Int. Med.* 1934; **7:** 861–867.

66 Wheeler E, White P, Reed E, Cohen M. Neurocirculatory asthenia (anxiety neurosis, effort syndrome, neurasthenia). *J. Am. Med. Assoc.* 1950; **142:** 878–889.

67 Jones J, Ray G, Minnich L, Hicks M, Kibler R, Lucas D. Evidence for active Epstein–Barr virus infection in patients with persistent, unexplained illnesses; elevated anti-early antigen antibodies. *Ann. Int. Med.* 1985; **102:** 1–7.

68 Behan P, Behan W. Postviral fatigue syndrome. *Crit. Rev. Neurobiol.* 1988; **4**: 157–179.

69 Joyce J, Hotopf M, Wessely S. The prognosis of chronic fatigue and chronic fatigue syndrome: a systematic review. *Q. J. Med.* **90**: 223–233.

70 Hellinger W, Smith T, Van Scoy R, Spitzer P, Forgacs P, Edson R. Chronic fatigue syndrome and the diagnostic utility of Epstein–Barr virus early antigen. *J. Am. Med. Assoc.* 1988; **260**: 971–973.

71 Gold D, Bowden R, Sixbey J, *et al.* Chronic fatigue: a prospective clinical and virologic study. *J. Am. Med. Assoc.* 1990; **264**: 48–53.

72 Sharpe M, Hawton K, Seagroatt V, Pasvol G. Follow up of patients with fatigue presenting to an infectious diseases clinic. *Br. Med. J.* 1992; **302**: 347–352.

73 Wilson A, Hickie I, Lloyd A, *et al.* Longitudinal study of the outcome of chronic fatigue syndrome. *Br. Med. J.* 1994; **308**: 756–760.

74 Vercoulen J, Swanink C, Fennis J, Galama J, van der Meer J, Bleijenberg G. Prognosis in chronic fatigue syndrome: a prospective study on the natural course. *J. Neurol. Neurosurg. Psychiatry* 1996; **60**: 489–494.

75 Ledingham J, Doherty S, Doherty M. Primary fibromyalgia syndrome: an outcome study. *Br. J. Rheum.* 1993; **32**: 139–142.

76 Felson D, Goldenberg D. The natural history of fibromyalgia. *Arth. Rheumat.* 1986; **29**: 1522–1526.

77 Henriksson C. Longterm effects of fibromyalgia on everyday life. *Scand. J. Rheum.* 1994; **23**: 36–41.

78 Norregaard J, Bulow P, Prescott E, Jacobsen S, Danneskiold-Samsoe B. A four-year follow-up study in fibromyalgia: relationship to chronic fatigue syndrome. *Scand. J. Rheum.* 1993; **22**: 35–38.

79 Nelson E, Kirk J, McHugo G, *et al.* Chief complaint fatigue; a longitudinal study from the patient's perspective. *Fam. Pract. Res.* 1987; **6**: 175–188.

80 Elnicki D, Shockcor W, Brick J, Beynon D. Evaluating the complaint of fatigue in primary care: diagnoses and outcomes. *Am. J. Med.* 1992; **93**: 303–307.

81 Kroenke K, Wood D, Mangelsdorff D, Meier N, Powell J. Chronic fatigue in primary care: prevalence, patient characteristics and outcome. *J. Am. Med. Assoc.* 1988; **260**: 929–934.

82 Ridsdale L, Evans A, Jerrett W, Mandalia S, Osler K, Vora H. Patients with fatigue in general practice: a prospective study. *Br. Med. J.* 1993; **307**: 103–106.

83 Granges G, Zilko P, Littlejohn G. Fibromyalgia syndrome: assessment of the severity of the condition two years after diagnosis. *J. Rheumatol.* 1994; **21**: 523–529.

84 Keller M, Shapiro R, Lavori P, Wolfe N. Relapse in major depressive disorder. *Arch. Gen. Psychiat.* 1982; **39**: 911–915.

85 Keller M. Depression: a long term illness. *Br. J. Psychiatry* 1994; **165(suppl 26)**: 9–15.

86 Bombardier C, Buchwald D. Outcome and prognosis of patients with chronic fatigue vs chronic fatigue syndrome. *Arch. Intern. Med.* 1995; **155**: 2105–2110.

87 Clark M, Katon W, Russo J, Kith P, Sintay M, Buchwald D. Chronic fatigue; risk factors for symptom persistence in a 2.5-year follow up study. *Am. J. Med.* 1995; **98**: 187–195.

88 Hinds G, McCluskey D. A retrospective study of chronic fatigue syndrome. *Proc. R. Coll. Phys. Edin.* 1993; **23**: 10–14.

8. CFS: muscles and nerves

When considering the history of neurasthenia, we have seen how the early models of the physical nature of the illness considered that fatigue was of peripheral, neuromuscular origin, but these were superseded by concepts of fatigue resulting from central nervous system dysfunction. At least part of the same progression can be observed in studies of CFS. Initially, particularly in the United Kingdom, suggested aetiologies of CFS revolved around possible neuromuscular dysfunction. This is not surprising – patients are clearly limited in the amount of physical activity they can undertake, and are 'only too aware of the muscle pain or ache located only too painfully in the muscle'[1]. It is therefore reasonable to suggest that such symptoms and disabilities have a primary neuromuscular cause. A considerable body of literature now exists to address this question.

8.1 Muscle pathology and biochemistry

Because patients with chronic fatigue and chronic fatigue syndrome can be so limited in terms of physical activity, and because they also frequently complain of pain located in their muscles, many investigators have been interested in the subject of possible neuromuscular dysfunction. Unlike the central nervous system, and, perhaps, the psyche, it is relatively easy to obtain samples of peripheral muscle for investigation. In consequence there is a large literature on the topic of muscle structure and function in CFS.

Is there a disorder of muscle structure?

In one of the earliest studies of muscle histology carried out in CFS, Behan and colleagues reported that all 20 of the muscle biopsies carried out were abnormal, with 15 showing single, widely scattered necrotic fibres[2]. There was a low Type I fibre prevalence, instead Type II fibres predominated. Type 1 fibres are aerobic, slow-twitch, red muscle fibres, whereas Type II are anaerobic, fast-twitch, white muscle fibres. Type I fibres, which are rich in mitochondria are more susceptible to disuse atrophy than Type II. Type II fibres develop both earlier fatigue and more profound acidosis than Type I fibres during heavy exercise, and are more susceptible to muscle cramps and exertional myalgia. In a later study the same group found mild to severe Type II atrophy in 39 out of 50 biopsies[3]. An Australian group reported mild non-specific atrophy of Type II fibres in another small series of biopsies[4,5]. A more recent study looked at less chronic, but still selected, referrals with post-viral fatigue[6]. Only 3 out of 23 had relatively mild Type II fibre atrophy, and the authors note that these were considered to have managed their disease poorly. Four showed Type II hypertrophy (in line with the original findings of Behan's group[2]). One possibility is that hypertrophy of one of the muscle fibre types is a response to atrophy of the other – but a subgroup have evidence of hypertrophy of both muscle fibre types[7].

The Liverpool group led by Richard Edwards reported an important study[8]. They found a range of changes in 81 per cent of muscle biopsies from patients with CFS. These included degenerative and regenerative changes, mitochondrial hyperplasia, increased single-fibre electromyographic activity and others. However, one-third of those from normal controls were similarly abnormal – the range of abnormalities resembling those of the cases. They concluded that there are no consistent changes in fibre size. Connolly and co-workers, in a study that deserves to be better known, found that in patients with typical symptoms of CFS, both with and without an apparent viral trigger, muscle biopsy and electrophysiology were essentially normal[9]. However, in a third group, in which symptoms of myalgia were prominent but not those of mental fatigue and fatigability, muscle biopsy abnormalities, albeit non-specific, were noted. The authors noted that this group made up only 2 per cent of those referred to the clinician concerned, who specializes in chronic fatigue. A Spanish group recorded that most muscle biopsies from CFS patients were normal, the others exhibiting minor changes, such as Type II hypertrophy, scattered fibre necrosis, abnormal oxidative pattern, and mild myofibrillar loss[10].

Meanwhile, studies of fibromyalgia are only a little less confusing – some claim an increase in Type I fibres[11]. Others report an increase in Type I fibres, but restricted to those with localized myalgia only, the rest being normal[12], and yet others report mild Type I and/or Type II fibre atrophy[13]. Electron microscopy has also revealed various pathological changes, but these were not confirmed by blinded, controlled studies[14,15]. The most recent reviews now assume that the frequency of Type I and Type II fibres is normal[16]. Rather than a global disorder of muscle histology, some samples of muscle tissue show areas of muscle microtrauma. This is a normal finding, the changes in fibromyalgia being quantitative rather than qualitative[17].

Is CFS a metabolic disorder?

No evidence has been found of an inflammatory response consistent with myositis. There is no evidence of increases in serum levels of skeletal muscle enzymes, such as creatine kinase, a sensitive indicator of muscle damage. Extensive biochemical studies have shown no evidence of abnormalities in mitochondrial or glycolytic enzymes[5]. Immunocytochemistry failed to show evidence of major histocompatibility complex 1 (MHC 1) products[10] – an observation of interest since such antigens are expressed in inflammatory myopathies such as dermatomyositis and polymyositis. This confirms the absence of a conventional inflammatory process, although it does not exclude viral persistence in which there is no MHC regulation (see below). Overall there is no evidence of widespread muscle cell damage when investigated by traditional histological methods[18].

Modern techniques now permit dynamic measures of muscle biochemistry in response to exercise. The first such investigation in CFS raised the possibility that symptoms may be the result of a metabolic myopathy. This was a single case report[19] that suggested such a defect in a doctor with prolonged fatigue after varicella infection. Conventional neurological examination was normal, but a muscle biopsy revealed scattered necrotic fibres and Type II fibre predominance. Using ^{31}P nuclear magnetic resonance spectroscopy as a non-invasive way of measuring intracellular muscle fibre pH and changes in intermediary metabolites, the researchers demonstrated early and severe acidification following prolonged ischaemic exercise. The conclusion was that the basis of the patient's fatigue was abnormal lactic acid accumulation as a result of excessive glycolytic activity. A subsequent larger study failed to replicate the original *Lancet* report, instead finding a tendency to slow recovery, as predicted, but no excess acidification, and no accumulation of inorganic phosphate[20]. Some groups continue to report seeing the occasional patient with early acidification (Natelson, personal communication) but most of the systematic studies fail to confirm the original observation. The San Francisco group also studied a sample of AIDS patients, potentially clinically relevant since they also frequently present with severe myalgia, and have a known persistent virus infection[21]. They and two other groups have failed to find any evidence of early acidosis or evidence of a metabolic myopathy in CFS[21–23]. Later attempts by the Oxford group responsible for the original case report to replicate their own findings were less successful[24]. Normal biochemical and metabolic responses to exercise have also been found in fibromyalgia[15,25,26] – a global alteration in energy metabolism is not thought to contribute to that condition either[15].

Lactate responses to exercise provide another, simpler, method of assessing muscle metabolism. The Liverpool researchers report that lactate response to exercise in CFS is either normal, or mildly increased compared with controls, but only towards the end of the test[27,28]. Researchers at Charing Cross Hospital have found a subgroup with an abnormal lactate response to submaximal exercise[29]. This group was less likely to have overt psychiatric disorder than those with normal lactate responses. They concluded that exercise intolerance might result from several different processes – psychiatric disorder, deconditioning, and impaired anaerobic metabolism.

There have also been claims of deficits in mitochondrial numbers, structure, and function. Byrne *et al.* described two patients with decreases in mitochondrial respiration[4], but later concluded that the abnormality was of dubious significance[30]. The Glasgow group reported that 35 out of 50 electron microscopic examinations revealed considerable structural abnormalities in the mitochondria[3], as did an Italian group, albeit in a smaller sample[31]. This would be compatible with the demonstration of reduced oxidative metabolism in CFS[32], but there remain objections to such a hypothesis. First, the frequent finding of normal physiological performance is incompatible with claims of a mitochondrial myopathy, as shown by the Oxford researchers[33]. Second, the potential role of inactivity must be considered. Edwards and his team demonstrated impaired mitochondrial function in a series of patients with unexplained muscle pain, labelled at that time as effort syndrome, but probably equally well described as CFS. However, they noted that activity levels have a significant effect on mitochondrial enzyme activity[34], so reductions in activity may be secondary to reduced muscle use[8,34], as may the finding of reduced muscle oxidative metabolism[32] (see below and Chapter 3). The importance of relating such findings to function is emphasized by the example of AIDS patients, in whom abnormalities of mitochondrial function coexist with normal physiological performance[21]. Third, a blind study found no difference in the prevalence of mitochondrial abnormalities as reported by the Glasgow group compared with normal controls[35].

Such findings are not entirely new. Going back to the effort syndrome literature both Maxwell Jones and Mandel Cohen found significantly greater rises in blood lactate following matched exercise protocols in subjects with effort syndrome/ neurocirculatory asthenia compared with normals[36]. As far back as 1900 excessive lactic acid production was noted in neurasthenia, but considered of secondary importance[37].

The suggestion that fatigue in CFS was the result of a myopathy has therefore not found widespread acceptance. Such findings have been difficult to replicate. The group that originally suggested such a process finally concluded that their findings 'do not support the hypothesis that any specific metabolic abnormality underlies fatigue in this syndrome, although abnormalities may be present in a minority of patients'[33].

Thus, even if these findings are confirmed, they may be a consequence, not a cause, of easy fatigability. Several authors argue their findings are the pattern seen in deconditioning[22,27]. Early acidosis also occurs in chronic hyperventilation (see below). Edwards and colleagues argue that findings such as those reported by Arnold and colleagues[19] are a normal response to decreased mitochondrial function consequent upon lack of activity[28], or a natural consequence of the predominance of Type II fibres[21] described in the original case report[19]. They are also non-specific.[31]P nuclear magnetic resonance spectroscopy of muscles gave a similar result in a case of schizophrenia[24].

Total RNA and total protein per cell has been shown to be reduced in muscle biopsies of CFS patients[7]. *In vivo* studies of whole body protein synthesis, and quadriceps muscle protein synthesis, were investigated using radiolabelled isotopes[6], and significant decreases found in CFS cases. Muscle RNA and protein synthesis was decreased[6]. These results confirm a reduced capacity for protein synthesis. One possibility is that persistent infection may interfere with the balance of protein synthesis and degradation as found in acute sepsis[38]. Another is that these findings are another result of inactivity – in both normal men with one month unilateral leg immobilization after tibial fracture, and patients with osteoarthritis atrophy of the quadriceps muscle, profound decreases in muscle protein synthesis, muscle RNA activity, accompanied by evidence of Type I muscle fibre atrophy (although there was no evidence of Type II fibre compensatory hypertrophy, as occasionally described in CFS). These changes were reversed by electrical stimulation[39,40].

Looking at all these studies of muscle structure and function together we conclude that a variety of abnormalities have been noted in CFS and fibromyalgia. Many represent normal variations, albeit at increased frequency. Specific abnormalities are found less frequently, and are a conflicting mixture of atrophy and hypertrophy of different fibre groups. No consensus exists as to their meaning. There is little to suggest a primary metabolic problem. The most recent commentators have concluded that both CFS and fibromyalgia are unlikely in the most part to be a primary muscle disorder, and that impaired muscle function and pain may be secondary phenomena[41,42].

8.2 Neurophysiology and neuromuscular function

Structural or biochemical deficits in the muscle appear unlikely to explain fatigue in CFS. What then is the physiological basis for fatigue in the condition? This question baffled investigators into neurasthenia, and remains a source of contention today. A useful conceptual framework is that of Richard Edwards, who divided fatigue into peripheral elements (caused by a failure at or beyond the neuromuscular junction) and central fatigue (caused by a failure of neural drive, reflected in an inability to sustain the necessary motor unit firing)[43]. Central fatigue may reflect deficits in the organization, integration, and initiation of motor activity (see Chapter 3). Like so much else, this is not a new concept. Over a hundred years ago Vivian Poore, a physician at Charing Cross, had previously divided fatigue into general fatigue, referable usually to the brain or nervous system, with systemic features, and local fatigue, referable mainly to the muscles[44]. Loss of power was a feature of local fatigue, but general fatigue has both physical and mental symptoms. Some people assume that central fatigue is a euphemism for abnormal motivation, but as we showed in Chapter 3 this is erroneous.

Early studies of the electromyograms (EMGs) of subjects involved in epidemics of so-called myalgic encephalomyelitis provided no evidence of peripheral mechanisms for excessive fatigability, although they were occasionally erroneously interpreted as so doing[45]. Rather crude studies of individual cases of 'pseudomyasthenia'[46] or 'asthenic syndrome'[47] also showed no evidence of peripheral fatigue, and were instead interpreted as proving poor motivation.

Is neuromuscular function abnormal?

There have been several studies looking at muscle strength and performance in CFS. Stokes *et al.* examined 30 patients with excessive fatigue, present for between 1 and 19 years, associated with severe morbidity and functional impairment[48]. They were compared with normal controls. Maximum isometric force, assessed in the quadriceps, was normal for all the males. Half of the females cases failed to achieve maximum force, but showed increases in force when twitches induced by electrical stimulation of the muscle were interpolated. This shows that the failure of force was not due to a peripheral mechanism, but to a reduction of central drive. This was not found in males. The Liverpool group also studied adductor pollicis brevis fatigability during arterial occlusion using a sphygmomanometer[48]. No significant differences emerged between cases and controls, nor were abnormalities found in maximal relaxation or the length of time for aerobic recovery.

From Australia, Andrew Lloyd, in collaboration with Simon Gandevia, a respected neurophysiologist, reported two studies of neuromuscular function in CFS. One feature of their studies is that they use samples defined on the basis of deficits in cell-mediated immunity. In the first[49] they studied endurance assessed by measurements of repeated maximal isometric contractions of elbow flexors. Maximum isometric strength was normal. Later they studied repetitive, submaximal exercise, which more closely approximates to the normal demands made on muscles in real life[50]. Maximal voluntary isometric strength was again normal, as were twitch interpolation studies, suggesting that there was no peripheral component to fatigue, and that central activation was also complete. Gandevia's group report similar findings in fibromyalgia[51]. The decline in force produced by submaximal isometric exercise was also normal, also noted in fibromyalgia. Fatigue index, a measure of the ratio of muscle endurance and maximal voluntary contraction, was reported as normal in CFS, in contrast to multiple sclerosis[52].

A similar reduction in isometric muscle strength but with increase force generation when electrical impulses were superimposed during maximal voluntary contraction has been noted in fibromyalgia[53], although a more recent study found normal muscle strength[51]. Also in fibromyalgia, investigators have reported reduced maximal voluntary contractions even when compared with sedentary controls[54]. The American study also showed that voluntary activation failure was present in CFS[20], in contrast to the reports from Liverpool and Sydney. Assessing the degree of voluntary activation is difficult, especially when voluntary activation is initially low, and may be influenced by such factors as pain.

A single Canadian study gives a different picture[55]. On exercise testing the CFS group had significantly lower exercise capacity than controls, as reported by several groups (see above). However, CFS patients had a slower acceleration of exercise heart rate. The authors interpret this in two ways – first an intrinsic defect in cardiac pacemaker function, and second a simultaneous dysfunction in skeletal muscle activity. They comment that deconditioning is an unlikely explanation, since that is associated with rapid rises in heart rate during exercise. However, another study found that CFS patients had significantly higher heart rates at submaximal exercise[27], and a third reports entirely normal responses[23].

Is CFS characterized by delayed fatigue?

Some of the above studies were occasionally criticized for not assessing prolonged recovery times, held to be characteristic of ME. Ramsay, for example, states that 'this phenomenon of muscle fatigability is the dominant and most persistent feature of the disease and in my opinion a diagnosis should not be made without it. Restoration of muscle power after exertion can take three to five days or more'[56]. Similar claims were made for neurasthenia. The Australian group did show some impairment of restoration of peak torque 10 minutes after the completion of the testing, but only in the males, and the authors did not feel this was a substantial finding[49]. By three hours recovery of function was normal. They concluded that 'the prominent subjective complaints of muscle fatigue in these patients contrasted with the relatively normal behaviour of their muscles during a controlled test'[49]. They later wondered if the prominent complaints of increased symptoms after exercise were related to excessive production of cytokines in response to exercise – they were not[57]. Another study also found no evidence of excessive production of cytokines post exercise, with the possible exception of a non-significant rise in tumour growth factor alpha[58]. Workers from the Liverpool group also studied delayed fatigue[59]. Chronically fatigued patients were exercised to exhaustion using cycle ergometry. They were restudied at 24 and 48 hours later. Both patients and controls demonstrated fatigability following maximal exercise. However, the rate of recovery of force was identical between the two groups, despite the fact that the patient group continued to complain of persistent weakness and fatigability even at 48 hours after exercise. An American study[32] retested subjects 48 hours after a single bout of strenuous exercise. Only one out of 15 subjects was unable to repeat the exercise test, and no differences in metabolic responses were noted. The same group went on to report that exercise caused a substantial increase in symptoms in only one patient, whilst for the majority subjective recordings of vigour and fatigue showed only minor changes[23].

Overall laboratory studies have failed to reveal evidence that exercise is associated either with an abnormal deterioration in performance, and/or evidence of 'relapse'[60]. This is in sharp contrast to the anecdotal reports of sufferers. We suspect the differences lie in the particular setting of the investigation, and that controlled studies in laboratory conditions with trained investigators fail to activate the particular cognitive responses to exercise that occur in the natural setting (see Chapter 12).

Viral infection and neuromuscular function

A different approach is to study the effects of viral infection on neuromuscular function. Studies have documented disturbances neuromuscular transmission occurring during acute viral infections, associated with a reduction in voluntary strength and endurance[61], although the same authors later suggested that impaired performance was influenced by subjective perception of the severity of symptoms rather than objective signs of illness[62]. Arguing by analogy, there were theoretical reasons for suspecting neurophysiological dysfunction in fatigue states arising after infective episodes. Rutherford and White studied a group of subjects with persistent fatigue after proven Epstein–Barr infection – a then unique group of subjects with definite post-infectious fatigue[63]. The pattern of results was similar to those observed by Lloyd and his colleagues, and the conclusions identical, that 'neither poor motivation nor muscle contractile failure is important in the pathogenesis of fatigue'[50].

Nerve conduction studies and CFS

Conventional recordings of motor and sensory nerve conduction studies are normal in CFS[64,65]. Somatosensory evoked potentials to median nerve stimulation are also normal[66]. Such results do not rule out abnormalities of thinly myelinated and demyelinated fibres, but these were excluded by later studies[18]. Jamal and Miller conclude that no evidence of sensory nerve dysfunction has been found[18] and that nerve conduction studies in CFS are essentially normal. Early reports of such abnormalities in studies of epidemic ME are not widely accepted, and may represent volitional disorders[67]. Abnormalities in conventional electromyography are not compatible with a diagnosis of CFS, and should prompt a search for an alternative explanation.

There is agreement that conventional neurophysiological studies provide no evidence for abnormalities in the structure and function of motor units. However, there is less agreement about the results of more sophisticated electrophysiological investigations, in particular single-fibre EMG (SF-EMG). This is a technique for studying the individual muscle fibre, and thus provides a more sensitive picture of the workings of individual motor units. It assesses the behaviour of individual muscle fibres within a 'motor unit', the group of muscle fibres supplied by a single motor axon, and in particular provides a measure of the 'jitter' or asynchrony between their activation, Sometimes one fibre may fail to be activated at all, suggesting 'impulse blocking'. Experienced investigators in Glasgow reported abnormal jitter values in 75 per cent of a selected sample[64]. However, impulse blocking, a feature of deficits in neuromuscular transmission, did not occur, nor did the results correlate with the presence of enteroviral RNA in muscle biopsies[68]. Others have argued that abnormal jitter alone cannot be related to fatigability[48,49], since there was no evidence of impulse blocking, which alone would indicate failure of the neuromuscular junction. Jamal himself responded by pointing out similar isolated abnormalities in cases of myasthenia which only later progress to show typical impulse blocking[69]. Nevertheless, such progression has not been demonstrated in CFS, despite the often long durations of illness, and an attempt at replication only demonstrated abnormal values of jitter in 4 out of 30 cases[70]. Another attempt at replication, which included studies before and after exercise in a small number of patients, was also unsuccessful[20] as was a German study[71].

CFS and the perception of effort

Neurophysiological and neuromuscular research has not shown any compelling evidence of a primary muscle disorder in CFS. If so, why are so many CFS patients so limited in terms of exercise tolerance? One theory is of a disorder of perception – that CFS patients rate themselves as subjectively more fatigued than the results of objective tests would indicate, and thus cease work at an earlier stage than indicated by the state of their muscles. Several investigators have studied the differences between perceived measures of work rate and exercise tolerance, and actual measures. Workers from Liverpool looked at exercise tolerance and perceived exertion using cycle ergometry[59]. They found that despite subjective evidence that maximum exercise had been achieved, this was not corroborated by the physiological findings. Riley *et al.*[27] also noted that ratings of perceived exertion differed between cases and both normal controls and those with irritable bowel syndrome (IBS). Similar findings have been noted in fibromyalgia[72,73]. CFS patients tended to over-rate both their premorbid exercise tolerance and their desired exercise tolerance, compared with both normal and IBS controls. Children with CFS and their parents likewise underestimate the child's actual level of activity[74]. Only the Australian group, using the same rating scale were unable to confirm differences in perceived exertion[50]. There is thus some evidence suggesting a dissociation between subjective experience of muscle fatigability and objective evidence, perhaps allied to a tendency to symptom monitoring. Remarkably, one study that used a frequent sampling technique to record activity throughout the day failed to document any differences in the amount of actual activity between CFS sufferers and normal controls[75], although a later study using an electronic measure of activity found, less surprisingly, that CFS patients were indeed less active than controls[76].

To summarize, some CFS patients have normal exercise responses, both physiologically and metabolically. Others have reduced endurance and an increase in the metabolic products of exercise. Yet others have a reduced exercise capacity, associated with a reduced heart rate. No single abnormality or explanation can link all these findings. Overall, the two most likely explanations are that many CFS patients have a completely normal exercise capacity, whilst others have a reduced capacity secondary to physical deconditioning. A third group fail to exercise to their apparent capacity, but whether or not this represents a reluctance to do so (because, for example, of a fear of pain, exhaustion, and relapse), or an inability to do so because of a reduced central drive, is unclear.

8.3 The roles of inactivity and fitness

We have already indicated that a major confounder in all studies of muscle function and structure is the influence of lack of activity. Reduced activity, whether secondary to injury, immobilization, or simple disuse, results in profound alterations in muscle structure and function (see Chapter 3). The effects of inactivity have been frequently described in the older medical literature[77,78]. Interest was reawakened by the research conducted into the effects of inactivity as part of the American space programme. It was found that complete bedrest produces muscle wasting, changes in the cardiovascular response to exertion, and consequent intolerance of activity. Other changes include impaired neuropsychological performance, altered autonomic regulation leading to deficits in postural blood pressure control, impaired balance and consequent dizziness on standing, and impaired thermoregulation[79-81]. Inactivity increases the sensation of fatigue and the sense of effort on exertion, but reduces the desire for exercise. The degree of inactivity required to produce these changes need not be great: they can be produced merely by enforced sitting in a chair for one week[82]. Changes in protein turnover can be detected after only six hours[83]. It is salutary to recall the wise words of Richard Asher who warned 'we should think twice about ordering a patient to bed and realize that beneath the comfort of the blanket there lurks a host of formidable dangers'[78].

Are CFS patients unfit? Some certainly are. In one study treadmill assessment revealed reduced work capacity, increased heart rate, and greater reported subjective effort, all consistent with physical unfitness[27]. Many fibromyalgia studies confirm the clinical impression of deconditioning[84,85], although there are exceptions[72]. The various changes in muscle metabolism and mitochondrial activity that have been reported might all be explained on the basis of physical deconditioning[22,28]. Increased subjective effort has also been observed in normal persons who are inactive[86]. Finally, both depression and anxiety are associated with reduced physical fitness and increased lactate responses to exercise[87-90].

Are such changes primary or secondary? The answer is unclear. Case–control designs, which at present make up almost all CFS studies, cannot answer this question. We can conclude that similar findings to those in CFS can be caused by lack of activity. Certainly CFS patients are characterized by inactivity – a substantial degree of functional impairment is necessary for the diagnosis in all of the current operational criteria. Only one prospective study sheds any light on the matter. In White's important cohort study of recovery from Epstein–Barr virus (White, personal communication), simple measures of unfitness taken within a few weeks of the onset of definite EBV infection were significantly associated with fatigue syndrome at four months.

Inactivity can therefore have profound effects on muscle function and structure. It results in physiological changes that reduce the capacity for activity and produce an increased sense of effort for a given level of activity, and causes changes in the functioning of the central and autonomic nervous system that may give rise to other symptoms typical of CFS. To what extent these processes are responsible for the symptoms of patients with CFS will require further investigation. However, the knowledge that physical training reverses the fatigue and cardiovascular changes induced in healthy volunteers by bedrest[91] suggests exercise training as a therapeutic intervention in CFS. This will be described in Chapter 17.

8.4 Myalgia

What about myalgia? CFS patients complain not only of fatigue but also of muscle pain. Whilst we have concluded above that muscle function is not compromised in CFS, could at least some of the pain be of muscular origin? Probably. The fibromyalgia literature suggests that muscle microtrauma, which consists of small scattered areas of focal necrosis and regeneration, is more common in cases than in normals. Evidence from fibromyalgia that exertional myalgia is abolished by epidural anaesthesia, and not by placebo, suggests some peripheral contribution to pain[92].

One theory is that these findings result from unaccustomed overexertion, in which eccentric contractions (when the muscle lengthens doing active work) cause microtrauma[93]. In Chapter 3 we described how this can lead to local pain, which develops between 24 and 48 hours later[94]. This pattern of delayed-onset muscle soreness (DOMS) is frequently described in the neurasthenia and CFS literature. It can be accompanied by transient elevations in creatine phosphokinase, indicating transient muscle injury. Such a theory is attractive, since it gives a physiological explanation for an otherwise perplexing symptom common to CFS and fibromyalgia. It also suggests that myalgia should be seen as a consequence, and not a cause, of chronic fatigue syndrome. Finally, it also suggests a therapeutic strategy, since eccentric contractions and local microtrauma can be prevented by physical training and increased fitness[95,96].

As usual research reveals a more complex picture. Biochemical and magnetic resonance spectroscopy studies of muscle in fibromyalgia patients fails to reveal the expected pattern of post-exertional muscle trauma[72,97]. Not all characteristics of CFS fit the hypothesis – for example myalgia at rest. Muscle soreness due to eccentric contractions tends to be localized to the involved muscle, rather than the diffuse myalgia that some patients experience.

Pain in fibromyalgia is not accompanied by increased electromyographic activity, measured when patients report pain, suggesting that the plausible concept that local pain results from local muscle tension is simplistic[98].

8.5 Effort syndrome

CFS is a disorder of effort. A similar disorder lay at the heart of another now anachronistic fatigue syndrome, the effort syndrome, also known as neurocirculatory asthenia, soldier's heart, or Da Costa's syndrome[99]. The clinical presentation of this syndrome is strikingly reminiscent of CFS, down to the frequent role of an infective trigger[100]. One particular set of studies, now rarely cited, are relevant to the current discussion.

These were carried out by Maxwell Jones at the Mill Hill Army Hospital, where 2324 soldiers with effort syndrome were seen during the Second World War[87,88]. Jones began studying the exercise tolerance and lactate response to activity in sufferers, anticipating the later detailed classic work by Mandel Cohen. Jones concluded that the key difference between anxiety and effort syndrome was not impaired exercise tolerance, present in both, nor early production of lactic acid, also present in both. Instead he wrote that effort syndrome patients were 'conscious of their poor exercise response and tend to associate there symptoms with physical effort (in fact develop an effort phobia); but in the anxiety group no such awareness is present and the somatic symptoms of anxiety are not correlated with exercise'.

Maxwell Jones is known to history as the founder of psychoanalytically based group therapy, but what he was describing was the manner in which cognitive and attributional factors played a role in mediating disability. Furthermore, despite his explicit orientation towards psychogenic perpetuating mechanisms, he also drew attention to the role of infection in triggering effort syndromes.

The exact nature of the haemodynamic disturbances induced by exercise in effort syndromes, and indeed anxiety disorders, remains a matter of continuing speculation. Modern researchers are now describing central mechanisms that bear some resemblance to those being postulated in CFS, such as the failure to increase cardiac output or heart rate during exercise[55,101], but the work of Maxwell Jones reminds us of the leitmotif of this chapter. There may well be an organically determined central mechanism underlying the symptoms of CFS, but the link between such dysfunction and the profound disability of CFS may lie in the cognitions of those afflicted, and the strategies that result.

8.6 Autonomic dysfunction

A new generation of researchers may be about to rediscover the classic investigations of effort syndrome, perhaps stimulated by the recent well publicized reports of an important role for cardiovascular dysfunction in CFS. A group at Johns Hopkins in Baltimore claim that neurally mediated hypotension, also known as vasovagal syncope, is associated with prolonged fatigue[102]. The term describes an abnormal cardiovascular reflex causing subjects to develop severe dizziness or even syncope (fainting) in response to orthostatic stress, such as suddenly standing up. The team first noted that a group of adolescents with vasovagal faints had similar symptoms to those of CFS, and that vasovagal faints could be induced in CFS patients. Upright tilt testing caused symptoms in nearly all the patients, of whom half fainted, with a lowering of both heart rate and blood pressure. The authors went on to speculate that the type of treatments that have been used for vasovagal fainting, such as fludrocortisone to increase blood volume, might have a role in CFS. Uncontrolled data were encouraging, and the authors are now carrying out a controlled clinical trial. The reported improvement showed by two CFS patients receiving venlafaxine[103], a mixed serotonin and noradrenaline re-uptake inhibitor, might also be related to improvement in postural hypotension[104].

This line of enquiry has been greeted with considerable enthusiasm in the United States, but before it is possible to accept autonomic dysfunction as a primary cause of CFS (rather than a secondary contributor to symptoms) it is essential that one important confounder is addressed. This is the role of inactivity. As we have already indicated, physical inactivity is a well known cause of postural hypotension, dizziness on standing, and blood pressure instability (see below).

Sympathetic dysfunction in response to stress has been found in CFS, and is similar to that observed in anxiety disorders, but dissimilar to that in depression[105]. The finding of a slower increase in heart rate in response to exercise[55] and also the finding of an increased heart rate in response to moderate exercise[27] both indicate that sympathetic dysfunction may be found in CFS, even if such findings are contradictory, and more likely to be explained by deconditioning. Vagal (parasympathetic) tone has also been noted to be reduced in CFS[106]. Lower heart rate response to exercise has also observed in fibromyalgia[107], which is not the expected finding in physical deconditioning, and might also suggest a reduction in sympathetic activity.

8.7 Conclusion

One reason for caution in accepting a primary neuromuscular cause is the clinical observation that in many patients pain occurs at rest, or immediately after waking up. Such myalgia cannot be accounted for by any known mechanism of muscle function[7]. Whereas patients with muscle diseases commonly complain of weakness leading to difficulties in specific actions, such as raising the arms above the head, tying shoe laces, and climbing stairs, and only rarely complained of feeling 'tired all the time', CFS patients are more likely to complain of a pervasive general fatigue and malaise[108]. However, the current authors have not noted such clear-cut differences.

Similarly, fatigue after mental exertion cannot be explained by a muscle defect either. The significance of mental fatigue and mental fatigability was investigated by Wessely and Powell[109] who showed that physical fatigue and fatigability was equally prominent in both affective disorders and peripheral neuromuscular disorders (such as myasthenia gravis), and hence its prominence in CFS has little pathophysiological significance, but the same was not true of mental fatigue and fatigability[109]. Whereas mental fatigue and fatigability occurred in the affective disorder controls, as one would expect, it only occurred in the neuromuscular controls when cases also had comorbid psychiatric disorder. In contrast, in the chronic fatigue subjects mental fatigue occurred in both those with and those without psychiatric disorder, although it was commoner in the former. The conclusion was that in the majority of the chronic fatigue cases, neuromuscular explanations were not possible if one assumes the more parsimonious conclusion of a single pathophysiology. A discriminant function analysis grouped most of the CFS cases with either affective disorders, or neuromuscular disorders with psychiatric morbidity – only 10 per cent were classified as pure neuromuscular cases.

We conclude that the fatigue in CFS is mediated by central rather than peripheral mechanisms, although the nature of these mechanisms remains obscure. Possibilities include aberration in circulatory regulation during exercise, as noted in neurocirculatory asthenia[101], the effects of inactivity on performance and centrally mediated disorders of perception and mood disorder. It is unlikely to represent abnormal muscle physiology at the level of the muscle, motor cortex, or motor neurones responsible for voluntary muscle activation[110]. Poor motivation is likely to be an explanation for only a small number of cases[51]. We will return to the theme of possible central mechanisms underlying the physical and psychological deficits of CFS in Chapter 11.

We therefore join the ranks of others, including those better qualified in this area, to conclude that overall CFS is not a neuromuscular disorder. There is probably a subgroup in whom primary neuromuscular mechanisms for abnormal fatigability do exist, but this will be a small minority of subjects. At present we would consider alternative neuromuscular diagnoses and/or mechanisms mainly in subjects presenting with symptoms such as fatigue and myalgia that are clearly exercise related, do not occur at rest, and are not accompanied by any particular symptoms of mental fatigability[9].

References

1 White P. Fatigue and chronic fatigue syndromes. In Bass C (ed.) *Somatization: Physical Symptoms and Psychological Illness.* Oxford, Blackwell Scientific, 1990: 104–140.
2 Behan P, Behan W, Bell E. The postviral fatigue syndrome: an analysis of the findings in 50 cases. *J. Infect.* 1985; **10**: 211–222.
3 Behan W, More I, Behan P. Mitochondrial abnormalities in the post-viral fatigue syndrome. *Acta Neuropathol.* 1991; **83**: 61–65.
4 Byrne E, Trounce I, Dennett X. Chronic relapsing myalgia (?post viral): clinical, histological, and biochemical studies. *Aust. NZ J. Med.* 1985; **15**: 305–8.
5 Byrne E, Trounce I. Chronic fatigue and myalgia syndrome: mitochondrial and glycolytic studies in skeletal muscle. *J. Neurol. Neurosurg. Psychiatry* 1987; **50**: 743–746.
6 Preedy V, Smith D, Salisbury J, Peters T. Biochemical and muscle studies in patients with acute onset post-viral fatigue syndrome. *J. Clin. Path.* 1993; **46**: 722–726.
7 Edwards R, Newham D, Peters T. Muscle biochemistry and pathophysiology in postviral fatigue syndrome. *Br. Med. Bull.* 1991; **47**: 826–837.
8 Edwards R, Gibson H, Clague J, Helliwell T. Muscle physiology and histopathology in chronic fatigue syndrome. In Kleinman A, Straus S (ed.) *Chronic Fatigue Syndrome.* Chichester, Wiley, 1993: 101–131.

9 Connolly S, Smith D, Doyle D, Fowler C. Chronic fatigue: electromyographic and neuropathological evaluation. *J. Neurol.* 1993; **240**: 435–438.

10 Grau J, Casademont J, Pedrol E, *et al.* Chronic fatigue syndrome: studies on skeletal muscle. *Clin. Neuropathol.* 1992; **11**: 329–332.

11 Kalyan Raman UP, Kalyan Raman K, Yunus MB, Masi AT. Muscle pathology in primary fibromyalgia syndrome: a light microscopic, histochemical and ultrastructural study. *J. Rheumatol.* 1984; **11**: 808–813.

12 Bengtsson A, Henriksson K. The muscle in fibromyalgia: a review of Swedish studies. *J. Rheumatol.* 1989; **16(suppl 19)**: 144–149.

13 Yunus MB, Kalyan Raman UP, Kalyan Raman K, Masi AT. Pathologic changes in muscle in primary fibromyalgia syndrome. *Am. J. Med.* 1986; **81**: 38–42.

14 Yunus MB, Kalyan Raman UP, Masi AT, Aldag JC. Electron microscopic studies of muscle biopsy in primary fibromyalgia syndrome: a controlled and blinded study. *J. Rheumatol.* 1989; **16**: 97–101.

15 Wortmann R. Searching for the cause of fibromyalgia: is there a defect in energy metabolism? *Arth. Rheumat.* 1994; **37**: 790–793.

16 Henriksson K, Bengtsson A, Lindman R, Thornell L. Morphological changes in muscle in fibromyalgia and chronic shoulder myalgia. In Vaeroy H, Merskey H, (ed.) *Progress in Fibromyalgia and Myofascial Pain*. Amsterdam, Elsevier, 1993: 61–73.

17 Jacobsen S, Bartels EM, Danneskiold-Samsoe B. Single cell morphology of muscle in patients with chronic muscle pain. *Scand. J. Rheumatol.* 1991; **20**: 336–343.

18 Jamal GA, Miller RG. Neurophysiology of postviral fatigue syndrome. *Br. Med. Bull.* 1991; **47**: 815–25.

19 Arnold DL, Bore PJ, Radda GK, Styles P, Taylor DJ. Excessive intracellular acidosis of skeletal muscle on exercise in a patient with a post-viral exhaustion/fatigue syndrome. A ^{31}P nuclear magnetic resonance study. *Lancet* 1984; **1**: 1367–1369.

20 Kent-Braun J, Sharma K, Weiner M, Massie B, Miller R. Central basis of muscle fatigue in chronic fatigue syndrome. *Neurology* 1993; **43**: 125–131.

21 Miller RG, Carson PJ, Moussavi RS, Green AT, Baker AJ, Weiner MW. Fatigue and myalgia in AIDS patients. *Neurology* 1991; **41**: 1603–1607.

22 Wong R, Lopaschuk G, Zhu G, *et al.* Skeletal muscle metabolism in the chronic fatigue syndrome. In vivo assessment by ^{31}P nuclear magnetic resonance spectroscopy. *Chest* 1992; **102**: 1716–1722.

23 Sisto S, MaManca J, Cordero D, *et al.* Metabolic and cardiovascular effects of a progressive exercise test in patients with chronic fatigue syndrome. *Am. J. Med.* 1996; **100**: 634–640.

24 Yonge R. Magnetic resonance muscle studies: implications for psychiatry. *J. R. Soc. Med.* 1988; **81**: 322–325.

25 Jacobsen S, Jensen KE, Thomsen C, Danneskiold-Samsoe B, Henriksen O. ^{31}P magnetic resonance spectroscopy of skeletal muscle in patients with fibromyalgia. *J. Rheumatol.* 1992; **19**: 1600–1603.

26 Jacobsen S, Danneskiold Samsoe B. Dynamic muscular endurance in primary fibromyalgia compared with chronic myofascial pain syndrome. *Arch. Phys. Med. Rehab.* 1992; **73**: 170–3.

27 Riley M, O'Brien C, McCluskey D, Bell N, Nicholls D. Aerobic work capacity in patients with chronic fatigue syndrome. *Br. Med. J.* 1990; **301**: 953–956.

28 Wagenmakers A, Coakley J, Edwards R. The metabolic consequences of reduced habitual activities in patients with muscle pain and disease. *Ergonomics* 1988; **31**: 1519–1527.

29 Lane R, Burgess A, Flint J, Riccio M, Archard L. Exercise responses and psychiatric disorder in chronic fatigue syndrome. *Br. Med. J.* 1995; **311**: 544–545.

30 Byrne E. Idiopathic chronic fatigue and myalgia syndrome: some thoughts on nomenclature and aetiology. *Med. J. Aust.* 1988; **148:** 80–82.

31 Vecchiet L, Montanari G, Pizzigallo E, *et al.* Sensory characterization of somatic parietal tissues in humans with chronic fatigue syndrome. *Neurosci. Lett.* 1996; **208:** 117–120.

32 McCully K, Natelson B, Iotti S, Sisto S, Leight J. Reduced oxidative muscle metabolism in chronic fatigue syndrome. *Muscle Nerve* 1996; **19:** 621–625.

33 Barnes P, Taylor D, Kemp G, Radda G. Skeletal muscle bioenergetics in the chronic fatigue syndrome. *J. Neurol. Neurosurg. Psychiatry* 1993; **56:** 679–683.

34 Brierley E, Johnson M, James O, Turnbull D. Effects of physical activity and age on mitochondrial function. *Q. J. Med.* 1996; **89:** 251–258.

35 Plioplys A, Plioplys S. Electron-microscopic investigation of muscle mitochondria in chronic fatigue syndrome. *Neuropsychobiology* 1995; **32:** 175–181.

36 Cohen M, Consolazio F, Johnson R. Blood lactate response during moderate exercise in neurocirculatory asthenia, anxiety neurosis or effort syndrome. *J. Clin. Invest.* 1947; **26:** 339–343.

37 Ladova R. The nature of neurasthenia: a study of the recent literature. *Medicine* 1900; **6:** 183–88.

38 Baracos V, Rodemann HP, Dunarello CA, Goldberg AL. Stimulation of muscle protein degradation and prostaglandin E2 release by leukocytic pyrogen (interleukin-1). A mechanism for the increased degradation of muscle proteins during fever. *New Engl. J. Med.* 1983; **308:** 553–558.

39 Gibson JN, Halliday D, Morrison WL, *et al.* Decrease in human quadriceps muscle protein turnover consequent upon leg immobilization. *Clin. Sci.* 1987; **72:** 503–509.

40 Gibson JN, Morrison WL, Scrimgeour CM, Smith K, Stoward PJ, Rennie MJ. Effects of therapeutic percutaneous electrical stimulation of atrophic human quadriceps on muscle composition, protein synthesis and contractile properties. *Eur. J. Clin. Invest.* 1989; **19:** 206–212.

41 Bennett RM, Jacobsen S. Muscle function and origin of pain in fibromyalgia. *Baillières Clin. Rheumatol.* 1994; **8:** 721–746.

42 Geel SE. The fibromyalgia syndrome: musculoskeletal pathophysiology. *Semin. Arthritis Rheum.* 1994; **23:** 347–53.

43 Edwards R. Human muscle function and fatigue. *Human Muscle Fatigue: Physiological Mechanisms.* London, Pitman Medical, 1981: 1–18.

44 Poore G. On fatigue. *Lancet* 1875; **i:** 163–164.

45 Thomas PK. Postviral fatigue syndrome. *Lancet* 1987; **i:** 218.

46 Fullerton D, Munsat T. Pseudomyasthenia gravis: a conversion reaction. *J. Nerv. Ment. Dis.* 1966; **142:** 78–86.

47 McQillen M, Jones R. Asthenic syndrome. *Arch. Neurol.* 1963; **8:** 52–57.

48 Stokes M, Cooper R, Edwards R. Normal strength and fatigability in patients with effort syndrome. *Br. Med. J.* 1988; **297:** 1014–1018.

49 Lloyd A, Hales J, Gandevia S. Muscle strength, endurance and recovery in the post-infection fatigue syndrome. *J. Neurol. Neurosurg. Psychiatry* 1988; **51:** 1316–1322.

50 Lloyd A, Gandevia S, Hales J. Muscle performance, voluntary activation, twitch properties and perceived effort in normal subjects and patients with the chronic fatigue syndrome. *Brain* 1991; **114:** 85–98.

51 Miller T, Allen G, Gandevia S. Muscle force, perceived effort, and voluntary activation of the elbow flexors assessed with sensitive twitch interpolation in fibromyalgia. *J. Rheumatol.* 1996; **23:** 1621-1627.

52 Djaldetti R, Ziv I, Achiron A, Melamed E. Fatigue in multiple sclerosis compared with chronic fatigue syndrome. *Neurology* 1996; **46:** 632–635.

53 Jacobsen S, Wildschiodtz G, Danneskiold Samsoe B. Isokinetic and isometric muscle strength combined with transcutaneous electrical muscle stimulation in primary fibromyalgia syndrome. *J. Rheumatol.* 1991; **18:** 1390–1339.

54 Vestergaard Poulsen P, Thomsen C, Norregaard J, Bulow P, Sinkjaer T, Henriksen O. ^{31}P NMR spectroscopy and electromyography during exercise and recovery in patients with fibromyalgia. *J. Rheumatol.* 1995; **22:** 1544–1551.

55 Montague T, Marrie T, Klassen G, Bewick D, Horacek B. Cardiac function at rest and with exercise in the chronic fatigue syndrome. *Chest* 1989; **95:** 779–784.

56 Ramsay M. *Postviral Fatigue Syndrome: The Saga of Royal Free Disease.* London, Gower Medical, 1986.

57 Lloyd A, Gandevia S, Brockman A, Hales J, Wakefield D. Cytokine production and fatigue in patients with chronic fatigue syndrome and healthy controls in response to exercise. *Clin. Infect. Dis.* 1994; **18 (suppl 1):** S142–146.

58 Peterson P, Sirr S, Grammith F, *et al.* Effects of mild exercise on cytokines and cerebral blood flow in chronic fatigue syndrome patients. *Clin. Diag. Lab. Immunol.* 1994; **1:** 222–226.

59. Gibson H, Carroll N, Clague JE, Edwards RH. Exercise performance and fatiguability in patients with chronic fatigue syndrome. *J. Neurol. Neurosurg. Psychiatry* 1993; **156:** 993–998.

60 McCully K, Sisto S, Natelson B. Use of exercise for treatment of chronic fatigue syndrome. *Sports Med.* 1996; **21:** 35–48.

61 Friman G. Effect of acute infectious disease on isometric muscle strength. *Scand. J. Lab. Clin. Invest.* 1977; **37:** 303–308.

62 Friman G, Wright JE, Ilback NG, *et al.* Does fever or myalgia indicate reduced physical performance capacity in viral infections? *Acta Med. Scand.* 1985; **217:** 353–361.

63 Rutherford O, White P. Human quadriceps strength and fatigability in patients with postviral fatigue. *J. Neurol. Neurosurg. Psychiatry* 1991; **54:** 961–964.

64 Jamal GA, Hansen S. Electrophysiological studies in the post-viral fatigue syndrome. *J. Neurol. Neurosurg. Psychiatry* 1985; **48:** 691–694.

65 Jamal G, Hansen S. Postviral fatigue syndrome: evidence for underlying organic disturbance in the muscle fibre. *Eur. J. Neurol.* 1989; **29:** 273–276.

66 Prasher P, Smith A, Findley L. Sensory and cognitive event-related potentials in myalgic encephalomyelitis. *J. Neurol. Neurosurg. Psychiatry* 1990; **53:** 247–253.

67 McEvedy C, Beard A. Royal Free epidemic of 1955; a reconsideration. *Br. Med. J.* 1970; **i:** 7–11.

68 Archard L, Bowles N, Behan P, Bell E, Doyle D. Postviral fatigue syndrome; persistence of enterovirus in muscle and elevated creatine kinase. *J. R. Soc. Med.* 1988; **81:** 326–329.

69 Jamal G. Neurophysiological findings in the post-viral fatigue syndrome (myalgic encephalomyelitis). In Jenkins R, Mowbray J (ed.) *Postviral Fatigue Syndrome.* Chichester, Wiley, 1991: 167–178.

70 Roberts L, Byrne E. Single fibre EMG studies in chronic fatigue syndrome: a reappraisal. *J. Neurol. Neurosurg. Psychiatry* 1994; **57:** 375–376.

71 Nix W. Normal neuromuscular transmission and 'central' muscle fatigue in chronic fatigue patients. *International Conference on Chronic Fatigue Syndrome,* 18–20 May 1994, Dublin.

72 Mengshoel A, Vollestad N, Forre O. Pain and fatigue induced by exercise in fibromyalgia patients and sedentary healthy subjects. *Clin. Exp. Rheumatol.* 1995; **13:** 477–482.

73 Norregaard J, Bulow P, Danneskiold-Samsoe B. Muscle strength, voluntary activation, twitch properties, and endurance in patients with fibromyalgia. *J. Neurol. Neurosurg. Psychiatry* 1994; **57:** 1106–1111.

74 Fry A, Martin M. Cognitive idiosyncrasies among children with the chronic fatigue

syndrome: anomalies in self-reported activity levels. *J. Psychosom. Res.* 1996; **41:** 213–223.

75 Stone A, Broderick J, Porter L, *et al.* Fatigue and mood in chronic fatigue syndrome patients: results of a momentary assessment protocol examining fatigue and mood levels and diurnal patterns. *Ann. Behav. Med.* 1994; **16:** 228–234.

76 Vercoulen J, Bazelmans E, Swanink C, *et al.* Physical activity in chronic fatigue syndrome: assessment and its role in fatigue. *J. Psychiat. Res.* 1997; **31,** 661–673.

77 Dock W. The evil sequelae of complete bed rest. *J. Am. Med. Assoc.* 1944; **125:** 1083–1085.

78 Asher R. The dangers of going to bed. *Br. Med. J.* 1947: **iv**: 966–8.

79 Zuber J, Wilgosh L. Prolonged immobilization of the body changes in performance and the electroencephalogram. *Science* 1963; **140:** 306–308.

80 Haines R. Effect of bed rest and exercise on body balance. *J. Appl. Physiol.* 1974; **36:** 323–327.

81 Greenleaf J, Kozlowski S. Physiological consequences of reduced physical activity during bed rest. *Exercise Sport Sci. Rev.* 1982; **10:** 84–119.

82 Lamb L, Stevens P, Johnson R. Hypokinesia secondary to chair rest from 4 to 10 days. *Aerosp. Med.* 1965; **36:** 755–763.

83 Booth F. Physiologic and biochemical effects of immobilization on muscle. *Clin. Orthopaed.* 1987; **10:** 15–20.

84 Klug G, McAuley E, Clark S. Factors influencing the development and maintenance of aerobic fitness: lessons applicable to the fibrositis syndrome. *J. Rheumatol.* 1989; **16(suppl 19):** 30–39.

85 Bennett R, Clark S, Goldberg L, *et al.* Aerobic fitness in patients with fibrositis. A controlled study of respiratory gas exchange and 133 Xenon clearance from exercising muscle. *Arth. Rheumat.* 1989; **32:** 454–460.

86 Hughes J, Crow R, Jacobs D, Mittelmark M, Leon A. Physical activity, smoking and exercise induced fatigue. *J. Behav. Med.* 1984; **7:** 217–230.

87 Jones M, Mellersh V. Comparison of exercise response in anxiety states and normal controls. *Psychosom. Med.* 1946; **8:** 180–187.

88 Jones M, Scarisbrick R. The effect of exercise of soldiers with neurocirculatory asthenia. *Psychosom. Med.* 1946; **8:** 188–192.

89 Hemphill R, Hall K, Crookes T. A preliminary report on fatigue and pain tolerance in depressive and psychoneurotic patients. *J. Ment. Sci.* 1952: 433–440.

90 Morgan W. A pilot investigation of physical working capacity in depressed and non depressed psychiatric males. *Res. Q.* 1969; **40:** 859–861.

91 Saltin B, Blomquist G, Mitchell J, Johnson R, Wildenthal K, Chapman C. Response to exercise after bed rest and training: a longitudinal study of adaptive changes in oxygen transport and body composition. *Circulation* 1968; **38(suppl 7):** 1–55.

92 Bengtsson M, Bengtsson A, Jorfeldt L. Diagnostic epidural opioid blockade in primary fibromyalgia at rest and during exercise. *Pain* 1989; **39:** 171–180.

93 Newham D. The consequences of eccentric contractions and their relationship to delayed onset muscle pain. *Eur. J. Appl. Physiol.* 1988; **57:** 353–359.

94 Editorial. Aching muscles after exercise. *Lancet* 1987, **ii**: 1123–1124.

95 Jones D, Round J. *Skeletal Muscle in Health and Disease. A Textbook in Muscle Physiology.* Manchester University Press, 1990.

96 Mair J, Mayr M, Muller E, *et al.* Rapid adaptation to eccentric exercise-induced muscle damage. *Int. J. Sports Med.* 1995; **16:** 352–356.

97 Jubrias S, Bennett R, Klug G. Increased incidence of a resonance in the phosphodiester region of 31P nuclear magnetic resonance spectra in the skeletal muscle of fibromyalgia patients. *Arth. Rheumat. 1994;* **37:** 801–807.

98 Zidar J, Backmann E, Bengtsson A, Henriksson K. Quantitative EMG and muscle tension in painful muscles in fibromyalgia. *Pain* 1990; **40:** 249–254.

99 Paul O. Da Costa's syndrome or neurocirculatory asthenia. *Br. Heart J.* 1987; **58:** 306–315.

100 Mackenzie J. Soldier's heart. *Br. Med. J.* 1916; **i:** 117–120.

101 Mantysaari MJ, Antila KJ, Peltonene TE. Blood pressure reactivity in patients with neurocirculatory asthenia. *Am. J. Hypertens.* 1988; **1:** 132–139.

102 Bou-Holaigah I, Rowe P, Kan J, Calkins H. The relationship between neurally mediated hypotension and the chronic fatigue syndrome. *J. Am. Med. Assoc.* 1995; **274:** 961–967.

103 Goodnick P. Treatment of chronic fatigue syndrome with venlafaxine. *Am. J. Psychiat.* 1996; **153:** 294.

104 Grubb B, Kosinki D. Preliminary observations on the effects of venlafaxine hydrochloride in the treatment of severe refractory orthostatic hypotension. *J. Serotonin Res.* 1996; **3:** 85–89.

105 Pagani M, Lucini D, Mela G, Langewitz W, Malliani A. Sympathetic overactivity in subjects complaining of unexplained fatigue. *Clin. Sci.* 1994; **87:** 655–661.

106 Sisto S, Tapp W, Drastai S, *et al.* Vagal tone is reduced during paced breathing in patients with the chronic fatigue syndrome. *Clin. Autonom. Res.* 1995; **5:** 139–143.

107 van Denderen J, Boersma J, Zeinstra P, Hollander A, van Neerbos B. Physiological effects of exhaustive physical exercise in primary fibromyalgia syndrome (PFS): Is PFS a disorder of neuroendocrine reactivity? *Scand. J. Rheum.* 1991; **21:** 35–37.

108 Wood G, Bentall R, Gopfert M, Edwards R. A comparative psychiatric assessment of patients with chronic fatigue syndrome and muscle disease. *Psychol. Med.* 1991; **21:** 619–628.

109 Wessely S, Powell R. Fatigue syndromes: a comparison of chronic 'postviral' fatigue with neuromuscular and affective disorder. *J. Neurol. Neurosurg. Psychiatry* 1989; **52:** 940–948.

110 McComas A, Miller R, Gandevia S. Fatigue brought on by malfunction of the central and peripheral nervous systems. In Gandevia S (ed.) *Fatigue.* New York, Plenum Press, 1995: 495–512.

9. Viruses, immunity, and CFS

The neurasthenia story showed how clinicians observed that fatigue syndromes could follow infective episodes, with the chief culprits assumed to be first the influenza virus, and second the typhoid bacillus. With the demise of neurasthenia, these clinical observations did not cease. Each of the general fatigue syndromes (neurasthenia, effort syndrome, chronic exhaustion) have at times been associated with infection, whilst such a link is implicit in the more specific syndromes, such as chronic brucellosis.

The new generation of fatigue studies and fatigue syndromes have also developed from the clinical observation of illnesses following infective episodes. Recent series continue to note that the majority of patients seen in specialist settings trace their illness to an infective episode, 72 per cent in the UK[1], 78 per cent in a Japanese series[2], 86 per cent in Holland[3], rising to 91 per cent in an American report[4]. The similarity of the symptoms of CFS to those of viral infection adds to the plausibility of such observations. In this chapter we will review the evidence for such an association, commencing with a brief consideration of the methodological problems that such attempts must overcome.

9.1 Viruses and CFS: establishing an association

Whilst there is considerable intuitive appeal in assuming a link between CFS and an infective agent, proving such an association is far from easy. Like all aetiological studies, the problems of bias, specificity, and confounding must be considered.

Bias

Most of the studies that we will review in this chapter use the same design, namely retrospective assessment of selected cases of CFS compared with normal controls. Causal links are then suggested between either the report of a precipitating infection or laboratory evidence of the same. However, such recall is subject to considerable bias.

Viral illnesses, like fatigue, are common events in the community. The average adult experiences between three and four such infections a year. Chance associations are thus common. The possibility of chance associations is magnified by what is known as recall bias or search after meaning. Because viral infections are so common, most of us rapidly forget them as soon as they are ended; try remembering the precise dates when you were 'down with a virus' more than one year ago. However, if by chance alone that time coincided with developing the onset of a chronic fatigue syndrome, then it is far more likely that the preceding infection will be recalled. It is interesting to note that although many patients initially state that a particular infective episode triggered their illness, on careful questioning they frequently recall a period of ill health preceding the infection[5,6]. The natural process of recall bias is further amplified by social and cultural factors of 'a virus'. This is the commonest explanation advanced for non-specific symptoms, and has the additional virtue of being neutral in terms of personal responsibility, a theme to which we will return. It is preferable to many of the alternatives, and in particular to the stigma of being labelled psychiatrically disordered – 'the victim of a germ infection is therefore blameless'[7].

Specificity

We will review in turn the evidence for different infective causes of CFS. However, this very diversity is itself a problem. Whilst each individual claim for an infective cause must be assessed on its merits, each must also be seen in the light of many similar claims made for other agents. Taken as a whole, it appears that identical clinical illnesses seem to appear after many infective illnesses, bacterial and even protozoal. A previous generation of doctors considered that neurasthenia was not just a sequela of influenza, but also of typhoid, syphilis, and many other non-viral agents. Such claims might have reflected misdiagnoses in the era before modern laboratory techniques reached their current level of sophistication, but recent authors continue to describe fatigue syndromes identical to CFS arising after many different viral agents[8,9], and also after non-viral infections such as giardia, mycoplasma, toxoplasmosis, Q fever, campylobacter, and borrelia[1,4,8,10,11]. Investigators unfamiliar with CFS have also described conditions with some resemblances to CFS after other infections, including schistosomiasis[12] and even tetanus[13]. With the exception of the claims for a novel enterovirus mentioned below, no one has suggested that on the minority of occasions when any one of these agents trigger a fatigue syndrome, it is a subtly different version of the agent from that encountered normally. Conversely, onset of fatigue after infection is not associated with any specific clinical features[14].

Confounding

Any apparent links between viral infection and chronic fatigue may be complicated by a series of confounders – anything that might also be related to both viral infection and chronic fatigue, and hence might be another explanation for the observed association. Immune status is one such confounder. Immune activation, which, as we shall see, is also associated with chronic fatigue, can lead to what is called an amnestic response, in which titres of antibodies to a wide variety of agents will rise non-specifically. This has been found by some investigators of CFS, with elevations in titres to Epstein – Barr virus, cytomegalovirus, human herpes virus, herpes simplex, and measles[15,16], but not others[14]. This antibody production may indicate either reactivation of latent virus, or alternatively some alteration in the regulation of immunoglobulin production.

Another cause of amnestic responses is stress and psychological disorder. A random sample of psychiatric inpatients were three times more likely to have high antibody titres to coxsackie B 1–5 than controls[17]. Similar increases have been demonstrated for Epstein – Barr virus (EBV) serology by some[18,19], but not others[20]. This brings us to the subject of the relationship between viral infection, immune disorder, stress, and psychiatric disorder, exemplified by the term 'psychoneuroimmunology'. This has many potentially important lessons for our understanding of CFS, which will be addressed later in this chapter. At this stage we will simply draw attention to the importance of these variables as possible confounders of any links between viral agents and CFS.

With these caveats in mind, we will now review the evidence linking specific viral agents and CFS. As the recent history of CFS began in the United States with reports of an association between chronic Epstein–Barr virus (EBV) infection and the illness. We will therefore start our review of the infective associations of CFS with EBV.

9.2 Epstein–Barr virus and CFS

Persistent fatigue after infectious mononucleosis was first described by Isaacs[21]. However, it was not until 1964 that the causative organism, the Epstein–Barr virus, a DNA virus belonging to the herpes family, was isolated, and linked to infectious mononucleosis. It is now known to be associated with a spectrum of both benign and malignant lymphoproliferative diseases.

In most countries EBV infection is universal by the age of three. However, amongst higher socio-economic groups in Western countries EBV infection may not occur until adolescence; for example, in the USA about 50 per cent of those entering college are uninfected[22]. A variety of antibodies are produced at different stages of infection. The initial antibody response to acute EBV infection produces IgM to the viral capsid antigen (VCA). This peaks within three weeks, and is usually undetectable by 12 weeks. It is succeeded by anti-VCA-IgG which persists indefinitely. Antibody to the early antigen (EBV-EA) also increases after infection, gradually declining over time. The final antibody produced is to the EBV nuclear antigen (anti-NA). It usually occurs after two to six months, and also persists for life. The patterns of these antibodies define the state of EBV infection in the normal person. A variety of humoral and cellular changes are also associated with acute infection. T-lymphocytes proliferate, but there is a preferential expansion of CD8 + (suppressor/cytotoxic) T-cells rather than CD4 + (helper) T-cells, hence the result is a reversal of the CD4:CD8 ratio.

After acute infection, the virus remains in a latent state within the host B-cells and salivary glands. Lymphocytes infected with EBV become long lived *in vivo*, and *in vitro* can be propagated indefinitely. Hence they are said to be 'immortalized'. EBV can be recovered from the saliva of many normal people. This figure rises if the host becomes immunocompromised. The virus can be recovered from 40 per cent of transplant and 100 per cent of AIDS patients[23].

There is one group of patients in whom there is no doubt that illness is related to chronic EBV infection. These are children with X-linked lymphoproliferative disorder (Duncan's syndrome). Children affected with this fortunately rare disorder have clear evidence of end organ dysfunction, such as pneumonitis, pancytoenia, and hepatitis. There is a high incidence of lymphoma, and mortality is high. EBV serology is grossly abnormal, with massive elevations of antibody production and viral replication[24]. Fatigue is a feature of the illness, but clinically it is easily distinguishable from those illnesses that are the subject of this book. It will not concern us further.

9.3 Chronic mononucleosis

The recent revival of interest in CFS followed a series of reports from Israel and USA of patients with fatigue, weakness, fevers, myalgias, and depression[25–28] (see Chapter 6). Clinically they were described as 'chronic neurasthenia'. However, researchers reported the presence of high titres to various EBV antigens, at that time assumed to be only found in acute EBV, including the restricted component of the EBV early antigen (anti-EA) and the viral capsid antigen (anti-VCA). The term 'chronic EBV' was also introduced, although the authors themselves were cautious in linking EBV to the disorder. They need not have bothered, since the consequence was a flood of new cases being referred to physicians[23].

Within two or three years doubts began to be cast on the relevance of the serological findings of exposure to EBV. It was already known most of the adult population has been exposed to the virus. It now became clear that some of the serological measures thought to indicate active infection in fact reflected previous exposure or were non-specific.

First, Horwitz and colleagues showed that asymptomatic individuals followed for up to eight years after recovery from EBV infection maintained EBV-EA antibodies well into the range previously thought to indicate chronic EBV[29]. Seroepidemiological studies have now established that the presence of antibodies to early antigen, and the absence of EBNA, is found in normal individuals[30,31]. Hellinger and colleagues at the Mayo Clinic, found that elevated antibodies to early antigen (anti-EBV-EA) did not distinguish between subgroups of CFS[32]. Furthermore, in asymptomatic blood donors 18 per cent had anti-EBV-EA, with substantial titres detected in 3 per cent. Although anti-EBV-EA was shown to be elevated in samples of CFS patients, it did not identify any particular subgroup, and it was neither sensitive nor specific[31].

Second, the new diagnosis was too common. Dedra Buchwald and colleagues, in the first of a series of important investigations reported a study of 'chronic mononucleosis' in primary care in Boston[33]. They found that 21 per cent of attenders fulfilled their criteria, with a median duration of illness of 16 months. This high prevalence surprised many investigators, although it was in keeping with the epidemiological studies reported in Chapter 3. Mean titres of IgM and IgG antibodies to VCA, early antigens, and EBNA did not differ between patients and controls.

Third, laboratory procedures were insufficiently rigorous. Merlin noted that laboratories were already advertising EBV serological tests for the diagnosis of 'chronic EBV'[22] It was suspected that these might be less than reliable, confirmed by a study from the CDC, showing up to fourfold differences both within and between laboratories[15]. Laboratory errors have been blamed for other 'pseudo-outbreaks' of infectious mononucleosis[34].

Fourth, antiviral agents such as aciclovir, which prevents EBV replication, are ineffective[35].

Finally, there was no correlation between symptoms and laboratory findings, nor any evidence of increased viral activity[36,37]. High antibody levels do not indicate either increased viral replication or diminished immune surveillance to EBV, arguing against both primary infection and reactivation[37]. The findings were not specific for EBV – Gary Holmes and colleagues from the CDC[15], in a case-control study of individuals from the Lake Tahoe epidemic (see below), found elevated antibodies not just to EBV, but also to cytomegalovirus, herpes simplex, and measles, although this has not been confirmed by others[38]. Buchwald *et al.* pointed out the importance of selection factors in the original reports, many patients being were referred on the basis of abnormal serological responses to EBV[33].

By 1989 Schooley, from Harvard Medical School, summed up the prevailing opinion: 'it is becoming increasingly unlikely that Epstein–Barr virus has an etiologic role in the pathogenesis of chronic fatigue'[39]. Similar sentiments were echoed by Straus[40] and Swartz[41].

Very recently there have been signs of yet another reappraisal of the role of EBV in CFS. The pendulum in the USA swung from enthusiastic espousal of the role of EBV to an almost total denial of any role. However, a few recent studies have begun to rehabilitate the virus, albeit in a more circumspect manner than before. We will consider the work of Peter White in London in the next section. However, James Jones in Denver has also begun to produce new evidence from molecular virology, with the intention of shifting from searching for evidence of the host response to virus, to the virus itself. Jones and his colleagues[42] looked at the different responses of B-lymphocytes to experimental manipulation. They used a variety of different healthy controls, based on their record of previous glundular fever and serological evidence of exposure to EBV. They were able to induce B-cell transformation, indicating active infection, in about 30 per cent of cases showing the early antigen, compared to between 5 and 10 per cent of the controls. However, looking at the characteristics of the viruses involved, they were unable to find substantial differences in the strains of virus between cases and controls, which implies that any deficit may be host, rather than virus, related. Jones does not claim to have proven that EBV is a causative agent in CFS, but instead has suggested that in a subset of CFS patients the host immunological surveillance system that suppresses circulating EBV-transformed cells may be diminished, permitting reactivation. When these results are taken with those of White discussed in the next section, it is clear that there is still life in some part of the EBV hypothesis.

9.4 Cohort studies of Epstein–Barr virus

In a prospective cohort, exposure is determined contemporaneously, and outcome assessed later. This is in contrast to cross-sectional or case–control studies in which the patient presents with the disease, and the researcher then looks backwards for evidence as to the causative agent. In principle, cohort studies offer several advantages; they can establish direction of causality and avoid recall and selection bias. This comes at a price – they are usually far more expensive than either cross-sectional or case – control studies.

In a brief communication Chang and Bittner reported their experience in a student health centre[43]. Of 337 students with proven glandular fever, only 1.5 per cent had chronic fatigue persisting beyond two months, or necessitating withdrawal from university. No relationship was found between poor outcome and either the severity of the initial infection (as judged by needing hospitalization) or to previous depression.

The most important study of EBV to date, which challenged both the above observations, was performed at St Bartholomew's Hospital by a team lead by Peter White. The sample consisted of all those seen by local general practitioners with possible glandular fever. Controls were those referred for testing, but negative for EBV, and a second series recruited by general practitioners with other viral illnesses not resembling glandular fever, such as upper respiratory tract infections. The subjects underwent extensive psychological and laboratory testing, and were then followed up at two and six months.

White showed that a fatigue syndrome did exist after glandular fever, and was both more common than, and distinct from, depression[44-46]. It was also commonest in those with glandular fever, followed by those with illnesses that were clinically similar, but actually consisted largely of adenovirus and influenza B (Table 9.1), confirming an earlier observation made in another student health centre[47]. The median duration of ill health was ten weeks in the post-glandular fever group, contrasted with four weeks in the other two.

Table 9.1 Prevalence of fatigue syndrome after viral infection (reproduced with permission from White[46])

	Onset	2 months	6 months
Glandular fever	58%	41%	10%
Glandular fever-like illnesses	44%	18%	4%
Upper respiratory tract infections	24%	4%	0%

A principal components analysis of the symptomatic data obtained using standardized interviews suggested that the fatigue syndrome consisted of the symptoms of fatigue, retardation, hypersomnia, and poor concentration, similar to the ICD-10 definition of neurasthenia. White was then able to compare those with and without a fatigue syndrome. A number of physical variables, such as the presence of cervical lymphadenopathy or pharyngitis on presentation and the absence of EB-VCA IgM, predicted fatigue two months later. However, by six months no physical variable was associated with fatigue, but those with a persisting fatigue syndrome were significantly less physically fit when tested at two months post-illness. Psychological variables, assessed retrospectively, were only weakly associated with persistent fatigue syndrome. However, very strong associations were noted between premorbid variables, such as past psychiatric history, introspection, and concurrent life events, and the development of post-EBV depression[48].

This is an important study. The results suggest that fatigue syndrome after EBV is a discrete entity, distinct from depression. Onset of post-infectious fatigue is related to a number of physical variables, including the severity of the illness, the nature of the infecting agent, and the immunological response. However, persistence at six months, when CFS is conventionally held to begin, is associated with decreased physical fitness. Finally, persistence of post-glandular fever depression might be associated with psychological risk factors.

9.5 Enteroviruses and CFS

In the United Kingdom events took a different course, and much of the attention devoted in the United States to EBV has been devoted to the enterovirus family.

What are the enteroviruses? They are RNA viruses and members of the family of picornaviridae, and include the coxsackie, echo, and polio viruses. About 70 have been identified. Clinically they usually cause innocuous infections – the ratio of non-serious to serious infections is about a thousand to one. In adults they can cause symptomatic infections such as Bornholm's disease and aseptic meningitis, illustrating their myotropic and neurotropic properties. These are usually also short-lived. Thus, following the elimination of polio from the developed world, the enteroviruses were no longer considered to cause serious infections in healthy adults.

How did enteroviruses become linked with fatigue, and CFS in particular? For an answer we make no apologies for returning to our historical theme and the origins of 'ME', since it was speculation concerning the involvement of polio in epidemics of 'myalgic encephalomyelitis' that began the pursuit of an enteroviral aetiology to CFS. The illness that affected the Los Angeles hospital in 1934 was called 'atypical poliomyelitis'. No organisms were identified in the 'mystery disease' at Akureyi, Iceland in 1948, which gave yet another synonym for CFS, 'Akureyi disease'. Astute observers noted that children in the areas affected by the epidemic later responded to poliomyelitis vaccination with higher levels of antibody than those in regions not affected[49]. The suggestion was that the children exposed to the Akureyi agent had developed some form of cross-immunity. Polio was also linked with the unusual epidemics in London hospitals seen in the 1950s.

All this now seems remote, and is of marginal concern to the topic of CFS. However, it was not marginal to a small group of observers, who had been interested in ME ever since the Royal Free epidemic of 1955, and continued to pursue possible links with enteroviruses. It must be pointed out that to do so required dedication, since the vast body of professional opinion was either ignorant, or sceptical of, this subject. It would have looked an unlikely area for those interested in obtaining research funding, or academic prestige.

After the end of the Royal Free epidemic the link between CFS (still known as ME) and enteroviruses was pursued by a small group of researchers. Much of the subsequent activity took place in Scotland. Between 1980 and 1981 doctors in a small practice in the west of Scotland reported 22 cases of a new illness, characterized by vague multisystem symptoms, accompanied by psychological symptoms such as anxiety and depression[50]. The authors themselves used the term 'protean' to describe the illness, and it is not clear who made the connection between this and ME, nor who decided to begin serological surveillance for the cocksackievirus. However, 82 per cent of the cases showed an association with coxsackie B exposure, judged by the high static titres of IgG antibody. Other studies of high static coxsackie B antibodies in patients with unusual symptoms started to appear[51,52].

These studies are not convincing. The issue of case definition was unresolved, as shown by a later study, also from the west of Scotland. This was a prospective study of the 'post-viral syndrome', which they attributed to the coxsackievirus, on the basis of serological exposure in 46 per cent of cases versus 35 per cent of controls[53]. However, the report stated that 28 per cent consulted less than 24 hours after the onset of symptoms, and in total 65 per cent had presented within a month, calling into question the definition of chronicity. None of the controls who were antibody positive had fatigue. At one year follow-up titres remained elevated in most of the cases, including all those who had improved. The results could be interpreted as showing that high static titres of antibody were of little significance. Similar methodology was used in a study of 50 sporadic cases seen in a specialist unit, in which elevated neutralizing antibodies were detected in 50 per cent of cases, compared with 17 per cent of normal controls[54].

Even at the time, it was acknowledged that interpretation of coxsackie B neutralizing antibody titres was problematic[54]. Thus the introduction of an IgM test, a better indication of recent infection, promised improved results. Using the new assay routine testing of cases of ME continued to show an association with exposure[17]. However, these results were challenged by a carefully planned case–control study[55]. Between 1985 and 1986 general practitioners in the Vale of Leven in Scotland were asked to refer for virological testing all suspected cases of post-viral fatigue and matched controls: 254 cases of post-viral fatigue of recent onset were referred for investigation. Age and sex matched controls were obtained from the same general practitioner at the same time. Analysis was blind. 24.4 per cent of cases and 22.6 per cent of controls were positive for coxsackie B IgM, and 56.2 per cent of cases positive for IgG, compared with 55.3 per cent of controls. In a further study no IgM antibody to coxsackie B4 was found in the cases[56]. Several further studies also failed to find any differences in enterovirus-specific IgM between cases and controls[14,57,58]. Another investigation of CFS patients found no evidence of intrathecally produced IgG antibodies in the cerebrospinal fluid[59].

The conclusion is that, in contrast to earlier claims, enterovirus serology, whether by the old IgG method, or the newer IgM ELISA test, has little role to play in the diagnosis of CFS[14,55]. The results of conventional serological testing offers no support for a role for enteroviruses in CFS, although it does not disprove it either. Instead, the results suggest considerable spatial and temporal changes in enteroviral serology.

A second line of enquiry implicating the enterovirus family was started by researchers at St Mary's Hospital, London[60]. Enteroviral infection was demonstrated by positive stool cultures in 22 per cent of patients referred with post-viral fatigue syndrome (PVFS), and again in 7 per cent one year later. In a second sample a group-specific enteroviral antigen (the VP-1 antigen) was found in 51 per cent, persisting in 45 per cent at four months. None was found in controls selected by the patients themselves. The study had a number of methodological problems. The definition of abnormal could be questioned – positivity was defined as more than 3 standard deviations above the same 36 controls. Not all patients chose controls. The case definition was inadequate; the authors state that 7 per cent had pericarditis, not normally part of the CFS spectrum (see above). The design was an example of ascertainment bias, with cases biased towards viral exposure, and controls the opposite. The study provided some evidence that 7 per cent of a selected sample of PVFS patients had persistent enteroviral infection, but its wider claims were questionable.

The initial optimism that greeted the introduction of the new test has not been justified. Halpin and Wessely sent blinded samples from CFS patient and neurological controls to the same laboratory[61]. The claim that controls were always negative could not be sustained, whilst the new test had low sensitivity and specificity[61]. Lynch and his colleagues at St Mary's cast further doubt on the relevance of VP-1 antigenaemia with similar levels being found in cases of CFS and controls with major depression[62,63]. Another study showed an overlap between the VP-1 antigen and a positive monospot associated with clinical glandular fever, again casting doubt on its specificity[64]. Mawle and colleagues from the Center for Disease Control were unable to replicate the presence of enteroviruses in stool specimens[58], as were Swanink and colleagues from the Netherlands[65]. The Dutch group also sent blinded samples to the St Mary's laboratory, and were unable to replicate the VP-1 findings[65]. No evidence could be produced in a number of studies of any clinical differences between those with, and those without, the antigen[61,64]. Despite all this, the test enjoyed enormous popularity, and played a key role in the acceptance of CFS in the United Kingdom (see Chapter 15). The test was withdrawn in 1991.

Just as the old tests became obsolete, the molecular revolution began to transform the identification of viruses in the laboratory, and it became possible to identify segments of viral genome in a variety of tissues. The first study of CFS to utilize the new technologies came from Len Archard and colleagues at Charing Cross[66]. Ninety-six subjects selected by the Glasgow team led by Peter Behan, later extended to 140, had muscle biopsies taken for molecular analysis. An enterovirus-specific probe was used, coding for the first two-thirds of the RNA-dependent RNA polymerase gene, which is highly conserved between various enteroviral serotypes. The resulting probe is thus enterovirus group-specific[67].

The St Mary's team were able to demonstrate enterovirus RNA about one-quarter of muscle biopsies taken from selected cases of PVFS[66]. When the group last reported in 1991 a total of 152 control samples have been analysed, from a variety of sources, and none were positive[67]. Work from the Glasgow group using the polymerase chain reaction confirmed the persistence of the enteroviral genome, finding it in 53 per cent of cases, but also found it in 16 per cent of controls[57].

Now this too looks doubtful. The Liverpool group were unable to detect any evidence of enteroviral infection in muscle biopsies from similar patients[68]. The Glasgow group were unable to replicate their own findings, finding similar amounts of enteroviral sequences in both cases and controls, and concluded that CFS was not 'dependent on persistent viral infection of muscle'[69]. No evidence was found of any enteroviral RNA in muscle biopsies from CFS patients in Sweden[59]. More specific difficulties relate to the extremely sensitive nature of the tests employed, which have been challenged on technical grounds[70,71]. Despite the tempting analogy between PVFS and inflammatory myopathy, the same techniques have failed to show any evidence of viral persistence, whether enteroviral or others, in the muscles of patients with true inflammatory myopathies, such as polymyositis or dermatomyositis[70,72]. At present the balance of evidence suggests that 'persistence of enteroviruses is unlikely to play a role in the development of CFS'[65] or that ' "enteroviral persistence" should not be used in connection with CFS'[73].

One of the problems in accepting a role for enterovirus in CFS is that the virus is so common, and usually mild or even innocuous. How can such a common, and frequently non-pathogenic virus give rise to such a severe illness in fit, healthy people? A further study from Charing Cross suggested one possible answer. Cunningham *et al.*[74] showed that in four out of eight cases of CFS, equal amounts of positive and negative (sometimes also called sense and anti-sense) enteroviral RNA were present, an abnormal finding (in normal infections the ratio should be 100:1). The authors propose this indicates that in CFS the persisting organism is a virus mutant that is defective in the control of viral genomic RNA replication. This possibility had also been considered for EBV, but in contrast Jones had failed to demonstrate any differences between the strains of EBV implicated in viral persistence[42]. The enterovirus findings were also not replicated in a larger sample[73]. Nevertheless, something similar was claimed by Geoff Clements and colleagues, also from Glasgow. They performed a blinded study that detected enteroviral-specific sequences in the serum of substantially more CFS patients than both healthy controls and those with acute viral infections[75]. They reported that such sequences indicated the presence of distinct novel enteroviruses[76]. However, another study using PCR has failed to find any evidence of enteroviral RNA in the sera or other specimens from either patients or controls[77].

A word of caution is necessary at this point. There is a tendency for those who, like the current authors, are not at home with the recent advances made in molecular biology, to be dazzled by the sophistication and ingenuity of studies using molecular techniques. However, despite the impressive medical technology, what is being performed is a case–control study, and can thus be looked at in exactly the same way as any other study reporting differences in exposure to a possible aetiological agent between cases and controls. The problems of selection and ascertainment bias outlined in Chapter 2 remain.

The second link with polio comes from the post-polio syndrome. During acute paralytic poliomyelitis the virus destroys the anterior horn cells of the spinal cord. A variety of adaptive mechanisms may follow, allowing at least some recovery. Fibre transformation takes place, from Type II to Type I, both sets of fibres show hypertrophy, and there is evidence of dendritic terminal sprouting. Nevertheless, some patients develop new symptoms many years after the original episode. Chief amongst these symptoms are fatigue, weakness, and muscle pain, manifest as new difficulties in walking or climbing stairs[78,79]. Various explanations have been proposed, many of which are directly relevant to the topic of CFS. It has been suggested that the virus persists, that further immune damage occurs, or that the increased demands upon the remaining motor units causes premature ageing[80]. The most likely pathophysiology is of ongoing motor neurone dysfunction which continues after the acute episode, but only becomes clinically apparent when the process of re-innervation can no longer compensate for the loss of motor neurones[81]. In a small number of cases it is possible that persistence of the enterovirus, perhaps in a mutated form, is responsible[82].

Post-polio syndrome is thus an example of a fatigue syndrome that is clearly post-viral, and may be due, in some cases, to viral persistence. However, there are important differences between CFS and post-polio syndrome. First, the symptoms of CFS are physical and mental fatigue and fatigability, rather than neuromuscular weakness. Second, although assiduously sought, there is no compelling evidence that enteroviruses trigger CFS, nor persist in an abnormal fashion. Third, unlike post-polio[83], there is no evidence of abnormal electrophysiological fatigability.

9.6 Cohort studies of the outcome of enterovirus infection

The longitudinal study of outcome of EBV infection has shown that, at least in the short term, EBV is a significant and specific risk factor for fatigue syndrome[44,45]. What is the situation regarding enteroviruses?

Scandinavian researchers followed up for between 2 and 12 years 238 patients diagnosed as having primary aseptic meningitis, many of which will have been due to enteroviruses[84]. Infection did not contribute to the risk of either mental illness or behavioural disturbance. As they were familiar with neurasthenia, and also gave rates of fatigability, it is likely they would not have overlooked cases fulfilling current CFS criteria. Lepow *et al.* followed up 306 cases of aseptic meningitis. At three months fatigue, poor concentration, and muscle tightness or weakness persisted in 32 per cent, but this had fallen to 3 per cent by two years[85]. This latter figure is well below what might have expected by chance alone, and suggests that follow-up was incomplete. However, neither study gives support to an increased risk of CFS-like syndromes after enteroviral infection, even associated with meningitis. Follow-up of patients, usually children, admitted to an infectious diseases unit with virus meningitis also confirmed that although symptoms persisted after discharge for a few weeks, none developed long-term morbidity[86]. Severe morbidity appears restricted to neonates and the immunologically compromised[87].

The only study to have looked specifically at post-viral fatigue after meningitis was a retrospective cohort study following 83 adults with presumed viral meningitis and comparing their outcome with 78 subjects who had suffered non-CNS non-enteroviral infection[88]. The results suggested a considerably higher prevalence of chronic fatigue and chronic fatigue syndrome than those reported in primary care settings, and following common viral infections[89]. There was no difference, though, in the rate of fatigue in the two groups, suggesting that viral meningitis was not a specific risk factor. Furthermore, CFS was predicted by previous psychiatric disorder and prolonged convalescence following the index illness.

9.7 Other viruses and CFS

The human herpes virus 6 (HHV-6), also known as human B-cell lymphotrophic virus, first isolated in lymphoproliferative diseases, has similarities with EBV, although unlike EBV it lyses, but does not transform, B-cells. It has been described as a virus in search of a disease, as the only condition which it has been linked to date is exanthema subitum, a common childhood illness. Attempts have been made to link it with CFS. Several groups have reported increased titres of HHV-6 antibodies[16,90–92] and evidence of active HHV-6 replication[93]. HHV-6 DNA has been detected in the lymphocytes of CFS patients[94]. When peripheral blood mononuclear cells from seven CFS patients were cultured *in vitro*, in three of the cases the cultures were strongly positive for HHV-6[95].

The main problem with interpreting such findings is that most people seroconvert to HHV-6 early in childhood, so antibodies to HHV-6 are almost universal. The prevalence of HHV-6 latency and reactivation in the population is not well established, making it difficult to be certain of the significance of this finding[96]. One group have linked HHV-6 with observed changes in the immune system (see below) – suggesting that HHV-6 is responsible for deleting a small subset of CD4+ cells that are primed to respond to soluble antigen[92]. Another possible link is that HHV-6 has the ability to infect and replicate in natural killer cells. More recently an Italian group was able to demonstrate both HHV-6 and HHV-7 in peripheral lymphocytes taken from CFS patients[97]. Normal controls gave similar results for both HHV-7 and the B variant of HHV-6, with differences only for the A variant. The significance of this observation remains to be determined.

The differences found in CFS patients reflect mean antibody titre, and, like other findings of increased antibodies to a variety of agents, may reflect non-specific polyclonal activation of antibody-producing plasma cells rather than recent infection[98]. The existence of group differences in HHV-6 serology is also disputed, since most studies have failed to find evidence implicating HHV-6[36,58,99–101]. The most convincing data against an important role for HHV-6 come from a recent study using a new polymerase chain reaction (PCR) marker for the detection of HHV-6 DNA in serum. Investigators were able to show a close association between HHV-6 and exanthema subitum (86 per cent), whilst none was detected in healthy adults. Only 1 out of 39 (2.6 per cent) patients with CFS tested positive[102]. Recent reviews suggest that either HHV-6 may be another infectious agent with the ability to trigger CFS[103], or that HHV-6 reactivation contributes to CFS symptoms[94] but in the absence of longitudinal data we remain unconvinced. It remains possible that HHV-6 reactivation occurs as a secondary phenomenon, and may thus contribute to symptoms.

Hepatitis, like glandular fever, is another condition for which a previous generation of physicians recognized that prolonged convalescence was a frequent outcome. At the end of the Second World War Benjamin and Hoyt reported on 200 soldiers with prolonged fatigue after hepatitis developing following immunization against yellow fever (post-vaccinal hepatitis). The principal symptoms, of extreme weakness, overpowering fatigue, multiple somatic symptoms, pain, and nervous irritability, made worse by activity, are more than reminiscent of CFS. Nearly all were considered to be 'psychoneurotic', although it was only in a minority that evidence existed of premorbid psychiatric disorder[104]. Since then fatigue after hepatitis has been surprisingly little studied. Some recent suggestions that CFS might be associated either with hepatitis C, or with hepatitis B vaccination, seem to have little foundation[105,106]. A follow-up study showed that patients admitted to an infective disease unit with either hepatitis A or B had more prolonged and severe post-infective fatigue than a series of controls with other infective episodes also requiring admission, such as meningitis or severe gastroenteritis[107]. Hence there is some suggestion that both hepatitis A and B should be added to the list of infective agents, like EBV, toxoplasmosis, Q fever[108], and CMV, with the capacity to cause slow recovery and prolonged fatigue. Less convincing evidence has been presented for many other viruses – for example, one well publicized case of CFS occurred in an English general practitioner who failed to recover from varicella[109]. In the community survey of Essen-Moller a case is described of life-long neurasthenia arising after an attack of zoster in adolescence[110].

Perhaps the single most publicized research in CFS, extensively reported by every major US newspaper, was a study from the prestigious Wistar Institute in Philadelphia implicating a novel human retrovirus, related to the human T-cell lymphotrophic virus (HTLV-II), in CFS[111]. Retroviruses, of which the most infamous are the human immunodeficiency virus (HIV) and the oncogenic human T-cell leukaemia virus (HTLV-1), use a reverse transcriptase to convert their own RNA into the corresponding DNA which is then integrated into the host cell. De Freitas reported that she found DNA sequences that were similar to those of HTLV-II in the majority of both adults and children studied. Antibodies to the virus were found in six out of twelve patients, and, surprisingly, three out of thirteen controls who had been exposed to the cases. These results caused a sensation[112]. However, there were also criticisms.

Although suggestive, these results did not prove a retroviral involvement. Insufficient clinical details were given. Most important has been the failure of several other groups to replicate the findings[58,113–116]. No differences in evidence of retroviral presence were found between several samples, including some patients who had taken part in the original studies, when tested under blind conditions[117]. None of the assays tested, and none of the laboratories, could differentiate between cases and controls.

The retrovirus story is thus a cautionary tale whenever one hears dramatic claims that any new infective agent is the 'cause' of CFS. The explanatory models that we espouse in this book indicate our considerable doubts that any so-called 'smoking gun' will be identified as the cause of the majority of cases of CFS.

9.8 Psychological vulnerability to infection and post-infectious fatigue

It is commonly believed that psychological stress increases vulnerability to viral infections, never better expressed than by Frank Loesser when he wrote 'Adelaide's lament' in 'Guys and Dolls'. However, the evidence for this observation has been, until recently, surprisingly scanty.

One of the earliest inquiries into the links between psychological disorder and a consequent vulnerability to both infection and a prolonged recovery from infection was the now classic study of John Imboden and colleagues. Prior to the 1957 Asian influenza epidemic they screened 600 Maryland civil servants using a psychological and personality inventory (the MMPI) and other clinical investigations and interviews[118]. The civil servants then became exposed to the epidemic, and 26 became infected. Those previously identified during the screening process as psychologically vulnerable were no more likely to become infected, but, having developed influenza, were ill for a longer period of time. The commonest symptom in the vulnerable group was tiredness and weakness. However, the period of follow-up was short, a few days.

The same group later replicated these findings in prospective studies of the effects of immunization[119] and an extraordinary study in which volunteers were given tularaemia[120]. In the previously described Scandinavian cohort study of aseptic meningitis[84], although no overall increase in fatigability was observed, the rate of post-exposure fatigue was twice as high in those rated premorbidly as anxious or depressed, a finding replicated by Hotopf and colleagues[88].

An association between psychological morbidity and recovery has been shown in non-epidemic infections as well. A 1947 study found a correlation between measures of psychological distress and length of stay in an army hospital after acute respiratory infections[121]. In a study using more modern methodology, depression was an independent variable predicting recovery from upper respiratory tract infection[122], but although the association was significant, the magnitude of the effect was small. The association was stronger for systemic (fever, headache, fatigue, nausea, etc.) than local symptoms (sore throat, cough, sneezing, etc.).

The herpes family has attracted much attention in this context. Many studies have addressed the question whether or not psychological stress predicts recurrence of herpes simplex virus (HSV) or the varicella zoster virus, which causes shingles and herpes zoster. A meta-analysis concluded that depressive symptoms were associated with a slightly increased risk of HSV recurrence[123]. Similarly, an elegant study of the aetiology of chronic pain, rather than chronic fatigue, after varicella zoster infection (shingles) showed that patients with higher anxiety and/or depression when first infected were more likely to develop chronic pain subsequently[124].

Overall, it has proved difficult to demonstrate that psychological morbidity predisposes to increased rates of infection, or even increased recall of infection. Married women report more colds and influenza[125], in keeping with the evidence that psychological morbidity is higher in married rather than single women. However, when one of us (SW) analysed data from the Health and Lifestyle Survey[126], no association was seen between psychological morbidity and the self-recall of colds/influenza. In Imboden's classic study (see above) those identified as psychologically vulnerable were no more likely to develop infections than the rest[118].

It is only in experimental situations that links between psychological vulnerability and susceptibility to infection have been demonstrated. The most convincing evidence came from the MRC Common Cold Unit before its untimely demise: 420 subjects first completed a variety of assessments concerning psychological factors, such as social support, life events, and current stress[127]. They were then inoculated with the common cold virus, and measures made of the rates of infection, determined both serologically and clinically. The results showed that there was a dose–response curve between the degree of psychological stress and the probability of developing an infection. This effect was visible for all five cold viruses tested. However, they were unable to replicate the previous report from the same unit of a link with introversion[128]. They were also unable to determine why stress should increase the risk of infection – it was not due to any measured immune parameters such as natural killer (NK) cell activity.

Cohen and colleagues provided the soundest evidence that psychological variables are associated with vulnerability to infection, and not just symptom reporting or illness behaviour. Cohen himself subsequently moved to Pittsburgh, where he recently was able to show that this vulnerability is related to social support – the greater the social support, the less the risk of infection. The results differed from Imboden's more naturalistic study in which psychological variables were only associated with symptom reporting and duration of illness[118]. Whether or not this represents a real difference between the response to influenza and the common cold, or is a reflection of methodological differences, is impossible to tell.

Specific studies of the relationship between psychological vulnerability and CFS were not carried out until very recently, partly because interest waned with the decline of both neurasthenia and other classic psychosomatic theories. The other more prosaic reason was that such studies are extremely expensive, and were not fundable until the current upsurge of interest in CFS.

Two such large-scale studies were recently reported. We have already drawn attention to the primary care cohort study of the outcome of over 1000 consultations for symptomatic viral infections[89]. The plan of that study (Fig. 9.1) shows that before the subjects were recruited, a large-scale postal screening exercise had been undertaken to record the experience of both fatigue and psychological distress. This survey, which has been referenced as part of the discussion of community studies of fatigue[129] (see Chapter 2), also provided measures of psychological vulnerability prior to exposure to infection, exactly the same design as that of Imboden and colleagues in their classic study. On this occasion, however, follow-up was six months later, and outcome variables included both chronic fatigue and CFS.

Those who rated themselves as significantly fatigued and/or psychologically distressed prior to presenting to the doctor with a viral infection were substantially more likely to go on to develop either chronic fatigue or chronic fatigue syndrome. Even in the fully adjusted analysis (Table 9.2) previous fatigue and previous psychological disorder both independently predicted chronic fatigue. The same study showed that getting a viral infection itself did not predict chronic fatigue. An association between psychological distress and subsequent 'post-viral' symptoms was demonstrated for general symptoms (headache, malaise, fatigue, and so on), but not for local symptoms (cough, sore throat, runny nose, and others), as shown 50 years previously[121]. Cope and colleagues also showed that fatigue had been a problem prior to developing a viral infection for most of those who were later classified as having 'post-viral' fatigue[6].

Table 9.2 Predictors of chronic fatigue after common viral injections in primary care

Variable	Odds ratio (95% confidence limits)	Probability
Prior fatigue	3.0 (1.9–4.7)	<.001
Prior GHQ case (stage 1)	1.8 (1.2–2.9)	.009
GHQ case (stage 2)	1.8 (1.1–2.8)	.01

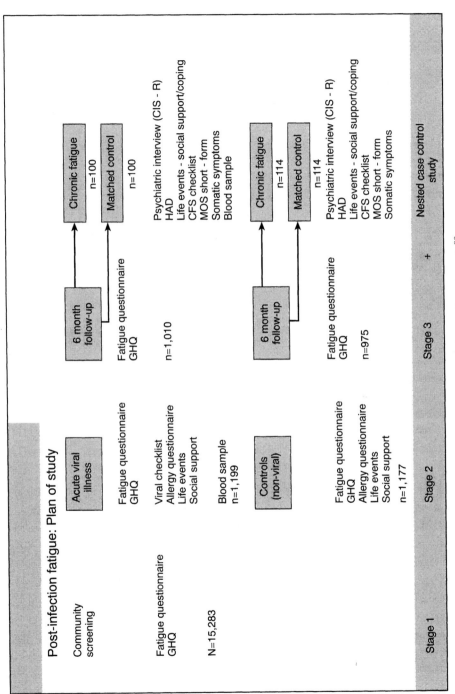

Fig. 9.1 Post-infection fatigue: plan of study[89].

9.9 Infection and psychological disorders

The preceding section has considered how psychological variables may affect vulnerability to infection and post-infectious fatigue (see also Section 9.18). We now turn to the converse possibility, that infection may predispose to psychological disorder.

We have seen how nearly all the medical authorities considered that infection was one cause of neurasthenia, with special emphasis on influenza and typhoid (Chapter 6). Whether or not these particular agents were specifically associated with neurasthenia cannot be determined, and the emphasis on these two at the expense of other agents may simply have reflected both their novelty, and contemporary concerns about their morbidity. However, the association between infective episodes and subsequent neurasthenia was rarely challenged.

The concept that infection could cause neurasthenia survived the demise of the latter illness, and continued to surface in the occasional paper on chronic exhaustion[130], or in papers with titles such as 'Tired, weak and toxic'. In Essen-Moller's famous Swedish epidemiological studies, a substantial proportion of 'acquired asthenia' was attributed to infection and encephalitis, as was adult neurosis[110]. Essen-Moller wrote that about half of the community cases of neurosis followed physical illness, of which infections were the major contributors. Psychiatric illness, mainly depression or anxiety, arising after glandular fever is a well known clinical phenomenon, particularly in women[131], whilst the combination of life stress and glandular fever is strongly associated with subsequent depression[48]. Patients admitted to hospital with 'non-specific viral infections' were between two and seven times more likely to receive psychiatric care in the year after the index admission – this increase gradually declining over the subsequent three years[132].

Can this relationship be further defined? It seems probable that infection involving the central nervous system has a greater propensity to cause fatigue. In Von Economo's classic studies of the outcome of encephalitis lethargica most attention has been paid to his descriptions of parkinsonian syndromes[133]. However, he also described neurasthenic states similar to CFS. Seven out of fourteen survivors of encephalitis surveyed by Essen-Moller in his population study were neurasthenic[110]. There are very few controlled studies of the outcome of adult encephalitis. However, a fourfold increase in the rate of abnormal fatigability was observed in the survivors of St Louis encephalitis[134], an arbovirus associated with substantial mortality. That the effect is specific to encephalitis is suggested by the failure of two studies of the outcome of aseptic meningitis to show increased rates of abnormal fatigability[84,85].

Why encephalitis should be a cause of CFS is speculative. Lishman[135] describes two methods by which viruses can cause organic brain syndromes – one is direct action of the virus within the CNS, the other is secondary to an autoimmune or hypersensitivity reaction to the virus either within or outside the CNS.

There is one further model of how viruses may alter central nervous system function that may have relevance to both psychiatric disorder and CFS. When viruses infect a host, they induce immune responses which in turn remove them, and destroy infected cells. Even if these are unsuccessful, and the virus manages to evade the host response, the immune system still responds in such a fashion which indicates the presence of the virus.

Recent evidence has suggested that viruses may evade the immune system and the host response in ways that either avoid a conventional response, or alter it in subtly. In particular, Oldstone has argued that viral infection can take place in the absence of specific signs of inflammation, in which the virus allows the basic function of the cell to continue, but alters its specialist ('luxury') function[136]. Viruses can escape the normal immunological surveillance, and then replicate in specialist cells without causing cell lysis[137]. Oldstone and his co-workers have managed to demonstrate this in animal models, for example by showing how infection by the lymphocytic choriomeningitis virus (LCMV) interferes with pituitary function in selected mouse strains. Even though pituitary function is substantially altered, the cells remain intact[138]. The mechanism appears to be that the virus does not directly destroy the relevant messenger RNA (mRNA), but instead appears to prevent transcription of the relevant pituitary hormone[139]. However, these experiments were performed in mice, not humans. In man evidence has been presented of persistent viral infection in pancreatic cells of some Type II diabetics and in the cardiac muscles of subjects with cardiomyopathies, neither associated with ordinary signs of continuing cell-mediated or humoral immune response[140].

Such models are seductive when considering CFS. They would explain why conventional studies of morphology are usually normal, whilst more dynamic studies, such as pituitary function, are not (see Chapter 11). A persistent virus infecting as yet unknown cells in the central nervous system to cause alteration in neurotransmitters is an interesting possibility, but is no more than that at the time of writing.

9.10 Viruses and CFS: conclusions

What can be concluded from this complex, contradictory, evidence? There can be little doubt that fatigue syndrome is a reality after certain infections. Some infections may be more liable to cause persistent neurasthenic sequelae than other, for example Epstein–Barr virus, Q fever, toxoplasmosis, and CMV. At least part of the risk of CFS comes from the nature of the precipitating infection.

Second, the risk of chronic fatigue is determined by other factors, among which appear to be personality and previous psychological vulnerability. Although not proven, such issues are particularly important with the commoner viruses, such as influenza and the enteroviruses. This risk increases with the duration of the fatigue state, a finding we will consider further.

Turning to the CFS literature, it becomes harder to discern a pattern. Testing for common viruses in CFS patients is clearly unprofitable, but certain viruses, most particularly EBV, can trigger the syndrome. As for the enteroviruses, the best that can be said is that the case is unproven. No definitive link has been established between evidence of exposure to infection, evidence of persistence, and evidence of relevant clinical abnormality.

The literature on psychological vulnerability, viral infection, and the development of post-infectious fatigue and/or psychiatric disorder is equally complex. We summarize it as follows. First, psychiatric disorder does not predispose to developing infection. Second, psychiatric disorder is a cause of persistent symptoms after infection, and in particular the more general symptoms such as fatigue and malaise with which we are concerned. Third, prior stress does affect the immune system, and either increases vulnerability to some viral infection, or causes reactivation of other infections, in particular the herpes viruses. The magnitude of this effect is unlikely to be substantial. Finally, there are many potential mechanisms by which viral infections may, either by direct or indirect actions within the central nervous system, cause psychological disorder, but confirmed examples of this are rare.

Finally, in the section on history we described how as each new infective agent was discovered, reports soon followed linking it with a neurasthenic condition. Our review shows this tendency shows no sign of abating – recent claims have been made for borna virus, spumavirus (another retrovirus), and parvovirus B19. We believe that the reasons for these many, and conflicting, claims, are twofold. The first is the intuitive appeal of infective agents as an explanation for CFS. Second, the relative ease with which such studies can be conducted.

9.11 Immunological abnormalities in CFS

In no area of CFS research does the literature change with such rapidity as in immunology. We will begin with a brief, simplistic guide to a few elements of the immune system that are frequently studied in CFS, for which we are much indebted to Andrew Lloyd. We will then review the claims made for immune abnormalities in the illness. We will not attempt a complete review of every study in the field. Comprehensive reviews of the immunology of CFS are provided by Buchwald and Komaroff[141], Lloyd et al.[142], and Strober[143].

T-lymphocytes

T-lymphocytes, so named because of the role of the thymus in their development, are critical to acquired immune responses and demonstrate antigen specificity and immunological memory. They display distinctive receptors on their cell surface, as well as a variety of other surface proteins. The function of the T-cell is the recognition of self and non-self determinants, and the direction of appropriate immune responses, some of which are cytotoxic. T-lymphocytes learn to discriminate self and non-self in the thymus. 'Self' is represented by molecules of the major histocompatibility complex (MHC). Recognition is mediated by a specific T-cell receptor (TCR) and the co-receptors CD3, CD4, and CD8, all of which are cell surface proteins. Mature T-cells express TCR, CD3, and either CD4 or CD8. The co-receptor expressed determines the MHC molecule (class I or II respectively). T-cells recognize antigens 'presented' to them on the surface of antigen-presenting cells such as Langerhans cells in the skin. CD4 T-cells recognize antigen displayed in associated with class II MHC molecules. CD8 T-cells respond to antigen presented in association with class I MHC molecules. CD4 lymphocytes are predominantly immunoregulatory cells, directing cytokine release, macrophage activation, antibody production by B-cells, and promoting cytotoxic responses. Accordingly CD4 T-cells are known as 'helper' or 'inducer' cells. Cytotoxicity, the killing of target cells (such as virally infected or cancerous cells), is a function most associated with CD8 + T-cells. Regulating the immune response, by restricting T-cell proliferation and inhibition of B-cell activities ('suppression') was thought to be another function of CD8 + cells (hence the name suppressor cells), although it is probably mediated by both subsets. However, CD8 cells are still known as 'cytotoxic' or 'suppressor' cells.

A brief word is necessary about the plethora of different codes and labels attached to various elements of the immune system. This reflects the complexity of the markers found on the surface of human leucocytes. These markers are numbered according to their ability to bind to certain monoclonal antibodies. These numbers are assigned at regular international workshops. When it is agreed that a specific cluster of mono-clonal antibodies react with the same antigen/epitope, the marker is given a CD (cluster of differentiation) number, of which there are already well over 100. The CD groups are antigenically, and not functionally, defined, which implies that their actual function in health, not to mention disease, is frequently unknown. However, they are frequently used to study lymphocyte populations in conditions in which the immune system is suspected of having a pathogenic role.

Natural killer (NK) cells

NK cells are large granular lymphocytes that lyse target cells, as do T-cells, but do so without being previously sensitized, and without antigen presentation in association with MHC molecules. In the current jargon they are not 'MHC restricted', and hence have a wide range of cytotoxic functions. NK cells are an important component of innate defence against a wide range of acute viral infections, and are increased during the initial phrase of such infections.

Cytokines

Cytokines are pleiotropic hormones which act as key messengers between cellular components of the host immune system. They amplify the immune response against viruses so it operates more effectively. They act via specific receptors on the target cells, such as T- or B-lymphocytes, which are to be stimulated. Among the rapidly growing list of cytokines (18 at the time of writing) are the interferons, interleukins, tumour necrosis factor, transforming growth factor, and others.

Particular attention has been devoted to the interleukins. Interleukin-1 (IL-1) is macrophage derived and acts as a potent inducer of the inflammatory response. Interleukin 2 (IL-2) is derived from activated T-cells and is a powerful stimulator of T-cell proliferation and activation. IL-1, IL-6, and TNFα are all initiators of the inflammatory process, including fever, hence their designation as endogenous pyrogens.

The three members of the interferon family are interferon-α (leucocyte derived), interferon-β (fibroblast derived), and interferon-γ (T-cell derived). The interferons promote the development of the so-called 'antiviral state', an important component of host defence against viral infection. In addition interferon-γ is a critical cytokine in T-cell responses.

9.12 Immunological studies in CFS: lymphocyte number and function

Some of the earliest reports of immune abnormalities in CFS concerned alterations in the numbers and proportions of T-cell subsets in the peripheral blood, especially the helper (CD4) and suppressor (CD8) cells. For example, Peter Behan was one of the first in the UK to study immune abnormalities, finding low levels of CD8 lymphocytes in those with short durations of illness, but low levels of CD4 in long-standing cases[54]. It is now accepted by most that absolute numbers of circulating total T-cells, and of both the CD4 (helper) and CD8 (suppressor) T-cells, are normal[16,91,92,144].

One line of inquiry has followed reports of impaired responsiveness of the immune system in CFS, crudely measured by *in vitro* tests of lymphocyte response to specific mitogens, and assumed to be indirect evidence of some impairment in the functional integrity of the immune system[54,145–147]. The most consistent evidence of such deficits has come from the Australian group led by Andrew Lloyd at the University of New South Wales. They have described abnormalities in delayed-type hypersensitivity, with allergy or hypoergy occurring in up to 50 per cent of cases[148]. This functional reduction in cellular immunity was accompanied by absolute reductions in total T-cells, and both helper/inducer (CD4), and suppressor/cytotoxic (CD8) subsets. They also found deficits in humoral immunity (see below). This pattern of reduction in helper cells (CD4) although not CD8, is found in HIV infection, as is depressed delayed-type skin reactivity. Unlike many groups, Lloyd and his colleagues have done considerable work in looking at both normal and clinically depressed populations, and recently reported that such responses occurred only in about 10 per cent of both normal and depressed controls[149]. Finally, the same group recently reported that abnormalities in cell-mediated immunity were common in Australian primary care, and not associated with chronic fatigue[150]. They conclude that cell-mediated immunity is extremely sensitive to relatively minor changes in both physical and emotional health.

Many of these initial findings could not be replicated. For example, Behan was unable to find similar abnormalities in a later series[8], whilst no difference in lymphocyte proliferation to coxsackie B4 and other antigens were reported by two other studies[56,151], which are not consistent with previous reports of differences in immune responsiveness.

Meanwhile, many American workers were producing evidence of immune activation. Although three studies[92,143,147] found that overall CD4 cell counts were within the normal range, the last two groups reported a decrease in one immunoregulatory subset, identified by studying isoforms of CD45, the leucocyte common antigen. Different isoforms (RA, RB, and RO) are expressed at different stages of maturation, but both groups found the deficit to be in the CD45 RA (immunologically 'naive') subset. This was interpreted as evidence of chronic immune stimulation, and was consistent with other findings of reduced *in vitro* lymphokine (IL-2) production[36,152]. Similar findings are noted in several autoimmune conditions, particularly during periods of illness exacerbation. The proportion of T-cells expressing intercellular adhesion molecule 1 (ICAM-1) was also increased[92]. This molecule, found on the CD4+ cell, is needed to permit cell to cell interactions before the T-cell can recognize and trigger the immune response. Its presence is another marker of immune activation.

One of the best known studies comes from the team lead by Jay Levy, an authority on the immunology of AIDS, at the University of California[16,153]. They too showed that a number of previously reported abnormalities, such as the number of the various T-cell subgroups, including the CD4 and CD8 classes, and the ratio of the CD4/CD8 (helper to suppressor cells) were normal. However, reflecting the ever-increasing sophistication of immunological analysis, they went on to study some of the cell markers that the CD8 cells express. They found that in the most severely affected group of CFS patients there were deficiencies in three cell markers. Landay and colleagues reported a reduction in the expression of CD11b molecules, although not everyone would agree that this adhesion molecule present on most leucocytes is equated with suppressor function. The second cell marker was an increase in CD38+ CD8+ T-cells, an activated cytotoxic population which Levy has argued is important in antiviral responses. Finally, they noted an increase in HLA-DR+ CD8+ markers. Taken as a whole, this pattern is evidence of immune activation, as seen in viral infection. However, other markers, such as CD25, CD57, and Leu8 antigens, were normal. This is surprising, since CD25+ is the IL-2 receptor, and is a marker of activation, since most resting T-cells are CD25-negative, and, if immune activation is indeed taking place as claimed, ought to be elevated. The abnormalities were only statistically significant for the most severely affected.

It is difficult to assess the full significance of these findings, especially for those whose background is outside immunology. A large number of comparisons were made, and there is no evidence to suggest that the reported abnormalities were those predicted. Given the number of comparisons, some significant differences can be expected by chance. Some previous findings were not replicated by Landay and colleagues, but have been replaced by new abnormalities. Most of the results in the cases are in the normal range – the differences reflect abnormalities of the mean. Given the rapid pace of immunology, there are inevitably gaps in our knowledge of the population norms, as well as the influence of the usual confounders, such as inactivity and depression. Although Landay and colleagues used a small number of depressed controls, and found significant differences between controls and CFS cases, other evidence continues to suggest that depression is an important confounder (see below). Replication of Landay's findings has been patchy. Two studies found no differences in the number and expression of cell activation markers (HLA-DR and IL-2 receptors)[151,154]. Another study did find a reduction in CD11b, but not CD38 or HLA-DR[155].

The picture is only a little less confusing when NK cell function is studied. As Table 9.3 indicates, there have been a number of conflicting claims of deficits in either absolute numbers or functional activity of NK cells. Morrison *et al.* showed that CFS patients had significant increases in four subsets of NK cells compared with normal controls, and that more expressed a high-affinity IL-2 receptor than controls. Another subset was decreased, whilst three others were normal[159]. Klimas and colleagues also found evidence of increase in CD56+ cells, another NK cell marker. It seems likely that many of these subsets are important in defence against minor viral infections, hence Morrison and colleagues explain their findings as further evidence in favour of viral persistence in CFS, and it is certainly true that latent viral infections, such as HIV, are associated with progressive decreases in NK cell activity. However, the evidence concerning NK cell numbers in CFS remains conflicting – a recent study finding that although 16 per cent of subjects had reduced NK numbers, in 40 per cent the numbers were increased[158]. One of us recently reported increased levels of NK cells in CFS, albeit not related to clinical status or outcome[162]. Some of these differences probably relate to the manner in which NK cells are defined, those defined by CD16 appearing reduced, but those defined by CD56 can be normal or even increased. There is more consensus about impairment of functional activity in CFS, but even then not everyone agrees (see Gold *et al.*[36]), and the significance of this impairment is unknown.

Table 9.3 Natural killer (NK) cell function and numbers

NK cell property	Authors
NK cells decreased	Behan *et al.*[54], Caligiuri *et al.*[156], Gupta and Vayuregula[92], Ho-Yen *et al.*[158], Morrison *et al.*[159], Masuda *et al.*[161]
NK cells normal	Miller *et al.*[55], Landay *et al.*[16], Straus *et al.*[157], Ho-Yen *et al.*[158], Rasmussen *et al.*[160]
NK cells increased	Gold *et al.*[36], Chao *et al.*[151], Ho-Yen *et al.*[158], Klimas *et al.*[147], Tirelli *et al.*[144], Peakman *et al.*[162]
NK function decreased	Kibler *et al.*[152], Caligiuri *et al.*[156], Klimas *et al.*[147], Morrison *et al.*[159], Masuda *et al.*[161], Barker *et al.*[153]
NK function normal	Borysiewicz *et al.*[145]
NK function increased	Gold *et al.*[36]

9.13 Immunological studies in CFS: humoral immune responses

Immunoglobulins

A few studies have reported either generalized or partial (particularly IgA and IgG) decreases in immunoglobulins. The partial deficiencies have been further divided. IgG is actually divided into four subclasses (although the first two, IgGI and IgG2, make up 90 per cent of the total IgG in normal subjects), and deficiencies of IgG subclasses have also been encountered – for example, both the Australian and Boston groups originally reported decreased subsets of IgG1 and IgG3, but not IgG2 or IgG4[163,164], whilst others found deficits restricted to IgG1 only[165]. IgG3 subclass deficiency would be particularly interesting, since it is associated with recurrent non-specific viral infections[142].

The measurement of immunoglobulin subclasses is notoriously difficult, and others have not confirmed these findings[16,54,92,145,166,167] reporting both normal overall immunoglobulins, as well as normal IgG subclasses. Similar results were obtained in fibromyalgia[168]. Even if immunoglobulin deficiencies were established, that could still be a secondary phenomenon to alterations in cytokine activity, and does not mean that an immune deficiency syndrome has been established. In a new study of

676 patients meeting the CDC criteria for CFS, IgG was actually higher in cases than controls[169]. The same group recently concluded that there were no significant differences in the level of any of the four IgG subsets (IgG1–4),[170] in contrast to an earlier report[164].

Immune complexes

Several authors now report increased levels of immune complexes in CFS[54,60,145], including in children[171]. Like the other immune abnormalities, this is not due to simple confounding by psychiatric disorder[172]. It has also not always been replicated. A case–control study used age and sex matched controls chosen by the general practitioner at the same time as the CFS subjects, the rate of immune complexes was certainly higher in the cases than expected, but was equally high in the controls[55]. A UK study also failed to find differences between cases and controls, although a greater number of cases scored above the 95 per cent range[56]. Immune complexes were not detected in a study of fibromyalgia[168], nor were any consistent abnormalities in cytokines or lymphocyte subsets. No evidence has ever been produced of clinical manifestations of immune complex disease, nor of low levels of complement, which might be expected[141]. Komaroff concluded that although there was an association between immune complexes and CFS, it was neither sensitive nor specific[172].

Cytokines

Excessive production of one or more of the cytokines is a tempting explanation of many of the features of CFS. Because of their effects in promoting inflammation, cytokines cause a variety of symptoms that are associated with immune activation (see Chapter 3). For example, IL-1 is associated with fatigue, fever, myalgia, and hypersomnia; IL-2 causes myalgia and insomnia; IL-6 lymphadenopathy; tumour necrosis factor causes headache, fever, and hypersomnia; interferon-α causes fever, myalgia, and lethargy; and finally interferon-γ is associated with myalgia and lymphadenopathy. Therapeutic use of interferon in the treatment of neoplastic disease and chronic hepatitis produces side effects which closely resemble the symptoms of both CFS and many psychiatric disorders[173,174], although, confusingly, *interferon* has also been used to treat CFS (see Chapter 17). Similar observations have been made after therapeutic use of other cytokines, such as IL-2 and tumour necrosis factor[175,176]. Central administration of cytokines to laboratory animals causes social withdrawal and general sickness behaviour.

It is therefore tempting to assume, and easy to comprehend, that CFS is due to excessive production of one or more cytokines. Some evidence has been produced. Serum levels of interferon-α were elevated in 3 out of 15 CFS subjects[177]. Elevation of IL-2 is also described[178]. Interleukin-1α, normally undetectable in most laboratories, has been reported as substantially elevated in 42 per cent of CFS cases entering a clinical trial[179]. Others have claimed elevations in IL-1β[180], IL-6[181], and several different cytokines[182]. Soluble IL-2 receptor, released from the membranes of activated T-cells and increased during the acute response to infectious acute mononucleosis[154], has been reported as elevated[183]. There are a large number of other immune modulators, and increases in at least one, transforming growth factor β, have also been observed[151].

As usual, nothing is so simple in CFS. Early claims of increases in IL-1β and IL-6 were subsequently withdrawn[151]. Soluble IL-2 receptor levels were normal in a case series[151] and a well controlled study[154]. Serum levels of interferon-α[184,185], interferon-γ[154,163,184–186], IL-1α[155,187], IL-1β[155,184,185,188], IL L-2[36,151,152,184], IL-4[151], IL-6[151,188], and tumour necrosis factor[155,187–189] were normal. A Swedish study found only modest elevations of IL-1α and IL-6, with only the former achieving statistical significance[154]. Even the study that reported elevations in five different cytokines[182] found that these only affected between 12 and 28 per cent of cases. Cytokine abnormalities have not been reported in fibromyalgia[168].

Similar abnormalities have also been reported in major depressive illnesses – for example, soluble IL-2 receptors are also elevated in severe depression[190] and are not reduced by dexamethasone administration. Normally glucocorticoids block T-cell proliferation. Although not clinically a confounder of CFS, the non-specificity of such finding is further emphasized by reports of similar elevations of IL-2 receptors in schizophrenia[191].

It is thus simplistic to expect that CFS would be explained by static abnormal serum cytokines. Low levels of cytokines do not necessarily mean low levels of activity. Low serum cytokines could be a feature of an immune system primed for an increased response to a novel stimulus, or alternatively could reflect genuine inhibition, or even an immune system chronically stimulated and exhausted. Dynamic testing of cytokine release from stimulated lymphocytes is one way of testing this. A low *in vitro* IL-2 response to T-cell stimulation by PHA (a T-cell mitogen) is one of the most consistent findings in CFS[27,36,152], but not by everyone[151,160]. *In vitro* production of monocyte-derived cytokines (IL-1α, IL-6, TNFα) is normal in one[160], but not another study[161]. Mowbray and Yousef discuss three cases in which oxypentifylline, a drug which blocks the release of cytokines such as TNF and IL-1 from macrophages, not only failed to alleviate symptoms, but made them worse in two of the three[189].

Attention has also been given to *in vitro* interferon response. These have been increased[193,195], normal[194], and decreased[147 152]. 2,5-oligoadenylate synthetase, an enzyme specifically induced by interferon, and hence induced during many acute viral infections[192], is another marker for interferon activity. Modest, but significant increases in this enzyme have been reported in CFS[25,27].

It has also been argued, with reason, that peripheral cytokine levels are unimportant, and that local production of cytokines within the central nervous system is a more plausible explanation of the aetiology of CFS[196]. However, CSF examinations for lymphokines, including IL-1β, TNFα, neopterin, interferon-α, and interferon-γ have been substantially normal[185,197]. This does not support such theories, but does not necessarily exclude them either. Another elegant hypothesis, also made by the innovative Sydney group, is that although resting levels of cytokines are normal, post-exertional symptoms could be due to excessive cytokine production after exercise. Several studies have shown moderate increases in plasma levels of various cytokines after submaximal exercise[198]. Unfortunately, this could not be substantiated in CFS[167,199]. Furthermore, a study that measured cytokine gene expression, a better marker than serum levels, found that acute exhausting exercise caused lower, rather than increased, production of cytokines[200]. Overall, no convincing evidence has been produced that excess circulating cytokines are important in causing symptoms.

9.14 Allergy and CFS

In selected hospital samples many patients report allergies to various substances. Allergy clinics regularly see patients with rhinitis, post-nasal discharge, sore throats, and chronic fatigue, who overlap with CFS[201]. Many patients report a history of allergies or atopy – 46 per cent in a recent series[202]. In a case–control study Straus and colleagues carried out skin testing with a variety of food or inhalant extracts[203]. Twelve (50 per cent) reacted to the food or inhalant extracts, compared with 20 to 30 per cent of the general population. An earlier paper[204] demonstrated increased *in vivo* lymphocyte responses to specific antigens, and increased numbers of IgE bearing B- and T-lymphocytes, all of which suggest an allergic contribution, although not in keeping with the pattern described by the Australian workers of decreased immune responsiveness, and decreased delayed hypersensitivity (see above). Despite the high frequency of reported allergy or atopy, it remains uncertain that this represents a true risk; in the most recent study of which we are aware, 66 per cent of the CFS cases reported such a history, but this proportion did not differ from matched community controls[188].

Allergy has attracted extraordinary attention in the popular literature. Allergy, especially in its more extreme forms such as multiple chemical sensitivity and 'twentieth-century disease', has become associated with CFS. However, there is little scientific evidence for these more extreme claims, which will be considered in Chapter 15.

9.15 Immune disorder and viral infection

Some authors have suggested that the observed immunological changes are not of pathological significance in their own right, but represent the normal immunological response to a persistent viral infection[159,189]. Levy *et al.*[205] argue that CFS reflects persistent activation of the peripheral white blood cells, particularly the CD8+ lymphocytes, which in turn fail to 'switch off'. The result is a sustained release of cytokines, which give rise to the symptoms of CFS. Finally, the chronically activated immune system reacts against the host, producing autoantibodies and increased cytotoxic T-cells.

This is the best articulated statement of a virological/immunological basis for CFS. There are, however, some inconsistencies. First, immune activation has not been universally demonstrated. Second, the overall picture in CFS is not that of acute viral infection. Certainly, viral infection is associated with immune changes[206]. Increased numbers of cells expressing certain antigens, such as CD11 or the CD57 group, is common in acute viral infections. Normally, changes such as decreased NK cell activity, lymphocyte activation, and so on last no longer than a few weeks[207]. Miller *et al.* found alterations in NK cells and B-cell numbers, but only in the acute post-viral cases, who had been ill for less than six months, and not in those with longer-lasting illnesses[55]. Viral infection decreases natural killer cell numbers, increases plasma IL-2 receptors, and so on, but only in the medium, not long term[206]. The best study to date, comparing patients with acute mononucleosis, those who had recovered from mononucleosis, and those with CFS, showed that major differences existed between the groups, with very little in the way of abnormal findings in CFS[154].

Third, the presumed final common pathway for symptom production and maintenance, elevated levels of a variety of cytokines, has not been shown. It remains plausible that some other mechanism exists linking a postulated transient cytokine rise with the production of longer-term clinical symptoms[208,209]. Modern psycho-neuroimmunological studies provide several possible pathways.

9.16 Immunological disturbances and clinical symptoms

One major hurdle in accepting that immunological factors play a primary role in CFS is that the laboratory results reported so far seemed to be divorced from clinical experience. For example, Lloyd and colleagues[148] reported occasionally severe deficits in CD4 cells, associated with significant impairment of cell-mediated immunity, down to a level at which there should be a substantial risk of opportunistic infections, but in a systematic review of outcome studies we were unable to find a single example. Measurement of peripheral blood T-cell subsets is neither a sensitive nor a specific marker of immunodeficiency.

Perhaps the most important question is whether or not any links exist between symptoms, disability, and immunological measures in CFS. Most immunological studies of CFS have not attempted to link immune and clinical measures, with some exceptions. Landay and colleagues found that the worst affected group tended to have the most abnormal values, and also noted that in two cases in which an improvement in symptoms occurred, this was 'accompanied by a return of normal of some immunological variables'[16]. Ojo-Amaize and colleagues also grouped subjects into three groups on the basis of severity, a composite measure of symptom duration. No appropriate statistical analysis was performed[210]. In contrast Straus's team from the National Institutes of Health, and Galama's team from Nijmegen in the Netherlands used a variety of measures of symptoms, emotional distress, and functional impairment[155,157]. There were no correlations between any immunological and clinical measure[155,157]. Two prognostic studies have also failed to link laboratory measures with clinical outcome. Wilson *et al.*[211,212] found no correlation between measures of cell-mediated immunity and outcome[213], whilst Clark *et al.* found no associations between outcome and either absolute number or percentage of CD4, CD8, CD11, or B4 lymphocytes, nor percentages of natural killer cells.

In a study specifically designed to look at this issue, subjects with CFS entering a randomized controlled trial of cognitive behaviour therapy for CFS[214] gave samples for immunological analysis before and after treatment[162]. There were no associations between clinical status and immunological measures at the start and completion of treatment, or between CFS subjects and normal controls. Percentage levels of total

CD3+ T-cells, CD4 T-cells, CD8 T-cells and activated subsets did not differ between CFS subjects and controls. Naive (CD45 RA+R0−) and memory (CD45 RA− R0+) T-cells did not differ between subjects and controls. Natural killer cells (CD16+/CD56+/CD3−) were significantly increased in CFS patients compared with controls, as was the percentage of CD11b+CD8 cells. There were no correlations between any immune variable and measures of clinical status, with the exception of a weak correlation between total CD4 T-cells and fatigue. There was a positive correlation between memory CD4 and CD8 T-cells and depression scores, and a negative correlation between naive CD4 T-cells and depression. No immune measures changed during the course of the study, and there was no link between clinical improvement as a result of the treatment programme and immune status. Immune measures did not predict response or lack of response to treatment.

It is possible to demonstrate links between clinical and immunological variables in other conditions – it is just that such links have not been found in CFS. For example, in HIV infection fatigue can be correlated with CD4+ cell numbers; the lower the number, the greater the fatigue[215]. This was related to elevations of interferon-α, IL-1, and TNF, which were assumed to be influencing fatigue by their effect on slow-wave sleep. In contrast, the paucity of such links in CFS is a weakness in primary immunological explanations of symptoms and disability in the illness.

9.17 Sample choice, selection bias, and confounders

The literature on CFS is beset by differences in samples, and the immunological literature is no exception. That duration may be a confounder was suggested by the results of one of the first studies in this field in which different lymphocyte profiles were noted in 'acute' and 'chronic' cases[54]. In many of the immune studies, patients were referred on the basis of elevated antibodies to various EBV antigens. It is thus possible that some of the immune abnormalities subsequently identified reflect this selection, and may not be clinically relevant. Others report only a subset of a larger sample, without giving information on how the subset was chosen. Only population-based studies will overcome this bias.

Little attention has been paid to possible confounders. Many drugs affect the immune response – non-steroidal anti-inflammatory drugs and antidepressants are frequently prescribed for patients with CFS. Both have substantial effects on measures of immune function. However, perhaps the most researched area of relevance to the subject of immune disturbance and CFS is the field of psychoimmunology. Many have argued that the observed immune changes in CFS are secondary to a disturbance of mood, or are the consequence of inactivity, sleep disturbance, or other confounders. This is the subject of the next section.

9.18 Mood, stress, and immune disorder

Looking at mood first, there is a large and detailed literature on the relationship between depression and immunity. Great claims have been made, but until recently there was no convincing demonstration of changes in cell-mediated immunity or T-cell number and function in most depressive illnesses (although B-cell functioning and cytokines remain relatively under-investigated). Many of the abnormalities reported in depression have been confounded by medication and the age of the subject, since immune abnormalities, like depression, become increasingly common with age (see Schieifer *et al.*[216]). Deficits in cell-mediated immunity are only established in the melancholic subtype of depression. For example, Ian Hickie and Andrew Lloyd have reported abnormalities in both *in vivo* and *in vitro* measures of cell-mediated immunity in unmedicated patients with melancholia[217]. These returned to normal after treatment, suggesting that the findings were state, not trait, markers. The same group, who have demonstrated decreases in lymphocyte response to PHA in CFS, also found similar decreases in depressed controls that just failed to reach significance[149]. They describe a general pattern in which outpatient depressives lie intermediate between normal controls and CFS patients on various measures of immune competence.

The literature on depression also reflects the inconsistencies of the literature on CFS, in that immune activation is also reported in both. Evidence of systemic immune activation, based on the presence of activated T-lymphocytes (both helper and memory cells and HLA-DR expression) has been found in severely depressed cases[218]. In CFS the expression of HLA-DR antigens has been reported as increasing in proportion to the severity of fatigue[16]; in depression expression of the same antigens is related to the severity of mood disorder[218].

Depression is far from the only psychosocial variable potentially associated with immunological changes. Acute psychosocial disturbance, usually covered by the catch-all term 'stress', is well established to be associated with alterations in immune function. Animal studies show that mice who have been stressed through various mechanisms are more likely to show signs of infection and weight loss when inoculated with viruses, including coxsackie B[219]. For example, Kiecolt-Glaser and colleagues have carried out a series of studies of the relationship between stress and immunological markers for EBV. Divorced and separated women have higher titres of EBV-VCA antibodies[220], as do those caring for relatives with Alzheimer's disease[221]. In students, four days of written disclosure of traumatic events led to increased T-cell proliferative response to PHA, maintained six weeks later[222]. This is, however, opposite to that found in some studies of CFS in which T-cell response to mitogens was impaired[54]. Medical students at the time of their examinations have both elevated EBV-VCA, CMV, and HSV-1 antibodies and decreased numbers of NK cells[223,224]. Thus there is convincing evidence that stress influences the immune system, but what is lacking is evidence that this has any effect on disease susceptibility[225].

The effect of both depression and stress on NK cell numbers and activity has been extensively studied. Irwin and colleagues have shown that in both depressed and non-depressed subjects, threatening life events are associated with a 50 per cent reduction in NK cell activity[226]. This large reduction is correlated with the number of depressive symptoms, but not with age, smoking, or alcohol. In a later longitudinal study the same group showed that the reduction of NK cell activity was related to the state of acute depression (i.e. it is a state, and not a trait, marker[227]), and is the principal immune change in both children[228] (see Chapter 13) and young adults with depression[229]. Natural killer cell activity is also reduced by even modest disturbances of sleep disturbance even in the absence of mood disorder[230,231]. Negative correlations have been demonstrated between scores on a personality rating scale (MMPI) scores and NK cell function[232]. On the other hand, active coping styles are positively correlated with NK cell function in asymptomatic HIV seropositive men[233]. There now seems little doubt that psychosocial factors are associated with impairments in NK cell activity[123]. As with CFS, the significance of NK cell reductions is unknown – there is no evidence of increased rates of infections in either CFS or depression[227], in contrast to the increased rates of reporting of the symptoms of infection.

Recent evidence has continued to add to the literature suggesting a relationship between immune and psychological function. Both aerobic exercise programmes and cognitive behaviour therapy reduced EBV-VCA and HHV-6 antibody production in a cohort of gay men[234]. Cognitive behaviour therapy also prevented decreases in mitogen responsivity and NK cell activity following a significant stressor (in this case notification of HIV status)[235]. Hence in CFS the occasional report[16,91] that immune abnormalities improved as clinical status improved does not prove that observed immune abnormalities are of aetiological significance.

The possible links between immune status, psychological function, and CFS seem complex enough. The role of the hypothalamo – pituitary – adrenal (HPA) axis is a further complication. Pituitary hormones influence the immune system. ACTH and cortisol are immunosuppresive, for example, preventing neutrophil adherence, and blocking cytokine-induced responses. *In vitro* lymphocyte response to stimulation is proportional to urinary cortisol excretion[236]. On the other hand, prolactin and growth hormone are more immune activating. Thus the exact nature of the immune disturbance secondary to neuroendocrine changes can be determined by subtle interactions. A recent review noted that if animals have anterior hypothalamic lesions the immune response is blunted, but augmented in posterior lesions[237]. Likewise, the hypothalamic response to stress, infective or otherwise, is very different in acute and chronic stress. Most experimental evidence concerns the former, but as clinicians we are more interested in the latter.

The actions of cytokines add to the subtlety (see Chapter 3). It is clear that cytokines have actions beyond the immune system, and in particular act within the central nervous system[238]. We know that neurones that respond to specific cytokines occur in the hypothalamus[239]. Animal studies have shown that viral infection can influence the production of steroid receptors. Interleukin-1 turns on the genes that control the release of corticotrophin releasing factor (CRF), which itself inhibits sleep[239,240]. Other cytokines, such as TNF, are sleep promoters[241].

Lack of exercise, an essential clinical feature of CFS, affects immune function. After exercise there is a substantial rise in the number and function of suppressor T-cells, cytotoxic T-cells, and NK cells[242]; perhaps lack of exercise is associated with a decrease in numbers.

This section on variables which may act as confounders in the relationship between immunity and CFS is only a sketch of the literature. Nevertheless, we trust the reader is now convinced that investigating possible abnormalities of the immune system in subjects who are likely to be inactive, taking antidepressants, sleeping badly or too much, depressed, or demoralized is a daunting task.

We therefore conclude our review of the possible interlinks between viral infection, immunity, psychiatric disorder, and chronic fatigue by noting that there are many plausible mechanisms by which acute viral infections may, via direct or indirect action on the central nervous system, cause psychiatric disorder. Nevertheless, confirmed examples of such actions are relatively rare. Similarly, the idea that acute stress may affect the immune system, and thus predispose to infection and/or post-infectious fatigue is a very common belief, and one with obvious attractions in terms of linking body and mind. It is also part and parcel of the new discipline of psychoimmunology, which has caught the popular imagination. The empirical literature on psychological vulnerability, viral infection, and subsequent post-infectious fatigue and/or psychiatric disorder does not readily support such simple models. There is little evidence that psychiatric disorder *per se* predisposes to infection – subjects with a range of psychiatric disorders do not appear to have increased rates of infection, even if they may show elevations of antibodies to a variety of infective agents. On the other hand, psychological disorder prior to infection does predict the duration of general symptoms such as fatigue and malaise after infection. Stress does affect the immune system and may predispose to infection or reactivation of certain viruses. The magnitude of this effect is unlikely to be substantial.

9.19 Genetics of CFS

At the beginning of the twentieth century most authorities favoured a distinction between inherited (genetic) and acquired neurasthenia. It was commonplace to observe that the illness ran in families, and could begin in early life. Such observations provided fuel for the popular theories of degeneration that influenced medical and psychiatric thought about many illnesses, not only neurasthenia.

The legacy of eugenics led to such ideas losing their attraction, and interest began to wane. A greater appreciation also developed of the methodological difficulties in separating congenital and acquired factors; for example, one of the last mentions of constitutional and acquired neurasthenia is by Essen-Moller in 1956, but only to admit to the unreliability of the label[110]. A role for genetics was never disproved, it became instead unfashionable and tainted. Only in the context of effort syndrome were careful studies performed, which did show a modest genetic contribution[243].

Such evidence was not conclusive of a genetic aetiology, and remained compatible with shared environmental factors. The methodology needed to separate nature and nurture, those of adoption and twin studies, was never utilized in studies of neurasthenia. Instead, most writers have used the Cohen and Wheeler studies as an introduction to a later generation of studies confirming a genetic contribution to the anxiety neuroses.

The previous generation of neurasthenia researchers did not have access to the modern genetic technologies. As yet few have applied these to CFS, but some contributions are being to appear. In one of the first, a group from Glasgow attempted to determine human lencocyte antigen (HLA) status in CFS[197]. They were hampered by difficulties in obtaining lymphocyte expression of HLA markers – an unusual situation. However, Middleton *et al.* did not experience similar difficulties, but reported no specific association of HLA class II antigens[244]. Nancy Klimas's group in Miami reported that the HLA-DQ3 and HLA-DR5 antigens were significantly associated with CFS[245]. However, working with our colleagues in immunology at King's College Hospital we have also been unable to replicate these findings. There are no published family history or twin studies on CFS to date, although the development of a twin register at the University of Washington and new Australian studies should remedy this.

A genetic contribution to CFS is not far-fetched. Such contributions are established for most psychiatric disorders. A genetic contribution to both susceptibility to, and recovery from, common viral infections, is possible, albeit yet to be demonstrated even outside the world of CFS. However, the lessons of psychiatric genetics must not be forgotten. Genetic susceptibility to a number of disorders is beyond doubt, but even the most ardent geneticist allows for strong environmental contributions.

9.20 Conclusion

At present we can only repeat the cautions offered by a number of authoritative reviewers[40,141,143,246]. There is evidence of some abnormalities of immune function, but such changes are inconsistent, non-specific, and rarely correlate with the clinical condition. As Walter Gunn, who used to be part of the CFS team at the Centers for Disease Control, noted 'What seems to show up in article after article is some kind of immune dysfunction. The problem is that the dysfunction is different in each article'[179].

Whereas Lloyd and his co-workers appear to be describing a syndrome associated with immune deficiency, or at least immune paresis, others produce evidence of immune activation. This is not necessarily contradictory, since deficits in cell-mediated immunity can coexist with evidence of immune activation, AIDS being the classic instance. Subtle changes in immunoregulatory subsets plus a tendency to activation of T- and B-cells are seen in a number of autoimmune diseases, such as Type I diabetes, Graves, disease, and chronic active hepatitis. One can argue that the immunoregulatory deficit could be a predisposing factor, and the activation a consequence of the disease – hence the presence of both immune paresis and activation is not *per se* contradictory. Nevertheless, the lack of a consistent single pattern remains a problem.

There is also no convincing mechanism to explain fatigue either; one should remember that it is not the decreasing numbers of T-cells that make HIV patients symptomatic, but the opportunistic infections that result, and these infections never occur in CFS. Finally, the problem of establishing cause or effect has barely begun.

The most recent and detailed reviews have therefore concluded that it is currently impossible to determine the significance of the observed changes in immunological status in CFS. One authority suggests that these changes are those of a hyperactive immune system secondary to viral infection[247]. Jay Levy[205] has argued that this chronically active immune system is thus reacting against the host as in autoimmune disorders. Recent research showing an increase in detectable autoantibodies supports this view[248]. As autoimmune diseases are commoner in women he further argues that this provides one explanation for the increased prevalence of CFS in women[205]. Another group of experts, prominent amongst them being Anthony Komaroff in Boston and Jim Jones in Denver, see the immunological changes as primary leading to secondary evidence of viral reactivation, hence CFS is a disorder of immune regulation of viral activity. A third view, articulated by Warren Strober at NIH, is that 'the possibility that the immunological findings in CFS are also found in more classic psychological diseases remains very much alive . . . perhaps secondary to subtle endocrine changes, characteristic of certain abnormal psychological states'[143]. We still have much to do.

References

1 Wessely S, Powell R. Fatigue syndromes: a comparison of chronic 'postviral' fatigue with neuromuscular and affective disorder. *J. Neurol. Neurosurg. Psychiatry* 1989; **52:** 940–948.
2 Hashimoto N, Kuraishi Y, Yokose T, *et al.* Chronic fatigue syndrome – 51 cases in the Jikei University School of Medicine. *Nippon Rinsho* 1992; **50:** 2653–64.
3 Vercoulen J, Swanink C, Fennis J, Galama J, van der Meer J, Bleijenberg G. Dimensional assessment of chronic fatigue syndrome. *J. Psychosom. Res.* 1994; **38:** 383–392.
4 Petersen P, Schenck C, Sherman R. Chronic fatigue syndrome in Minnesota. *Minnesota Med.* 1991; **74:** 21–26.
5 Gunn W. In Kleinman A, Straus S (ed.) *Chronic Fatigue Syndrome.* Chichester, Wiley, 1993: 288.
6 Cope H, Mann A, Pelosi A, David A. Psychosocial risk factors for chronic fatigue and chronic fatigue syndrome following presumed viral infection: a case control study. *Psychol. Med.* 1996; **26:** 1197–1209.
7 Helman C. Feed a cold and starve a fever. *Cul. Med. Psychol.* 1978; **7:** 107–137.
8 Behan P, Behan W. Postviral fatigue syndrome. *Crit. Rev. Neurobiol.* 1988; **4:** 157–179.
9 Lloyd A, Hickie I, Boughton R, Spencer O, Wakefield D. Prevalence of chronic fatigue syndrome in an Australian population. *Med. J. Aust.* 1990; **153:** 522–528.
10 Salit I. Sporadic post-infectious neuromyasthenia. *Can. Med. Assoc. J.* 1985; **133:** 659–663.
11 Levine P, Jacobson S, Pocinki A, *et al.* Clinical, epidemiologic, and virologic studies in four clusters of the chronic fatigue syndrome. *Arch. Intern. Med.* 1992; **152:** 1611–1616.
12 Frank J. Emotional reactions of American soldiers to an unfamiliar disease. *Am. J. Psych.* 1946; **102:** 631–640.
13 Luisto M. Outcome and neurological sequelae of patients after tetanus. *Acta Neurol. Scand.* 1989; **80:** 504–511.
14 Buchwald D, Umali J, Pearlman T, Kith P, Ashley R, Wener M. Post infectious chronic fatigue: a distinct syndrome? *Clin. Infect. Dis.* 1996; **23:** 385–387.
15 Holmes G, Kaplan J, Stewart J, Hunt B, Pinsky P, Schonberger S. A cluster of patients with a chronic mononucleosis-like syndrome: is Epstein – Barr virus the cause? *J. Am. Med. Assoc.* 1987; **257:** 2297–2303.
16 Landay A, Jessop C, Lennette E, Levy J. Chronic fatigue syndrome: clinical condition associated with immune activation. *Lancet* 1991; **338:** 707–712.
17 Bell E, McCartney R, Riding M. Coxsackie B viruses and myalgic encephalomyelitis. *J. R. Soc. Med.* 1988; **81:** 329–331.

18 Allen AD, Tilkian SM. Depression correlated with cellular immunity in systemic immunodeficient Epstein–Barr virus syndrome (SIDES). *J. Clin. Psychiatry* 1986; **47**: 133–135.

19 Delisi L, Nurnerger J, Goldin L, Simmons-Alling S, Gershon E. Epstein–Barr virus and depression. *Arch. Gen. Psychiat.* 1986; **43**: 815–816.

20 Amsterdam J, Henle W, Winokur A, Wolkowitz O, Pichar D, Paul S. Serum antibodies to Epstein–Barr virus in patients with major depressive disorder. *Am. J. Psych.* 1986; **143**: 1593–1596.

21 Isaacs R. Chronic infectious mononucleosis. *Blood* 1948; **3**: 858–861.

22 Merlin TL. Chronic mononucleosis: pitfalls in the laboratory diagnosis. *Hum. Pathol.* 1986; **17**: 2–8.

23 Jones J, Straus S. Chronic Epstein – Barr virus infection. *Am. Rev. Med.* 1987; **38**: 195–209.

24 Okano M, Thiele GM, Purtilo DT. Severe chronic active Epstein–Barr virus infection syndrome and adenovirus type-2 infection. *Am. J. Pediatr. Hematol. Oncol.* 1990; **12**: 168–173.

25 Tobi M, Morag A, Ravid Z, *et al*. Prolonged illness associated with serological evidence of persistent Epstein–Barr virus infection. *Lancet* 1982; **i**: 61–64.

26 Dubois R, Seeley J, Brus I, *et al*. Chronic mononucleosis syndrome. *South. Med. J.* 1984; **77**: 1376–1382.

27 Straus S, Tosato G, Armstrong G, *et al*. Persisting illness and fatigue in adults with evidence of Epstein–Barr virus infection. *Ann. Int. Med.* 1985; **102**: 7–16.

28 Jones J, Ray G, Minnich L, Hicks M, Kibler R, Lucas D. Evidence for active Epstein–Barr virus infection in patients with persistent, unexplained illnesses; elevated anti-early antigen antibodies. *Ann. Int. Med.* 1985; **102**: 1–7.

29 Horwitz CA, Henle W, Henle G, Rudnick H, Latts E. Long-term serological follow-up of patients for Epstein–Barr virus after recovery from infectious mononucleosis. *J. Infect. Dis.* 1985; **151**: 1150–1153.

30 Sumaya C. Serologic and virologic epidemiology of Epstein–Barr virus: relevance to chronic fatigue syndrome. *Rev. Infect. Dis.* 1991; **13(suppl 1)**: S 19–25.

31 Woodward C, Cox R. Epstein–Barr virus serology in the chronic fatigue syndrome. *J. Infect.* 1992; **24**: 133–139.

32 Hellinger W, Smith T, Van Scoy R, Spitzer P, Forgacs P, Edson R. Chronic fatigue syndrome and the diagnostic utility of Epstein–Barr virus early antigen. *J. Am. Med. Assoc.* 1988; **260**: 971–973.

33 Buchwald D, Sullivan J, Komaroff A. Frequency of 'Chronic active Epstein–Barr virus infection' in a general medical practice. *J. Am. Med. Assoc.* 1987; **257**: 2303–2307.

34 Anon. Pseudo-outbreak of infectious mononucleosis-Puerto Rico, 1990. *MMWR* 1991; **40**: 552–555.

35 Straus S, Dale J, Tobi M, *et al*. Acyclovir treatment of the chronic fatigue syndrome: lack of efficacy in a placebo-controlled trial. *New Engl. J. Med.* 1988; **319**: 1692–1698.

36 Gold D, Bowden R, Sixbey J, *et al*. Chronic fatigue: a prospective clinical and virologic study. *J. Am. Med. Assoc.* 1990; **264**: 48–53.

37 Swanink C, van der Meer J, Vercoulen J, Bleijenberg G, Fennis J, Galama J. Epstein–Barr virus (EBV) and the chronic fatigue syndrome: normal virus load and normal immunological reactivity in the EBV regression assay. *Clin. Infect. Dis.* 1995; **20**: 1390–1392.

38 Hotchin N, Read R, Smith D, Crawford D. Active Epstein–Barr virus infection in post-viral fatigue syndrome. *J. Infect.* 1989; **18**: 143–150.

39 Schooley R. Epstein–Barr virus. *Curr. Opin. Infect. Dis.* 1989; **2**: 267–271.

40 Straus S. The chronic mononucleosis syndrome. *J. Infect.* 1988; **157**: 405–412.

41 Swartz M. The chronic fatigue syndrome-one entity or many? *New Engl. J. Med.* 1988; **319:** 1726–1728.

42 Jones J, Streib J, Baker S, Heberger M. Chronic fatigue syndrome: I. Epstein–Barr virus immune response and molecular epidemiology. *J. Med. Virol.* 1991; **33:** 151–158.

43 Chang R, Bittner W. Chronic fatigue syndrome. *J. Am. Med. Assoc.* 1991; **265:** 337.

44 White P, Thomas J, Amess J, Grover S, Kangro H, Clare A. The existence of a fatigue syndrome after glandular fever. *Psychol. Med.* 1995; **25:** 907–916.

45 White P, Grover S, Kangro H, Thomas J, Amess J, Clare A. The validity and reliability of the fatigue syndrome that follows glandular fever. *Psychol. Med.* 1995; **25:** 917–924.

46 White P, Thomas J, Amess J, Crawford D, Grover S, Kangro H. The incidence, prevalence and prognosis of the fatigue syndrome which follows Epstein–Barr virus infection. *Br. J. Psych.*, in press.

47 Lambore S, McSherry J, Kraus A. Acute and chronic symptoms of mononucleosis. *J. Fam. Pract.* 1991; **33:** 33–37.

48 Bruce-Jones W, White P, Thomas J, Clare A. The effect of social disadvantage on the fatigue syndrome, psychiatric disorders and physical recovery, following glandular fever. *Psychol. Med.* 1994; **24:** 651–659.

49 Sigurdsson B, Gudnadottir M, Petursson G. Response to poliomyelitis vaccination. *Lancet* 1958; **i:** 370–371.

50 Fegan K, Behan P, Bell E. Myalgic encephalomyelitis: report of an epidemic. *J. R. Coll. Gen. Pract.* 1983; **33:** 335–337.

51 Keighley B, Bell E. Sporadic myalgic encephalomyelitis in a rural practice. *J. R. Coll. Gen. Pract.* 1983; **33:** 339–341.

52 Calder B, Warnock P. Coxsackie B infection in a Scottish general practice. *J. R. Coll. Gen. Pract.* 1984; **35:** 15–19.

53 Calder B, Warnock P, McCartney R, Bell E. Coxsackie B viruses and the post-viral syndrome: a prospective study in general practice. *J. R. Coll. Gen. Pract.* 1987; **37:** 11–14.

54 Behan P, Behan P, Bell E. The postviral fatigue syndrome: an analysis of the findings in 50 cases. *J. Infect.* 1985; **10:** 211–222.

55 Miller H, Carmichael H, Calder B, *et al.* Antibody to coxsackie B virus in diagnosing postviral fatigue syndrome. *Br. Med. J.* 1991; **302:** 140–143.

56 Milton J, Clements G, Edwards R. Immune responsiveness in chronic fatigue syndrome. *Postgrad. Med. J.* 1991; **67:** 532–537.

57 Gow J, Behan W, Clements G, Woodall C, Riding M, Behan P. Enteroviral RNA sequences detected by polymerase chain reaction in muscle of patients with postviral fatigue syndrome. *Br. Med. J.* 1991; **302:** 692–696.

58 Mawle A, Nisenbaum R, Dobbins J, *et al.* Seroepidemiology of chronic fatigue syndrome: a case control study. *Clin. Infect. Dis.* 1995; **21:** 1386–1389.

59 Lindh G, Samuelson A, Hedlund I, Evengard B, Lindquist L, Ehrnst A. No findings of enterovirus in Swedish patients with chronic fatigue syndrome. *Scan. J. Infect. Dis.* 1996; **28:** 305–308.

60 Yousef G, Bell E, Mann G, Murugesan V, McCartney R, Mowbray J. Chronic enterovirus infection in patients with postviral fatigue syndrome. *Lancet* 1988; **i:** 146–150.

61 Halpin D, Wessely S. VP-1 antigen in chronic postviral fatigue syndrome. *Lancet* 1989; **ii:** 1028–1029.

62 Lynch S, Seth R. Postviral fatigue syndrome and the VP-1 antigen. *Lancet* 1989; **ii:** 1160–1161.

63 Lynch S, Seth R, Main J. Monospot and VP-1 tests in chronic fatigue syndrome and depression. *J. R. Soc. Med.* 1992; **85:** 537–540.

64 Bowman S, Brostoff J, Newman S, Mowbray J. Postviral syndrome – how can a diagnosis be made? *J. R. Soc. Med.* 1989; **82**: 712–716.

65 Swanink C, Melchers W, van der Meer J, *et al.* Enteroviruses and the chronic fatigue syndrome. *Clin. Infect. Disc.* 1994; **19**: 860–864.

66 Archard L, Bowles N, Behan P, Bell E, Doyle D. Postviral fatigue syndrome; persistence of enterovirus in muscle and elevated creatine kinase. *J. R. Soc. Med.* 1988; **81**: 326–329.

67 Cunningham L, Bowles NE, Archard LC. Persistent virus infection of muscle in postviral fatigue syndrome. *Br. Med. Bull.* 1991; **47**: 852–71.

68 McArdle A, McArdle F, Jackson M, Page S, Fahal I, Edwards R. Investigation by polymerase chain reaction of enteroviral infection in patients with chronic fatigue syndrome. *Clin. Sci.* 1996; **90**: 295–300.

69 Gow J, Behan W, Simpson K, McGarry F, Keir S, Behan P. Studies of enteroviruses in patients with chronic fatigue syndrome. *Clin. Infect. Dis.* 1994; **18(suppl 1)**: S126–S129.

70 Leon Monzon M, Dalakas MC. Absence of persistent infection with enteroviruses in muscles of patients with inflammatory myopathies. *Ann. Neurol.* 1992; **32**: 219–222.

71 Kleinman A, Straus S (ed.) *Chronic Fatigue Syndrome.* Chichester, Wiley, 1993.

72 Leff RL, Love LA, Miller FW, *et al.* Viruses in idiopathic inflammatory myopathies: absence of candidate viral genomes in muscle. *Lancet* 1992; **339**: 1192–1195.

73 Gow J, Behan P. Viruses and chronic fatigue syndrome. *J. Chronic Fatigue Syndrome* 1996; **2**: 67–83.

74 Cunningham L, Bowles NE, Lane RJ, Dubowitz V, Archard LC. Persistence of enteroviral RNA in chronic fatigue syndrome is associated with the abnormal production of equal amounts of positive and negative strands of enteroviral RNA. *J. Gen. Virol.* 1990; **71**: 1399–1402.

75 Clements G, McGarry F, Nairn C, Galbraith D. Detection of enterovirus-specific RNA in serum: the relationship to chronic fatigue. *J. Med. Virol.* 1995; **45**: 156–161.

76 Galbraith D, Narin C, Clements G. Phylogenic analysis of short enteroviral sequences from patients with chronic fatigue syndrome. *J. Gen. Virol.* 1995; **76**: 1701–1707.

77 Straus S. Chronic fatigue syndrome. *Br. Med. J.* 1996; **313**: 831–832.

78 Agre JC, Rodriquez AA, Sperling KB. Symptoms and clinical impressions of patients seen in a postpolio clinic. *Arch. Phys. Med. Rehab.* 1989; **70**: 367–370.

79 Agre JC. The role of exercise in the patient with post-polio syndrome. *Ann. Acad. Sci.* 1995; **753**: 321–334.

80 Agre JC, Rodriquez AA, Tafel JA. Late effects of polio: critical review of the literature on neuromuscular function. *Arch. Phys. Med. Rehab.* 1991; **72**: 923–931.

81 Dalakas MC. The post-polio syndrome as an evolved clinical entity. Definition and clinical description. *Ann. NY Acad. Sci.* 1995; **753**: 68–80.

82 Leon Monzon ME, Dalakas MC. Detection of poliovirus antibodies and poliovirus genome in patients with the post-polio syndrome. *Ann. NY Acad. Sci.* 1995; **753**: 208–18.

83 Rodriquez AA, Agre JC, Harmon RL, Franke TM, Swiggum ER, Curt JT. Electromyographic and neuromuscular variables in post-polio subjects. *Arch. Phys. Med. Rehab.* 1995; **76**: 989–993.

84 Muller R, Nylander I, Larsson L, Widen L, Frankenhauser M. Sequelae of primary aseptic meningo-encephalitis. A clinical, sociomedical, electroencephalographic and psychological study. *Acta Psychiatr. Neurol. Scand.* 1958; **33(suppl 126)**: 1–115.

85 Lepow M, Coyne N, Thompson L, Carver D, Robbins F. A clinical, epidemiological and laboratory investigation of aseptic meningitis during the four-year period, 1955–1958: II. The clinical disease and its sequelae. *New Engl. J. Med.* 1962; **266**: 1188–1193.

86 Todd W, MacMillan M, Gray J. Echo virus type 30 meningitis in Edinburgh. *Scot. Med. J.* 1983; **28**: 160–163.

87 Rotbart H. Enteroviral infections of the central nervous system. *Clin. Infect. Dis.* 1995; **20:** 971–981.

88 Hotopf M, Noah N, Wessely S. Chronic fatigue and minor psychiatric morbidity after viral meningitis: a controlled study. *J. Neurol. Neurosurg. Psychiatry* 1996; **60:** 504–509.

89 Wessely S, Chalder T, Hirsch S, Pawlikowska T, Wallace P, Wright D. Post infectious fatigue: a prospective study in primary care. *Lancet* 1995; **345:** 1333–1338.

90 Ablashi DV, Zompetta C, Lease C, *et al.* Human herpesvirus 6 (HHV6) and chronic fatigue syndrome (CFS). *Can. Dis. Weekly Rep.* 1991; **17:** 33–40.

91 Read R, Larson E, Harvey J, *et al.* Clinical and Laboratory findings in the Paul-Bunnell negative glandular fever-fatigue syndrome. *J. Infect.* 1990; **21:** 157–165.

92 Gupta S, Vayuvegula B. A comprehensive immunological analysis in chronic fatigue syndrome. *Scand. J. Immunol.* 1991; **33:** 319–327.

93 Buchwald D, Cheney P, Peterson D, *et al.* A chronic illness characterized by fatigue, neurologic and immunologic disorders, and active human herpes type infections. *Ann. Int. Med.* 1992; **116:** 103–116.

94 Ablashi D, Ablashi K, Kramarsky B, Bernbaum J, Whitman J, Pearson G. Viruses and chronic fatigue syndrome: current status. *J. Chronic Fatigue Syndrome* 1995; **1:** 3–22.

95 Josephs S, Henry B, Balachandran N, *et al.* HHV-6 reactivation in chronic fatigue syndrome. *Lancet* 1991; **337:** 1346–1347.

96 Hay J, Jenkins F. Human herpesviruses and chronic fatigue syndrome. In Straus S (ed.) *Chronic Fatigue Syndrome.* New York, Dekker, 1994: 181–198.

97 Di Luca D, Zorzenon M, Mirandola P, Colle R, Botta G, Cassai E. Human herpesvirus 6 and human herpesvirus 7 in chronic fatigue syndrome. *J. Clin. Microbiol.* 1995; **33:** 1660–1661.

98 Klonoff D. Chronic fatigue syndrome. *Clin. Infect. Dis.* 1992; **15:** 812–823.

99 Marshall G, Gesser R, Yamanishi K, Starr S. Chronic fatigue in children: clinical features, Epstein–Barr virus and human herpesvirus 6 serology and long term follow up. *Pediatr. Inf. Dis. J.* 1991; **10:** 287–290.

100 Smith M, Mitchell J, Corey L, McCauley E, Glover D, Tenover F. Chronic fatigue in adolescents. *Pediatrics* 1991; **88:** 195–201.

101 Swanink C, Vercoulen J, Bleijenberg G, Fennis J, Galama J, Van Der Meer J. Chronic fatigue syndrome: a clinical and laboratory study with a well matched control group. *J. Intern. Med.* 1995; **237:** 499–506.

102 Secchiero P, Carrigan DR, Asano Y, *et al.* Detection of human herpesvirus 6 in plasma of children with primary infection and immunosuppressed patients by polymerase chain reaction. *J. Infect. Dis.* 1995; **171:** 273–80.

103 Fekety R. Infection and chronic fatigue syndrome. In Straus S (ed.) *Chronic Fatigue Syndrome.* New York, Dekker, 1994: 101–180.

104 Benjamin J, Hoyt R. Disability following post-vaccinal (yellow fever) hepatitis: a study of 200 patients manifesting delayed convalescence. *J. Am. Med. Assoc.* 1945; **128:** 319–324.

105 Dale J, Bisceglie A, Hoofnagle J, Straus S. Chronic fatigue syndrome: lack of association with hepatitis C virus infection. *J. Med. Virol.* 1991; **34:** 119–121.

106 Delarge G, Salit I, Pennie R, Alary M, Duval B, Ward B. Rélation eventuelle entre le vaccination contre l'hepatitis B et le syndrome de fatigue chronique. *L'Union Med. Can.* 1993; **122:** 278–279.

107 Berelowitz G, Burgess A, Thanabalasingham T, Murray-Lyon I, Wright D. Post-hepatitis syndrome revisited. *J. Viral. Hep.* 1995; **2:** 133–138.

108 Marmion B, Shannon M, Maddocks I, Strom P, Penttila I. Protracted fatigue and debility after acute Q fever. *Lancet* 1996; **347:** 977–978.

109 Arnold DL, Bore PJ, Radda GK, Styles P, Taylor DJ. Excessive intracellular acidosis of skeletal muscle on exercise in a patient with a post-viral exhaustion/fatigue syndrome. A 31P nuclear magnetic resonance study. *Lancet* 1984; **1:** 1367–1369.

110 Essen-Moller E. Individual traits and morbidity in a Swedish rural population. *Acta Psychiat. Scand.* 1956 **(suppl 100):** 1–160.

111 DeFreitas E, Hilliard B, Cheney P, *et al.* Retroviral sequence related to human T-lymphotropic virus type II in patients with chronic fatigue immunodysfunction syndrome. *Proc. Nat. Acad. Sci. USA* 1991; **88:** 2922–2926.

112 Johnson H. *Osler's Web: Inside the Labyrinth of the Chronic Fatigue Syndrome Epidemic.* New York, Crown, 1996.

113 Gow J, Simpson G, Schliephake A, *et al.* Search for retrovirus in chronic fatigue syndrome. *J. Clin. Pathol.* 1992; **45:** 1058–1061.

114 Honda M, Kitamura K, Nakasone T, *et al.* Japanese patients with chronic fatigue syndrome are negative for known retrovirus infections. *Microbiol. Immunol.* 1993; **37:** 779–784.

115 Khan A, Heneine W, Chapman L, *et al.* Assessment of a retrovirus sequence and other possible risk factors for the chronic fatigue syndrome in adults. *Ann. Intern. Med.* 1993; **118:** 241–245.

116 Heneine W, Woods TC, Sinha SD, *et al.* Lack of evidence for infection with known human and animal retroviruses in patients with chronic fatigue syndrome. *Clin. Infect. Dis.* 1994; **18:** S121–S125.

117 Anon. Inability of retroviral tests to identify persons with chronic fatigue syndrome, 1992. *J. Am. Med. Assoc.* 1993; **269:** 1779–1780.

118 Imboden J, Canter A, Cluff L. Convalesence from influenza: a study of the psychological and clinical determinants. *Arch. Intern. Med.* 1961; **108:** 393–399.

119 Canter A, Cluff L, Imboden J. Hypersensitive reactions to immunization inoculations and antecedent psychologic status. *J. Psychosom. Res.* 1972; **16:** 99–101.

120 Canter A. Changes in mood during incubation of acute febrile illness and the effects of pre-exposure psychologic status. *Psychosom. Med.* 1972; **34:** 424–430.

121 Brodman K, Mittelmann B, Wechsler D, Weider A, Wolff H. The relationship of personality disturbances to duration of convalescence from acute respiratory infections. *Psychosom. Med.* 1947; **9:** 37–44.

122 Barsky AJ, Goodson JD, Lane RS, Cleary PD. The amplification of somatic symptoms. *Psychosom. Med.* 1988; **50:** 510–9.

123 Zorrilla M, McKay J, Luborsjy L, Schmidt K. Relation of stressors and depressive symptoms to clinical progression of viral illness. *Am. J. Psychiat.* 1996; **153:** 626–635.

124 Dworkin R, Hartstein G, Rosner H, Walther R, Sweeney E, Brand L. A high-risk method for studying psychosocial antecedents of chronic pain: the prospective investigation of herpes zoster. *J. Abnorm. Psychol.* 1992; **101:** 200–205.

125 Briscoe M. *Sex Differences in Psychological Well-being.* Cambridge University Press, 1982.

126 Cox B, Blaxter M, Buckle A, *et al. The Health and Lifestyle Survey.* London, Health Promotion Research Trust, 1987.

127 Cohen S, Tyrrell D, Smith A. Psychological stress and susceptibility to the common cold. *New Engl. J. Med.* 1991; **325:** 606–612.

128 Totman R, Kiff J, Reed S, Craig J. Predicting experimental colds in volunteers from different measures of recent life stress. *J. Psychosom. Res.* 1980; **24:** 155–163.

129 Pawlikowska T, Chalder T, Hirsch S, Wallace P, Wright D, Wessely S. A population based study of fatigue and psychological distress. *Br. Med. J.* 1994; **308:** 743–746.

130 Dowden C, Johnson W. Exhaustion states. *J. Am. Med. Assoc.* 1929; **93:** 1702–1706.

131 Cadie M, Nye F, Storey P. Anxiety and depression after infectious mononucleosis. *Br. J. Psychiatry* 1976; **128:** 559–561.

132 Mayou R, Seagroatt V, Goldacre M. Use of psychiatric services by patients in a general hospital. *Br. Med. J.* 1991; **303:** 1029–1032.

133 Von Economo C. *Encephalitis Lethargica – Its Sequelae and Treatment.* Oxford University Press, 1931.

134 Lawton A, Rich T, McLendon S, Gates E, Bond J. Follow up studies of the St Louis encephalitis in Florida: reevaluation of the emotional and health status of the survivors five years after the acute illness. *South. Med. J.* 1970; **63:** 66–71.

135 Lishman WA. *Organic Psychiatry: The Psychological Consequences of Cerebral Disorder.* Oxford, Blackwell Scientific, 1987.

136 Oldstone MB. Viruses can cause disease in the absence of morphological evidence of cell injury: implication for uncovering new diseases in the future. *J. Infect. Dis.* 1989; **159:** 384–389.

137 Lipkin WI, Battenberg EL, Bloom FE, Oldstone MB. Viral infection of neurons can depress neurotransmitter mRNA levels without histologic injury. *Brain Res.* 1988; **451:** 333–339.

138 Klavinskis LS, Oldstone MB. Lymphocytic choriomeningitis virus selectively alters differentiated but not housekeeping functions: block in expression of growth hormone gene is at the level of transcriptional initiation. *Virology* 1989; **168:** 232–235.

139 de la Torre JC, Oldstone MB. Selective disruption of growth hormone transcription machinery by viral infection. *Proc. Natl. Acad. Sci. USA* 1992; **89:** 9939–9943.

140 Bowles NE, Rose ML, Taylor P, *et al.* End-stage dilated cardiomyopathy. Persistence of enterovirus RNA in myocardium at cardiac transplantation and lack of immune response. *Circulation* 1989; **80:** 1128–1136.

141 Buchwald D, Komaroff A. Review of laboratory findings for patients with chronic fatigue syndrome. *Rev. Infect. Dis.* 1991; **13(suppl 1):** 12–18.

142 Lloyd AR, Wakefield D, Hickie I. Immunity and the pathophysiology of chronic fatigue syndrome. In Kleinman A, Straus S (ed.) *Chronic Fatigue Syndrome.* Chichester, Wiley, 1993: 176–187.

143 Strober W. Immunological function in chronic fatigue syndrome. In Straus S (ed.) *Chronic fatigue Syndrome.* New York, Dekker, 1994: 207–240.

144 Tirelli U, Marotta G, Improta S, Pinto A. Immunological abnormalities in patients with chronic fatigue syndrome. *Scand. J. Immunol.* 1994; **40:** 601–608.

145 Borysiewicz L, Haworth S, Cohen J, Mundin J, Rickinson A. Epstein – Barr virus-specific immune defects in patients with persistent symptoms following infectious mononucleosis. *Q. J. Med.* 1986; **58:** 111–121.

146 Tosato G, Straus S, Henle W, Pike SE, Blaese RM. Characteristic T cell dysfunction in patients with chronic active Epstein – Barr virus infection (chronic infectious mononucleosis). *J. Immunol.* 1985; **134:** 3082–3088.

147 Klimas N, Salvato F, Morgan R, Fletcher M. Immunologic abnormalities in chronic fatigue syndrome. *J. Clin. Microbiol.* 1990; **28:** 1403–1410.

148 Lloyd A, Wakefield D, Broughton C, Dwyer J. Immunological abnormalities in the chronic fatigue syndrome. *Med. J. Aust.* 1989; **151:** 122–124.

149 Lloyd A, Hickie I, Hickie C, Dwyer J, Wakefield D. Cell mediated immunity in patients with chronic fatigue syndrome, healthy control subjects and patients with major depression. *Clin. Exper. Immunol.* 1992; **87:** 76–79.

150 Hickie I, Koojer A, Hadzi-Pavlovic D, Bennett B, Wilson A, Lloyd A. Fatigue in selected primary care settings: socio-demographic and psychiatric correlates. *Med. J. Aust.* 1996; **164:** 585–588.

151 Chao C, Janoff E, Hu S, *et al.* Altered cytokine release in peripheral blood mononuclear cell cultures from patients with the chronic fatigue syndrome. *Cytokine* 1991; **3:** 292–298.

152 Kibler R, Lucas D, Hicks M, Poulos B, Jones J. Immune function in chronic active Epstein – Barr virus infection. *J. Clin. Invest.* 1985; **5**: 46–54.

153 Barker A, Fujimura S, Fadem M, Landay A, Levy J. Immunologic abnormalities associated with chronic fatigue syndrome. *Clin. Infect. Dis.* 1994; **18(suppl 1)**: S136–S141.

154 Linde A, Andersson, B, Svensen S, *et al.* Serum levels of lymphokine and soluble cellular receptors in primary Epstein–Barr virus infection and in patients with chronic fatigue syndrome. *J. Infect. Dis.* 1992;**165**: 994–1000.

155 Swaninck C, Vercoulen J, Galama J, *et al.* Lymphoctye subsets, apoptosis and cytokines in patients with chronic fatigue syndrome. *J. Infect. Dis.* 1996; **173**: 460–463.

156 Caliguri M, Murray C, Buchwald D, *et al.* Phenotypic and functional deficiency of natural killer cells in patients with chronic fatigue syndrome. *J. Immunol.* 1987; **139**: 3303–3313.

157 Straus S, Fritz S, Dale J, Gould B, Strober W. Lymphocyte phenotype and function in the chronic fatigue syndrome. *J. Clin. Immunol.* 1993; **13**: 30–40.

158 Ho-Yen D, Billington R, Urquhart J. Natural killer cells and the post-viral fatigue syndrome. *Scand. J. Infect. Dis.* 1991; **23**: 711–716.

159 Morrison L, Behan W, Behan P. Changes in natural killer cell phenotype in patients with post-viral fatigue syndrome. *Clin. Exper. Immunol.* 1991; **83**: 441–446.

160 Rasmussen A, Nielsen H, Andersen V, *et al.* Chronic fatigue syndrome: a controlled cross sectional study. *J. Rheumatol.* 1994; **21**: 1527–1531.

161 Masuda A, Nozoe S, Matsuyama T, Tanaka H. Psychobehavioral and immunological characteristics of adult people with chronic fatigue and patients with chronic fatigue syndrome. *Psychosom. Med.* 1994; **56**: 512–518.

162 Peakman M, Deale A, Field R, Mahalingam M, Wessely S. Clinical improvement in chronic fatigue syndrome is not associated with lymphocyte subsets of function or activation. *Clin. Immunol. Immunopath.* 1997; **82**: 83–91.

163 Lloyd A, Abi-Hanna D, Wakefield D. Interferon and myalgic encephalomyelitis. *Lancet* 1988; **i**: 471.

164 Komaroff A, Geiger A, Wormsely S. IgG subclass deficiencies in chronic fatigue syndrome. *Lancet* 1988; **i**: 1288–1289.

165 Read R, Spickett G, Harvey J, Edwards AJ, Lason HE. IgG1 subclass deficiency in patients with chronic fatigue syndrome. *Lancet* 1988; **i**: 241–242.

166 Hilgers A, Krueger G, Lembke U, Ramon A. Postinfectious chronic fatigue syndrome: case history of thirty-five patients in Germany. *In Vivo* 1991; **5**: 201–206.

167 McCluskey D. Pharmacological approaches to the therapy of chronic fatigue syndrome. In Kleinman A, Straus S (ed.) *Chronic Fatigue Syndrome.* Chichester, Wiley, 1993: 280–297.

168 Wallace D, Peter J, Bowman R, Wormsley S, Silverman S. Fibromyalgia, cytokines, fatigue syndromes and immune regulation. *Adv. Pain Res. Therapy* 1990; **17**: 277–287.

169 Bates D, Buchwald D, Lee J, *et al.* Clinical laboratory test findings in patients with chronic fatigue syndrome. *Arch. Intern. Med.* 1995; **155**: 97–103.

170 Komaroff A, Fagioli L. Medical assessment of fatigue and chronic fatigue syndrome. In Demitrack M, Abbey S (ed.) *Chronic Fatigue Syndrome: An Integrative Approach to Evaluation and Treatment.* New York, Guilford Press, 1996: 154–184.

171 Kminek A, Simunek I, Janatkova I. Chronic fatigue syndrome, complement and infection with Epstein – Barr virus in children. *Complement Inflamm.* 1990; **7**: 125.

172 Komaroff A. Clinical presentation of chronic fatigue syndrome. In Straus S, Kleinman A (ed.) *Chronic Fatigue Syndrome.* Chichester, Wiley, 1993: 43–61.

173 McDonald E, Mann A, Thomas H. Interferons as mediators of psychiatric morbidity. An investigation in a trial of recombinant alpha-interferon in hepatitis-B carriers. *Lancet* 1987; **ii**: 1175–1178

174 Adams F, Quesada JR, Gutterman JU. Neuropsychiatric manifestations of human leukocyte interferon therapy in patients with cancer. *J. Am. Med. Assoc.* 1984; **252:** 938–941.

175 Chapman PB, Lester TJ, Casper ES, *et al.* Clinical pharmacology of recombinant human tumor necrosis factor in patients with advanced cancer. *J. Clin. Oncol.* 1987; **5:** 1942–1951.

176 Moldofsky H. Fibromyalgia, sleep disorder and chronic fatigue syndrome. In Kleinman A, Straus S (ed.) *Chronic Fatigue Syndrome.* Chichester; Wiley, 1993: 262–279.

177 Ho-Yen DO, Carrington D, Armstrong AA. Myalgic encephalomyelitis and alpha-interferon. *Lancet* 1988; **1:** 125.

178 Cheney P, Dorman S, Bell D. Interleukin-2 and the chronic fatigue syndrome. *Ann. Intern. Med.* 1989; **110:** 321.

179 Cotton P. Treatment proposed for chronic fatigue syndrome: research continues to compile data on disorder. *J. Am. Med. Assoc.* 1991; **266:** 2667–2668.

180 Dawson J. Brainstorming the postviral fatigue syndrome. *Br. Med. J.* 1988; **297:** 1151.

181 Chao C, Gallagher M, Phair J, Peterson P. Serum neopterin and interleukin 6 levels in chronic fatigue syndrome. *J. Infect. Dis.* 1990; **162:** 1412–1413.

182 Patarca R, Klimas NG, Lugtendorf S, Antoni M, Fletcher MA. Dysregulated expression of tumor necrosis factor in chronic fatigue syndrome: interrelations with cellular sources and patterns of soluble immune mediator expression. *Clin. Infect. Dis.* 1994; **18:** S147–S153.

183 Coyle P, Krupp L, Mohr K, Doscher C, Mehta P. Immune activation markers in neurological patients with symptomatic chronic fatigue. *Ann. Neurol.* 1991; **30:** 306.

184 Straus SE, Dale JK, Peter JB, Dinarello CA. Circulating lymphokine levels in the chronic fatigue syndrome. *J. Infect. Dis.* 1989; **160:** 1085–1086.

185 Lloyd A, Hickie I, Brockman A, Dwyer J, Wakefield D. Cytokine levels in serum and cerebrospinal fluid in patients with chronic fatigue symptomatic and control subjects. *J. Infect. Dis.* 1991; **164:** 1023–1024.

186 McDonald E, Mann A. Interferon in viral illness and myalgic encephalomyelitis. In Jenkins R, Mowbray J (ed.) *Postviral Fatigue Syndrome.* Chichester, Wiley, 1991: 195–202.

187 Behan PO, Behan WM, Horrobin D. Effect of high doses of essential fatty acids on the postviral fatigue syndrome. *Acta Neurol. Scand.* 1990; **82:** 209–216.

188 MacDonald K, Osterholm M, LeDell K, *et al.* A case control study to assess possible triggers and cofactors in chronic fatigue syndrome. *Am. J. Med.* 1996; **100:** 548–554.

189 Mowbray JF, Yousef GE. Immunology of postviral fatigue syndrome. *Br. Med. Bull.* 1991; **47:** 886–894.

190 Maes M, Bosmans E, Suy E, Vandervorst C, DeJonckheere C, Raus J. Depression-related disturbances in mitogen-induced lymphocyte responses and interleukin-1 beta and soluble interleukin-2 receptor production. *Acta Psychiatr. Scand.* 1991; **84:** 379–386.

191 Rapaport MH, McAllister CG, Pickar D, Nelson DL, Paul SM. Elevated levels of soluble interleukin 2 receptors in schizophrenia. *Arch. Gen. Psychiat.* 1989; **46:** 291–229.

192 Schattner A, Merlin G, Bregman V, *et al.* (2'–5') Oligo A synthetase in human poly-morphonuclear cells increased activity in interferon treatment and in viral infections. *Clin. Exper. Immunol.* 1984; **57:** 265–70.

193 Altmann C, Larratt K, Golubjatnikov R, Kirmani N, Rytel M. Immunologic markers in the chronic fatigue syndrome. *Clin. Res.* 1988; **36:** 845A.

194 Morte S, Castilla A, Civeira MP, Serrano M, Prieto J. Gamma-interferon and chronic fatigue syndrome. *Lancet* 1988; **ii:** 623–624.

195 Lever AM, Lewis DM, Bannister BA, Fry M, Berry N. Interferon production in postviral fatigue syndrome. *Lancet* 1988; **ii:** 101.

196 Hickie I, Lloyd A, Wakefield D, Parker G. The psychiatric status of patients with chronic fatigue syndrome. *Br. J. Psychiatry* 1990; **156:** 534–540.

197 Behan PO, Bakheit AM. Clinical spectrum of postviral fatigue syndrome. *Br. Med. Bull.* 1991; **47**: 793–808.

198 Dufaux B, Order U. Plasma elastase-a, antitrypsin, neopterin, tumor necrosis factor, and soluble interleukin-2 receptor after prolonged exercise. *Int. J. Sports Med.* 1989; **10**: 434–438.

199 Lloyd A, Gandevia S, Brockman A, Hales J, Wakefield D. Cytokine production and fatigue in patients with chronic fatigue syndrome and healthy controls in response to exercise. *Clin. Infect. Dis.* 1994; **18(suppl 1)**: S142–S146.

200 Natelson B, Zhou X, Ottenweller J, *et al.* Effect of acute exhausting exercise on cytokine gene expression in men. *Int. J. Sports Med.* 1996; **17**: 299–302.

201 Treadwell E, Metzger W. Chronic fatigue: psyche or sleep? *Arch. Intern. Med.* 1990; **150**: 1121.

202 Bates D, Schmitt W, Lee J, Kornish R, Komaroff A. Prevalence of fatigue and chronic fatigue syndrome in a primary care practice. *Arch. Intern. Med.* 1993; **153**: 2759–2765.

203 Straus S, Dale J, Wright R, Metcalfe D. Allergy and the chronic fatigue syndrome. *J. Allergy Clin. Immunol.* 1988; **81**: 791–795.

204 Olson GB, Kanaan MN, Gersuk GM, Kelley LM, Jones JF. Correlation between allergy and persistent Epstein–Barr virus infections in chronic-active Epstein–Barr virus-infected patients. *J. Allergy Clin. Immunol.* 1986; **78**: 308–14.

205 Levy J, Landay A, Jessop C, Lennette E. Chronic fatigue syndrome; is it a state of chronic immune activation against an infectious virus? *Contemp. Issues Infect. Dis.* 1993; **10**: 127–145.

206 Griffin DE. Immunologic abnormalities accompanying acute and chronic viral infections. *Rev. Infect. Dis.* 1991; **13**: S129–33.

207 Notkins A, Mergenhagen S, Howard R. Effect of viral infections on the function of the immune system. *Ann. Rev. Microbiol.* 1970; **24**: 525–540.

208 Hickie I, Lloyd A. Are cytokines associated with neuropsychiatric syndromes in humans? *Int. J. Immunopharmacol.* 1995; **17**: 677–683.

209 Kreuger J, Majde J. Cytokines and sleep. *Int. Arch. Allergy Immunol.* 1995; **106**: 97–100.

210 Ojo-Amaize E, Conley E, Peter J. Decreased natural killer cell activity is associated with severity of chronic fatigue syndrome immune dysfunction syndrome. *Clin. Infect. Dis.* 1994; **18**: S157–S159.

211 Wilson A, Hickie I, Lloyd A, *et al.* Longitudinal study of the outcome of chronic fatigue syndrome. *Br. Med. J.* 1994; **308**: 756–760.

212 Wilson A, Hickie I, Lloyd A, Hadzi Pavlovic D, Wakefield D. Cell-mediated immune function and the outcome of chronic fatigue syndrome. *Int. J. Immunopharmacol.* 1995; **17**: 691–694.

213 Clark M, Katon W, Russo J, Kith P, Sintay M, Buchwald D. Chronic fatigue; risk factors for symptom persistence in a 2.5-year follow up study. *Am. J. Med.* 1995; **98**: 187–195.

214 Deale A, Chalder T, Marks I, Wessely S. A randomised controlled trial of cognitive behaviour versus relaxation therapy for chronic fatigue syndrome. *Am. J. Psych.* 1997: 154: 408–414

215 Darko DF, McCutchan JA, Kripke DF, Gillin JC, Golshan S. Fatigue, sleep disturbance, disability, and indices of progression of HIV infection. *Am. J. Psychiatry* 1992; **149**: 514–520.

216 Schleifer SJ, Keller SE, Bond RN, Cohen J, Stein M. Major depressive disorder and immunity. Role of age, sex, severity, and hospitalization. *Arch. Gen. Psychiatry* 1989; **46**: 81–87.

217 Hickie I, Hickie C, Lloyd A, Silove D, Wakefield D. Impaired *in vivo* immune responses in patients with melancholia. *Br. J. Psychiatry* 1993; **162**: 651–657.

218 Maes M, Jacobs J, Lambreckhts J. Evidence for a systemic immune activation during depression; results of leucocyte enumeration by flow cytometry in conjunction with antibody staining. *Psychol. Med.* 1992; **22:** 45–53.

219 Johnson T, Lavender J, Hultin E, Rasmussen A. The influence of avoidance-learning stress of resistance to Coxsackie B virus in mice. *J. Immunol.* 1963; **91:** 569–579.

220 Kiecolt Glaser JK, Fisher LD, Ogrocki P, Stout JC, Speicher CE, Glaser R. Marital quality, marital disruption, and immune function. *Psychosom. Med.* 1987; **49:** 13–34.

221 Kiecolt Glaser JK, Glaser R, Shuttleworth EC, Dyer CS, Ogrocki P, Speicher CE. Chronic stress and immunity in family caregivers of Alzheimer's disease victims. *Psychosom. Med.* 1987; **49:** 523–535.

222 Pennebaker JW, Susman JR. Disclosure of traumas and psychosomatic processes. *Soc. Sci. Med.* 1988; **26:** 327–32.

223 Kielcolt-Glaser J, Garner W, Speigher C, Penn G, Holliday J, Glaser R. Psychosocial modifiers of immunocompetence in medical students. *Psychosom. Med.* 1984; **46:** 7–14.

224 Glaser R, Rice J, Sheridan J, *et al.* Stress-related immune suppression: Health implications. *Brain. Behav. Immunol.* 1987; **1:** 7–20.

225 Cohen S, Williamson G. Stress and infectious disease in humans. *Psychol. Bull.* 1991; **109:** 5–24.

226 Irwin M, Patterson T, Smith TL, *et al.* Reduction of immune function in life stress and depression. *Biol. Psychiat.* 1990; **27:** 22–30.

227 Irwin M, Lacher U, Caldwell C. Depression and reduced natural killer cytotoxicity: a longitudinal study of depressed patients and control subjects. *Psychol. Med.* 1992; **22:** 1045–50.

228 Bartlett J, Schleifer S, Demetrikopoulos M, Keller S. Immune differences in children with and without depression. *Biol. Psychiat.* 1995; **38:** 771–774.

229 Schleifer SJ, Keller SE, Bartlett JA, Eckholdt HM, Delaney BR. Immunity in young adults with major depressive disorder. *Am. J. Psychiatry* 1996; **153:** 477–482.

230 Cover H, Irwin M. Immunity and depression: insomnia, retardation, and reduction of natural killer cell activity. *J. Behav. Med.* 1994; **17:** 217–323.

231 Irwin M, Mascovich A, Gillin JC, Willoughby R, Pike J, Smith TL. Partial sleep deprivation reduces natural killer cell activity in humans. *Psychosom. Med.* 1994; **56:** 493–498.

232 Heisel J, Locke S, Kraus L, Williams R. Natural killer cell activity and MMPI scores of a cohort of college students. *Am. J. Psychiat.* 1986; **143:** 1382–1386.

233 Goodkin K, Blaney NT, Feaster D, *et al.* Active coping style is associated with natural killer cell cytotoxicity in asymptomatic HIV-1 seropositive homosexual men. *J. Psychosom. Res.* 1992; **36:** 635–650.

234 Esterling BA, Antoni MH, Schneiderman N, *et al.* Psychosocial modulation of antibody to Epstein–Barr viral capsid antigen and human herpesvirus type-6 in HIV-1-infected and at-risk gay men. *Psychosom. Med.* 1992; **54:** 3543–71.

235 Antoni MH, Baggett L, Ironson G, *et al.* Cognitive-behavioral stress management intervention buffers distress responses and immunologic changes following notification of HIV-1 seropositivity. *J. Consult. Clin. Psychol.* 1991; **59:** 906–915.

236 Maes M, Bosmans E, Suy E, Minner B, Raus J. A further exploration of the relationships between immune parameters and the HPA-axis activity in depressed patients. *Psychol. Med.* 1991; **21:** 313–320.

237 Arnason B. Nervous system–immune system communication. *Rev. Infect. Dis.* 1991; **13 (suppl 1):** S134–S137.

238 Sternberg E. Emotions and disease: From balance of humours to balance of molecules. *Nat. Med.* 1997; **3:** 264–267.

239 Breder CD, Dinarello CA, Saper CB. Interleukin-1 immunoreactive innervation of the human hypothalamus. *Science* 1988; **240:** 321–324.

240 Sapolsky R, Rivier C, Yamamoto G, Plotsky P, Vale W. Interleukin-1 stimulates the secretion of hypothalamic corticotropin-releasing factor. *Science* 1987; **238:** 522–524.

241 Krueger J, Karnovsky M. Sleep and the immune response. *Ann. NY Acad. Sci.* 1987; **496:** 510–516.

242 Murray DR, Irwin M, Rearden CA, Ziegler M, Motulsky H, Maisel AS. Sympathetic and immune interactions during dynamic exercise. Mediation via a beta 2-adrenergic-dependent mechanism. *Circulation* 1992; **86:** 203–213.

243 Wheeler E, White P, Reed E, Cohen M. Familial incidence of neurocirculatory asthenia ('anxiety neurosis', 'effort syndrome'). *J. Clin. Invest.* 1948: **27:** 562–82.

244 Middleton D, Savage D, Smith D. No association of HLA class II antigens in chronic fatigue syndrome. *Dis. Markers* 1991; **9:** 47–49.

245 Keller RH, Lane JL, Klimas N, *et al.* Association between HLA class II antigens and the chronic fatigue immune dysfunction syndrome. *Clin. Infect. Dis.* 1994; **18:** S154–S156.

246 Shafran S. The chronic fatigue syndrome. *Am. J. Med.* 1991; **90:** 730–739.

247 Levy J. Introduction; viral studies of chronic fatigue syndrome. *Clin. Infect. Dis.* 1994; **18 (suppl 1):** S117–S120.

248 Konstantinov K, von Mikecz A, Buchwald D, Jones J, Gerace L, Tan E. Autoantibodies to nuclear envelope antigens in chronic fatigue syndrome. *J. Clin. Invest.* 1996; **98:** 1888–1896.

10. CFS and psychiatric disorders

10.1 Introduction

We have previously looked at the epidemiology of fatigue (Chapter 2) and the epidemiological evidence for an association between fatigue and psychological distress (Chapter 4). We now turn to fatigue syndromes and their possible associations with discrete psychiatric disorders. Later chapters will consider the role of broader social, cultural, and psychological factors, with specific reference to the aetiology of disability.

Many have commented on the high prevalence of symptoms traditionally associated with psychiatric disorders in subjects labelled as CFS or its equivalents. In one series of 500 patients emotional symptoms were observed in 80 per cent of cases, namely 'mild depression, often accompanied by anxiety, intense introspection and hypochondriasis'[1]. Others write that emotional symptoms are 'cardinal'[2] or 'characteristic'[3], or that depression is 'invariable'[4]. Dowsett reported emotional lability, including depression, elation, and frustration in 98 per cent, and cognitive disturbance in 80 per cent[5].

Psychological symptoms are thus common, but what about psychiatric disorders? All the above authors who reported a high prevalence of psychological symptoms were united in their belief that such observations did not imply a high proportion of psychiatric diagnoses. Before we consider whether or not this was confirmed by systematic research, it is important to review the concept of psychiatric disorder, and its limitations.

Psychiatric diagnosis and medically unexplained syndromes

CFS is only one of a number of common medically unexplained syndromes (see Chapter 14). Such illnesses are problematic because of the prevailing dualism that continues to surround issues of diagnosis[6,7]. By making psychiatric diagnoses one is implicitly subscribing to the idea that illnesses can be separated as physical or mental, and that a psychiatric diagnosis implies the latter. Such views inevitably lead to moralistic judgements, such as that psychiatric diagnoses imply blame or personal weakness (see Chapters 12 and 15). However, such divisions fail to understand the nature of psychiatric diagnosis. In the context of CFS Kendell has pointed out that 'the statement that someone has a depressive illness is merely a statement about their symptoms. It has no causal implications'[8]. A psychiatric diagnosis such as depression or panic disorder is made when the patient describes certain symptoms that are classified under those respective headings – no more and no less. All the other bag and baggage of physical versus mental, blame, responsibility, culpability, and so on is what society and prejudice has added on. The explicit division between physical and mental illness is criticized by nearly everyone who writes about it, yet seems unshakeable.

In the area that is the subject matter of this book, the situation is even worse. The dualistic attitude to classification is even more problematic, since medically unexplained syndromes such as CFS appear in both medical and psychiatric classification systems, but sit comfortably in neither. This confusion is reflected in the current ICD-10 classification. Post-viral fatigue syndrome (with myalgic encephalomyelitis as a synonym) comes under neurology, whereas neurasthenia (with chronic fatigue syndrome as a synonym) comes under psychiatry. However, the descriptions of the two are as near as makes no difference identical[9]. Subsequent clarifications from the World Health Organization made it clear that this was not made on the basis of any evidence of any fundamental distinctions between the two categories, nor to endorse any particular aetiological view of these syndromes. Instead, it was in recognition of the fundamental divide that exists within current views of the syndrome, and hence to enable those on both sides of the divide to record a diagnosis when faced with the chronically fatigued patient. Such a 'solution' emphasizes the weakness of the current classification systems in this area.

At present the medical approach to these disorders sees them as organic diseases, albeit usually of functional rather than structural nature. The psychiatric approach sees them as psychiatric disorders, such as depression and anxiety, albeit often presenting atypically and/or somatoform disorders in which psychogenesis is also presumed. But what if both are correct – the patient having a disorder of function, such as irritable bowel syndrome, but also meeting criteria for depression? Is this medical or psychiatric?

Clearly there is no correct answer to this question. All classification systems are compromises. Although the intellectual case for multi-axial classification, particularly in the area of medically unexplained syndromes, is overwhelming[10], neither doctors nor patients will ever shift from the need to give a single answer to the question 'what is wrong with me or my patient?'. In these circumstances it is necessary to accept the importance of diagnostic systems, not least because they may convey valuable information on outcome and appropriate treatment.

Table 10.1 shows that psychiatric disorders are frequently diagnosed in CFS. Different investigators have used different instruments and different criteria; but a pattern can be discerned. Depressive disorders are common, followed by somatization disorder and anxiety disorders. However, a substantial minority do not fulfil criteria for any psychological disorder. This pattern is consistent, even when either fatigue[11], or other symptoms held to be characteristic of CFS[12–14] are excluded from the criteria used for diagnosing psychiatric disorder. We will consider each category in turn.

Table 10.1 Psychiatric symptoms in fatigued patients. Updated from David[65] with permission

Reference	Setting	No. of subjects with chronic fatigue or % of sample	Assessment	Psychiatric morbidity (fatigued vs non-fatigued)
A: Patients in primary care				
Morrison[133]	Colorado	176/7600 fatigue main complaint (2.3%)	GP records	41% psychological (18% depression) 39% physical (20% virus)
Buchwald et al.[134]	Boston	105 (21%) (of 500)	Interview	78% depressed 60% anxious
Kroenke et al.[135]	Army Primary Care (US)	24% (of 1159) 28% F; 19% M fatigue a major problem >30 days	BDI MSPQ MBHI	56% vs 0% depression 57% vs 12% anxiety
Cathebras et al.[136]	Canada	93/686 13.5%	DIS SCL-90 CES-D	45% lifetime psych. diag. vs 28% controls 17% current major depression vs 8.8 controls 1.1 vs 1.0 SD
McDonald et al.[56]	UK	77/686 (11%) CF	CIS-R	72% any ICD-9 diagnosis 36% neurotic depression
Cope et al.[113]	UK	64 post-infectious fatigue	CIS-R BDI STAI	76% any ICD-9 diag. 48% BDI cases vs 8% controls
Ridsdale et al.[137]	UK	220 CF	GHQ-12	CF 3 times more likely to have previons depresion or anxiety
Wessely et al.[57]	UK	214 CF and CFS	GHQ-12 HAD CIS	CF; 60% current psych. vs 19% control (OR 6.4) CFS: 75% current psych. (OR 5.5)

Table 10.1 (*contd*)

Reference	Setting	No. of subjects with chronic fatigue or % of sample	Assessment	Psychiatric morbidity (fatigued vs non-fatigued)
Hickie et al.[138]	Australia	398/1593 (25%)	GHQ CIDI	Odds ratio (psych disorder) for fatigued vs non-fatigued cases = 6.2 21% current depression (30% lifetime) 16% current anxiety (34% lifetime)
B: Patients in hospital settings				
Manu et al.[50]	Fatigue clinic (US)	100	DIS	66% any current psych. diagnosis: 36% depression
Millon et al.[139]	Allergy clinic (US)	20 past EBV	HAM-D POMS	95% scored >20 = mod. depression
Valdini et al.[140]	New York health centre	22	SCL-90	68% 'depressed'
Kruesi et al.[12]	Tertiary care (US) (clinical trial)	28 'chronic EBV'	DIS	75% psych. diag. 46% MDE
Manu et al.[141]	Fatigue clinic (US)	71	DIS	73% psych. diag. 68% depression
Schweitzer et al.[142]	Fatigue clinic (US)	40	IBQ GHQ	67% GHQ cases
Lane et al.[143]	Fatigue clinic (US)	43	PSE	42% any current psych. diag. (33% depression)
Shanks and Ho-Yen[23]	Infectious clinic (Scotland)	64	SADS GHQ HAD	45% psych. diag.
Bombardier and Buchwald[144]	CFS clinic (US)	445	DIS	Current: CF 20% MDE, 7% panic CFS 21% MDE 11% panic Lifetime: CF 65% MDE, 21% SD CFS 74% MDE, 32% SD

Table 10.1 (*contd*)

Reference	Setting	No. of subjects with chronic fatigue or % of sample	Assessment	Psychiatric morbidity (fatigued versus non-fatigued)
Clark et al.[49]	CFS clinic (US)	98	DIS IDD-L GHQ	Current: 41% any psych. disorder (10% MDE, 9% panic, 24% SD, 17% GAD) Lifetime: (76% any psych disorder 70% MDE, 29% panic, 33% GAD)
C: Patients in hospital settings including normal or medical controls				
Taerk et al.[108]	Fatigue clinic (Canada)	24	DIS	67% lifetime major depress vs 29% controls
Wessely and Powell[11]	Neurological hospital (UK)	47	SADS	72% psych. diag. (67% MDE) vs 36% neurological controls
Hickie et al.[110]	Australia Fatigue clinic (clinical trial)	48	SCID IBQ	46% major depression 2% SD
Gold et al.[109]	Viral clinic (US)	26	DIS	42% current MDE 73% lifetime MDE
Wood et al.[14]	Fatigue clinic (UK)	34	PSE	41% 'cases' 23.5% depression: medical controls 15% (15% MDE)
Katon et al.[13]	Fatigue clinic (US)	98	DIS	45% current psych. diag. (15% MDE, 11% panic, 20% SD): medical controls 6% 86% lifetime psych. diag.: medical controls 48%
Blakely et al.[46]	Fatigue clinic (New Zealand)	58	GHQ MMPI BDI WOC	Males; 63% GHQ cases vs 16% controls: 63% Beck cases vs 13% controls Females: GHQ case 57% vs 11%: Beck 48% vs 10%
Pepper et al.[85]	Fatigue Clinic (US)	45	SCID CES-D MCMI	51% lifetime psych. diag. vs 32% controls 23% current psych. diag. vs 8% controls

Table 10.1 (*contd*)

Reference	Setting	No. of subjects with chronic fatigue or % of sample	Assessment	Psychiatric morbidity (fatigued vs non-fatigued)
Vercoulen *et al.*[145]	Fatigue clinic (Netherlands)	298	SCL-90 BDI	36% depression
Swanink *et al.*[146]	Fatigue clinic (Netherlands)	88	BDI	Depression: 18% CFS vs 18% controls
Farmer *et al.*[34]	Fatigue clinic (UK)	100	SCAN	34% somatoform vs 0% controls 34% current depression vs 8% 23% anxiety vs 18% 97% neurasthenia vs 2% any psych. disorder: OR = 2.5
Johnson *et al.*[17]	Fatigue clinic (USA)	48	DIS BDI	45% any psych. disorder 35% depression (psych. disorder prior to onset excluded)
Fischler *et al.*[35]	Fatigue clinic (Belgium)	53	SCID	Any current disorder: 77% CFS vs 50% medical controls 30% MDE vs 10% medical controls 57% GAD vs 14% medical controls

Abbreviations:
BDI: Beck Depression Inventory
CES-D: Center for Epidemiologic Studies Depression Scale
CF: chronic fatigue
CFS: chronic fatigue syndrome
CIDI: Composite International Diagnostic Interview
CIS-R: Revised Clinical Interview Schedule
DIS: Diagnostic Interview Schedule
GAD: generalized anxiety disorder
HAD: Hospital Anxiety and Depression Scale
HAM-D: Hamilton Rating Scale for Depression
IBQ: Illness Behaviour Questionnaire
IDD-L: Inventory to Diagnose Depression
MBHI: Millon Behavioural Health Inventory

MCMI: Millon Clinical Multiaxial Inventory
MDE: major depressive episode
MMPI: Minnesota Multiphasic Personality Inventory
MSPQ: Modified Somatic Perception Questionnaire
OR: odds ratio
PILL: Pennebaker Inventory of Limbic Languidness
POMS: Profile of Mood States
PSE: Present State Examination
SADS: Schedule for Affective Disorders and Schizophrenia
SCAN: Schedule for Clinical Assessment in Neuropsychiatry
SCID: Structured Clinical Interview for DSM-IIIR
SD: somatization disorder
STAI: Spielberger Trait Anxiety Inventory
SCL-90: Symptom Checklist
WOC: ways of coping.

10.2 CFS and depression

In Chapter 4 we noted that fatigue is a common symptom of low mood. It is not the only one, but it is striking that the other symptoms routinely complained of by depressed subjects are similar to those encountered in CFS, not just in their nature but also in the relative frequency with which they occur[15]. Lists of symptom frequencies provided[16] could easily be substituted for those found in both professional and popular articles on CFS. When direct comparisons are made, CFS patients and those with major depression had a similar range of somatic symptoms[11,17], differences only being evidence for muscle pain at rest[11] or after exercise[18]. The epidemiology of depression, with its over-representation of women and peak prevalence in young adults between 25 and 44, is similar to that claimed for CFS. Given the overlap in both symptoms and epidemiology, the frequency with which operationally defined affective disorder is found in samples of CFS is not unexpected (see Table 10.1).

Clinicians are therefore right to point out there are many patients who present with chronic fatigue and/or a label of CFS but in whom a diagnosis of major depression is a more parsimonious label conveying relevant information about likely aetiology, treatment, and prognosis. On the other hand, clinicians who, like the authors, have experience of both CFS and conventional psychiatric clinics are also aware that even if operational criteria emphasize the common ground between CFS and depression, there are also differences that are as revealing as the similarities. Some of these differences will be considered in the subsequent chapter on the neurobiology of CFS (Chapter 11). Others relate to the heterogeneity of depression as a concept.

One of these grey areas is the concept of atypical depression. A specific lack of 'physical energy' is one of the criteria for atypical depression, which can be diagnosed when a subject has mood change associated with two or more of the following features – extreme fatigue, overeating, oversleeping, and chronic oversensitivity to rejection[19]. An overlap with CFS can thus be expected. Indeed, the question in the SCID (a standardized interview used to make DSM-IIIR diagnoses) concerning atypical depression reads as follows: 'Do your arms and legs sometimes feel heavy, as though they were full of lead? Is it ever a physical effort to climb stairs or get out of bed?'. To date only one report has addressed this problem – Demitrack and colleagues found that 63 per cent of their CFS sample fulfilled criteria for major depressive disorder, of whom nearly all were atypical in presentation. However, only 14 per cent of a group of DSM-IIIR atypical depressives met full CDC criteria for CFS[20].

A closer inspection of the phenomenology of CFS and classic major depression reveals other areas of difference. Although the somatic symptoms of depression closely resemble the somatic symptoms of CFS, the same may not be true of the more cognitive ones. Powell *et al.* contrasted the symptomatology of depressed inpatients in a psychiatric hospital with that of a sample of CFS patients, largely outpatients, in a neurological centre[21]. The hypothesis that CFS patients would show less evidence of such cognitive features as low self-esteem, suicidal ideation, and hopelessness was confirmed, as others have observed before[22] and since[17,23,24]. The authors interpreted this as indicating that, when confronted by the same core symptoms, an individual's cognitive and attributional style affects these expressions of pathological guilt, and that external attribution to a virus (implicit in the self-diagnosis of ME which nearly all had made) protects self-esteem, but at the expense of self-control and personal efficacy. Thus CFS patients believing their symptoms to be the result of a virus, and not their own actions, will be protected from self-blame and guilt, but at the cost of increased helplessness in the face of an invisible, external adversary (Chapter 12). On the other hand, it is also argued that these differences are simply more direct expressions of a different psychopathological process[17], and that perceived helplessness and loss of control, whilst present, is not related to depression[25]. At the moment the argument is unresolved, but it does highlight how plastic is the phenomenology of both CFS and depression. The strength of the association between depression and CFS is determined by which concepts of both depression and CFS are employed. If depression is defined in a manner emphasizing such cognitive features as guilt and suicidal intention, then it will be less common in CFS, whereas a definition emphasizing more biological features, less influenced by personality, will result in increased rates.

Much of the dispute about the links between CFS and depression is a consequence of a failure to recognize how fluid are the boundaries of depression, and the modern tendency to ignore the nuances of phenomenology in favour of rigid adherence to psychiatric diagnostic classification, reflected in a tendency to lump all these different feelings as dysphoric mood. An older literature points out that depression is accompanied by the feeling of fatigue on slightest exertion, as described in CFS, but in a primary depressive illness this sense of fatigue is accompanied by a loss also of pleasure, both in anticipation of the act, and after its fulfilment[26,27]. This may be observed for both physical and mental effort[28]. There remain many difficulties in assessing mood disorder (see Chapter 16). Many CFS patients state that what they experience is a feeling different from sadness, which they recognize as emotional distress, and more like something 'physical'[29]. They also frequently emphasize not a loss of interest in activity, but frustration at not being able to undertake any. Diurnal variation also seems to differ between CFS and classic depression[30]. As Healy points out[31], psychiatrists should be the professionals most interested in paying attention to the patient's own description of feelings. Healy goes on the blame this on the

Freudian legacy – a disinclination to take the patient's own explanations at face value. CFS provides an opportunity for both psychiatrists and physicians to rediscover the importance of phenomenology[32].

10.3 CFS and anxiety

There are many reasons why anxiety disorders might occur with CFS. The intense experience of somatic symptoms such as fatigue, headache, dizziness, and chest pain characterizes panic disorder. The diagnosis of generalized anxiety disorder (GAD) requires at least three symptoms from a list including easy fatigue, difficulty concentrating, irritability, poor sleep, and muscle tension. Avoidance behaviour is the defining characteristic of phobic disorders. Avoidance behaviour is often encountered in CFS as a strategy to reduce symptoms (although it can be hard to separate it from exercise intolerance). The early studies of psychiatric morbidity make surprisingly little mention of the anxiety disorders, but this is probably because nearly all used diagnostic systems such as the DSM-III, RDC, and CATEGO that insist on the primacy of mood over anxiety disorders.

The picture has started to change. In one study of 200 patients with a chief complaint of fatigue, 13 per cent fulfilled criteria for current panic disorder, which almost always preceded or was concurrent with the onset of chronic fatigue[33]. Three recent studies suggested an increased role for anxiety disorders, with about 20 per cent fulfilling criteria for one or more anxiety disorders[34,35]. Specifically a Belgian study reported an eightfold increased risk of generalized anxiety disorder (GAD) compared with medical controls[35].

Another area in which CFS and anxiety disorders might overlap is via the process of hyperventilation. Hyperventilation is an abnormality of respiratory control, and is defined as breathing in excess of metabolic requirements[36]. It causes a fall in arterial carbon dioxide levels, which in turn produces a wide variety of somatic symptoms, including fatigue[37]. It is a process, rather than a diagnosis, and can have a number of causes, both psychological and physical.

Interest in a possible link between CFS and hyperventilation pre-dates the current revival of fatigue syndromes, and can be found in both previous and recent writings on effort syndromes (see Chapters 6 and 14). However, in this country it has been championed by a cardiological team at Charing Cross Hospital led by Peter Nixon[38,39]. Nixon and his colleagues have claimed that 'all the patients . . . previously diagnosed by physicians as suffering from myalgic encephalomyelitis or postviral fatigue and then referred to us turned out to have effort syndrome (exhaustion and hyperventilation)'[33]. They went on to diagnose chronic hyperventilation in 93 out of 100 consecutive referrals[39].

Nixon uses a homeostatic model of the body, and views CFS as the result of excessive and prolonged arousal, with the individual continually striving beyond the limits of his or her physiological and psychological tolerance. According to this somewhat anachronistic model the result is chronic hyperventilation[40]. That chronic hyperventilation can cause symptoms that are close to those in CFS is certainly true[41] – the question is just how often does this occur in practice?

The answer is not as frequently as Nixon claims. There are no specific symptoms for hyperventilation, and the methods used to diagnose hyperventilation in these and other studies have been criticized[36]. An American study noted that ventilatory responses to carbon dioxide were normal, but that resting pCO_2 was lower in the CFS patients than controls[42] suggesting mild hyperventilation at rest. In a series of consecutive patients examined at King's College Hospital only 13 per cent fulfilled definite and 16 per cent borderline criteria for hyperventilation[43]. Riley and colleagues also studied exercise capacity and found no evidence for hyperventilation[44].

Even in those in whom hyperventilation is confirmed, the pathophysiology of fatigue is not clear: Folgering and Snik noted that subjective fatigue did not correlate with EMG measures of fatigability, and concluded that fatigue is not simply due to hyperventilation-induced changes in muscle performance[37]. In a series of patients with 'behavioural breathlessness', a syndrome corresponding to the old concept of effort syndrome (see Chapter 14) and overlapping with CFS, breathing retraining improved measures of hyperventilation, but not depression, anxiety, or fatigue[45]. Hyperventilation may play an important role in a subset of patients with CFS, but care must be taken not to exaggerate its role.

10.4 CFS, somatic symptoms, and somatization disorder

Somatic symptoms and CFS

Whereas studies of CFS usually find subjects scoring midway between normal and psychiatric controls on most measures, such as the Beck Depression Inventory, the General Health Questionnaire, and so on, there is one exception. CFS patients endorse more somatic symptoms than either psychiatric or medical controls[13,25,46,47]. In a study conducted at the National Hospital for Neurology CFS patients had a mean number of 14 somatic symptoms, compared with 8 for neurological and 11 for depressed controls[11]. The number of somatic symptoms is related to functional impairment and prognosis – the more, the worse are both[48,49].

Somatization disorder and CFS

It has already been suggested that the majority of those seen in the CFS clinic fulfil criteria for psychiatric disorder, whatever that means. Somatization is thus relevant on two levels. First, most of those seen in specialist care believe they have a physical illness (see below). If they also fulfil criteria for known psychiatric disorders they hence fulfil the Goldberg criteria for somatization. Second, a subgroup will fulfil criteria for the specific category of somatization disorder.

Rates of somatization disorder

Whereas psychiatric disorder is common in CFS settings, somatization disorder is not. In one of the earliest studies Manu and colleagues reported a prevalence of 15 per cent[50]. Manu's group diagnosed the condition in 5 per cent of fatigued cases not meeting CDC criteria, but 28 per cent of those fulfilling the criteria for CFS[51]. Most studies find between 10 and 20 per cent of patients fulfil criteria (see Clark and Katon[52] and Table 10.2). One criticism that can be made of this finding is the problem of tautology, since the definitions of both CFS and somatization disorder require multiple symptoms[53]. When Lane and colleagues compared those with CFS with chronically fatigued patients who did not fulfil the criteria for CFS, one of chief differences between them was that the former were more likely to fulfil criteria for somatization disorder[51]. They concluded that the multiple symptom criteria for CFS actively select for somatization disorder. When those symptoms that were included in both the definitions of CFS and SD were excluded, the prevalence of SD fell from 46 to 20 per cent[13].

Table 10.2 Prevalence of somatization disorder in hospital samples of chronic fatigue syndrome

Reference	Prevalence (%)
Bombardier and Buchwald[144]	32
Clark et al.[49]	24
Farmer et al.[34]	34 (all ICD-10 somatoform disorders); 15 (DSM-IIIR)
Fiedler et al.	12
Fischler et al.[35]	11
Hickie et al.[110]	0
Katon et al.[13]	20
Kruesi et al.[12]	7
Lane et al.[51]	28
Johnson et al.[53]	6
Manu and Matthews[50]	15
Wessely and Powell[11]	15
Wood et al.[14]	6

Somatization disorder is thus found in CFS clinics, but it is not common. Somatization disorder is also not unique to CFS clinics, and a similar situation exists in general medical clinics. The best survey to date, carried out by Van Hemert and colleagues in Utrecht[54], found a prevalence in all new medical outpatients of 8 per cent, rising to 14 per cent in those with doubtful medical diagnoses, not dramatically different from the prevalence in CFS clinics.

On the other hand, somatization disorder is uncommon in samples of chronically fatigued patients identified in general practice – with a prevalence of 0.6 per cent in the ECA sample[55]. No cases were found in two UK community samples[56,57]. It is also very uncommon in the community – the expected community prevalences range from 0.03 to 0.3 per cent[58].

The relevance of somatization disorder to CFS

Does this matter? If it is simply a question of swapping labels, then why not simply replace somatization disorder with CFS, which is certainly more acceptable to patients. One reason for caution is that to do so would turn one's back on the considerable research that already exists concerning somatization disorder, which has been shown to have some validity in terms of prognosis, genetics, and treatment response, even if its aetiology remains unclear. We feel that the concept of somatization disorder, whilst not without its weaknesses, can be of use.

Somatization disorder is part of medical life, rather than something intrinsic to CFS. Donna Stewart documented how one sample of patients with 'twentieth-century disease', also known as total allergy syndrome, had at various times also been labelled as having candidiasis, hypoglycaemia, food allergy, and now chronic fatigue syndrome[59]. In a CFS clinic complaints of food intolerance were associated with the presence of somatization disorder[60]. Many would have consistently fulfilled criteria for somatization disorder throughout their illness careers, even if their own disease attribution changed. A cadre of such patients now appears in the guise of chronic fatigue syndrome, and can be sighted in the self-help or media literature. Such patients may not shed much light on the nature of chronic fatigue syndrome as it exists in general practice, but may illuminate our understanding of the sociology of illness and illness behaviour (see Chapter 15).

Various groups have started to recognize this problem. Australian researchers have presented data showing that a minority of those seen in a CFS clinic can be differentiated from the majority by such variables as duration, prognosis, psychological morbidity, and disability, and also an index of immunological dysfunction[61]. They argue that the minority group should be classified under the somatoform disorders, reserving the label CFS for those with shorter duration, fewer more 'typical' symptoms, and less disability. The UK consensus criteria[62] also suggest that CFS should not be diagnosed if the subject fulfils criteria for somatization disorder (whereas depression or anxiety are still compatible with a diagnosis of CFS). Acknowledging the concept of somatization disorder is beneficial to researchers who wish to further the understanding of CFS – it seems likely that distinguishing between chronically fatigued patients with and without somatization disorder will assist research into the nature of the former.

Moving from research to clinical practice, the utility of excluding somatization disorder from CFS becomes less clear. Many patients who fulfil criteria for somatization and attend CFS clinics hold strong convictions regarding their diagnosis, and it is rarely, if ever, fruitful to challenge them. Providing the diagnosis is recognized by the clinician, it may be more helpful to manage the patient using the strategies currently advocated for the treatment of somatization disorder[63] whilst retaining the label of CFS.

A multidimensional approach to somatization

We emphasize that we take a wide view of the process of somatization and its relevance to chronic fatigue syndrome. We have discussed in this section somatization either as a process (the Goldberg view) or a discrete disorder (the DSM-IV view). However, somatisation has further meanings[64]. In other sections of this book we consider the pathophysiology of somatic symptoms and the role of such factors as sleep, hyperventilation, and inactivity on the experience of chronic fatigue. In Chapter 12 we will explore the role of cognitions, behaviours, and attributions on the experience, reporting, and persistence of somatic symptoms in general, and chronic fatigue in particular.

10.5 CFS and hysteria

Given the well known difficulties with the concept and diagnosis of hysteria, which have led many authorities to propose it should cease to be used, we are tempted to avoid the issue altogether. Nevertheless, the label of 'hysteria' has so often been attached to CFS and CFS-like conditions that some comment is necessary.

Physicians, both in the past and present, have described individual patients as hysterical. Perhaps the only change over the years is that doctors are less likely to do so in public. Usually the word is used in its pejorative sense, as an alternative for malingering, difficult, argumentative, histrionic, and so on. On the other hand, the specific use of the term 'hysteria', meaning a conversion disorder, in which psychological distress and/or conflicts are 'converted' or expressed as a loss of physical function, is largely restricted to psychiatric practice. Systematic studies have failed to show a firm association between conversion disorder and CFS. Although all the current psychiatric diagnostic systems include a category for hysteria/conversion disorder, only one paper reported a single case[11] and that was from Queen Square, London, the traditional home of hysteria. We agree with Anthony David[65] who writes that it seems unlikely that psychiatrists currently use the 'H' word in the context of CFS. This is confirmed by the evidence of controlled studies.

Some studies find that some CFS patients show abnormal fatigue or weakness in the testing situation, but when electrically stimulated the muscles behave normally (see Chapter 8). Such findings are compatible with an hysterical origin to symptoms in some patients. However, by no means all studies report this finding, and other explanations are possible for the failure of central drive.

Thus hysteria, used properly as meaning conversion disorder, is rarely a tenable explanation for CFS. Three caveats are necessary. First, in the context of epidemic forms of ME, explanations involving transmitted emotional distress ('mass hysteria'), merit attention. However, as we and others have also shown[66], such examples have little to do with CFS. Second, the term 'Briquet's hysteria' is sometimes used to describe somatization disorder (see above). Finally, there is a modest overlap between current concepts of conversion disorder used by both child psychiatrists and paediatricians, and CFS in children (see Chapter 13).

10.6 CFS and hypochondriasis

Hypochondriasis describes a syndrome in which the person's main concern is with the possibility of suffering from an organic disease and has implications for psychological management, especially as regards reassurance[67]. However, hypochondriasis implies fear of illness – in our experience most CFS patients have already, for whatever reason and from whatever source, identified the illness they are suffering from, and hence hypochondriasis is usually an inappropriate label or concept.

10.7 CFS and eating disorders

Behan and Bakheit[68] report that the 'psychiatric status in a small number of patients has progressed to a definite disturbance of eating, most commonly anorexia nervosa. Several patients indeed have a clinical condition indistinguishable from severe anorexia nervosa with depression'. From the other perspective researchers from Edinburgh[69] reported four patients with anorexia nervosa who claimed their illness began with a viral-like illness and speculate that if CFS results from a deficiency of corticotrophin releasing hormone (CRH; see Chapter 11) then anorexia might result from an excess. There are also overlaps between immunological findings in anorexia and CFS[70]. However, case series that attempt to link common events such as viral infection with specific disorders must be regarded with considerable caution.

10.8 CFS, stress, and life events

It is often anecdotally claimed that the onset of CFS is associated not only with infection, but also with stressful life events. We have already drawn attention to the Victorian literature on neurasthenia that made a similar observation (Chapters 5 and 6). In the modern era one-third of patients in one series reported a stressful event prior to onset[14] rising to 95 per cent in another[71]. However, such observations are strongly affected by recall bias, and need confirmation by standardized methods of inquiry.

Perhaps surprisingly such confirmation has been hard to acquire. In a small series self-reported stressful life events were commoner in the year prior to the onset of illness in 25 CFS sufferers compared with controls. On the other hand, a life events checklist showed no differences between subjects with CFS, those with irritable bowel syndrome, and normal controls[72]. The best evidence so far comes from studies that used the time-consuming and detailed life events methodology developed by George Brown and the Bedford College group. Researchers led by Peter White at St Bartholomew's Hospital prospectively studied patients in primary care presenting with acute infectious mononucleosis[73]. The coincidence of a life event and infection was strongly associated with development of post-infectious psychiatric disorder, and in particular depression. However, social adversity did not influence the development of a pure fatigue syndrome, which White has elsewhere argued can be distinguished from depression after glandular fever[74]. On the other hand, Hatcher and colleagues in Leeds found that 60 per cent of CFS patients had a severe life event or difficulty in the nine months prior to the onset of illness, compared with 20 per cent of controls (Hatcher, personal communication). Life events classified as 'dilemmas' made up much of this excess.

There is more evidence to suggest that life stress influences outcome. In a study of CFS that used a life events schedule Collette Ray and her colleagues found negative life events were associated not with chronic fatigue *per se*, but with emotional distress[75]. Social stress was similarly associated with psychiatric morbidity rather than chronic fatigue in a primary care study[56]. Negative life events predict a poor outcome in fibromyalgia patients[76]. On the other hand positive experiences did improve both fatigue and impairment[75]. A natural experiment was provided by the coincidence of Hurricane Andrew and the large group of CFS patients followed up by the Miami group[77]. The experience of the hurricane produced a worsening of symptoms in the patients, particularly in those emotionally distressed by the disaster. The San Francisco earthquake had a similar effect on neurasthenia sufferers[78].

One particular life event that is becoming increasingly controversial is the trauma of road accidents. The reason for the prominence of this particular stressor is clear – the potential involvement of the courts. Do road accidents trigger CFS? The answer is we don't know. The only data of which we are aware comes from Canada, where Salit noted that 4 per cent of his specialist sample report a link with trauma. No aetiological conclusions can be drawn from such observations, nor does Salit attempt any. A similar and more long-standing problem exists in the USA, where the category of post-traumatic fibromyalgia attracts considerable attention and controversy[79], particularly in the medicolegal arena[80–82].

The particular prominence of CFS and road traffic accidents arises from the lead case of Page versus Smith, during which one of the authors (SW) gave expert testimony. Mr Page was the blameless victim of a road traffic accident, when his car was in collision with another vehicle. He had a history of what had first been called chronic neurotic disorder, and later changed to post-viral fatigue. He was recovering from one such episode at the time of the collision. He suffered no physical injury in the accident, but within hours had experienced many of his old symptoms again.

No virological or neurological process could explain this sequence of events, but it was argued on Mr Page's behalf by the author that the best explanation was analogous to the sequence of events leading to post-traumatic stress – in other words it was, to use the legal term, nervous shock, that had precipitated the relapse of his condition. Whether one chose to label it as post-viral fatigue, depression, or somatization did not matter, although it mattered considerably to Mr Page. His previous illness thus rendered him vulnerable to such a reaction after an accident which would leave most of us unscathed. The argument thus depended on the legal adage 'you take your victim as you find him or her', or the concept of the egg-shell skull/personality.

Mr Page won, but not without making legal history. The judgment went through the Court of Appeal, to the House of Lords, and back to the Court of Appeal. The reason was not to establish the existence of CFS, as some erroneously thought, but to establish the concept of foreseeability and vulnerability. The decision had far-reaching implications for the field of personal injury litigation, not all of them beneficial[83]. However, these need not concern us. Did the judgment establish that nervous shock i.e. traumatic life events can cause CFS?

The answer is no. First, the case was about relapse, not causation. Second, the court in its wisdom decided to accept the anecdotal observations of Mr Page's doctors, including the author, that they had encountered, in routine clinical practice, similar cases before. Courts are entitled to make that judgment, but that does not make it true. We have already discussed at length the problems in relating the onset of CFS to the occurrence of viral infection. All of these epidemiological and methodological problems apply equally to attempts to determine the link, if any, between trauma and CFS, with the added spice of the medicolegal colossus.

In general we have reservations about some of the claims made both for and against the role of stress and CFS. This partly reflects the reluctance of research-minded psychiatrists and epidemiologists to use the term, because of its imprecise, subjective nature, and difficulties in assessment. It is indeed an 'unreliable word best used sparingly'[84].

10.9 CFS, personality, and personality disorder

For some psychiatrists, personality means personality disorder – stable abnormalities of personality development. Various classifications exist in the literature, and a few researchers have attempted to match these descriptions in clinical studies of CFS. The results have not been dramatic. Personality disorders (known as Axis II disorders to distinguish them from Axis I symptom-based diagnoses such as depression or anxiety) are not a prominent feature of CFS. Some studies have shown a variety of personality disorders in CFS patients, including obsessive-compulsive, avoidant, borderline, and histrionic, but no more than in controls with multiple sclerosis or depression[85,86], emphasizing the effect both mood disorder and chronic illness have on personality. We think it unlikely that further study of personality disorder will shed more light on the nature of CFS. However, the concept of personality and CFS is very much alive, not least in the accounts of the sufferers themselves.

Our experience, shared by many others, is that CFS patients as seen in our clinics are particularly likely to give a history of being fit and athletic prior to becoming ill[44,87–89]. The behavioural models of CFS that we espouse would predict that such patients would be at risk of rapid physical deconditioning after a period of enforced rest, more so than those, who, like one of the current authors (SW), have long since abandoned any pretensions of keeping fit. Similarly, many patients say that when they first became ill, they were likely to adopt overaggressive early attempts at exercise. The popular literature strongly reinforces this image: sufferers are prone to be overactive, unlikely to take things easy, 'the last types to take time of work for no good reason'[90]. 'It seemed like a bad bout of flu from which (as usual) I did not allow myself proper time to recover'[91], or 'I refused to admit something was wrong'[92]. Another blamed her relapse because 'I am a workaholic, the old demon took over'[93]. Sufferers 'work until they drop, whilst everyone else creeps to bed with the slightest headache or sniffle . . . lazy people don't get ME'[94].

This leads into the area of personality and CFS[95]. In a later chapter we will note how the popular, and indeed self, image of the typical sufferer is frequently that of the conscientious, successful, dedicated person with high standards and responsibilities. We will also suggest that such observations assist in understanding why sufferers might succumb to stressors or triggers that might not have such an influence on less conscientious individuals, and how such observations are also in keeping with a cognitive behavioural model of the illness (Chapter 12).

Such observations, whilst a valuable insight into the perceptions of the sufferer as described in the literature and encountered in the clinic, are anecdotal, and subject to a number of biases. What does the literature show? Two recent studies provided support for the frequent clinical observation that some sufferers seen in specialist centres report premorbid personalities and lifestyles characterized by a tendency to 'oversubscribe to social norms that dictate exhaustion as a way of life'[96], mirrored in particularly strenuous work and social lives[97]. Clinicians rated another series of patients as having 'high self imposed expectations'[35]. When medical anthropologists Norma Ware and Arthur Kleinman studied 50 CFS patients attending the practice of Anthony Komaroff in Boston, they found that 'a desire for accomplishment and success, underwritten by exacting standards for personal performance, impelled these individuals always to try harder, go further, in an attempt to meet the expectations that had set for themselves at work, home and school'. The recorded interviews were full of such phrases as 'hyper', 'always on the go', 'workaholic', and so on[96,98]. On the other hand, although in another series sufferers rated themselves as more 'hard driving' than controls, and to have more outside activities prior to illness, so did patients with irritable bowel syndrome[72]. Similarly, a study of 100 patients attending the fatigue clinic at King's College Hospital and controls with rheumatoid arthritis failed to show any substantial differences between the two groups[99].

We are not surprised that there exist inconsistencies in the research literature. All such accounts are retrospective assessments, usually by the sufferer themselves, of their personality before the onset of illness. Any retrospective account of personality is subject to recall bias, but we suspect such forces are particularly active in CFS. Why is personality so emphasized in the narratives of CFS sufferers? One reason is that is how CFS sufferers are, but there are other possibilities. We believe that such histories give an insight into the broader social factors that lie behind the current interest in CFS, and to which we will devote more attention in Chapter 15. The importance of the repeated observation of the particular personality characteristics of sufferers might be to emphasize the non-psychiatric nature of CFS. The current president of the ME Association stated that one of the distinctive differences between ME sufferers and depressives is that those with ME are highly motivated achievers – 'they almost have too much willpower, whereas depressives have virtually none'[100].

If depression, hysteria, and so on occur in malingerers, shirkers, and those with low moral fibre, then establishing that the CFS sufferer has none of these characteristics is a necessary part of legitimization. Sufferers are more likely to 'have a good premorbid personality and work record'[101]; indeed, 'the fact that they were all known to have good premorbid personalities made us consider an organic cause for their illness'[2]. Good premorbid personality does not prevent psychiatric disorder, but many believe it does. It is plausible that sufferers, in circumstances where they perceive the possibility of receiving a psychiatric diagnosis, emphasize those aspects of personality and behaviour which appear to provide evidence against psychiatric disorder.

The role of personality and achievement is thus confusing. As with the alleged excess of medical personnel among sufferers, one must not neglect the role of selection bias. Relevant factors may be illness behaviour, access to medical care, and so on. Our own intuition is that, once the dust has settled, CFS sufferers will be found to have personalities neither better nor worse than anyone else.

10.10 Why might psychiatric disorders be associated with CFS?

The evidence for some association between psychiatric disorder and CFS is convincing. We now turn to possible explanations of this association, for which there are several[65,102,103]. We have already considered the possible links between fatigue and psychiatric disorder (Chapter 4); we will now only consider those with particular relevance to CFS:

(1) misdiagnosis;

(2) simple physical illness model – a reaction to disability;

(3) complex physical illness model – helplessness, status ambiguity, etc.;

(4) comorbidity (joint causation of physical and psychological disorder);

(5) misdiagnosis of psychological disorder as CFS;

(6) selection bias.

Methodology

A common criticism of the studies linking psychiatric disorder and CFS is the overlap between the symptoms of CFS and those of depression. We discussed this in Chapter 2, but a particular issue when considering CFS is that of the measurement of depression in the physically ill. The overlap between the symptoms of depression and those of physical illness is a constant concern for psychiatrists working in the area of general medicine. Many physical illnesses are associated with poor sleep, anorexia, weight loss, and fatigue. These symptoms mimic those of depressive illness, and can lead to either over- or underdiagnosis of depression in the physically ill[104]. Many common diagnostic assessments include questions on physical symptoms such as sleep, appetite, and so on. For that reason estimates of the rates of psychiatric illness in medical patients vary widely, from 10 to 80 per cent.

One solution is to use assessments that avoid the somatic symptoms of depression, but concentrate on other features of depressive illness that are not so easily confounded. For example, the Hospital Anxiety and Depression Scale (HAD[105]) is designed for use in medical patients, and is specifically designed to record anhedonia, or loss of pleasure, which the authors claim most closely represents the concept of depression. However, CFS subjects have higher HAD scores than chronic neurological controls, but lower than depressed inpatients in a psychiatric ward[11]. An alternative is to remove one or more symptoms held to be common to both depression and CFS from the diagnostic criteria employed for psychiatric disorder – although to a certain extent this prejudges the issue in question. Nevertheless, this has been adopted by several groups[11,14], without any substantial change in the pattern of results.

A second methodological limitation is information bias due to the lack of 'blinding' of the psychiatric interviewer in all published studies. Bias is reduced, but not eliminated, by using standardized interviews, and the absence of a structured interview is a serious flaw. One study attempted to ensure that psychiatric interviewing was blind to diagnosis[14] but only a study of fibromyalgia appears to have maintained 'blindness'[106]. This showed little difference in psychiatric morbidity between fibromyalgia cases, and two groups of controls, either normal or with rheumatoid arthritis, the only exception being somatization disorder, commoner in fibromyalgia. Similar studies are needed in CFS.

Despite these difficulties, some external validity for existing studies is suggested by the results of self-report questionnaires. These have included the General Health Questionnaire, Hospital Anxiety and Depression Scale, Beck Depression Inventory, Spielberger Anxiety Scales, MMPI, Profile of Mood States, SCL-90, and the Zung Self Rating Depression Scale. The consensus appears to be substantial increases in most scores compared with normative data or physical illness control groups, although not to the same extent as found in 'psychiatric' controls, with the exception of measures of somatization or somatic symptoms. Overall, no matter what the psychiatric instrument, CFS patients lie midway between those with chronic medical illness and those with formal psychiatric disorder in their respective specialist settings.

'Normal' reaction to physical illness

If it is not solely a measurement problem, then the next explanation lies in the association between physical and psychiatric disorder. Physical illness is strongly associated with psychiatric disorder; those with physical illness have between two to three times the risk of developing a psychiatric disorder compared with those without. The variables associated with high rates of psychiatric disorder in physical illness are also present in CFS. The illness, at least in hospital practice, is severe and chronic. It is disabling, and associated with multiple symptoms affecting multiple organ systems. It is associated with chronic pain, which both causes and amplifies psychiatric disorder[107].

It is therefore plausible to suggest that this is the simplest explanation for the close association between CFS and psychiatric disorder. The easiest way to answer this question is to compare those with other chronic disabling medical conditions with CFS samples (see Table 10.3). Wessely and Powell compared cases with controls with chronic neuromuscular diseases, and found that the risk of psychological disorder was twice as great in the cases[11]. A study using a similar design[14] reported an even higher relative risk compared with chronic muscle disease (and in that study the neuromuscular controls had more enduring and long-lasting illness), whilst CFS patients were six times more likely to fulfil psychiatric diagnostic criteria than controls with rheumatoid arthritis[13]. The increased rates of psychiatric disorder are not simply a reaction to the stress of physical disability or chronicity.

Table 10.3 Current psychiatric disorder in CFS compared with medical controls

Reference	Control group	Psychiatric disorder: CFS (%)	Psychiatric disorder: controls (%)	Relative risk of psychiatric disorder in CFS compared with controls
Wessely and Powell[11]	Neuromuscular	72	36	2.0
Katon et al.[13]	Rheumatoid arthritis	45	6	7.5
Wood et al.[14]	Myopathy	41	12.5	3.3
Pepper et al.[85]	Multiple sclerosis	23	8	2.9
Fischler et al.[35]	ENT/dermatology	77	50	3.4
Johnson et al. [17, 86]	Multiple sclerosis	45	16	2.8

The temporal relationship between fatigue and psychiatric symptoms can also provide some information. If psychological distress is a reaction to physical morbidity, then one expects it to post-date the onset of illness. Very little evidence has been found to substantiate this, and instead the commonest pattern is for either psychological morbidity to precede the onset of CFS[13,51], or for both fatigue and psychological morbidity to start together[14]. Similarly, rates of previous psychiatric disorder have been considerably elevated[12,13,71,108,109] or slightly elevated[11,35]. Only one study is discrepant, finding no difference in the rates of previous disorder between cases and controls[110]. However, all these studies are subject to complex biases of recall and referral, and do not permit any definitive conclusions about the role of past psychiatric illness and predisposition to CFS. A further problem is that, as we discussed in Chapter 2, the natural history of depression in the community is that fatigue is a common early symptom before the onset of typical mood disorder. Hence showing that fatigue precedes mood disorder may simply reflect the natural history of the condition, and not any 'cause and effect' relationship.

In all these studies selection biases are present. It is possible that general practitioners are less likely to refer patients with CFS-like illnesses to hospital if they are aware of a significant past psychiatric history. Alternatively, patients with previous psychiatric morbidity may be more likely to self-refer to physicians, or to be referred because of overt psychological distress. It is plausible that the presence of past psychiatric history has an influence on the probability of referral. A further problem is that one influential definition of CFS[111] excludes cases with a previous psychiatric history. If these criteria are rigorously applied (something we think is in practice unusual) it would be impossible to assess the role of past psychiatric vulnerability on the development of CFS. Finally, somatic symptoms such as fatigue are a common prodrome of affective disorder (see Chapter 4), so CFS-like symptoms preceding the onset of mood disorder may still be part of a single process, and do not prove that the latter is simply secondary to the former.

Retrospective studies of CFS patients in hospital settings, looking for differences in rates of previous psychiatric history, are not satisfactory. The role of psychiatric disorder as a risk factor for the development of CFS can only be ascertained in either population-based case–control studies, or prospective studies of vulnerability. No true examples of the former exist, although studies in UK primary care, which come close, have shown that prior psychiatric disorder is associated with the onset of chronic fatigue and/or CFS. These and other studies of the development of chronic fatigue and chronic fatigue syndrome after one defined trigger (viral infection) show that previous psychological disorder increases the risk of subsequent chronic fatigue and CFS[112–114].

Status ambiguity

The above studies used chronic illness controls. However, illnesses such as rheumatoid arthritis and myasthenia gravis may not be totally satisfactory comparisons. These disorders are well established, accepted, usually associated with visible disability, and not a source of any particular controversy. None of these apply to CFS. On the other hand, those with many chronic physical illnesses also suffer from uncertainty, for example about prognosis and (especially in many muscle disorders) the risk of transmitting the disorder to their children. Bridges and Goldberg found no evidence that neurological patients lacking a definite diagnosis had increased rates of psychiatric disorder[115] – although other authors have found that the absence of a physical diagnosis is associated with high rates of psychiatric problems. The cognitive schema described above, of guilt and low self-esteem, are not found in CFS[17,21]. We will consider issues such as status ambiguity and stigma in Chapters 12 and 15. Whilst these may impede recovery and contribute to physical and social impairment and are clearly a further source of distress, we do not believe such factors alone account for the excess psychopathology seen in CFS.

Comorbidity

The next explanation is that both the psychological disorder and CFS arise from a common pathology. This is not tenable if one adheres to a neuromuscular pathogenesis, but if CFS is thought to have some association with central nervous dysfunction, then a comorbidity explanation becomes relevant. This possibility has often been ignored by psychiatrists, who can be justly accused of thinking 'brainlessly', just as physicians all too often think 'mindlessly'[116]. It is beyond dispute that lesions within the central nervous system can be associated with increased rates of psychopathology, although rarely in a specific way. This is an important link between psychiatric disorder and CFS, and is the main subject of the next chapter.

Comorbidity may also play a part in explaining the finding that psychiatric disorder predicts the development of CFS after defined events such as viral infection. Because CFS and psychiatric disorder are so closely linked, it might be that 'like predicts like' – in other words rather than psychiatric disorder predicting CFS, it is associated with the development of the comorbid psychiatric disorder rather than CFS itself. Only very large prospective studies can answer this question, but some suggestion that this might be the case comes from the primary care studies already discussed[112]. The finding that life events at the time of developing glandular fever are strongly associated with post-EBV depression but not post-EBV fatigue is also suggestive[73].

Misdiagnosis

In this model psychiatric disorder is assumed to cause CFS. It suggests that CFS is an emotional illness, manifested by fatigue, and is not due to a viral infection (except perhaps as a non-specific stressor analogous to a life event). Evidence in favour of this includes studies that show that psychological vulnerability precedes the onset of CFS, or that psychological symptoms and fatigue begin together (although this would also be compatible with comorbid explanations). Evidence of response to psychological treatments would also favour this model, but should be interpreted with caution, since it is possible that such factors may be effective in alleviating variables concerned with prognosis, rather than onset.

There is little doubt that misdiagnosis is common in samples of patients with the label of CFS. We have encountered patients with the diagnosis, both self and professionally made, who were suffering from other disorders, including schizophrenia, benzodiazepine withdrawal, alcohol abuse, and others. Some would also argue that somatization disorder is another disorder often misdiagnosed as CFS. These diagnoses are now accepted as being incompatible with the current concepts of CFS[62].

It is in the area of affective and somatic symptoms that problems still arise. One doctor's severe CFS is another's severe depression[117]. As we have been at pains to point out, both conditions are essentially symptomatic, and not aetiological, descriptions. The differentiation between the two can become a matter of operational criteria, and reflects cultural and semantic differences as much as symptomatic profiles. We are thus reluctant to claim that depression is frequently misdiagnosed as CFS, since that implies a greater understanding of mood disorder than is the case. On the other hand, there is no escaping the considerable overlap between depression and chronic fatigue syndrome[118]. We will draw attention to these overlaps in sections on symptoms, immunology, neuropsychology, neuroimaging, and elsewhere.

Selection bias

The next possibility is that the high rates of psychiatric morbidity seen in CFS represents the phenomenon of selection bias, since it is true that all the original studies of psychiatric disorder and CFS took place in the specialist setting. Psychiatric disorder is a powerful promoter of illness behaviour – perhaps people went to the doctor, and eventually to the specialist clinic, not because of their chronic fatigue, but because of their psychological distress. Studies in this setting would therefore give a false impression of the strength of the association between chronic fatigue and psychopathology.

There is a well known example of this process in the literature on another syndrome with strong overlaps with CFS, irritable bowel syndrome (IBS). IBS researchers have exploited the possibilities of epidemiology to determine whether or not the strong association between psychiatric disorder and CFS is in fact a product of selection bias. The answer is a qualified yes.

Like CFS, the excess of psychiatric illness in hospital samples of patients with IBS is well known[119]. Higher frequencies of depression, anxiety, somatization, and personality disturbance have been reported in IBS[119]. When patients presenting with IBS were compared with those with peptic ulcers, those with IBS had greater numbers of somatic symptoms, increased consultation rates for minor illnesses, were more likely to view colds and 'flu' as serious, and had increased rates of unusual illness behaviour in childhood[120]. All of these suggest an association with consultation behaviour.

The picture changes in general practice and the community. Sandler *et al.* noted that 62 per cent of community cases of IBS never consulted a doctor. Those that did were distinguished by more severe symptoms[121]. Medical consultation was also more likely if other symptoms were present, among which were fatigue, weakness, and myalgia. Furthermore, presentation with IBS was associated with a pattern of presentation for other symptoms, suggesting that medicalization of problems was associated with a general help-seeking tendency, and a tendency to symptom focusing. Other studies have confirmed that community cases of IBS were not significantly different from controls on psychological variables, but did differ from patient samples. One interesting finding was that the community IBS controls had lower levels of psychological distress, but also lower levels of psychological denial[122,123]. Only one study is inconsistent, finding increased somatic distress in both hospital attenders and community controls with IBS[124].

Thus in IBS the evidence suggests that presentation is closely associated with psychological distress and the tendency to medicalize problems. Overt psychological symptoms did not distinguish IBS patients from those with organic gastrointestinal illnesses – both scoring higher on measures of depression, somatization, and disease conviction than normal controls[125].

A recent study used the same strategy to answer the same questions about fibromyalgia[126]. Clinic patients had more psychiatric diagnoses, more psychological distress, more pain, and more fatigue than people who had fibromyalgia but had not sought medical treatment. The controls were recruited after a newspaper advertisement, which is not ideal, but the results are similar to the conclusions of the IBS literature.

But does the same apply to CFS? This time the answer is a qualified no. When subjects with CFS identified in a systematic survey of primary care were compared with those seen in a specialist clinic, certain differences were present[127]. The primary care patients rarely used phrases such as ME or CFS to describe their problems, and did not conform to any social class stereotype. However, psychological distress did not differ between the two groups.

The conclusion is that two of the apparent mysterious features of fatigue syndromes, the high rate of psychiatric disorders and the excess of upper social classes and in particular health service professionals, may partly reflect how and why people seek care, rather than intrinsic features of the disorder itself. However, the association with psychological disorder is not determined by selection bias, unlike IBS and perhaps fibromyalgia.

The similarities between CFS, and both IBS and fibromyalgia, emerge from the conclusions of Drossman and Thompson in their review of IBS. None are simple, somatic expressions of psychiatric disorders[128]. However, psychosocial factors influence how the illness is experienced, and its prognosis[49,129,130]. Most patients seen by specialists have refractory illness and psychosocial disturbance.

10.11 Conclusion

A large number of those receiving labels such as CFS satisfy criteria for psychiatric diagnoses. We have already considered possible explanations for this finding. We shall conclude with a few warnings about what it does *not* mean. It does not mean that symptoms are factitious or hysterical in origin, which is still an issue in the media, even though never considered by serious investigators of CFS. Nor does it mean that psychiatric disorders are necessarily the cause of CFS. Komaroff noted 'One problem is that CFS is defined by a group of symptoms, without any objective abnormalities on physical examination or laboratory testing that readily establish the diagnosis. Another problem is that the same is true of depression and somatization disorder'[131]. So-called 'organic' factors may be equally important in those who do fulfil psychiatric criteria, and 'psychological' factors can still be important in those who do not[132].

We also conclude that CFS is not associated with any single psychiatric disorder. The early literature, including contributions from the current authors, emphasized the importance of depression. Subsequent work has turned the spotlight on the anxiety and somatoform disorders. CFS and the anxiety disorders are more congruent in terms of neuroendocrinology (Chapter 11), illness beliefs and behaviours (Chapter 12), and treatment response (Chapter 17) than CFS and depression.

So far we have looked rather narrowly at the of subject of psychiatric disorders and CFS. We have concluded that many subjects fulfil criteria for psychiatric diagnoses, but what this means is unclear. We have also concluded that a substantial number do not. However, psychiatric disorder is not synonymous with psychological problems. Our own treatment approach depends less upon making a formal psychiatric diagnosis, and far more on an understanding of social, cognitive, behavioural, and physiological factors.

References

1 Behan P, Behan W. Postviral fatigue syndrome. *Crit. Rev. Neurobiol.* 1988; **4:** 157–179.
2 Fegan K, Behan P, Bell E. Myalgic encephalomyelitis: report of an epidemic. *J. R. Coll. Gen. Pract.* 1983; **33:** 335–337.
3 Bell E, McCartney R, Riding M. Coxsackie B viruses and myalgic encephalomyelitis. *J. R. Soc. Med.* 1988; **81:** 329–331.
4 Behan W, More I, Behan P. Mitochondrial abnormalities in the post-viral fatigue syndrome. *Acta Neuropathol.* 1991; **83:** 61–65.
5 Dowsett E, Ramsay A, McCartney R, Bell E. Myalgic encephalomyelitis—a persistent enteroviral infection? *Postgrad. Med. J.* 1990; **66:** 526–530.
6 Mayou R, Sharpe M. Diagnosis, illness and disease. *Q. J. Med.* 1995; **88:** 827–831.
7 Sharpe M. Chronic fatigue syndrome. *Psychiat. Clin. North Am.* 1996; **19:** 549–573.
8 Kendell R. Chronic fatigue, viruses and depression. *Lancet* 1991; **337:** 160–162.
9 David A, Wessely S. Chronic fatigue, ME and ICD-10. *Lancet* 1993; **342:** 1247–1248.
10 Mayou R, Bass C, Sharpe M. Overview of epidemiology, classification and aetiology. In Mayou R, Bass C, Sharpe M (ed.) *Treatment of Functional Somatics Symptoms.* Oxford University Press, 1995: 42–65.
11 Wessely S, Powell R. Fatigue syndromes: a comparison of chronic 'postviral' fatigue with neuromuscular and affective disorder. *J. Neurol. Neurosurg. Psychiatry* 1989; **52:** 940–948.
12 Kruesi M, Dale J, Straus S. Psychiatric diagnoses in patients who have chronic fatigue syndrome. *J. Clin. Psychol.* 1989; **50:** 53–56.
13 Katon W, Buchwald D, Simon G, Russo J, Mease P. Psychiatric illness in patients with chronic fatigue and rheumatoid arthritis. *J. Gen. Intern. Med.* 1991; **6:** 277–285.
14 Wood G, Bentall R, Gopfert M, Edwards R. A comparative psychiatric assessment of patients with chronic fatigue syndrome and muscle disease. *Psychol. Med.* 1991; **21:** 619–628.
15 Wessely S. Myalgic encephalomyelitis: a warning. *J. R. Soc. Med.* 1989; **82:** 215–216.
16 Mathew R, Weinman M, Mirabi M. Physical symptoms of depression. *Br. J. Psychiatry* 1981; **139:** 293–296.
17 Johnson S, DeLuca J, Natelson B. Depression in fatiguing illness: comparing patients with chronic fatigue syndrome, multiple sclerosis and depression. *J. Affect Disord.* 1996: **38**: 21–30.
18 Komaroff A, Fagioli L, Geiger A, *et al.* An examination of the working case definition of chronic fatigue syndrome. *Am. J. Med.* 1996; **100:** 56–64.

19 Liebowitz M, Quitkin F, Stewart J, *et al.* Antidepressant specificity in atypical depression. *Arch. Gen. Psychiat.* 1988; **45:** 129–137.

20 Zubieta J, Engleberg N, Yargic L, Pande A, Demitrack M. Seasonal variation in patients with chronic fatigue; comparison with major mood disorders. *J. Psychiat. Res.* 1994; **28:** 13–22.

21 Powell R, Dolan R, Wessely S. Attributions and self-esteem in depression and chronic fatigue syndromes. *J. Psychosom. Res.* 1990; **34:** 665–673.

22 Oppenheim H. *Text-book of Nervous Diseases for Physicians and Students,* 5th edn. London, Foulis, 1908.

23 Shanks M, Ho-Yen D. A clinical study of chronic fatigue syndrome. *Br. J. Psychiat.* 1995; **166:** 798–801.

24 Carter B, Edwards J, Kronenberger W, Michalczyk L, Marshall G. Case control study of chronic fatigue in pediatric patients. *Pediatrics* 1995; **95:** 179–186.

25 Vercoulen J, Hommes O, Swanink C, *et al.* The measurement of fatigue in patients with multiple sclerosis: a multidimensional comparison with patients with chronic fatigue syndrome and healthy subjects. *Arch. Neurol.* 1996; **46:** 632–635.

26 Shands H, Finesinger J. A note on the significance of fatigue. *Psychosom. Med.* 1952; **14:** 309–314.

27 Beck A. *Depression: Clinical, Theoretical and Experimental Aspects.* Philadelphia, University of Pennsylvania Press, 1967.

28 Karno M, Hoffman R. The pseudoanergic syndrome. In Kiev A (ed.) *Somatic Manifestations of Depressive Disorders. Excerpta Medica,* 1974: 55–85.

29 Wheeler B. Feminist and psychological implications of chronic fatigue syndrome. *Femin. Psychol.* 1992; **2:** 197–203.

30 Stone A, Broderick J, Porter L, *et al.* Fatigue and mood in chronic fatigue syndrome patients: results of a momentary assessment protocol examining fatigue and mood levels and diurnal patterns. *Ann. Behav. Med.* 1994; **16:** 228–234.

31 Healy D. *The Suspended Revolution: Psychiatry and Psychotherapy Re-examined.* London, Faber and Faber, 1990.

32 David A, Wessely S, Pelosi A. Post-viral fatigue: time for a new approach. *Br. Med. J.* 1988; **296:** 696–699.

33 Manu P, Matthews D, Lane T. Panic disorder among patients with chronic fatigue. *South. Med. J.* 1991; **84:** 451–456.

34 Farmer A, Jones I, Hillier J, Llewelyn M, Borysiewicz L, Smith A. Neuraesthenia revisited: ICD-10 and DSM-III-R psychiatric syndromes in chronic fatigue patients and comparison subjects. *Br. J. Psychiatry,* 1995; **167:**503–506.

35 Fischler B, Cluydts R, De Gucht V, Kaufman L, DeMeirleir K. Generalised anxiety disorders in chronic fatigue syndrome. *Acta Psychiat. Scand.* 1997: **95:** 405–13.

36 Gardner W. The pathophysiology of hyperventilation disorders. *Chest* 1996; **109:** 516–534.

37 Folgering H, Snik A. Hyperventilation syndrome and muscle fatigue. *J. Psychosom. Res.* 1988; **32:** 165–171.

38 Rosen S, King J, Nixon P. Brainstorming the postviral fatigue syndrome. *Br. Med. J.* 1988; **297:** 1543.

39 Rosen SD, King JC, Wilkinson JB, Nixon PGF. Is chronic fatigue syndrome synonymous with effort syndrome? *J. R. Soc. Med.* 1990; **83:** 761–764.

40 Nixon PG. The grey area of effort syndrome and hyperventilation: from Thomas Lewis to today. *J. R. Coll. Physicians* 1993; **27:** 377–83.

41 Bass C, Garnder W. Respiratory and psychiatric abnormalities in chronic symptomatic hyperventilation. *Br. Med. J.* 1985; **290:** 1387–1390.

42 Lavietes M, Natelson B, Cordero D, Ellis S, Tapp W. Does the stressed patient with chronic fatigue syndrome hyperventilate? *Int. J. Behav. Med.* 1996; **3:** 70–83.

43 Saisch S, Deale A, Gardner W, Wessely S. Hyperventilation and chronic fatigue syndrome. *Q. J. Med.* 1994; **87**: 63–67.

44 Riley M, O'Brien C, McCluskey D, Bell N, Nicholls D. Aerobic work capacity in patients with chronic fatigue syndrome. *Br. Med. J.* 1990; **301**: 953–956.

45 Tweeddale P, Rowbottom I, McHardy G. Breathing retraining: effect on anxiety and depression scores in behavioural breathlessness. *J. Psychosom. Res.* 1994; **38**: 11–22.

46 Blakely A, Howard R, Sosich R, Murdoch J, Menkes D, Spears G. Psychological symptoms, personality and ways of coping in chronic fatigue syndrome. *Psychol. Med.* 1991; **21**: 347–362.

47 Carter B, Marshall G. New developments: diagnosis and management of chronic fatigue in children and adolescents. *Curr. Probl. Pediatr.* 1995; **25**: 281–293.

48 Manu P, Affleck G, Tennen H, Morse P, Escobar J. Hypochondriasis influences quality of life outcomes in patients with chronic fatigue. *Psychother. Psychosom.* 1996; **65**: 76–81.

49 Clark M, Katon W, Russo J, Kith P, Sintay M, Buchwald D. Chronic fatigue; risk factors for symptom persistence in a 2.5-year follow up study. *Am. J. Med.* 1995; **98**: 187–195.

50 Manu P, Matthews D. The mental health of patients with a chief complaint of chronic fatigue: a prospective evaluation and follow-up. *Arch. Intern. Med.* 1988; **148**: 2213–2217.

51 Lane T, Manu P, Matthews D. Depression and somatization in the chronic fatigue syndrome. *Am. J. Med.* 1991; **91**: 335–344.

52 Clark M, Katon W. The relevance of psychiatric research on somatization to the concept of chronic fatigue syndrome. In Straus S (ed.) *Chronic Fatigue Syndrome.* New York, Dekker, 1994: 329–349.

53 Johnson S, Deluca J, Natelson B. Assessing somatization disorder in the chronic fatigue syndrome. *Psychosom. Med.* 1996; **58**: 50–57.

54 Van Hemert A, Hengeveld M, Bolk J, Rooijmans H, Vandenbroucke J. Psychiatric disorder in relation to medical illness among patients of a general medical out-patient clinic. *Psychol. Med.* 1993; **23**: 167–173.

55 Walker E, Katon W, Jemelka R. Psychiatric disorders and medical care utilisation among people who report fatigue in the general population. *J. Gen. Intern. Med.* 1993; **8**: 436–440.

56 McDonald E, David A, Pelosi A, Mann A. Chronic fatigue in general practice attenders. *Psychol. Med.* 1993; **23**: 987–998.

57 Wessely S, Chalder T, Hirsch S, Wallace P, Wright D. The prevalence and morbidity of chronic fatigue and chronic fatigue syndrome: a prospective primary care study. *Am. J. Publ. Health*; 1997: **87**: 1449–55.

58 Escobar J, Burnam A, Karno M, Forsythe A, Golding J. Somatization in the community. *Arch. Gen. Psychiat.* 1987; **44**: 713–718.

59 Stewart D. The changing face of somatisation. *Psychosomatics* 1990; **31**: 153–158.

60 Manu P, Matthews D, Lane T. Food intolerance in patients with chronic fatigue. *Int. J. Eating Disorders* 1993; **13**: 203–209.

61 Hickie I, Lloyd A, Hadzi-Pavlovic D, Parker G, Bird K, Wakefield D. Can the chronic fatigue syndrome be defined by distinct clinical features? *Psychol. Med.* 1995; **25**: 925–935.

62 Sharpe M, Archard L, Banatvala J, *et al.* Chronic fatigue syndrome: guidelines for research. *J. R. Soc. Med.* 1991; **84**: 118–121.

63 Bass C, Benjamin S. The management of chronic somatisation. *Br. J. Psychiatry* 1993; **162**: 472–480.

64 Sharpe M, Bass C, Mayou R. An overview of the treatment of functional somatic symptoms. In Mayou R, Bass C, Sharpe M (ed.) *Treatment of Functional Somatic Symptoms.* Oxford University Press, 1995: 66–86.

65 David AS. Postviral fatigue syndrome and psychiatry. *Br. Med. Bull.* 1991; **47**: 966–988.

66 Briggs N, Levine P. A comparative review of systemic and neurological symptomatology in 12 outbreaks collectively described as chronic fatigue syndrome, epidemic neuro-myasthenia and myalgic encephalomyelitis. *Clin. Infect. Dis.* 1994; **18(suppl 1):** 32–42.

67 Warwick HM, Salkovskis PM. Reassurance. *Br. Med. J.* 1985; **290:** 1028.

68 Behan PO, Bakheit AM. Clinical spectrum of postviral fatigue syndrome. *Br. Med. Bull.* 1991; **47:** 793–808.

69 Park R, Lawrie S, Freeman C. Post-viral onset of anorexia nervosa. *Br. J. Psychiatry* 1995; **166:** 386–389.

70 Pomeroy C, Eckert E, Hu S, *et al.* Role of interleukin-6 and transforming growth factor-b in anorexia nervosa. *Biol. Psychol.* 1994; **36:** 836–839.

71 Dobbins J, Natelson B, Brassloff I, Drastal S, Sisto S. Physical, behavioral and psycho-logical risk factors for chronic fatigue syndrome: a central role for stress? *J. Chronic Fatigue Syndrome* 1995; **1:** 43–58.

72 Lewis S, Cooper C, Bennett D. Psychosocial factors and chronic fatigue syndrome. *Psychol. Med.* 1994; **24:** 661–671.

73 Bruce-Jones W, White P, Thomas J, Clare A. The effect of social disadvantage on the fatigue syndrome, psychiatric disorders and physical recovery, following glandular fever. *Psychol. Med.* 1994; **24:** 651–659.

74 White P, Thomas J, Amess J, Grover S, Kangro H, Clare A. The existence of a fatigue syndrome after glandular fever. *Psychol. Med.* 1995; **25:** 907–916.

75 Ray C, Jefferies S, Weir W. Life events and the course of chronic fatigue syndrome. *Br. J. Med. Psychol.* 1995; **68:** 323–331.

76 Wigers S. Fibromyalgia outcome: the predictive value of symptom duration, physical activity, disability pension, and critical life events – a 4.5 year prospective study. *J. Psychosom. Res.* 1996; **41:** 235–244.

77 Lutgendorf S, Antoni M, Ironson G, *et al.* Physical symptoms of chronic fatigue syndrome are exacerbated by the stress of Hurricane Andrew. *Psychosom. Med.* 1995; **57:** 310–323.

78 Tuckey C. Treatment of neurasthenia by hypnotism and suggestion. *Practitioner* 1911: 185–192.

79 Waylonis GW, Perkins RH. Post-traumatic fibromyalgia. A long-term follow-up. *Am. J. Phys. Med. Rehabil.* 1994; **73:** 403–12.

80 Capen K. The courts, expert witnesses and fibromyalgia. *Can. Med. Assoc. J.* 1995; **153:** 206–208.

81 Bohr T. Problems with myofascial pain syndrome and fibromyalgia syndrome. *Neurology* 1996; **46:** 593–597.

82 Wolfe F. The fibromyalgia syndrome: a consensus report on fibromyalgia and disability. *J. Rheumatol.* 1996; **23:** 534–537.

83 Wessely S. Liability for psychiatric illness. *J. Psychosom. Res.* 1995. **39:** 659–69.

84 Wilkinson G. Stress: another chimera. *Br. Med. J.* 1991; **302:** 191–2.

85 Pepper C, Krupp L, Friedberg F, Doscher C, Coyle P. A comparison of neuropsychiatric characteristics in chronic fatigue syndrome, multiple sclerosis and major depression. *J. Neuropsychol. Clin. Neurosci.* 1993; **5:** 200–205.

86 Johnson S, DeLuca J, Natelson B. Personality dimensions in the chronic fatigue syn-drome: a comparison with multiple sclerosis and depression. *J. Psychiat. Res.* 1996; **30:** 9–20.

87 Wessely S, David A, Butler S, Chalder T. The management of chronic 'post-viral' fatigue syndrome. *J. R. Coll. Gen. Pract.* 1989; **39:** 26–29.

88 Eichner E. Chronic fatigue syndrome; how vulnerable are athletes? *Physician Sports Med.* 1989; **16:** 157–160.

89 MacDonald K, Osterholm M, LeDell K, *et al.* A case control study to assess possible triggers and cofactors in chronic fatigue syndrome. *Am. J. Med.* 1996; **100:** 548–554.
90 Shepherd C. *Living with M.E. A self-help guide.* London, Cedar, 1989.
91 Roeber J. Industry of anxiety. *Vogue,* August 1989: 178–179.
92 Flett K. Why ME? *Arena,* March 1990.
93 Dryden W. The counsellor and ME. In Dryden W (ed.) *The Dryden Interviews: Dialogues on the Psychotherapeutic Process.* 1992: 100–109.
94 Bragg P. Kilroy was here. *Interaction* 1989; **3:** 503.
95 Abbey S. Somatization, illness attribution and the sociocultural psychiatry of chronic fatigue syndrome. In Kleinman A, Straus S (ed.) *Chronic Fatigue Syndrome.* Chichester, Wiley, 1993: 238–261.
96 Ware N. Society, mind and body in chronic fatigue syndrome: an anthropological view. In Kleinman A, Straus S (ed.) *Chronic Fatigue Syndrome.* Chichester, Wiley, 1993: 62–82.
97 Van Houdenhove B, Onghena P, Neerinckx E, Hellin J. Does high 'action-proneness' make people more vulnerable to chronic fatigue syndrome? A controlled psychometric study. *J. Psychosom. Res.* 1995; **39:** 633–640.
98 Ware N. Suffering and the social construction of illness: the delegitimisation of illness experience in chronic fatigue syndrome. *Med. Anthropol. Q.* 1992; **6:** 347–361.
99 Wood B, Joyce J, Wessely S. Personality characteristics in chronic fatigue syndrome and rheumatoid arthritis. *submitted.*
100 Stacey S. Tired and tested. *Harpers and Queen,* October 1990.
101 Dowsett EG. Conversation piece. *Postgrad. Med. J.* 1992; **68:** 63–5.
102 Ray C. Chronic fatigue syndrome and depression: conceptual and methodological ambiguities. *Psychol. Med.* 1991; **21:** 1–9.
103 Abbey S, Garfinkel P. Chronic fatigue syndrome and the psychiatrist. *Can. J. Psychiat.* 1990; **35:** 625–633.
104 Silverstone P. Measuring depression in the physically ill. *Int. J. Method Psychiat. Res.* 1991; **1:** 3–12.
105 Zigmond A, Snaith R. The Hospital Anxiety and Depression Scale. *Acta Psychiat. Scand.* 1983; **67:** 361–370.
106 Ahles T, Khan S, Yunus M, Spiegel D, Masi A. Psychiatric status of patients with primary fibromyalgia, patients with rheumatoid arthritis, and subjects without pain: a blind comparison of DSM-III diagnoses. *Am. J. Psychol.* 1991; **148:** 1721–1726.
107 Von Korff M, Simon G. The relationship between pain and depression. *Br. J. Psychiatry* 1996; **168(suppl 30):** 101–108.
108 Taerk G, Toner B, Salit I, Garfinkel P, Ozersky S. Depression in patients with neuro-myasthenia (benign myalgic encephalomyelitis). *Int. J. Psychiat. Med.* 1987; **17:** 49–56.
109 Gold D, Bowden R, Sixbey J, *et al.* Chronic fatigue: a prospective clinical and virologic study. *J. Am. Med. Assoc.* 1990; **264:** 48–53.
110 Hickie I, Lloyd A, Wakefield D, Parker G. The psychiatric status of patients with chronic fatigue syndrome. *Br. J. Psychiatry* 1990; **156:** 534–540.
111 Holmes G, Kaplan J, Gantz N, *et al.* Chronic fatigue syndrome: a working case definition. *Ann. Intern. Med.* 1988; **108:** 387–389.
112 Wessely S, Chalder T, Hirsch S, Wallace P, Wright D. Psychological symptoms, somatic symptoms and psychiatric disorder in chronic fatigue and chronic fatigue syndrome: a prospective study in primary care. *Am. J. Psychiat.* 1996; **153:** 1050–1059.
113 Cope H, Mann A, Pelosi A, David A. Psychosocial risk factors for chronic fatigue and chronic fatigue syndrome following presumed viral infection: a case control study. *Psychol. Med.* 1996; **26:** 1197–1209.

114 Hotopf M, Noah N, Wessely S. Chronic fatigue and minor psychiatric morbidity after viral meningitis: a controlled study. *J. Neurol. Neurosurg. Psychiatry* 1996; **60:** 504–509.

115 Bridges KW, Goldberg DP. Psychiatric illness in inpatients with neurological disorders: patients' views on discussion of emotional problems with neurologists. *Br. Med. J.* 1984; **289:** 656–8.

116 Eisenberg L. Mindlessness and brainlessness in psychiatry. *Br. Med. J. Psychiatry* 1986; **148:** 497–508.

117 Levine P, Kreuger G, Straus S. Postviral chronic fatigue syndrome: a round table. *J. Infect. Dis.* 1989; **160:** 722–724.

118 Abbey S, Garfinkel P. Chronic fatigue syndrome and depression: cause, effect or covariate. *Rev. Infect. Dis.* 1991; **13(suppl 1):** S73–S83.

119 Drossman D, Creed F, Fava G, *et al.* Psychosocial aspects of the functional gastro-intestinal disorders. *Gastroenterol. Int.* 1995; **8:** 47–90.

120 Whitehead W, Winget C, Fedoravicius A, Wooley S, Blackwell B. Learned illness behavior in patients with irritable bowel syndrome and peptic ulcer. *Digest. Dis. Sci.* 1982; **27:** 202–208.

121 Sandler RS, Drossman DA, Nathan HP, McKee DC. Symptom complaints and health care seeking behavior in subjects with bowel dysfunction. *Gastroenterology* 1984; **87:** 314–8.

122 Drossman DA, McKee DC, Sandler RS, *et al.* Psychosocial factors in the irritable bowel syndrome. A multivariate study of patients and nonpatients with irritable bowel syndrome. *Gastroenterology* 1988; **95:** 701–8.

123 Whitehead W, Bosmajian L, Zonderman A, Costa P, Schuster M. Symptoms of psychologic distress associated with irritable bowel syndrome: comparison of community and medical clinic samples. *Gastroenterology* 1988; **95:** 709–714.

124 Welch GW, Hillman LC, Pomare EW. Psychoneurotic symptomatology in the irritable bowel syndrome: a study of reporters and non-reporters. *Br. Med. J.* 1985; **291:** 1382–4.

125 Smith R, Greenbaum D, Vancouver I, *et al.* Psychological factors are associated with health care seeking rather than diagnosis in irritable bowel syndrome. *Gastroenterology* 1990; **98:** 293–301.

126 Aaron LA, Bradley LA, Alarcon GS, *et al.* Psychiatric diagnoses in patients with fibromyalgia are related to health care-seeking behavior rather than to illness. *Arthritis Rheum.* 1996; **39:** 436–45.

127 Euba R, Chalder T, Deale A, Wessely S. A comparison of the characteristics of chronic fatigue syndrome in primary and tertiary care. *Br. J. Psychiatry* 1996; **168:** 121–126.

128 Drossman D, Thompson W. The irritable bowel syndrome; review and a graduated, multicomponent treatment approach. *Ann. Intern. Med.* 1992; **116:** 1009–1016.

129 Wilson A, Hickie I, Lloyd A, *et al.* Longitudinal study of the outcome of chronic fatigue syndrome. *Br. Med. J.* 1994; **308:** 756–760.

130 Vercoulen J, Swanink C, Fennis J, Galama J, van der Meer J, Bleijenberg G. Prognosis in chronic fatigue syndrome: a prospective study on the natural course. *J. Neurol. Neurosurg. Psychiatry* 1996; **60:** 489–494.

131 Komaroff A. Clinical presentation of chronic fatigue syndrome. In Straus S, Kleinman A (ed.) *Chronic Fatigue Syndrome.* Chichester, Wiley, 1993: 43–61.

132 Mayou R, Bass C, Sharpe M (ed.) *The Treatment of Functional Somatic Symptoms.* Oxford University Press, 1995.

133 Morrison J. Fatigue as a presenting complaint in family practice. *J. Fam. Pract.* 1980; **10:** 795–801.

134 Buchwald D, Sullivan J, Komaroff A. Frequency of 'chronic active Epstein–Barr virus infection' in a general medical practice. *J. Am. Med. Assoc.* 1987; **257:** 2303–2307.

135 Kroenke K, Wood D, Mangelsdorff D, Meier N, Powell J. Chronic fatigue in primary care: Prevalence, patient characteristics and outcome. *J. Am. Med. Assoc.* 1988; **260:** 929–934.

136 Cathebras P, Robbins J, Kirmayer L, Hayton B. Fatigue in primary care: prevalence, psychiatric comorbidity, illness behaviour and outcome. *J. Gen. Intern. Med.* 1992; **7:** 276–286.

137 Ridsdale L, Evans A, Jerrett W, Mandalia S, Osler K, Vora H. Patients with fatigue in general practice: a prospective study. *Br. Med. J.* 1993; **307:** 103–106.

138 Hickie I, Koojer A, Hadzi-Pavlovic D, Bennett B, Wilson A, Lloyd A. Fatigue in selected primary care settings: socio-demographic and psychiatric correlates. *Med. J. Aust.* 1996; **164:** 585–588.

139 Millon C, Salvato F, Blaney N, *et al.* A psychological assessment of chronic fatigue syndrome/chronic Epstein–Barr virus patients. *Psychol. Health* 1989; **3:** 131–141.

140 Valdini A, Steinhardt S, Jaffe A. Demographic correlates of fatigue in a university family health center. *Fam. Pract.* 1987; **4:** 103–107.

141 Manu P, Lane T, Matthews D. Idiopathic chronic fatigue: depressive symptoms and functional somatic complaints. In Demitrack M, Abbey S (ed.) *Chronic Fatigue Syndrome: An Integrative Approach to Evaluation and Treatment* New York, Guilford Press, 1996: 36–47.

142 Schweitzer R, Robertson D, Kelly B, Whiting J. Illness behaviour of patients with chronic fatigue syndrome. *J. Psychosom. Res.* 1994; **38:** 41–50.

143 Lane R, Burgess A, Flint J, Riccio M, Archard L. Exercise responses and psychiatric disorder in chronic fatigue syndrome. *Br. Med. J.* 1995; **311:** 544–545.

144 Bombardier C, Buchwald D. Outcome and prognosis of patients with chronic fatigue vs chronic fatigue syndrome. *Arch. Intern. Med.* 1995; **155:** 2105–2110.

145 Vercoulen J, Swanink C, Fennis J, Galama J, van der Meer J, Bleijenberg G. Dimensional assessment of chronic fatigue syndrome. *J. Psychosom. Res.* 1994; **38:** 383–392.

146 Swanink C, Vercoulen J, Bleijenberg G, Fennis J, Galama J, Van Der Meer J. Chronic fatigue syndrome: a clinical and laboratory study with a well matched control group. *J. Intern. Med.* 1995; **237:** 499–506.

11. The neurobiology of CFS

11.1 Neuropsychology of CFS

Are there neuropsychological deficits in CFS?

Clinicians dealing with neurasthenia had no doubt that the illness affected not only the subject's physical performance, but also the mental performance. Beard wrote that 'memory is often temporarily weakened, and consecutive thought and sustained mental activity frequently impossible'[1]. When Janet singled out psychasthenia from the overburdened concept of neurasthenia, he drew attention to the psychological deficits that were at the core of the illness. 'Tiredness and a horrible sense of fatigue is caused in psychasthenics by the least physical or psychological effort . . . fatigue rapidly affects sensations and perceptions, intellect and movement'[2]. Edward Cowles defined an early symptom of the disease as the inability to sustain 'prolonged effort at attention'[3]. All the authorities recognized that mental effort exacerbated symptoms, and that various mental processes were affected.

With the revival of interest in CFS, the clinical observations made by Janet and his contemporaries were restated. In modern terms CFS patients have been described as having mental fatigue and fatigability, or 'cognitive disturbances', a term that simply refers to difficulties in thinking. Given the prominence of these and other complaints, many investigators have attempted to clarify these deficits by using modern neuropsychological testing.

Most patients with CFS experience a variety of symptoms suggestive of marked cognitive disturbance[4,5]. Questionnaire studies confirm these clinical observations. Studies using questionnaire measures of cognitive symptoms confirm the range and severity of subjective cognitive difficulties in CFS[6,7].

There have been a series of preliminary reports claiming profound neuropsychological impairment in CFS. For example, Bastien reported pronounced deficits in attention, concentration, sequencing, spatial perception, and verbal memory, as well as a fall in IQ. She concluded that CFS produces an 'atypical organic brain syndrome'[8]. Another American study reported finding severe memories deficits, indicative of organic lesions within the limbic system[9]. Others have failed to find any evidence of abnormality. Altay and colleagues from Toronto found that CFS patients scored better than a group of controls on a range of neuropsychological tests[10]. Researchers at the University of Miami using the Mini Mental State examination and the Wechsler Memory Scale, found no overall impairment compared with normative data[4].

The first rigorous study came from the Cognitive Neurosciences group at the National Institutes of Health (NIH)[7]. They administered a variety of neuropsychological tests, lasting eight hours over two days, in a subgroup of 20 patients. General intellectual performance was normal. Measures of reaction time and other timed tasks were also normal. Tests of planning, problem solving, digit span, and extensive tests of semantic and verbal memory were also normal. Specific deficits were noted only on tests of complex visual reproduction. One unusual finding was that subjects demonstrated more impaired performance on cued, than on free recall, as was also noted by others[9]. This is the opposite to the situation in most organic brain conditions.

Problems remain with this study. Only normal controls were used. The sample was highly selected, and represented the severe end of the CFS spectrum. Not all of the tests were equally validated. However, others have reached similar conclusions, Global intellectual functioning is normal. Processing of sensory information is normal[11]. Memory, both verbal and visual, is usually normal, except when assessed using more complex paradigms involving interference or greater mental effort[12]. Global intellectual and higher mental functioning is also unimpaired.

Neuropsychological abnormalities in CFS are therefore relatively restricted to more sophisticated tests of complex functioning, and in particular attention. Professor Andrew Smith was one of the earliest psychologists to suggest impairments not of short-term memory, but of sustained attention[13]. Simple tests of attention, such as digit span, are usually normal. Studies using the PASAT, a more complex attentional task, find that CFS patients perform worse than controls[14-16]. Results on the Stroop test, a visual attentional task that includes an assessment of the effect of interference by irrelevant stimuli, and is thus another complex attentional test, also suggest that CFS patients usually perform worse than controls[17,18]. Joyce *et al.* studied primary care patients developing chronic fatigue syndrome after viral infections using a computerized test battery (CANTAB)[19]. The results showed reduced attentional capacity, which resulted in impaired performance on effortful cognitive tasks. Impairment is thus greatest when rapid cognitive processing is required[19,20].

The role of depression

What are the explanations for these findings? The first possibility is that the observed complaints are related to mood disorder. It is well known that a number of psychiatric disorders are associated with substantial cognitive impairment. For example, Watts and Sharrock showed that depressed patients have two types of subjective complaints, namely 'going blank', and complaints that their minds are wandering[21]. Both of these are frequently reported by CFS patients. Conversely, CFS patients rate themselves as clumsy, lethargic, mentally slow, depressed, and so on, complaints frequently encountered in depression[13]. Previously held views that depression was associated with only minor impairments in psychological test performance are now regarded as false[22]. Depression is now known to be associated with a generalized impairment on more stringent tests of memory and learning, associated with abnormalities in concentration and attention[22,23]. Automatic processing, such as recognition memory, is relatively unaffected. Weingartner has shown that depressed patients experience difficulties in effortful processing. The more effortful the task, the greater the impairment. He also showed a strong correlation between impairment in both motor and memory tasks, especially those requiring sustained effort[24]. Being able to link cognitive difficulties and mood disorder with a reduction of sustained motor power has clear relevance to the problem of CFS.

It is therefore reasonable to suspect that the cognitive complaints encountered in CFS are related to mood disorder. Wessely and Powell showed that symptoms of 'mental fatigue' were severe in CFS patients, but were equally severe in a depressed control group[25]. Several groups using formal neuropsychological testing have noted considerable overlap between the findings in CFS and depression[15,18,20,26]. The NIH group found a consistent, and strong, correlation between the severity of mood disturbance and the number and severity of memory complaints[7]. CFS patients frequently report difficulties in reading and recalling what they have read – severity of complaints about reading problems is related to the severity of depressed mood[27].

A study from the Institute of Psychiatry looked at neuropsychological functioning in a non-selected primary care sample of chronically fatigued subjects. As reported elsewhere, there was a strong association between subjective complaints of cognitive difficulty and affect[28]. However, the link between subjective fatigue and poor performance on effortful memory processing persisted even when the sample was restricted to non-depressed CFS cases only. Anxiety was not associated with impaired cognitive performance. They suggest that the link between CFS, psychological disorder, and cognitive function is partly, but not fully, confounded by mood disorder, and is not related to anxiety. Krupp and colleagues continued the same observations, finding that abnormalities on memory testing in CFS subjects were accounted for by elevated depression scores[26]. Not all studies confirm this[29,30], perhaps because of methodological differences, but this remains the most probable interpretation[12]. Despite the above findings, the role of anxiety on more complex attentional tasks cannot be excluded either.

Other possible confounders

Another group suggested that somatic vigilance may underlie the subjective complaints of cognitive disturbance; CFS patients, as part of a general pattern of symptom monitoring and awareness of somatic symptoms (see Chapter 12) are thus more aware of symptoms that might then be interpreted as cognitive failure[18]. This hypothesis has the advantage of linking the results of neuropsychological testing with assessments in other domains. It has already been noted that cognitive complaints are closely correlated with somatic complaints[31].

Andrew Smith has suggested another important confounder, namely sleep disturbance. Common sense and experience tells us that poor sleep is associated with various subjective symptoms such as difficulties in sustained attention. Smith and colleagues have used the sensitive Stroop test to demonstrate the link between problems in attention and sleep disturbance[32]. Smith now suggests that much of the cognitive impairment seen in CFS is a physiological consequence of acute fatigue resulting from such factors as sleep disturbance.

The question of sleep reminds us that neuropsychological testing in general is critically dependent upon such factors as attention and arousal and that such functions as memory are closely related to the general level of alertness[33]. Arousal is that state of physiological excitement which improves the efficiency of task performance. It has several different components, correlated with specific neuro-transmitter systems. Each component has 'enabling' functions, acting as a mediator of arousal[22]. Disturbances in these mechanisms would result in inefficient perfor-mance of certain tasks, leading to fatigue, distractibility, poor concentration, and so on. Functions such as memory are thus closely related to the general level of alertness, so that a drowsy, fatigued, sleepless, medicated, or uncooperative person may well have substantial deficits on neuropsychological testing not indicative of 'brain' pathology. It is generally easier for neuropsychologists to measure discrete problems, such as aphasia, rather than the vague, subjective problems of CFS.

Neuropsychology and CFS: summary

It is therefore concluded that the neuropsychological deficits in CFS are relatively modest, and disproportionate to the severity of the subjective complaints[12,18,31]. Some aspects of neuropsychological dysfunction are reminiscent of the findings on neuromuscular disorder and CFS (Chapter 7), in which it was concluded that there was a disassociation between subjective and objective reports of muscle dysfunction. Likewise, despite claims that mental effort was associated with delayed detrimental effect, much as was suggested for the delayed effects of physical exertion, this has not yet been confirmed[20].

Overall, the complaints of impaired recall and concentration experienced by CFS patients probably relate to the effects of mood disorder[34]. Nevertheless, not all the cognitive difficulties found in CFS can be explained by mood disorder, and care should be taken not to confuse subjective complaints (correlated with mood disorder) with objective performance deficit (not necessarily mood related). Experimental findings of difficulties in sustained attention are less likely to be explained by mood disorder. The issue is, however, which are the more important? Patients complain of symptoms, which are the source of their distress, and the reasons why they consult. It remains to be seen whether or not the abnormalities noted by some groups are clinically relevant or not. White and colleagues studied neuropsychological function prospectively in their cohort of people recovering from acute mononucleosis. Im-paired attention, as measured by the PASAT, was present, but correlated with premorbid intelligence. On the other hand, poor concentration correlated with psychiatric morbidity and subjective mental fatigue[35].

11.2 Viruses and the neuropsychiatry of fatigue

In Chapter 9 we considered the epidemiological evidence linking viral infection with CFS. We concluded that the Epstein–Barr virus could trigger CFS, but was not responsible for prolonged fatigue syndromes. Only with true encephalitis could we find reasonable evidence for a direct link between viral agents and chronic fatigue syndromes. Serious viral infections such as encephalitis are fortunately rare, and are unlikely ever to explain more than a small fraction of existing cases of CFS. Follow-up studies of the outcome of viral infections give only weak support to a role of infective agents in the production of long-term fatigability, even after viral meningitis (see Chapter 9). However, epidemiological data do suggest that the risk of neur-asthenic syndromes is considerably increased in the survivors of some encephali-tides[36]. We have already drawn attention to similar observations in Von Economo's classic clinical studies of the outcome of encephalitis lethargica[37].

Of greater potential relevance is the possibility of more common and subtle dysfunction occurring after infection with less serious agents. Many common viruses reach the central nervous system. For example, both the measles virus and measles vaccine virus produce transient neurophysiological disturbance within the central nervous system[38]. Modest EEG changes have been noted in CFS samples, although it should be emphasized there is no suggestion of any epileptic phenomena, nor any similarities to the EEG features of the encephalitides[39]. Different viruses have differing affinities for the various regions and/or cell types of the brain whilst experimental evidence is accumulating of the ability of viral agents to interfere with the production of specific neurotransmitters, sometimes without producing the characteristic patterns of inflammation and cellular damage that are usually asso-ciated with infection (see Chapter 9).

The neuropsychological consequences of acute infection have been elegantly documented by Smith and colleagues at the late lamented MRC Common Cold Unit. They have demonstrated information-processing deficits after infection with the common cold or influenza virus, with the former causing impairments on a motor task, the latter on a visual search task[40]. These performance impairments can persist after the clinical symptoms have resolved[41], and can be reproduced by giving interferon[42]. Influenza does not affect memory or reasoning[43]. Studies of acute glandular fever found a similar range of deficits[44]. However, the duration of these deficits is still measured in days, rather than months, and caution should be observed before extrapolating these studies to the subject of CFS.

11.3 Neurophysiology

Another approach to the assessment of the cognitive difficulties so frequently mentioned by CFS patients is to measure cortical evoked potentials. Scalp electrodes are used to measure underlying brain activity after particular stimuli, which may be visual, auditory, or cognitive. Cognitive event potentials are therefore records of the neural activity resulting from particular stimuli, and are a measure of functional brain activity. The waveforms that are generated during the performance of particular cognitive tasks can be dissected into components reflecting the differing stages of information processing. Of particular interest are the long-latency evoked potentials. One subset of these, the N2–P3 complex, has been extensively studied in neurology and psychiatry, since it is thought to reflect both attentional and memory processes.

Prasher *et al.* studied cortical evoked potentials in a series of CFS subjects[45]. Somatosensory, auditory, and visual evoked potentials were normal. This, and the small study of central motor conduction time[46], firmly rules out the occasional analogy between CFS and multiple sclerosis. In contrast, about half the sample showed abnormalities in either the P3 waveform or the time taken to respond to the target stimulus. The potentials were either reduced in amplitude, or delayed. Could these findings be influenced by psychiatric disorder? Similar findings occur in schizophrenia, but what about affective disorder? Prasher *et al.* did not assess mood disorder, but on the basis of a literature review considered that their findings were not explained by depression. Others have questioned this interpretation[47]. The amplitude of the P300 evoked potential is affected by a number of different factors, including task difficulty, expectancy, and so on, as well as both age and fatigue. A recent study found that subjects with major depression did show abnormally long P3 latencies for spatial tasks, which was related to the intensity of sleep disturbance[48].

The Prasher findings have also not been replicated by a group working at the NIH in Washington[11]. Thirteen CFS patients and controls completed a series of extremely demanding cognitive tasks. Electrophysiological measures, including the N1, P2, N2, and P300 components of the event-related brain potentials, were normal. Perceptual, attention, and short-term memory processes were unaffected, and differences were restricted to reaction times[11]. One potential difference between the studies, however, was that positive findings related to auditory tasks[45], but the negative findings related to visual processing[11].

11.4 Neuroimaging

Scanning of the central nervous system can be divided into two types – structural and functional. Structural scanning of the CNS is usually performed either by computerized tomography (CT), or by nuclear magnetic resonance imaging (MRI). We are unaware of any claims of abnormalities on CT scanning. The first study using MRI was published in 1992[49]. They report MRI abnormalities in 78 per cent of 144 patients studied as part of the controversial 'Lake Tahoe' epidemic in Nevada. These abnormalities, frequently labelled 'UBOs' ('unidentified bright objects'), appear in a variety of diseases, and even normal subjects, and indeed were found in 21 per cent of the controls of the Lake Tahoe study. However, the epidemiology of the study is unclear[50]. The case definition must be questioned, as a separate report of the same cohort noted that the cases had 'more severe neurological symptoms including seizures, psychosis, dementia and the loss of fine motor skills'[51]. Buchwald and colleagues report seven cases of primary seizures, and ten of profound acute ataxia[49]. Such cases would be excluded from all the current definitions of CFS.

A later well conducted study found abnormalities in 27 per cent, falling to 22 per cent when three cases who went on to develop alternative diagnoses were excluded[52]. The most recent studies of subjects with chronic fatigue or CFS found no increase in MRI abnormalities[53,54]. Findings of white matter abnormalities require careful interpretation, since it is a sensitive technique and may reveal 'abnormalities' of little consequence. White matter abnormalities occur in a number of settings, including affective disorder, and their significance remains to be determined[49,55,56].

Although structural abnormalities of the CNS seem unlikely in most subjects, there is a very convincing rationale for undertaking studies of CNS function. Our historical survey showed that the concept of a functional disorder, in the true sense of the word, in CFS has been discussed for many years. However, only recently have scanning techniques capable of studying brain function become available.

In essence functional scans of the CNS depend upon labelling a compound with radio tracer, and then monitoring its distribution on a detection system. There are two such systems currently in use: single-positron emission tomography (SPET), and positron emission tomography (PET). The latter is the more expensive and complex, but has better spatial resolution.

SPET has become established for the measurement of relative cerebral blood flow and regional blood volume. Measuring cerebral blood flow is useful, because brain physiology and brain blood flow are usually (although not always) correlated ('coupled'). However, although simple to describe, in practice it is extremely complex, since such variables as task, motivation, environment, etc. must all be considered. There are also age and gender differences – women, for example, have higher blood flows than men. SPET is also developing into a method for measuring neurotransmitter receptor numbers.

What has been shown so far in CFS? Early studies, some still incompletely reported, suggest a range of abnormalities, with no visible single pattern. Frontal and temporal lobe hypoperfusion was found in a study of 46 CFS patients[57]. A British team[58] found patchy frontal and parietal deficits in just under half of 40 cases. Temporal asymmetry was reported in another[59]. In contrast a Belgian group report a positive correlation between cognitive deficits and increased frontal blood flow[60].

Probably the most publicized study, from the Middlesex group, found that brainstem perfusion was significantly reduced in CFS subjects compared with controls, with depressed patients showing intermediate values[61]. However, other groups do not report brainstem perfusion values because of the technical difficulties of imaging this small structure[62], whilst there is little clinical evidence of any symptoms or signs suggestive of brainstem dysfunction in CFS patients[63]. Another methodological problem is that this and other studies make comparisons between areas of the brain and a reference region, namely the cerebellum. This assumes that blood flow to the cerebellum is unaffected, a conclusion that is not justified in depression[64]. The report of brainstem hypoperfusion requires independent replication[63].

It seems reasonable to conclude that cerebral blood flow is altered in CFS, but how much is this due to depression and/or anxiety? The Canadian group concludes that the SPET findings in CFS are similar to those encountered in major psychiatric illnesses[65], reinforced by other studies that have failed to find any consistent differences with major depression[59,60,66]. Schwartz *et al.* found that the number of tracer update defects was increased in CFS compared with normal subjects, but did not differ from controls with major depression[67]. There are now over 20 studies using either SPET and PET in the depressive or anxiety disorders[22,68]. Several studies show global reduction in cortical blood flow in affective disorder, and are tending to confirm abnormalities in the frontal cortex, associated with changes in the temproparietal association cortices[68]. These appear to be related not to the subtype of depression, but to depressed mood *per se*. Laterality effects are also reported, but are inconsistent. Of relevance to CFS is the finding that in depression retardation and low mood correlated negatively with rCBF in the left dorsolateral frontal cortex, whilst cognitive difficulties correlated positively with rCBF in the left medial prefrontal cortex[69]. Also relevant are studies reporting a reduction in cerebral glucose uptake in the caudate nucleus of depressed subjects (see Robbins *et al.*[22] and Goodwin[68]), which has also been observed in fibromyalgia[70]. Thus some consistency is emerging between the results of neuroimaging and neuropsychology, suggesting that a disturbance of the frontostriatal axis has a part to play in affective disorder. At present there seems to be considerable overlap between the results of neuroimaging studies in CFS and affective disorder, with evidence of heterogeneity in both conditions.

In general, the application of the dynamic neuroimaging to complex conditions such as CFS has happened in advance of establishing the full range of normal variation within the population. Even in such a small literature variations in results are already observable, and it is at present impossible to come to any firm conclusions. The conclusion of a recent study seems sensible: 'findings are neither sufficiently sensitive nor specific to allow its use as a diagnostic tool, although it may have a role in understanding the pathophysiology of the disease'[62].

11.5 Neuroendocrinology and neurochemistry

Background

The investigation of the neuroendocrine system has become increasingly popular for two reasons. First, because of the insights it provides into the workings of the neuroendocrine system itself, and second because it provides a method ('window') of assessing the central nervous neurotransmitter systems regulating endocrine activity.

The hypothalamic–pituitary–adrenal axis (HPA) plays a central role in the body's response to stress, whether physical or psychological (see Fig. 11.1). The axis itself is regulated by a complex system of long and short feedback loops. Activation of the HPA axis is ultimately terminated by specific glucocorticoid receptors, which operate quickly ('fast feedback') in response to minute-by-minute variations in plasma cortisol, and a more delayed pathway responding to chronic elevations of cortisol, and involves inhibition of the transcription of those genes responsible for hormone biosynthesis.

One of the key hormones involved in the HPA axis is CRH (corticotrophin releasing hormone). CRH functions both as a hypothalamic releasing factor and a neurotransmitter in cortex and limbic regions. It is released from the paraventricular nucleus of the hypothalamus, and then stimulates specific receptors in the anterior pituitary which lead to the release of adrenocorticotrophin releasing hormone (ACTH). CRH is thus the initiator of the HPA-mediated stress response. Increased central drive resulting from hypersecretion of CRH is currently a favoured hypothesis for the pathogenesis of major affective disorder[71,72]. As well as initiating the release of ACTH it also increases sympathetic nervous function.

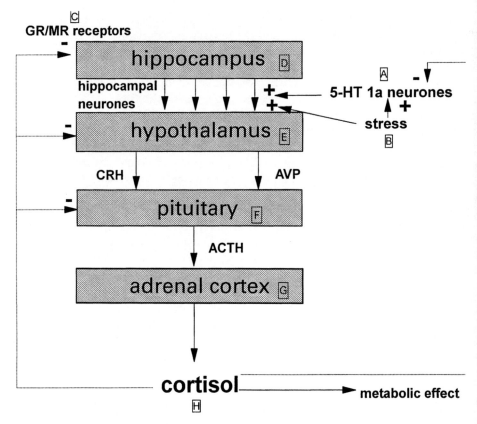

Fig. 11.1 Components of the HPA axis, and directions of positive and negative feedback loops. Abbreviations CRH (corticotrophin releasing hormone); ACTH (adrenocortico-trophin); AVP (arginine vasopressin); MR (mineralocorticoid receptors); GR (glucocorticoid receptors). Abnormalities in the axis are marked by letters A–H; details of these are listed below:

A: Increased 5-HT$_{1a}$ neuronal function

B: Increased psychological or physical stress

C: Impaired hippocampal negative feedback

D: Previous hippocampal damage from depression- or chronic stress-induced hypercortisolaemia

E: Reduced central drive to HPA axis

F: Impaired pituitary response to CRH or stress

G: Abnormal adrenal cortex response to ACTH

H: Hypocortisolism

Several lines of inquiry have led to the current surge of interest in the relationship of HPA activity to CFS. The first is the many similarities between depression and CFS, and the known neuroendocrine abnormalities in the latter. The second comes from the parallels between clinical conditions characterized by lack of cortisol, such as Addison's disease, and early clinical observations of cortisol deficiency in chronic fatigue states. Confusingly, some lines of inquiry rely on the resemblance both clinically and endocrinologically between depression and CFS, whilst others draw from the opposite, namely the differences between the two conditions.

One of the fundamental observations of modern biological psychiatry was that a proportion of those with major depression show excess production of ACTH, and hence cortisol, together with the failure of dexamethasone to suppress endogenous cortisol production, the dexamethasone suppression test (DST). More recent work has centred on the role of CRH. CRH itself, when administered centrally, has behavioural activation properties, which may underlie the agitation and increased arousal of some depressive states[73]. Depression, linked to excessive CRH, might thus be, in neuroendocrine terms, an over-exuberant stress response. Given both the overlap between depression and CFS, and the clinical role for stress so frequently commented upon, it was not surprising that workers had hypothesized a similar role for hypothalamic disorder as a final common pathway for the generation of CFS-like symptoms such as mood disorder, fatigue, sleep, and appetite disturbance[25,74]

However, there were also early hints that the neurobiology of CFS and that of depression might show some differences. For example, abnormal dexamethasone suppression was an easy marker to study, and might be expected to show the same phenomenon of non-suppression as in depression. However, this was not to be the case, as two studies, one of CFS the other of fibromyalgia, found that dexamethasone non-suppression is surprisingly unusual[75,76].

Another potentially aberrant finding, suggestive of differences between major depression and CFS, was anticipated in one of the first papers on the subject of persistent fatigue after glandular fever[77,78]. This proposed that chronic fatigue states might be characterized not by high, but by low cortisol[77]. Another early paper[79] suggested a similar link.

The classic clinical syndrome of glucocorticoid deficiency is Addison's disease, which is indeed associated with fatigue and generalized somatic symptoms. Chronic fatigue was also the commonest complaint in a recent outcome study of the survivors of bilateral adrenalectomies[80]. Glucocorticoid withdrawal has been reported to precipitate fibromyalgia[81]. Thus low cortisol, linked to central CRH deficiency, might also underlie the failure of attention found in CFS and 'atypical' depression*. Lack of CRH might also be associated with an inability to 'respond to the stressors, or, more simply, the demands of everyday life'[71]. Thus a good theoretical case can be made for linking low central CRH, low peripheral cortisol, and some of the symptoms of CFS. However, proving this is less easy. Central CRH deficiency is impossible to demonstrate directly in humans, and there is no animal model of CFS, hence evidence to support this hypothesis comes mainly from indirect measures.

---

* We place atypical in inverted commas because atypical depression is not atypical. It is the agitated, hyperaroused depressive state that is unusual. Mood disorder with increased sleep and general lethargy is far more commoner in the community. Psychiatric classification, and often psychiatric thinking, is based on what is encountered in specialist psychiatric settings. Such disorders are often profoundly atypical themselves

Neuroendocrine investigations of CFS and fibromyalgia

The most comprehensive investigation of HPA function in CFS was carried out at the National Institutes of Health (NIH), in Washington. Mark Demitrack and colleagues studied 30 CFS cases and 72 normal controls[82]. The intention was to test the integrity of the HPA axis. Two methods were used, one to study the normal diurnal variation in indices of cortisol activity, the other to look at dynamic responses to challenge by corticotrophin releasing hormone (CRH) and adrenocorticotrophic hormone (ACTH).

Demitrack and colleagues found, as Isaacs[77] had predicted, that free plasma cortisol levels were low in the CFS patients, as was the basal evening cortisol level, but plasma levels of basal evening ACTH were elevated. The adrenal glands appeared to have initially enhanced sensitivity to ACTH (thus excluding a primary adrenal cause), but the maximal response was blunted. The ability of CRF to stimulate ACTH release was also reduced, as in affective disorder, but on this occasion the attenuated response could not be explained by negative feedback from high glucocorticoid levels. Basal ACTH was correlated with both fatigue and depression. The authors interpret this as evidence of a mild, centrally induced adrenal insufficiency which is, in turn, secondary to CRF deficiency of unknown origin. Cerebrospinal fluid levels of CRF were normal, which is unusual, given the low cortisol levels.

Thus although neuroendocrine alterations occur in major depression, and depressed individuals show a similar attenuated ACTH response to CRH, the fact that the NIH group[82] found evidence of hypocortisolism, rather than hypercortisolism, suggests that the results were not simply due to confounding by depression, although the same series of patients were known to have high rates of operationally defined depressive disorders[83].

In a small study of non-depressed CFS patients the King's College, London group showed attenuated prolactin responses to insulin hypoglycaemia, but no change in other stress hormone (such as growth hormone) responses[84], suggesting a possible impairment of hypothalamic–pituitary response to stress.

Researchers studying fibromyalgia have also reported low 24-hour urine cortisol with loss of diurnal variation[85,86] as in CFS, but did not find elevated evening ACTH levels. The pituitary response to exogenous CRH also differed from that observed in CFS. Two groups report a blunting of the cortisol response to either CRH stimulation or insulin-induced hypoglycaemia[86,87]. A reduced cortisol response to exercise has been found in fibromyalgia[88]. The findings in fibromyalgia thus resemble in some ways, but are not identical to, those reported for CFS[85,89]. They have been interpreted as evidence of a reduced central drive to the HPA axis, but it must be emphasized that the literature is by no means clear-cut, and that it is possible to argue that the perturbations in the HPA axis so far observed in CFS and fibromyalgia may represent factors operating at many different sites in the axis, including hypothalamus, pituitary, and adrenal. Only further research, including larger samples, is likely to resolve these issues.

The pattern of abnormalities described by Demitrack and colleagues is not specific to CFS. As the authors made clear, similar results have been found not only in post-operative cases of Cushing's syndrome, but also fibromyalgia, hypothyroidism, seasonal affective disorder, and post-traumatic stress disorder (PTSD)[90,91]. Two out of three studies of PTSD suggest low urinary cortisol, with a consistent increase in the number of lymphocyte glucocorticoid receptors. Rachel Yehuda and her colleagues have gone on to show that dexamethasone suppression is abnormal in some PTSD patients, but in the opposite direction to that encountered in major depression. She has argued that PTSD is characterized by an enhanced sensitivity of the HPA feedback mechanism.

A different neuroendocrine mechanism has been suggested following claims that insulin-like growth factor (IGF-1), also known as somatomedin-C, is decreased in fibromyalgia[92] and post-polio syndrome[93]. This is an intriguing finding, since IGF-1 is a mediator of growth hormone activity, which in turn is responsible for muscle homeostasis. Growth hormone is produced during stage 4 sleep. An attractive model can be made linking sleep disturbance with functional muscle symptoms via a disruption of the growth hormone axis. Unfortunately, like other tantalizing findings, it has not been replicated[94].

Neurotransmitter function in CFS

What basic mechanisms might underlie the observed alterations in HPA function? The answers may come from studies of central neurotransmitter pathways, and in particular those involving the serotonin (5-hydroxytryptamine or 5-HT) pathways. These are involved in the regulation of a number of hypothalamic functions. Serotonin fibres innervate hypothalamic nuclei, and form synapses with CRF immunoreactive neurones[95]. A variety of serotonin agonists, including fenfluramine and buspirone, stimulate the release of pituitary hormones[96].

There are obvious difficulties in direct measurement of serotonin in humans. Cerebrospinal and plasma metabolites can be measured, although researchers who have done so find that levels of the principal metabolites are essentially normal, with the exception of an increase in 5-HIAA, the serotonin metabolite[97]. However, not even the most ardent enthusiast can claim that either cerebrospinal or plasma measures give much indication of central activity. Instead, investigators have to rely on indirect measures, using neuroendocrine probes to stimulate central receptors and measure the response – a 'window' into brain function as the strategy is sometimes described. In the first study using this strategy the response to buspirone, a $5\text{-}HT_{1A}$ receptor agonist, in 15 CFS patients, was compared with normal and depressed controls[74]. Little difference was found between the two control groups, but there was a significantly increased early rise in prolactin levels after buspirone challenge in the CFS patients. Because prolactin release after buspirone is blocked by, among others, serotonin antagonists, the authors suggested that the results demonstrate increased sensitivity of central 5-HT receptors in CFS, consistent with a reduction in central serotonin activity. They later also reported attenuated ACTH response to the selective 5-HT_{1A} agonist, ipsapirone[98], perhaps explaining why CRH and ACTH fail to respond even in the presence of increased 5-HT function. However, without knowledge of the growth hormone and prolactin responses this does not discriminate between a general pituitary hyper-responsiveness or a selective receptor problem. This was highlighted by the results of the Oxford group, who also used buspirone in male CFS patients and controls[99]. Patients had significantly higher prolactin responses to the challenge, but the growth hormone response did not differ. This was interpreted as evidence against an increase in hypothalamic $5\text{-}HT_{1A}$ receptor sensitivity. In a preliminary study the King's group used *d*-fenfluramine, a more selective 5-HT agonist, but found a blunted prolactin response, although their choice of controls was not ideal[84].

A second, more extensive, study from the King's group gave interesting results[100]. Again using *d*-fenfluramine to target the 5-HT$_2$ receptor, they compared CFS subjects repeatedly screened to exclude depression, depressed patients from the Maudsley, and normal controls. All were medication free. Depressed patients showed lower 5-HT responses, and higher cortisol levels, as expected. The normals were normal. However, the CFS patients, screened to exclude depression, showed higher 5-HT-mediated responses than controls, with lower circulating cortisol levels than controls (Fig. 11.2). These results confirm that CFS cannot be considered a form of masked depression (see Chapter 10). The Oxford group recently replicated the *d*-fenfluramine findings in chronically fatigued males[101].

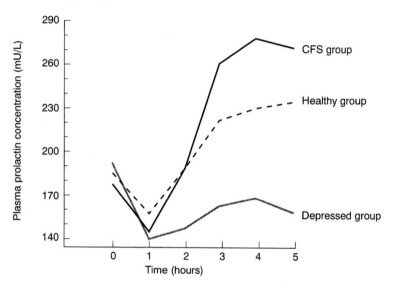

Fig. 11.2 Mean plasma prolactin concentrations after oral *d*-fenfluramine (30 mg) at 0 h in depressed patients ($n = 10$), CFS patients ($n = 10$), and healthy controls ($n = 20$).

Summary

Depression is associated with hypercortisolism. It seems likely that CFS is associated with the reverse. Depression may be associated with reduced 5-HT function, and there is some, albeit contradictory, evidence that CFS might be associated with the reverse. The relationship between these two variables, cortisol and 5-HT function, remains very unclear. Increased 5-HT activity could be the cause of the observed low cortisols in CFS, but the reverse is also possible (i.e., 5-HT upregulation could be secondary to the low cortisol).

It is tempting to speculate that at least some of the symptoms of CFS are due to a functional deficit of CRH. It is equally tempting to speculate on the relationship between these abnormalities and infection, since it is now known that neurones that respond to specific cytokines occur in the hypothalamus[102]. It is also reasonable to draw attention to the link between central serotinergic receptors, CRH synthesis in the hypothalamus, and the HPA axis[95]. Low cortisol could explain those studies showing evidence of a global, non-specific immune activation in CFS, because cortisol has a general property of damping down the immune response. CRH administered centrally (but not peripherally) also reduces peripheral NK cell activity[103], a frequent finding in CFS studies (Chapter 9). Ur and colleagues have suggested that the various manifestations of CFS and depression, both in their similarities and differences, may reflect the relative contribution of IL-1 and CRF[104].

Neuroendocrinology may also provide a link with the evidence reviewed in the previous chapter linking a past history of depression with subsequent onset of CFS. Depression is associated with hypercortisolaemia and chronic social stress. Animal studies have shown that chronic stress-induced hypercortisolaemia causes permanent loss of neurones in the hippocampal regions of the brain, and long-standing abnormalities in HPA axis function[105]. In humans, hypercortisolaemic depressed patients show reduced hippocampal volumes, while chronic stress such as sexual abuse may cause HPA axis perturbations long after the stress has resolved[106]. Thus it may be that previous episodes of depression or chronic stress leave so called 'endocrine scars', increasing the risk of subsequent CFS or depression.

The links between infection, cytokines, central neurotransmitters, and the HPA axis are thus a rich source of possible hypotheses concerning the pathophysiology of CFS[104,107], but a number of caveats must be made. Serotonin is but one among many amines and peptides that participate in the regulation of pituitary corticotrophin function[96]. Stress-induced activation of CRF neurones is complex, being mediated by many neuronal and hormonal factors. The results could also be non-specific: dexamethasone non-suppression of cortisol could be induced in normal subjects by weight loss and sleep deprivation[108]. Weight loss is not a prominent feature of CFS, so it is possible that the absence of weight loss and presence of hypersomnia accounts for the opposing neuroendocrine findings between CFS and depression. Workers from Liverpool were able to produce the same neuroendocrine findings as Demitrack and colleagues by studying normal subjects after five days of night-shift work[109]. They concluded that neuroendocrine findings in CFS may be the consequence of disrupted sleep and social routine.

Just as serotonin appears in many other sites, CRF is also not confined to the hypothalamus. It is widely distributed in the brainstem, limbic system, and cortex[110]. Areas of the brain such as the amygdala, stria terminalis, and raphe nuclei have particularly high concentrations of CRF, all of which areas are traditionally associated with control of a variety of behaviours and of affect[73]. CRF functions not only as a hypothalamic releasing factor regulating pituitary adrenal activity, but has many other roles, including that of a neurotransmitter.

Finally, we are aware of only one population-based study to address these issues. Finnish researchers were unable to find any differences between basal and post-DST cortisol between fatigued cases and controls[111]. Post-DST serum cortisol did not predict fatigue once adjustment had been made for age, gender, body mass, social status, and depression. As we have said so often during this book, it may be inappropriate to draw conclusions about the majority of chronic fatigue cases in the community from investigations of the minority in specialist settings.

In conclusion, a model in which CFS is due to CRF deficiency, and depression is due to CRF excess, is seductive, as is one simply contrasting the up- and down-regulation of serotonergic neurotransmission. It may explain some of the symptomatic differences between at least some forms of depression and CFS, but ignores the equally important similarities. Furthermore, both the recent studies contrasting depression and CFS seem to suggest a greater degree of homogeneity in the neurobiology of affective disorder than is justified. Investigators have struggled, and failed, to come up with a single unifying hypothesis for the neurobiological substrate of depression, and the literature is scattered with casualties. Most now agree that a single explanation of a deficit in either noradrenaline or serotonin (the monoamine hypothesis) is untenable, and it would be a pity if CFS investigators fail to learn from this experience. It would also be a pity if researchers in CFS fail to profit from the problems encountered from a large number of small studies, each carrying a substantial risk of missing significant findings.

Putting this together, it seems likely that some abnormality in CRF metabolism underlies both depression and CFS, and that serotonin function may well be abnormal in both, but in different ways. We suspect that a simple neurobiological distinction between the two will be hard to sustain, but that further investigation will reveal differences between subtypes of depression, some of which (e.g. the atypical depression complex) will link with CFS, and others may not. We share Demitrack's view that what is being witnessed is the final common pathway of chronic exhaustion, rather than a discrete disease entity. We also share his view that the CFS represents the end of complex unfolding of physiological and behavioural events, and that a single biological descriptor is most unlikely to explain the behavioural abnormalities that characterize the syndrome[112].

11.6 Serotonin, and other fatigue syndromes

Abnormalities of the serotonergic system may not be specific to either mood disorder or CFS. There is evidence that cerebral serotonergic abnormalities are associated with almost all pain syndromes[113], non-ulcer dyspepsia[114], irritable bowel syndrome[115,116], and premenstrual syndrome[117]. Similar abnormalities in fibromyalgia are particularly relevant to CFS. Abnormalities of brain serotonin have been suggested as being of importance in fibromyalgia[118], and serum serotonin and serotonin re-uptake receptors have been reported as reduced[119,120]. Yunus *et al.* extended their analysis to plasma tryptophan, the serotonin precursor, and its transport ratio, a more meaningful index of entry into the central nervous system[121]. Both were abnormal in fibromyalgia patients compared with normal controls. A study which reported low levels of serotonin metabolites in the cerebrospinal fluid of patients with fibromyalgia is consistent with this observation[122], although it has not been found in CFS patients[97]. Russell has proposed that a central reduction in 5-HT activity underlies the experience of pain, fatigue, and sleep disturbance in fibromyalgia[123].

11.7 CFS, fibromyalgia and sleep

The nature of sleep, its measurement, and the effect of abnormalities of sleep on fatigue were reviewed in Chapter 3. In this section we are concerned specifically with abnormalities of sleep in patients with the defined fatigue syndromes of CFS. Although the focus of this book remains CFS, because so much of the sleep literature derives from samples of patients labelled as suffering from fibromyalgia (FM), we shall draw attention to the fibromyalgia literature as well. We must acknowledge the uncertainty that exist as to whether or not findings from the fibromyalgia literature are directly applicable to CFS, although we think the similarities outweigh the differences (see Chapter 14).

Definition of fatigue in CFS and FM

When considering the role of sleep disorder we must return to the problem of definition (see Chapter 1). What exactly is meant by fatigue in the definitions of these syndromes? Whilst there is general agreement that the fatigue of CFS and FM is defined as a feeling state rather than as a performance decrement, the precise nature of that feeling state is often less clear (see Chapter 1). The current case definition for CFS does point out that fatigue should be predominantly a feeling of 'lack of energy or exhaustion', rather than 'sleepiness'[124]. Furthermore an early study using an objective test of sleepiness (the multiple sleep latency test or MSLT) in patients with CFS reported that although fatigued, they were not especially sleepy[125]. Despite these attempts to define fatigue more clearly, the findings reviewed below suggest that most investigators are rather imprecise when assessing patients for studies. This is important because whilst 'sleepiness' or 'somnolence' may be described as fatigue, it is likely to have different associations with sleep than lack of energy[126].

Sleep and CFS

Problems with sleeping are so common amongst patients with CFS they are listed as a subsidiary symptom in most case definitions, but only a small number of studies have explored these complaints in detail. These are reviewed under the heading of subjective reports and polysomnographic studies.

Subjective complaints

Surveys have confirmed that subjective complaints about the nature and quality of sleep are common amongst patients with CFS[127]. A questionnaire assessment of 93 patients found that approximately 70 per cent complained of problems with sleep[128]. The most common complaints reported in this and other studies were of unrefreshing, disturbed, or poor quality sleep[128,129]. Other common sleep complaints are of difficulty falling asleep, and an increased need for sleep[128–130].

Objective measurements of sleep

A small number of studies have actually measured the sleep of patients with CFS using polysomnograph recording (see Chapter 3). This is usually done by having the subjects spend several nights in a 'sleep laboratory' whilst they have their sleep recorded. More recently the development of miniaturized recorders has made more naturalistic home recording possible.

Several of these studies have highlighted an apparently high prevalence of major sleep disorders in patients with CFS. This finding are all the more remarkable in the light of the fact that narcolepsy and sleep apnoea are exclusionary criteria from the current case definition[124]. For example three Australian patients have been described with a diagnosis of CFS in whom a diagnosis of narcolepsy was made after sleep recording[131]. However, as the paper notes that the patients' principal complaint was of daytime sleepiness this may tell us more about the diagnostic assessment of these patients than about CFS. Similar considerations are raised by other studies of patients with prominent sleep complaints. Dedra Buchwald from Seattle found that almost half of a sample of patients with CFS selected on the basis of having symptoms suggestive of sleep problems had sleep apnoea, though in most cases only to a 'mild' degree[132]. Lauren Krupp in New York[129] reported that one-quarter of a similarly selected sample had periodic leg movement disorder. Peter Manu in the USA reported that 10 of 30 consecutive referrals had either narcolepsy, sleep apnoea syndrome, or periodic leg movements[133]. These studies raise the important issue of sleep disorder as a differential diagnosis of CFS. They do not, however, help us answer the question of whether carefully selected consecutive series of patients with CFS have abnormal sleep and what role abnormalities of sleep may play in the aetiology of their symptoms.

One of us has carried out two studies of sleep in consecutive series of carefully assessed patients with CFS. In the first study[128] we recruited 12 patients with CFS but who did not meet criteria for major depressive disorder or have symptoms suggestive of sleep apnoea or narcolepsy. They were compared with age and sex matched healthy controls. Both groups completed sleep diaries and two nights' home polysomnography. The patients with CFS reported spending longer in bed and sleeping less well (with frequent nocturnal awakenings). The polysomnograph records largely supported these subjective reports showing that the patients woke more often during the night than the healthy comparison group. No major sleep disorders were found. More recently we repeated the study using a new and larger sample of consecutive referrals meeting criteria for CFS[134]. This time we also excluded any patients who met criteria for dysthymia, depression, or anxiety disorder. The findings were similar; patients spent longer in bed, tended to nap during the day, and many, but not all, had interrupted sleep.

In conclusion patient populations labelled as CFS may include a relatively high proportion of individuals with specific and treatable sleep disorders. More carefully selected samples do not. Carefully selected patients do, however, report excessive time in bed, daytime napping, and fragmented, inefficient sleep, reports that are confirmed by polysomnographic recording.

Sleep and FM

As with CFS several studies of patients with FM, who were selected as having a high likelihood of sleep disorder, have found a number of cases of narcolepsy[135], sleep apnoea[136,137], and periodic limb movement disorder. A more recent study on an unselected sample has also suggested an association with restless legs syndrome[138]. However, although these findings are clinically important, they do not address the mechanism of fatigue in the majority of patients with FM. Pertinent to this issue is the proposal that a specific sleep abnormality underlies FM. This hypothesis is the result of observations made by Harvey Moldofsky of Toronto more than 20 years ago[139]. Of ten patients with FM (then called fibrositis) he noted that seven had unusual alpha (fast 7.5–11 Hz) waves appearing during periods of non-rapid eye movement (NREM) sleep. This abnormality had been previously noted in fatigued patients and had been called 'alpha–delta' sleep[140]. Moldofsky and colleagues referred to it as the 'alpha EEG NREM sleep abnormality'[139] and hypothesized that this abnormality produced the pain and possibly the fatigue of patients with FM. The Toronto laboratory has subsequently replicated the abnormality in other samples of patients with FM[141]. Although the finding and theory has been persuasively presented, a number of questions remain unanswered: can the abnormality be reproduced in other laboratories, is it specific to FM, and what is its causal significance?

The attempts of other laboratories to replicate this finding has met with mixed success, being found by some investigators[142–145] but not others[133,146,147]. One possible explanation for this discrepancy is a technical point concerning EEG electrode position[146]. However, even if this explanation is correct, it remains unclear whether a valid observation is being missed by some investigators, or an artefact of muscle activity misinterpreted by others. The status of the abnormality therefore remains uncertain.

Are the sleep abnormalities specific to CFS and FM?

The sleep fragmentation observed in patients with CFS is certainly not specific to the diagnosis and has also been observed in patients with emotional disorder. Both dysthymic and anxious patients have poor sleep continuity including difficulty falling asleep, difficulty staying asleep, and spending longer in bed to obtain the same duration of sleep (reduced sleep efficiency)[148,149]. It is notable in this regard that subjectively reported sleep disorder in patients with CFS was found in one study to be correlated with degree of anxiety[150]. Given the overlap between fibromyalgia, CFS, and disorders of affect[151] these are clear confounding variables.

The specificity of the alpha–delta abnormality to FS is also in doubt. There is evidence that a similar abnormality can be found in patients with arthritis[152], as well as in patients with a diagnosis of CFS. Does this reflect a shared pathophysiology of pain and fatigue, or simply a common non-specific abnormality[147], perhaps associated with nocturnal vigilance[153] or anxiety[147]?

Does abnormal sleep cause the symptoms of CFS and FM?

Thus far we have noted that sleep abnormalities are common in patients with CFS and FM, but the specificity of these abnormalities is in doubt. We will now consider whether there is any evidence that problems with sleep contribute to the symptoms or putative biological abnormalities of CFS and FM. Two experimental approaches have been attempted. The first is to try to induce the syndrome by creating the sleep abnormality, and the second is to see if the syndrome can be effectively treated by interventions that selectively reduce or remove the sleep disorder.

Sleep disruption experiments

Volunteers who agree to deprive themselves of sleep feel fatigued, although this fatigue is usually characterized by predominant sleepiness (see Chapter 3). Experimental disruption of sleep to produce a fragmented EEG pattern also makes subjects fatigued and sleepy the next day[154]. One report suggests that whilst any disruption of sleep results in weakness, fatigue, and muscular pain, these symptoms are more severe when it is stage 4 NREM sleep that is disrupted. This requires replication. None of these investigations of sleep disruption were of patient samples, and there must therefore be doubt over whether the actual syndromes of CFS and FS were being reproduced, or simply similar non-specific symptoms with altogether different aetiologies. We must therefore ask does treatment of the sleep abnormality reduce pain and fatigue in patients with CFS and FM?

Treatment studies

There are no studies of intervention into sleep published in CFS, although it is the authors' clinical impression that reduction of prolonged sleep and/or normalization of a chaotic sleep/wake patterns does contribute to improvement in patients with CFS.

In patients with FM, Moldofsky[155] has reported that chlorpromazine (100 mg at night) increased the number of slow waves on a sleep EEG and also reduced fatigue and pain. It is not clear whether this effect was medicated via sleep or by another mechanism such as reduction in anxiety. A more recent study evaluated the effect of a low dose of amitriptyline (25 mg at night) in fibromyalgia[156]. Although about one-quarter of the patients reported a reduction in pain and fatigue this was not associated with any changes in the amount of alpha-NREM sleep. However, the alpha-NREM abnormality was only identified in a minority of patients at baseline.

Conclusion

So what can we conclude? Sleep deprivation or disruption can cause fatigue but this is usually characterized by predominant sleepiness. Major sleep disorders such as sleep apnoea and narcolepsy have been frequently reported in patients diagnosed as having CFS, despite these condition being excluded by the case definition. The nature and importance of more subtle sleep disorders in CFS and FM remains uncertain. There is sufficient evidence to suggest that disrupted sleep, whether or not of the specific alpha-NREM variety, may contribute to fatigue, muscle pain, and poor concentration[157]. It is also of interest that altered sleep/wake pattern may contribute to the biological abnormalities reported in CFS[82,109]. It seems unlikely, however, that sleep disorder is more than a contributing factor to the aetiology of these syndromes and that other factors including inactivity, emotional distress, illness beliefs, and neuroendocrine abnormalities also play a role.

References

1 Beard G. *A Practical Treatise on Nervous Exhaustion (Neurasthenia): its Symptoms, Nature, Sequences, Treatment*. New York, William Wood, 1880.

2 Janet P. *Les Obsessions et la Psychasthénie*, Vol. 1. Paris, Alcan, 1919.

3 Cowles E. The mental symptoms of fatigue. *NY Med. J.* 1893; **57**: 345–352.

4 Millon C, Salvato F, Blaney N, *et al*. A psychological assessment of chronic fatigue syndrome/chronic Epstein–Barr virus patients. *Psychol Health* 1989; **3**: 131–141.

5 Ray C, Weir W, Cullen S, Phillips S. Illness perception and symptom components in chronic fatigue syndrome. *J. Psychosom. Res.* 1992; **36**: 246–256.

6 Smith A. Cognitive changes in myalgic encephalomyelitis. In Jenkins R, Mowbray J (ed.) *Postviral Fatigue Syndrome*. Chichester, Wiley, 1991: 179–194.

7 Grafman J, Schwartz V, Scheffers M, Houser C, Straus S. Analysis of neuropsychological functioning in patients with chronic fatigue syndrome. *J. Neurol. Neurosurg. Psychiatry* 1993; **56**: 684–689.

8 Bastien S. Patterns of neuropsychological abnormalities and cognitive impairment in adults and children. *Cambridge International Symposium on Myalgic Encephalomyelitis*. 1990: 6.

9 Sandman C, Barron J, Nackoul K, Goldstein J, Fidler F. Memory deficits associated with chronic fatigue immune dysfunction syndrome. *Biol. Psychiat.* 1993; **33**: 618–623.

10 Altay H, Abbey S, Toner B, Salit I, Brooker H, Garfinkel P. The neuropsychological dimensions of post infectious neuromyasthenia (chronic fatigue syndrome): a preliminary report. *Int. J. Psychiat. Med.* 1990; **20**: 141–149.

11 Scheffers M, Johnson R, Grafman J, Dale J, Straus S. Attention and short-term memory in chronic fatigue syndrome patients: an event-related potential analysis. *Neurology* 1992; **42**: 1667–1675.

12 Moss-Morris R, Petrie K, Large R, Kydd R. Neuropsychological deficits in chronic fatigue syndrome: artifact or reality? *J. Neurol. Neurosurg. Psychiatry* 1996; **60**: 474–477.

13 Smith A. Chronic fatigue syndrome and performance. In Smith A, Jones D (ed.) *Handbook of Human Performance*. London, Academic Press, 1992: 261–278.

14 Deluca J, Johnson S, Natelson B. Information processing efficiency in chronic fatigue syndrome and multiple sclerosis. *Arch. Neurol.* 1993; **50**: 301–304.

15 Deluca J, Johnson S, Beldowicz D, Natelson B. Neuropsychological impairments in chronic fatigue syndrome, multiple sclerosis, and depression. *J. Neurol. Neurosurg. Psychiatry* 1995; **58**: 38–43.

16 Johnson S, DeLuca J, Diamond B, Natelson B. Selective impairment of auditory processing in chronic fatigue syndrome: a comparison with multiple sclerosis and healthy controls. *Percept. Motor Skills* 1996; **83**: 51–62.

17 Smith A, Behan P, Bell W, Millar K, Bakheit M. Behavioural problems associated with the chronic fatigue syndrome. *Br. J. Psychol.* 1993; **84**: 411–423.

18 Schmaling K, DiClementi J, Cullum M, Jones J. Cognitive functioning in chronic fatigue syndrome and depression: A preliminary comparison. *Psychosom. Med.* 1994; **56**: 383–388.

19 Joyce E, Blumenthal S, Wessely S. Memory, attention and executive function in chronic fatigue syndrome. *J. Neurol. Neurosurg. Psychiatry* 1996; **60**: 495–503.

20 Marshall P, Forstot M, Callies A, Peterson P, Schenck C. Cognitive slowing and working memory difficulties in chronic fatigue syndrome. *Psychosom. Med.* 1997; **59**:58–66

21 Watts F, Sharrock R. Description and measurement of concentration problems in depressed patients. *Psychol. Med.* 1985; **15** :317–326.

22 Robbins T, Joyce E, Sahakian B. Neuropsychology and imaging. In Paykel E (ed.) *Handbook of Affective Disorders.* Edinburgh, Churchill Livingstone, 1992: 289–308.

23 Brown RG, Scott LC, Bench CJ, Dolan RJ. Cognitive function in depression: its relationship to the presence and severity of intellectual decline. *Psychol. Med.* 1994; **24**: 829–47.

24 Cohen R, Weingartner H, Smallberg S, Pickar D, Murphy D. Effort and cognition in depression. *Arch. Gen. Psychiat.* 1982; **39**: 593–597.

25 Wessely S, Powell R. Fatigue syndromes: a comparison of chronic 'postviral' fatigue with neuromuscular and affective disorder. *J. Neurol. Neurosurg. Psychiatry* 1989; **52**:940–948.

26 Krupp L, Sliwinski M, Masur D, Freidberg F, Coyle P. Cognitive functioning and depression in patients with chronic fatigue syndrome and multiple sclerosis. *Arch. Neurol.* 1994; **51**:701–710.

27 Wearden A, Appleby L. Cognitive performance and complaints of cognitive impairment in chronic fatigue syndrome. *Psychol. Med.* 1997; **27**:81–90.

28 McDonald E, Cope H, David A. Cognitive impairment in patients with chronic fatigue: a preliminary study. *J. Neurol. Neurosurg. Psychiatry* 1993; **56**:812–815.

29 Michiels V, Cluydts R, Fischler B, Hoffman G, Le Bon O, De Meirleir K. Cognitive functioning in patients with chronic fatigue syndrome. *J. Clin. Exper. Neuropsychol.* 1996; **18**:666–677.

30 Marcel B, Komaroff A, Fagioli L, Kornish J, Albert M. Cognitive deficits in patients with chronic fatigue syndrome. *Biol. Psychiat.* 1996; **40**:535–541.

31 Ray C, Phillips L, Weir W. Quality of attention in chronic fatigue syndrome; subjective reports of everyday attention and cognitive difficulty, and performance on tasks of focused attention. *Br. J. Clin. Psychol.* 1993; **32**:357–364.

32 Smith A, Pollock J, Thomas M, Llewelyn M, Borysiewicz L. The relationship between subjective ratings of sleep and mental functioning in healthy subjects and patients with chronic fatigue syndrome. *Human Psychopharmacol.* 1996; **11**:161–167.

33 Eysenck M. *Attention and Arousal.* Berlin, Springer, 1982.

34 Wearden A, Appleby L. Research on cognitive complaints and cognitive functioning in patients with chronic fatigue syndrome (CFS): what conclusions can we draw? *J. Psychosom. Res.* 1996; **41**:197–211.

35 White P, Dash A, Thomas J. Concentration and the ability to sustain attention after glandular fever. *submitted.*

36 Lawton A, Rich T, McLendon S, Gates E, Bond J. Follow up studies of the St Louis encephalitis in Florida: reevaluation of the emotional and health status of the survivors five years after the acute illness. *South. Med. J.* 1970; **63**:66–71.

37 Von Economo C. *Encephalitis Lethargica–Its Sequelae and Treatment.* Oxford University Press, 1931.

38 Pampliglioni G, Griffiths A, Bramwell E. Transient cerebral changes after vaccination against measles. *Lancet* 1971; **ii**:5–8.

39 Jamal G. Neurophysiological findings in the post-viral fatigue syndrome (myalgic encephalomyelitis). In Jenkins R, Mowbray J (ed.) *Postviral Fatigue Syndrome.* Chichester, Wiley, 1991:167–178.

40 Smith A, Tyrrell D, Al-Nakib W, *et al.* The effects of experimentally induced respiratory virus infections on performance. *Psychol. Med.* 1988; **18**: 65–71.

41 Smith A. A review of the effects of colds and influenza on human performance. *J. Soc. Occup. Med.* 1989; **39**: 65–68.

42 Smith A, Tyrrell D, Coyle K, Higgins P. Effects of interferon alpha on performance in man: a preliminary report. *Psychopharmacology* 1988; **96**: 414–416.

43 Smith A, Thomas M, Brockman P, Kent J, Nicholson K. Effect of influenza B virus infection on human performance. *Br. Med. J.* 1993; **306**: 760–761.

44 Hall S, Smith A. Behavioural effects of infectious mononucleosis. *Neuropsychobiology* 1996; **33**: 202–209.

45 Prasher P, Smith A, Findley L. Sensory and cognitive event-related potentials in myalgic encephalomyelitis. *J. Neurol. Neurosurg. Psychiatry* 1990; **53**: 247–253.

46 Waddy H, Wessely S, Murray N. Central motor conduction studies in chronic 'postviral' fatigue syndrome. *Electroencephalogr. Clin. Neurophysiol.* 1990 **(suppl 73)**: S160.

47 David AS. Postviral fatigue syndrome and psychiatry. *Br. Med. Bull.* 1991; **47**: 966–988.

48 Bruder G, Towey J, Stewart J, Friedman D, Tenke C, Quitkin F. Event-related potentials in depression: influence of task, stimulus hemifield and clinical features on P3 latency. *Biol. Psychiat.* 1991; **30**: 233–246.

49 Buchwald D, Cheney P, Peterson D, *et al.* A chronic illness characterized by fatigue, neurologic and immunologic disorders, and active human herpes type 6 infection. *Ann. Intern. Med.* 1992; **116**: 103–116.

50 Holmes G, Kaplan J, Stewart J, Hunt B, Pinsky P, Schonberger S. A cluster of patients with a chronic mononucleosis-like syndrome: is Epstein–Barr virus the cause? *J. Am. Med. Assoc.* 1987; **257**: 2297–2303.

51 Daugherty S, Henry B, Peterson D, Swarts R, Bastien S, Thomas R. Chronic fatigue syndrome in Northern Nevada. *Rev. Infect. Dis.* 1991; **13(suppl 1)**: S39–S44.

52 Natelson B, Cohen J, Brassloff I, Lee H-J. A controlled study of brain magnetic resonance imaging in patients with the chronic fatigue syndrome. *J. Neurol Sci.* 1994; **120**: 213–217.

53 Cope H, Pernet A, Kendall B, David A. Cognitive functioning and magnetic resonance imaging in chronic fatigue. *Br. J. Psychiatry* 1995; **167**: 86–94.

54 Greco A, Tannock C,,Brostoff J, Costa D. Brain MR in chronic fatigue syndrome. *Am. J. Neuroradiol.* 1997; **18**: 1265–69.

55 Dupont R, Jernigan T, Butlers N. Subcortical abnormalities detected in bipolar affective disorder. *Arch. Gen. Psychiat.* 1990; **47**: 55–59.

56 Brown FW, Lewine RJ, Hudgins PA, Risch SC. White matter hyperintensity signals in psychiatric and nonpsychiatric subjects. *Am. J. Psychiat.* 1992; **149**: 620–625.

57 Mena I, Villanueva-Mayer J. Study of cerebral perfusion by NEUROSPECT in patients with chronic fatigue syndrome. In Hyde B (ed.) *The Clinical and Scientific Basis of ME/CFS.* Ottawa: Nightingale Research Foundation

58 Troughton A, Blacker R, Vivian G.[99m]Tc HMPAO SPECT in the chronic fatigue syndrome. *Clin. Radiol.* 1992; **45**: 59.

59 Simon T, Cowden E, Seastrunk J, Weiner E, Hickey D. Chronic fatigue syndrome: flow and functional abnormalities seen with SPECT. *Radiology* 1991; **181(suppl)**: 173.

60 Fischler B, D'Haenen H, Cluydts R, *et al.* Comparison of[99m] HMPAO SPECT scan between chronic fatigue syndrome, major depression and healthy controls: an exploratory study of clinical correlates of regional cerebral blood flow. *Neuropsychobiology* 1996; **34**: 175–183.

61 Costa D, Tannock C, Brostoff J. Brainstem perfusion is impaired in patients with myalgic encephalomyelitis/chronic fatigue syndrome. *Q. J. Med.* 1995; **88**: 767–773.

62 Patterson J, Aitchinson F, Wyper D, Hadley D, Majeed T, Beham P. SPECT brain imaging in chronic fatigue syndrome. *Rev. Immunol. Immunofarmacol.* 1995; **15**: 53–58.

63 Cope H, David A. Neuroimaging in chronic fatigue syndrome. *J. Neurol. Neurosurg. Psychiatry* 1996; **60:** 471–473.

64 Bench CJ, Friston KJ, Brown RG, Scott LC, Frackowiak RS, Dolan RJ. The anatomy of melancholia—focal abnormalities of cerebral blood flow in major depression. *Psychol. Med.* 1992; **22:** 607–15.

65 Ichise M, Salit S, Abbey S, *et al.* Assessment of regional cerebral perfusion by ^{99}Tc HMPAO SPECT in chronic fatigue syndrome. *Nucl. Med. Commun.* 1992; **13:** 767–772.

66 Goldstein J, Mena I, Jouanne E, Lesser I. The assessment of vascular abnormalities in late life chronic fatigue syndrome by brain SPECT; comparison with late life major depressive disorder. *J. Chronic Fatigue Syndrome* 1995; **1:** 55–79.

67 Schwartz R, Komaroff A, Garada B, *et al.* SPECT imaging of the brain: comparison of findings in patients with chronic fatigue syndrome, AIDS dementia complex, and major unipolar depression. *Am. J. Roentgenol.* 1994; **162:** 943–951.

68 Goodwin G. Functional imaging, affective disorder and dementia. *Br. Med. Bull.* 1996; **52:** 495–512.

69 Bench C, Friston K, Brown R, Frackowiak R, Dolan R. Regional cerebral blood flow in depression measured by positron emission tomography: the relationship with clinical dimensions. *Psychol. Med.* 1993; **23:** 579–590.

70 Mountz J, Bradley L, Modell J, *et al.* Fibromyalgia in women: abnormalities of regional cerebral blood flow in the thalamus and the caudate nuclus are associated with low pain threshold levels. *Arth. Rheumat.* 1995; **38:** 926–938.

71 Michelson D, Licinio J, Gold P. Mediation of the stress response by the hypothalamic–pituitary–adrenal axis. In Friedman M, Charney D, Deutsch A (ed.) *Neurobiological and Clinical Consequences of Stress; from Normal Adaption to PTSD.* Philadelphia, Lippincott-Raven, 1995: 225–238.

72 Checkley S. The neuroendocrinology of depression and chronic stress. *Br. Med. Bull.* 1996; **52:** 597–617.

73 Nemeroff CB. The role of corticotropin-releasing factor in the pathogenesis of major depression. *Pharmacopsychiatry* 1988; **21:** 76–82.

74 Bakheit A, Behan P, Dinan T, Gray C, O'Keane V. Possible upregulation of hypothalamic 5-hydroxytryptamine receptors in patients with postviral fatigue syndrome. *Br. Med. J.* 1992; **304:** 1010–1012.

75 Taerk G, Toner B, Salit I, Garfinkel P, Ozersky S. Depression in patients with neuromyasthenia (benign myalgic encephalomyelitis). *Int. J. Psychiat. Med.* 1987; **17:** 49–56.

76 Hudson JI, Pliner LF, Hudson MS, Goldenberg DL, Melby JC. The dexamethasone suppression test in fibrositis. *Biol. Psychiatry* 1984; **19:** 1489–1493.

77 Isaacs R. Chronic infectious mononucleosis. *Blood* 1948; **3:** 858–861.

78 Kleinman A, Straus S (ed.) *Chronic Fatigue Syndrome.* Chichester, Wiley, 1993.

79 Poletiakhoff A. Adrenocortical activity and some clinical findings in chronic fatigue. *J. Psychosom. Res.* 1981; **25:** 91–95.

80 Riordain D, Farley D, Young W, Grant C, van Heerden J. Long term outcome of bilateral adrenalectomy in patients with Cushing's syndrome. *Surgery* 1994; **116:** 1088–1093.

81 Disdier P, Harle J, Brue T, *et al.* Severe fibromyalgia after hypophysectomy for Cushing's disease. *Arth. Rheumat.* 1991; **34:** 493–495.

82 Demitrack M, Dale J, Straus S, *et al.* Evidence for impaired activation of the hypothalamic–pituitary–adrenal axis in patients with chronic fatigue syndrome. *J. Clin. Endocrinol. Metabol.* 1991; **73:** 1224–1234.

83 Kruesi M, Dale J, Straus S. Psychiatric diagnoses in patients who have chronic fatigue syndrome. *J. Clin. Psychiat.* 1989; **50:** 53–56.

84 Bearn J, Allain T, Coskeran P, *et al.* Neuroendocrine responses to D-fenfluramine and insulin-induced hypoglycaemica in chronic fatigue syndrome. *Biol. Psychiat.* 1995; **37:** 245–252.

85 McCain G, Tilbe K. Diurnal hormone variation in fibromyalgia syndrome: a comparison with rheumatoid arthritis. *J. Rheumatol.* 1989; **16(suppl 19):** 154–157.

86 Crofford L, Pillemer S, Kalogeras K, *et al.* Hypothalamic–pituitary–adrenal axis perturbations in patients with fibromyalgia. *Arth. Rheumatol.* 1994; **37:** 1583–1592.

87 Griep E, Boersma J, de Kloet R. Altered reactivity of the hypothalamic–pituitary–adrenal axis in the primary fibromyalgia syndrome. *J. Rheumatol.* 1993; **20:** 469–474.

88 van Denderen J, Boersma J, Zeinstra P, Hollander A, van Neerbos B. Physiological effects of exhaustive physical exercise in primary fibromyalgia syndrome (PFS): Is PFS a disorder of neuroendocrine reactivity? *Scan. J. Rheumatol.* 1991; **21:** 35–37.

89 Ferraccioli G, Cavalieri F, Salaffi F, *et al.* Neuroendocrinologic findings in primary fibromyalgia (soft tissue chronic pain syndrome) and in other chronic rheumatic conditions (rheumatoid arthritis, low back pain). *J. Rheumatol.* 1990; **17:** 869–873.

90 Mason JW, Giller EL, Kosten TR, Ostroff RB, Podd L. Urinary free-cortisol levels in posttraumatic stress disorder patients. *J. Nerv. Ment. Dis.* 1986; **174:** 145–9.

91 Yehuda R, Southwick S, Nussbaum G, Wahby V, Giller E, Mason J. Low urinary cortisol excretion in patients with posttraumatic stress disorder. *J. Nerv. Ment. Dis.* 1990; **176:** 366–369.

92 Bennett R, Clark S, Campbell S, Burckhardt C. Low levels of somatomedin C in patients with fibromyalgia. *Arth. Rheumatol.* 1992; **35:** 1113–1116.

93 Gupta KL, Shetty KR, Agre JC, Cuisinier MC, Rudman IW, Rudman D. Human growth hormone effect on serum IGF-I and muscle function in poliomyelitis survivors. *Arch. Phys. Med. Rehab.* 1994; **75:** 889–894.

94 Buchwald D, Umali J, Stene M. Insulin-like growth factor-l (somatomedin C) levels in chronic fatigue syndrome and fibromyalgia. *J. Rheumatol.* 1996; **23:** 739–742.

95 Liposits Z, Phelix C, Paull WK. Synaptic interaction of serotonergic axons and corticotropin releasing factor (CRF) synthesizing neurons in the hypothalamic paraventricular nucleus of the rat. A light and electron microscopic immunocytochemical study. *Histochemistry* 1987; **86:** 541–9.

96 Delbende C, Delarue C, Lefebvre H, *et al.* Glucocorticoids, transmitters and stress. *Br. J. Psychiatry* 1992 **(suppl 15):** 24–35.

97 Demitrack M, Gold P, Dale J, Krahan D, Kling M, Straus S. Plasma and cerebrospinal fluid monoamine metabolism in patients with chronic fatigue syndrome: preliminary findings. *Biol. Psychiat.* 1992; **32:** 1065–1077.

98 Majeed T, Dinan T, Behan P. Ipsapirone induced ACTH release – evidence for impaired activation of the hypothalamic–pituitary–adrenal axis in patients with chronic fatigue syndrome. *First World Congress on Chronic Fatigue Syndrome and Related Disorders,* 1995, Brussels: 103.

99 Sharpe M, Clements A, Hawton K, Young A, Sargent P, Cowen P. Increased prolactin response to buspirone in chronic fatigue syndrome. *J. Affect. Disord.* 1996; **41:** 71–76.

100 Cleare A, Bearn J, Allain T, *et al.* Contrasting neuroendocrine responses in depression and chronic fatigue syndrome. *J. Affect. Disord.* 1995; **35:** 283–289.

101 Sharpe M, Hawton K, Clements A, Cowen P. Increased brain serotonin function in men with chronic fatigue syndrome. *Br. Med. J.* 1997; **315:** 164–5.

102 Breder CD, Dinarello CA, Saper CB. Interleukin-1 immunoreactive innervation of the human hypothalamus. *Science* 1988; **240:** 321–324.

103 Irwin M, Vale W, Rivier C. Central corticotropin-releasing factor mediates the suppressive effect of stress on natural killer cytotoxicity. *Endocrinology* 1990; **126:** 2837–2844.

104 Ur E, White P, Grossman A. Hypothesis: cytokines may be activated to cause depressive illness and chronic fatigue syndrome. *Eur. Arch. Psychiat. Clin. Neurosci.* 1992; **241:** 317–322.

105 McEwen B. Neuroendocrine Interactions. In Bloom F, Kupfer D (ed.) *Psychopharmacology: the Fourth Generation of Progress.* New York, Raven Press, 1995: 705–718.

106 De Bellis M, Chrousos G, Dorn L, *et al.* Hypothalamic–pituitary–adrenal axis dysregulation in sexually abused girls. *J. Clin. Endocrinol. Metabol.* 1994; **78:** 249–255.

107 Hickie I, Lloyd A. Are cytokines associated with neuropsychiatric syndromes in humans? *Int. J. Immunopharmacol.* 1995; **17:** 677–683.

108 Mullen P, Linsell C, Parker D. Influence of sleep and calorie restriction on biological markers for depression. *Lancet* 1986; **ii:** 1051–1055.

109 Leese G, Chattington P, Fraser W, Vora J, Edwards R, Williams G. Short-term night-shift, working mimics the pituitary-adrenocortical dysfunction of chronic fatigue syndrome. *J. Clin. Endocrinol. Metabol.* 1996; **81:** 1867–1870.

110 Fisher LA, Brown MR. Central regulation of stress responses: regulation of the autonomic nervous system and visceral function by corticotrophin releasing factor-41. *Baillières Clin. Endocrinol. Metabol.* 1991; **5:** 35–50.

111 Hyyppa M, Lindholm T, Lehtinen V, Puukka P. Self-perceived fatigue and cortisol secretion in a community sample. *J. Psychosom. Res.* 1993; **37:** 589–594.

112 Demitrack M. The psychobiology of chronic fatigue: the central nervous system as a final common pathway. In Demitrack M, Abbey S (ed.) *Chronic Fatigue Syndrome: An Integrative Approach to Evaluation and Treatment.* New York, Guilford Press, 1996: 72–112.

113 Hampf G. Effects of serotonin antagonists on patients with atypical facial pain. *J. Craniomandibular Disord.* 1989; **3:** 211–212.

114 Chua A, Keating J, Hamilton D, Keeling PW, Dinan TG. Central serotonin receptors and delayed gastric emptying in non-ulcer dyspepsia. *Br. Med. J.* 1992; **305:** 280–282.

115 Dinan TG, Barry S, Ahkion S, Chua A, Keeling PW. Assessment of central noradrenergic functioning in irritable bowel syndrome using a neuroendocrine challenge test. *J. Psychosom. Res.* 1990; **34:** 575–580.

116 Gorard DA, Dewsnap PA, Medbak SH, Perry LA, Libby GW, Farthing MJ. Central 5-hydroxytryptaminergic function in irritable bowel syndrome. *Scand. J. Gastroenterol.* 1995; **30:** 994–999

117 Rapkin A. The role of serotonin in premenstrual syndrome. *Clin. Obstet. Gynaecol.* 1992; **35:** 629–636.

118 Moldofsky H, Warsh J. Plasma tryptophan and musculoskeletal pain in nonarticular rheumatism ('fibrositis syndrome'). *Pain* 1978; **5:** 65–71.

119 Yunus MB, Dailey JW, Aldag JC, Masi AT, Jobe PC. Plasma and urinary catecholamines in primary fibromyalgia: a controlled study. *J. Rheumatol.* 1992; **19:** 95–97.

120 Russell IJ, Michalek JE, Vipraio GA, Fletcher EM, Javors MA, Bowden CA. Platelet 3H-imipramine uptake receptor density and serum serotonin levels in patients with fibromyalgia/fibrositis syndrome. *J. Rheumatol.* 1992; **19:** 104–109.

121 Yunus MB, Dailey JW, Aldag JC, Masi AT, Jobe PC. Plasma tryptophan and other amino acids in primary fibromyalgia: a controlled study. *J. Rheumatol.* 1992; **19:** 90–94.

122 Houvenagel E, Forzy G, Leloire O, *et al.* Cerebrospinal fluid monoamines in primary fibromyalgia. *Rev. Rheum. Mal. Osteartric.* 1990; **57:** 21–3.

123 Russell IJ. Neurohormonal: abnormal laboratory findings related to pain and fatigue in fibromyalgia. *J. Musculoskel. Pain* 1995; **3:** 59–65.

124 Fukuda K, Straus S, Hickie I, Sharpe M, Dobbins J, Komaroff A. The chronic fatigue syndrome: a comprehensive approach to its definition and study. *Ann. Intern. Med.* 1994; **121:** 953–959.

125 Mahowald M, Nicol S, Culliton P, Brummit C, Peterson P. Chronic Epstein–Barr virus syndrome: objective measurement of night time sleep and day time somnolence. *Sleep Res.* 1988; **17**: 308.

126 Horne J. Dimensions to sleepiness. In Monk T (ed.) *Sleep, Sleepiness and Performance.* New York, Wiley, 1991: 169–195.

127 Schaefer KM. Sleep disturbances and fatigue in women with fibromyalgia and chronic fatigue syndrome. *J. Obstet. Gynecol. Neonatal Nursing* 1995; **24**: 229–233.

128 Morriss R, Sharpe M, Sharpley A, Cowen P, Hawton K, Morris J. Abnormalities of sleep in patients with the chronic fatigue syndrome. *Br. Med. J.* 1993; **306**: 1161–1164.

129 Krupp L, Jandorf L, Coyle P, Mendelson W. Sleep disturbance in chronic fatigue syndrome. *J. Psychosom. Res.* 1993; **37**: 325–331.

130 Sharpe M, Hawton K, Seagroatt V, Pasvol G. Follow up of patients with fatigue presenting to an infectious diseases clinic. *Br. Med. J.* 1992; **302**: 347–352.

131 Ambrogetti A, Olson L. Consideration of narcolepsy in the differential diagnosis of chronic fatigue syndrome. *Med. J. Aust.* 1994; **160**: 426–429.

132 Buchwald D, Pascualy R, Bombardier C, Kith P. Sleep disorders in patients with chronic fatigue. *Clin. Infect. Dis.* 1994; **18**: S68–72.

133 Manu P, Lane T, Mathews D, Castriotta R, Watson R, Abeles M. Alpha-delta sleep in patients with a chief complaint of chronic fatigue. *South. Med. J.* 1994; **87**: 465–490.

134 Sharpley A, Clements A, Hawton K, Sharpe M. Do patients with 'pure' chronic fatigue syndrome (neurasthenia) have abnormal sleep? *Psychosom. Med.*; 1997; **59**:592–596.

135 Disdier P, Genton P, Bolla G, *et al.* Clinical screening for narcolepsy/cataplexy in patients with fibromyalgia. *Clin. Rheumatol.* 1994; **13**: 132–134.

136 Molony R, MacPeek D, Schiffman P, *et al.* Sleep, sleep apnoea and the fibromyalgia syndrome. *J. Rheumatol.* 1986; **13**: 797–800.

137 May K, West S, Baker M, Everett D. Sleep apnoea in male patients with the fibromyalgia syndrome. *Am. J. Med.* 1993; **94**: 505–508.

138 Yunus M, Aldag J. Restless legs syndrome and leg cramps in fibromyalgia syndrome: a controlled study. *Br. Med. J.* 1996; **312**: 1339.

139 Moldofsky H, Scarisbrick P, England R, Smythe H. Musculoskeletal symptoms and non-REM sleep disturbances in patients with 'fibrositis syndrome' and healthy subjects. *Psychosom. Med.* 1975; **37**: 341–351.

140 Hauri P, Hawkins H. Alpha-delta sleep. *Electroencephalogr. Clin. Neurophysiol.* 1973; **34**: 233–237.

141 Moldofsky H. Fibromyalgia, sleep disorder and chronic fatigue syndrome. In Kleinman A, Straus S (ed.) *Chronic Fatigue Syndrome.* Chichester, Wiley, 1993: 262–279.

142 Simms R, Gunderman J, Howard G, Goldenberg D. The alpha-delta sleep abnormality in fibromyalgia. *Arth. Rheumat.* 1988; **31**: S100.

143 Silva A, Bertorini T, Lemmi H. Polysomnography in idiopathic muscle pain syndrome (fibrositis). *Arq. Neuropsiquiatr.* 1991; **49**: 437–441.

144 Branco J, Atalaia A, Paiva T. Sleep cycles and alpha-delta sleep in fibromyalgia syndrome. *J. Rheumatol.* 1994; **21**: 1113–1117.

145 Drewes A, Gade K, Neilsen K, Bjerregad K, Taagholt S, Svendsen L. Clustering of sleep electroencephalographic patterns in patients with the fibromyalgia syndrome. *Br. J. Rheumatol.* 1995; **34**: 1151–1156.

146 Flanigan MJ, Morehouse RL, Shapiro CM. Determination of observer-rated alpha activity during sleep. *Sleep* 1995; **18**: 702–6.

147 Horne J, Shackell B. Alpha-like EEG activity in non-REM sleep and the fibromyalgia (fibrositis) syndrome. *Electroencephalogr. Clin. Neurophysiol.* 1991; **79**: 271–276.

148 Reynolds C, Shaw D, Newton T, Coble P, Kupfer D. EEG sleep in outpatients with generalized anxiety: a preliminary comparison with depressed outpatients. *Psychiat. Res.* 1983; **8**: 81–89.

149 Arriaga F, Rosado P, Paiva T. The sleep of dysthymic patients: a comparison with normal controls. *Biol. Psychiat.* 1990; **74**: 649–657.

150 Chambers M, Kim J. The role of state-trait anxiety in insomnia and daytime restedness. *Behav. Med.* 1993; **19**: 42–46.

151 Hudson J, Pope H. The concept of affective spectrum disorder: relationship to fibromyalgia and other syndromes of chronic fatigue and chronic muscle pain. *Baillières Clin. Rheumatol.* 1994; **8**: 839–856.

152 Hirsch M, Carlander B, Verge M, *et al.* Objective and subjective sleep disturbances in patients with rheumatoid arthritis: a reappraisal. *Arth. Rheumat.* 1994; **37**: 41–49.

153 Anch A, Lue F, MacLean A, Moldofsky H. Sleep physiology and psychological aspects of the fibrositis (fibromyalgia) syndrome. *Can. J. Psychiat.* 1991; **45**: 179–184.

154 Martin S, Engleman H, Deary I, Douglas N. The effect of sleep fragmentation on daytime function. *Am. J. Respirol. Crit. Care Med.* 1996; **153**: 1328–1332.

155 Moldofsky H, Lue F. The relationship of alpha and delta EEG frequencies to pain and mood in 'fibrositis' patients treated with chlorpromazine and L-tryptophan. *Electroencephalogr. Clin. Neurophysiol.* 1980; **50**: 71–80.

156 Carrette S, Oakson G, Guimont C, Steriade M. Sleep electroencephalography and the clinical response to amitriptyline in patients with fibromyalgia. *Arth. Rheumat.* 1995; **38**: 1211–1217.

157 Affleck G, Urrows S, Tennen H, Higgins P, Abeles M. Sequential daily relations of sleep, pain intensity, and attention to pain among women with fibromyalgia. *Pain* 1996; **68**: 363–368.

158 Cleare A, Wessely S. Chronic fatigue syndrome: an update. *Postgrad. Update* 1996; **52**: 61–69.

12. The role of psychological factors in CFS

In Chapter 10 we considered the role of emotional disorders in CFS. We concluded that whilst they may be important, and sometimes adequate, explanations for the symptoms of CFS, other factors have to be considered for a more complete understanding of the illness. We then reviewed possible neurobiological mechanisms, concluding that whilst an exciting line of inquiry, the findings so far are only just beginning to add to our knowledge. In this chapter we focus on the role of psychosocial variables and their influence on CFS. In particular we consider the nature and origin of patients' beliefs about the illness, and their importance in determining its expression and outcome.

12.1 The nature and origin of patients' beliefs about CFS

We start where the patient starts, with an attempt to make sense of the otherwise incoherent and confusing symptoms they are experiencing. In particular we begin by considering the nature of the label that CFS patients choose to make sense of their condition — their attribution. We will consider what attributions patients with CFS make, why they come to the conclusions they do, and the implications of these conclusions.

Patients attending specialist medical services with CFS typically attribute their symptoms to a *physical disease process*, regardless of whether or not physicians are able to find any evidence of relevant physical pathology[1-8]. Furthermore they are typically resistant to the suggestion that psychological and emotional factors are important factors in the aetiology of the illness. A series of in-depth interviews with patients attending an infectious disease clinics with CFS found that almost all believed their illness to be physical in nature, and that the most appropriate diagnosis was ME (myalgic encephalomyelitis). When asked to elaborate most believed viruses to be the aetiological agent, for example 'a viral induced illness'. Other patients offered more diverse ideas on the notion of infection, for example '. . . my tonsils were still infectious when I had them removed — I sort of just got flooded with it (the infection)'. Physical factors were commonly considered not only as precipitating the illness, but also perpetuating it by persistence, for example '. . . a virus that is locked in the body cells' or damage, for example '. . . the virus has affected my immune system'[9]. Although almost half the patients believed social stressors had also played a part these were regarded to have acted by exacerbating a physical disease process, rather than by causing emotional distress. Two mechanisms were proposed. First, that stress had weakened the immune system, thus making the body more vulnerable to infection: 'Things like stress at work . . . weaken the system. . . . It seems to me that perhaps a virus, not necessarily a very harmful one on its own, might get below the body's defences because of the weaknesses'. Second, that stress worsened the already existing physical disease process: 'Without the stress the virus would not have affected me so badly'. Not only were emotional factors conspicuous by their absence but a significant minority of patients took time to point out to the interviewer what they believed the cause of the illness was *not*. Without exception these patients believed that cause was *not* 'psychological' which typically meant being imaginary, 'psychiatric' or in some way their fault, for example 'It [the illness] hit me at a time of life when I couldn't have been more fulfilled. So at no time must anyone dare tell me that it's all in the mind'. A similar qualitative investigation of the concerns and beliefs of patients attending a specialist CFS clinic in the USA obtained similar findings[10].

A recent study that compared the illness beliefs in CFS and multiple sclerosis found that the degree of conviction in the presence of an organic disease process expressed by patients with CFS was equal to that of sufferers from multiple sclerosis[8]. This is a remarkable finding when one considers the differences between these groups, most particularly in terms of their experiences with, and information they are likely to have received from, a medical profession deeply sceptical of the reality and physical basis of CFS. We have previously discussed the research evidence for physical disease processes in CFS and concluded that the subject is indeed one of uncertainty. Similarly, whilst the evidence does not suggest that CFS is a *mental* illness as the term is commonly understood, there is good evidence that psychosocial factors are of importance in its development and outcome. Hence the pro-physical disease and anti-psychogenesis attribution of many patients with CFS is both striking and potentially important. Why do patients develop these attributions, and why does it matter?

Ambiguity and bias

CFS is an illness of ambiguous status and uncertain cause. This ambiguity is problematic because it allows a wide range of beliefs, ideas, and fears to flourish, some of which may be inaccurate and unhelpful. Jerome Frank, the noted American psychotherapist, suggested a range of psychological responses to account for the chronic fatigue and emotional disorders he encountered in soldiers in the United States making slow recoveries from a mysterious infection, later found to be schistosomiasis. Frank detailed a variety of psychological reactions impeding recovery. Anxiety about the future, ignorance of the basic facts of the disease, lack of trust in their doctors, and a feeling that they would never recover, were all common[11]. He concluded that 'Patients suffering from unfamiliar diseases tend to develop emotional reactions which impede recovery, such as anxiety, resentment and confusion'. Aronowitz has made similar observations about the early epidemics of ME[12].

ME: mystery and uncertainty

Controversy concerning CFS is clearly rife. Unlike patients with multiple sclerosis or rheumatoid arthritis, the illness status of the potential CFS patient is uncertain. Why can they not work and are they really ill? They are consequently open to accusation and blame for not fulfilling duties. This ambiguity in turn leads to frequent conflict with relatives, employers, and the medical profession (we will consider these factors in the wider context of modern illness in Chapter 15). Furthermore, having vague, ill-defined symptoms such as fatigue, headache, poor sleep, and so on, for which no one can supply a satisfactory explanation, may lead to subjects blaming themselves for the disorder. Enquiry of fibromyalgia sufferers reveals similar concerns. They have apprehensions about having an illness of unknown cause, dissatisfaction with medical care, and concerns that others might not believe the intensity of their pain[13,14]. Patients are therefore under considerable social and personal pressure to offer a plausible explanation for their incapacity to others and to themselves and avidly seek any information they feel is relevant to help them in this process[9,15,16].

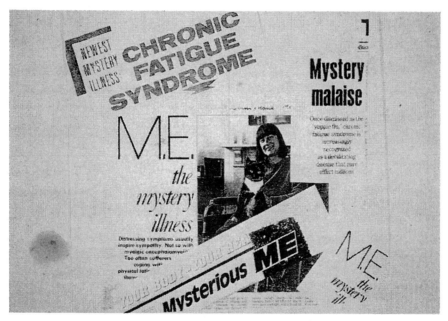

Fig. 12.1 ME: mystery and uncertainty.

Bias and attribution

As we saw above, one of the most common specific illness beliefs adopted by patients with CFS is that of a viral or post-viral condition. We have reviewed the evidence implicating viral agents in the aetiology of CFS, and concluded that overall it is not compelling (Chapter 9). Why then do patients come to such clear conclusions? The most likely reason is the person's recollection of experiencing symptoms consistent with infection at the onset of their illness. Although understandable, this attribution may be influenced by a number of biases.

First, viruses are very common – factors such as recall bias and search after meaning may lead to excessive aetiological weight being placed on the virus that happened to be around at that time (see Chapter 9). Second, the symptoms arising after non-specific infection may be remarkably similar to those occurring during episodes of mood disorder[17,18]. Although one contribution to a recent book on the subject is subtitled 'You don't get a temperature with a nervous breakdown'[19], both chills and fevers are not uncommon presentations of psychiatric disorder[20,21]. It is very easy to confuse the symptoms of one with the other. Symptoms of an emotional stress response may therefore be confused with those of infection. Third, whilst the attribution of the initial illness to viral infection may or may not have been correct, the adoption of the same attribution for ongoing symptoms is a different question. In many conditions the balance of physical and psychosocial causes in aetiology changes over time. One example is so-called post-concussional syndrome[22]. Precipitating causes are not necessarily perpetuating causes, although confirmatory bias may result in the initial explanation being adhered to long after the virus has done its work.

Patients' attributions may also be influenced by the information they receive from others about the illness. In this respect they may find themselves in double jeopardy: on the one hand there is an absence of meaningful information concerning the nature of their illness, its management, and outcome, and on the other some available information is potentially misleading and even deleterious to their well-being. It was notable in the aforementioned study[9] that health professionals reportedly had relatively little influence on the development of patients beliefs. Furthermore, in most cases their influence was simply to confirm a viral explanation, for example '. . . I was told by my doctor that I probably had a virus to begin with and that, for some unknown reason triggered off the chronic fatigue'. Another patient reported '. . .I don't want to believe the theory that my GP has, that it is all my fault because of my lifestyle'.

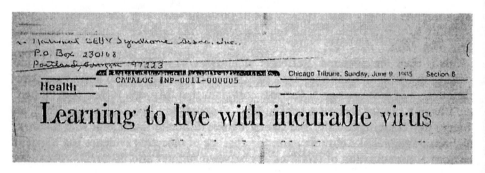

Fig. 12.2 Learning to live with incurable virus, (Chicago *Tribune*).

Correspondingly patients turn to and are influenced by the written material provided by journalists, patient associations, and the authors of self-help books. As one patient put it '. . . reading from campaign groups – which is all the information there is I suppose'. Unfortunately this information itself may be biased toward simple physical explanations of the illness that minimize the role of psychological factors and portray the illness as uncontrollable and even incurable[23,24]. Could the perception of CFS, ME, CFIDS, and related illnesses as incurable become a self-fulfilling prophecy, as suggested by one iconoclastic observer of the fatigue scene[25]? Certainly the patient's 'self-efficacy', the judgement of how successful one believes one will be in executing any course of action, is a crucial determinant of whether or not activity is attempted[26,27]. We think it probable that the general atmosphere promoted by some of the CFS literature may have a deleterious effect.

Attributions made by patient and doctor thus matter. We have shown how symptomatically there is little to separate the concepts of ME, neurasthenia, and CFS; the clinical descriptions are interchangeable. In a well respected text the best that can be offered for those with ME is 'sympathy and moral support'[28]. However, when the same symptoms are listed under the psychiatry section, this time as neurasthenia, the advice is active rehabilitation, cognitive therapy, and antidepressant medication[28]. Similarly, when CFS is seen as a viral problem, then there is 'no effective agent to treat the viral agent(s) of CFS . . . patients should be advised to obtain sufficient rest as required and avoid exercise'[29].

Socially acceptable explanations for illness

Why is information about the nature of the illness so polarized, and some explanations more acceptable than others? We have seen that whilst a proportion of the CFS sufferers interviewed do acknowledge that stress as well as infection may have played a part in the aetiology of their illness, it was considered to act through a physical (such as weakening immunity) rather than emotional mechanisms[9,30]. Patients reject the idea of psychogenesis, a concept seemingly accepted by patients seen in psychiatric clinics with depression[1]. This apparent contradiction between an acceptance of 'stress' and a rejection of psychogenesis reflects the social meaning of these explanations; illness acquired through external agency such as stress and viral illness is commonly seen as *blameless*[31], whereas a role for psychological factors raises doubts about both the *reality of the illness* (and hence eligibility to the sick role)[32], and the *character of the sufferer*[33]. In other words it is their own fault.

This is then the dilemma. Sufferers of illnesses like CFS and fibromyalgia look healthy, and have no abnormal tests, or other evidence to enable to occupy a sick role without loss of face or stigma. Patients complain that 'My skin is clear and tanned. I don't have a plaster cast on a broken leg . . . people say "you look so well" '[34], and observe that 'looking healthy and strong' causes difficulty in dealings with doctors[35]. In chronic fatigue, like chronic pain, the absence of objective evidence is a barrier to the normal organization of relationships between sufferer and doctor[36-8]. Because of this doctors turn to labels perceived by the patient (and also by the doctor) as pejorative, with the patient feeling both rejected and stigmatized[36]. The absence of objective evidence of ill health can have similar effects on relationships between patient and friends – many sufferers report their illness had altered their social relationships because 'no one understood what my illness was'[39]. Such complaints are neither new, nor specific, to CFS, but are an important part of the negative experience of patients with any chronic but ambiguous illness.

Alice Evans, from the US Public Health Service treated patients with brucellosis and researched the causes of 'chronic brucellosis' for many years (see Chapter 14). She championed the cause of the patients, perhaps because she believed she had the disease[40]. She wrote that 'it is a severe trial for the brucellosis patient, which contributes largely to the mental depression characteristic of the disease, that when he appeals for medical aid he is told that his illness is only imaginary and that all that is necessary for his recovery is to acquire the proper mental attitude'[41]. In our own time there are countless examples of similar sentiments in which the wider controversy about CFS, and in particular the suggestion that psychological or psychosocial factors may play a part, is interpreted by the individual sufferer as both disconfirming of the illness and distressing.

Others who have examined the attributions of patients in detail have come to similar conclusions. At the beginning of the century Ballet wrote about sufferers from neurasthenia that they 'spoke abundantly about their headaches and their muscular weakness, but deliberately concealed their emotionalism, symptoms it would offend their self-esteem to confess'[42]. At the end of the century Donna Greenberg wrote 'Patients who suffer from unrelenting fatigue fear they have a serious, occult medical problem and worry that people will think they had a mental problem or a blameworthy characterological weakness of will'[43]. Perhaps the strongest theme to emerge from the self-help literature and the individual writings of sufferers is just how stigmatizing and hateful is a label of any psychological disorder [23, 44]. The cultural beliefs underpinning this stigmatization are deeply rooted in the prevailing assumption of a mind–body dichotomy. The dilemma is eloquently expressed by Norma Ware, a Harvard anthropologist as follows:

Mind is the seat of reason and volition, body the locus of 'natural' biological processes that lie largely outside the realms of rationality agency and intention. The task and the challenge of mind is to exercise dominance over the body, to bring it under rational control. With control and volition come responsibility. We are held accountable for what we command or intend. Thus paradoxically, sickness of mind ('loss of reason') signifies not only failure of will and loss of control, but a failure of will and loss of control *we brought on ourselves*. It follows that we are responsible; psychological disorder is 'our own fault'.

The person who acknowledges psychogenesis is vulnerable to the accusation of being to blame. We may then ask whether some persons are more vulnerable to this pressure than others.

Personally acceptable explanation for illness

The typical case history given of sufferers frequently fulfils the image of conscientious, successful, dedicated person with high standards and responsibilities. CFS sufferers are often described using adjectives such as 'successful', 'high achievers', doers', 'dedicated' 'conscientious', 'hard working', and even 'overachiever', 'lifestyle dominated' or 'overactive' are frequently encountered[45–50]. Typical sufferers might be 'career women who push themselves to attain goals, working long hours and not eating properly'[51] or a '26 year old successful hard working stock broker . . . healthy, cheerful, social and energetic, often working 12 or more hours a day but none the less enthusiastically filling her remaining hours with plenty of sport or parties'[52]. Even children must be 'enthusiastic, energetic, positive-minded people who try too hard when they are ill'[53]. Such descriptions probably lie behind one of the less acceptable synonyms for CFS, 'yuppie flu'.

Similar attitudes were elicited during cognitive therapy of patients with CFS recruited from an infectious disease clinic in Oxford. The most common were high personal standards and perfectionism, with the implication that failure to live up to standards would mean failure as a person[15]. Such persons might be expected to be vulnerable to situations in which they are unable to live up to their personal expectations. When such failures happen, self-esteem may be threatened. It is therefore plausible that the physical disease attribution acts to protect the psychologically vulnerable patient from a threat to their self-esteem. In support of this hypothesis is the observation that, even when meeting diagnostic criteria for depressive illness, patients with CFS or post-infectious fatigue syndromes have been found to manifest both an absence of guilt, and a preserved self-esteem[17, 54–56]. The process of blaming a physical cause for the symptoms and incapacity may therefore deflect the blame and allow the person to preserve their self-image as strong responsible individuals with an immense ability to cope with adversity – 'not the sort of person to become depressed'[15,30,54,57].

Such ideas mesh well with one sociological explanation for the rise of CFS in the 1980s[58]. The general emphasis on achievement that was part of the *Zeitgeist* of the 1980s increases the risk that vulnerable persons will be under pressure to perform. At the same time these personal and societal pressures fostered both an increased sense of failure and self-blame when unable to perform at previously high levels, coupled with a reluctance to acknowledge any internal reasons why this might be so, lest they be interpreted as signs of weakness[33, 59]. Similar observations have been made about the aetiology of CFS in children[60].

Illness identity and patient groups

Perhaps in part as a reaction to a perceived lack of social and medical acknowledgement of their suffering, many patients with CFS come to see the illness as the central problem in their lives and even as a cause to be championed[7]. Linked with this conviction is a strong sense of community with other sufferers. This can be seen on the macro level, with the emergence of support, fund-raising, and lobby groups[61]. We shall discuss these wider social forces in Chapter 15. On the individual level it is reflected in the language of sufferers.

In a study of the language used by support groups on the Internet[44], CFS sufferers were found to have very high rates of 'self-reference' ('my disease') compared those with diabetes or cancer who were more likely to talk of 'the disease' or 'that disease'. Of all the illness groups on the Internet, the CFS patients wrote the longest replies, attesting to the importance of such communication. This profound identification with the illness as a 'cause' can become almost mystical. An editorial in a patients' magazine entitled 'Belief in ourselves' commented that 'We are standard bearers . . . We know that somehow, somewhere, out there, a mistake has been made. We know we are in the right . . . Every sufferer's experience helps us bear witness to the truth . . . One day we shall prevail'[62].

It is hard to ignore the effect of such passionate rhetoric and conviction, which must have beneficial effects on group identity, coherence, and perhaps the self-esteem of those who read it. But are there adverse effects as well? One controversial finding is that in two studies[4, 63], but not a third[64], membership of a self-help group was independently associated with either poor prognosis or poor compliance with treatment. One interpretation is that membership is associated with longer illness duration and greater illness severity. Another is that membership of a self-help group is associated with certain beliefs and illness behaviours, such as symptom reinforcement, anti-mental health biases and an adherence to certain ways of coping with the illness (see below). 'A potential danger of group support is an unwillingness to tolerate multiple conceptualisations and coping strategies. Such intolerance reduces the kind of information available to group members'[44].

Another possible drawback of a strong illness identity implicit in group membership lies in the information conveyed about outcome. Self-help groups are likely to attract the most chronically ill and the most disabled. In our clinical experience when patients improve they leave the group scene in order to resume their lives. Many report on the negative and demoralizing effect of interacting with sufferers with often profound disability. The information conveyed on outcome in the popular literature is gloomy – the disease has 'an alarming tendency to chronicity'[65],[66] and sufferers must make 'very significant changes in their life style'[65].

12.2 The importance of illness beliefs

We have examined the nature of patients' beliefs about the illness and the factors which may shape them. But do they matter? We argue that they do, and that irrespective of the biology of CFS they have important effects on the presentation of the illness, the type of help sought, and even the eventual outcome.

Outcome

The evidence that patients' attributions actually predict the outcome of their illness is strong. Several prognostic studies have found that the rather crudely measured psychological variable of disease conviction is associated with a worse outcome for patients attending hospital services[4,67,68]. Even in the community, believing symptoms were due to 'ME' was associated with more fatigue and disability, even when initial duration and severity of symptoms was controlled for[30]. In contrast, laboratory variables associated with hypothetical disease processes do not predict outcome at all[67,69,70].

Why might patients' beliefs about their illness predict outcome? There are several possibilities. First, the patients who believe most strongly in a physical attribution may be correct – they have a more malign disease process (but one that is beyond conventional laboratory measurement) that yields a worse outcome. This seems unlikely, however, because when measurable physical variables were controlled the association between attribution and outcome persisted[67]. Second, there may be a common variable such as personality that leads to both poor outcome and a somatic attribution. That is a possible explanation but it does not offer us any insight into the mechanism involved. Third, the patients' beliefs themselves may influence the outcome. In particular, the relevant cognitions are not that the illness is physical, but that it is serious and beyond control. These last possibilities are of considerable interest because if true, it implies that changes in belief may led to improvements in outcome.

In order to explore the role of illness beliefs in illness perpetuation we must widen the scope of our discussion to include a wider range of illness-related cognitions. It is normal for people to have thoughts about all aspects of their illness, and not just about the cause or diagnosis[71]. We suggest that such illness-related cognitions could provide a link between the crude concept of simple illness attribution and clinical outcome, and that the mechanism involves their effect on the patient's emotions and choice of coping strategies.

Emotion

The simple statement that many patients with CFS believe their illness to be physical fails to convey the meanings and texture of the beliefs. Some patients convey *implicit* assumptions about the meaning of symptoms via their choice of language – ME means that 'a virus is locked in my body cells'[9], or more elaborately 'these living viruses are erratic and unpredictable. The prickly-edged ones pierce their way into the body cells. If disturbed by the patient's activity they become as aggressive as a disturbed wasps' nest, and can be felt giving needle-like jabs (or stimulating the nerves to do so)'[72]. The disease attribution of CFS also conveys certain *explicit* meanings, such as the assumption that the illness is incurable, or associated with other even worse outcomes. Hence CFS means 'not just "hyperfatigue", but also significant neurological impairment and perhaps even death'[73]. In what is almost certainly the best known and most influential popular article on the subject a sufferer said that her symptoms meant 'an endless mononucleosis with a touch of Alzheimer'[74]. She continued that CFS was 'a package of misery', as well as a harbinger of 'serious damage. . . cancer, brain lesions. . . whether or not anyone recovers from CEBV is an issue mired in a depressing debate'[74]. A recent British book talked about 'deaths from ME . . . cardiac deaths, there are tumour deaths, there are liver deaths, all kind of deaths'[75]. Patients' illness beliefs are thus not simply neutral statements about probable aetiology, but are potent causes of fear, anxiety, and depression. This is an important point. We emphasize that the belief that CFS is a physical illness is neither inaccurate nor problematic – it is only when physical attributions act as a proxy for broader illness representations, and in particular the set of beliefs that CFS is chronic, severe, intractable, and uncontrollable, that problems develop.

The symptoms of distress may in turn be misinterpreted as further evidence of physical disease. For example subjective difficulties in thinking and alertness that may arise as a result of sleep disturbance, anxiety, and depression[76,77] could be blamed on brain damage, 'organic destruction of the nervous system'[78] or 'CFS dementia'[79]. Feelings of malaise arising because of depression and inactivity could be due to viral infection. Some of the beliefs are so potentially aversive and anxiogenic in their consequences that they are labelled 'catastrophic cognitions'. These might include the fear that any activity which causes an increase in fatigue is damaging or impossible; that 'doing too much' causes permanent muscle damage; and that CFS is irreversible or untreatable. In chronic pain catastrophizing is closely related to fear of movement, depression, and avoidance[80,81]. Catastrophic beliefs are equally common in CFS patients, and are associated with greater disability[82]. The role of catastrophic cognitions emphasizes that the attribution of unexplained symptoms to CFS is not neutral in its meanings and implications, but carries with it a set of other beliefs and assumptions, chief amongst which are that symptoms mean damage, that minimizing them is necessary, that the best way of doing this is via rest, and that failure to do so will have tragic consequences. We suggest that it is this link between attribution, the meanings of that attribution, and the promotion of a pattern of behavioural avoidance that may be the most likely explanation for the empirical finding of an association between physical attribution and poor outcome.

Coping behaviour

What would we predict as be the consequence of these beliefs for the patient's coping behaviour? It would be to promote the restriction of activity and avoidance of stimulation, both mental and physical. Studies have indeed found that the commonest coping strategy used by patients attending hospital clinics is avoidance[4, 9, 30, 68]. If patients understand that their symptoms are the result of discrete pathological processes, and if they also believe that such symptoms are warning signs which, if ignored, will lead to worse or even permanent disability, taking every precaution to reduce such symptoms becomes rational and understandable. There can be little doubt that many CFS sufferers consciously adopt coping strategies based upon avoiding activities that their experience has shown are associated with an exacerbation of symptoms. This might include reducing physical activity, but also reducing mental activity such as reading or watching television, social activities involving friends, or even certain foods[4]. A study of activity-related cognitions and actual physical activity found that such cognitions were related to reduced physical activity in CFS sufferers, but not in a control sample of multiple sclerosis sufferers[83].

Such strategies are also advocated by readily available information. The popular literature frequently emphasizes rest/avoidance as a coping strategy (see Chapter 15). For example, 'Always remember, until an exciting medical announcement is made, that there is no one drug to cure ME. The only cure is rest and keeping the affected parts of the body rigid so as to improve the body's defences'[72] or 'the only hope is that one day some substance will be isolated that has the power to zap the ME virus', and until then 'the most doctors can do is to advise patients to rest, and wait for the ME to go away'[84]. The beneficial effect of rest and the deleterious effect of activity is so much a part of the concept of ME that the person who did the most to advance the case for ME in this country wrote that 'if some doctors get beneficial effects after exercise, then their patients are not suffering from ME'[85].

What might happen if such advice is not heeded? A self-help book tells sufferers that they must only do 'seventy five percent of what you are capable of . . . unless you want to plummet down with another relapse soon, you really must follow the rule of doing less than you think you can'[86]. Another frequent theme of the literature is the cost of ignoring such advice. The original fact sheets produced by one of the self-help groups for CFS sufferers stated in bold type 'For the majority of M.E. sufferers, physical and mental exertion is to be avoided, and adequate rest essential. Important: if you have muscle fatigue do not exercise, this could cause a severe relapse' (M.E. Action Campaign 1989) although it is a pleasure to record that the patients' organizations themselves now regard such stark advice as simplistic. Nevertheless, encouraging children back to school might be harmful, 'especially because of the possibility of heart complications'[87]. A newsletter published for young sufferers tells them that 'Up to 30 per cent of patients may suffer from cardiac complications, depending upon the strain of infecting virus. There is therefore a danger of pushing a child too far physically'[88]. The same publication goes on to state that only 25 per cent of sufferers (i.e children) make a complete recovery. Similarly, 'cardiac complications are the commonest terminal event in ME'[89].

The link between attribution and avoidance has been supported by the results of a recent Dutch study which compared patients with CFS and patients with multiple sclerosis. As might be expected both groups attributed their symptoms to a physical cause[90], and in both groups the perception of lack of control over symptoms and symptom monitoring was associated with disability, confirming that these are *general* processes rather than specific factors in CFS. However, it was only in CFS that there was a relationship between attributing fatigue to a physical cause and lack of physical activity, and between lack of physical activity and severity of fatigue, suggesting that in CFS it is the *specific* illness beliefs that determine the pattern of behavioural avoidance, and contribute to the experience of fatigue.

Once rest/avoidance strategies have been adopted patients continue to use them because they work, or at least they appear to. In the immediate aftermath of a viral infection, which is how most current sufferers say their illness commenced, the immediate symptoms of fatigue, myalgia, pain, and sleep disturbance do indeed force people to rest. Furthermore, research has shown that those most likely to experience such acute symptoms intensely are those who have had previous episodes of emotional disorder[91]. Although no compelling evidence has been presented, we also think it probable that people who have been unusually physically fit prior to an acute infection also experience particularly intense physical symptoms, perhaps because they experience more rapid and profound physical deconditioning than others. The unusually athletic might also be prone to monitor their internal sensations more closely than most. In this context it is notable that those who develop CFS have an increased likelihood of a previous episode of emotional disorder (see Chapter 11), and also often report being particularly physically fit prior to their illness[92, 93].

Rest is also chosen because the opposite (i.e exercise) has been found to be ineffective. The literature contains numerous examples of abrupt attempts to return to dramatic physical activity which fail[94]. We will later argue that such efforts were either excessive in the light of current (as opposed to past) capabilities, or too brief. None the less, there can be little doubt that by the time patients reach specialist clinics, they will, for whatever reason, have consciously determined to reduce their amount of activity for fear of exacerbating their symptoms, and will continue to monitor both activity and its immediate consequences in order to avoid 'relapse'. The question is whether such strategies are the most effective in the long term. We think they are not.

The issue is therefore one of short term symptom reduction versus long term recovery: resting to reduce symptoms may be effective in minimizing symptoms in the short term, but only at a long term cost. We have already reviewed (Chapters 3 and 8) the deleterious effects of lack of activity on neuromuscular, neurological, cardiac, and respiratory function. This evidence alone should give pause for thought before recommending rest as a coping strategy in CFS. A decade ago Robert Schooley of Harvard Medical School observed 'there is no evidence that forced rest or inactivity ameliorates the illness or that physical activity worsens the underlying process'[95]. Empirical research confirms the adverse consequences of such strategies. We also draw attention to the only two relevant trials of which we are aware. The first, a randomized trial of bedrest for students suffering from acute mononucleosis, showed that those whose activity was unrestricted recovered more quickly than those who received bedrest[96]. The second is a trial of exercise versus rest for soldiers recovering from hepatitis which confirmed the benefits of early exercise[97].

In CFS there is evidence that those patients who maintain activity and distract themselves from symptoms are less functionally impaired than those who avoid activity or focus on symptoms[98–101]. In a prospective study behavioural disengagement predicted worse disability[113]. Symptom monitoring in normal individuals is associated with increased illness fears and increased somatic symptoms[102]. It is particularly noted in CFS[90, 100]. Concern about the meaning and significance of symptoms (which are often interpreted as 'warning signals') is heightened by the unpredictable nature of CFS. Another consequence of increased sensitivity to bodily sensations may be the greater sense of effort required to carry out both physical and mental tasks (see Chapters 8 and 11).

12.3 A cognitive behavioural model of CFS

We have seen that among patients attending specialist services certain illness-related beliefs and cognitions are particularly common. Such beliefs do not arise in a vacuum, but are the end result of an integration of individual attitudes, previous experience, available information, and the wider set of cultural and social pressures to which we have drawn attention.

These beliefs influence the person's emotional, behavioural, and via these, their physiological state. Thus the belief 'I'm damaging myself' causes anxiety whilst 'it's hopeless, I'll never get better' may lead to depression. The idea that activity 'only makes the illness worse' favours coping by avoidance of activity. Finally both emotional arousal and inactivity can influence physiology. These may be some of the ways in which illness beliefs play a role in perpetuating the illness.

Belief, emotion, physiology, and behaviour interact in mutually reinforcing vicious circles, an idea first outlined 80 years ago[103, 104]. The experience of symptoms, and fears about their meaning, interfere with the normal physiological and psychological processes required for effortful activity or cognitive processes. The consequence of increased concern is heightened awareness, selective attention, and 'body watching', which can then intensify both the experience and perceived frequency of symptoms, thereby confirming illness beliefs and reinforcing illness behaviour. This in turn contributes to a vicious circle of increasing symptomatic distress and increasing restriction of activity in order to cope with such symptoms. The more activity is avoided, the worse are the symptoms whenever it is attempted, thus providing further validation of the accuracy of the person's illness beliefs. Episodic attempts to be active merely serve to strengthen the patient's belief conviction of suffering from an insurmountable disease and leads to further concern about symptoms.

CFS and chronic pain

As we and others[105] have noted, there are many similarities between patients with chronic fatigue and those with chronic pain. Many illness beliefs of patients with CFS are similar to those of patients with chronic pain. These might include 'I should rest in bed'. 'I am damaging myself by doing too much'. Others are more specific to CFS: 'I have only a limited supply of energy', 'my immune system is damaged'.

The chronic pain literature also emphasizes the role of avoidance in perpetuating disability[106]. In chronic pain there is little dissent from the observation that fear of symptoms provokes and fuels avoidance behaviour, and that operant conditioning may account for symptom persistence[106]. As the patient's expectation that pain will follow activity increases, so do the precautions taken to avoid such symptoms. If these prove unsuccessful, fear increases. Stimuli that are anticipated, but unpredictable and uncontrollable, are particularly likely to lead to the final stage, when fear becomes fixed by the development of phobic anxiety. Avoidance of situations, including work, social activity, and travel, may result in the development of a phobic response on re-exposure. This is signalled by anxiety which in turn exacerbates pain (see Chapter 3), a further vicious circle.

We argue that perpetuation of CFS is based on a similar process in which where strategies such as rest, effective in the short term, may be maladaptive in the long term. Similarly, by the time the illness has become chronic, fear of activity itself may be sufficient to provoke symptoms. The implications of this model for treatment are considerable and would suggest the role for cognitive and behavioural interventions. These are outlined in Chapter 18.

12.4 Conclusion

The core message of this chapter is that what triggers an episode of chronic fatigue and/or chronic fatigue syndrome may not be what keeps it going. Just as chronic pain leads to major changes in lifestyle, activity, and behaviour that are independent of the original stimulus[107], so does chronic fatigue. We make a critical distinction between predisposing, precipitating, and perpetuating factors. We suggest that attributions do matter and may be important illness perpetuating factors. The good news is that all are, in theory, amenable to change. How this might happen is the subject of Chapter 18.

12.5 Caveat

This chapter is concerned with the tragic plight of what may be a small group of people – those who have the symptoms of CFS, the belief that their illness is called CFS or ME, and who show considerable disability and/or a need to make substantial accommodation to their illness. They are not representative of the population of patients with chronic fatigue[108, 109], and may not be representative even of those who use the term CFS or its variants to describe their illness[110]. In primary care, somatic attribution of fatigue was not associated with more physical symptoms[111], less psychological distress[111], or a worse outcome[112]. We know little about the illness representations of this group: this is an important area of investigation, particularly, if as we suspect, such people experience less disability than those who attend specialist clinics.

References

1 Wessely S, Powell R. Fatigue syndromes: a comparison of chronic 'postviral' fatigue with neuromuscular and affective disorder. *J. Neurol. Neurosurg. Psychiatry* 1989; **52:** 940–948.

2 Hickie I, Lloyd A, Wakefield D, Parker G. The psychiatric status of patients with chronic fatigue syndrome. *Br. J. Psychiatry* 1990; **156:** 534–540.

3 Lane T, Manu P, Matthews D. Depression and somatization in the chronic fatigue syndrome. *Am. J. Med.* 1991; **91:** 335–344.

4 Sharpe M, Hawton K, Seagroatt V, Pasvol G. Follow up of patients with fatigue presenting to an infectious diseases clinic. *Br. Med. J.* 1992; **302:** 347–352.

5 Ray C, Weir W, Cullen S, Phillips S. Illness perception and symptom components in chronic fatigue syndrome. *J. Psychosom. Res.* 1992; **36:** 246–256.

6 Vercoulen J, Swanink C, Fennis J, Galama J, van der Meer J, Bleijenberg G. Dimensional assessment of chronic fatigue syndrome. *J. Psychosom. Res.* 1994; **38:** 383–392.

7 Schweitzer R, Robertson D, Kelly B, Whiting J. Illness behaviour of patients with chronic fatigue syndrome. *J. Psychosom. Res.* 1994; **38:** 41–50.

8 Trigwell P, Hatcher S, Johnson M, Stanley P, House A. 'Abnormal' illness behaviour in chronic fatigue syndrome and multiple sclerosis. *Br. Med. J.* 1995; **311:** 15–18.

9 Clements A, Sharpe M, Simtin S, Borrill J, Hawton K. Illness beliefs of patients with chronic fatigue syndrome: a quantitative investigation. *J. Psychosom. Res.* 1997; **42:** 615–24.

10 Ware N. Society, mind and body in chronic fatigue syndrome: an anthropological view. In Kleinman A, Straus S (ed.) *Chronic Fatigue Syndrome.* Chichester, Wiley, 1993: 62–82.

11 Frank J. Emotional reactions of American soldiers to an unfamiliar disease. *Am. J. Psychiat.* 1946; **102:** 631–640.

12 Aronowitz R. From myalgic encephalitis to yuppie flu: a history of chronic fatigue syndrome. In Rosenberg C, Golden J (ed.) *Framing Disease.* New Brunswick, Rutgers University Press, 1992: 155–181.

13 Gaston Johansson F, Gustafsson M, Felldin R, Sanne H. A comparative study of feelings, attitudes and behaviors of patients with fibromyalgia and rheumatoid arthritis. *Soc. Sci. Med.* 1990; **31:** 941–7.

14 Robbins J, Kirmayer L, Kapista M. Illness worry and disability in fibromyalgia. *Int. J. Psychiat. Med.* 1990; **20:** 49–64.

15 Surawy C, Hackmann A, Hawton K, Sharpe M. Chronic fatigue syndrome: A cognitive approach. *Behav. Res. Ther.* 1995; **33:** 535–544.

16 Woodward R, Broom D, Legge D. Diagnosis in chronic illness: disabling or enabling – the case of chronic fatigue syndrome. *J. R. Soc. Med.* 1995; **88:** 325–329.

17 Imboden J, Canter A, Cluff L. Brucellosis: III. Psychologic aspects of delayed convalescence. *Arch. Intern. Med.* 1959; **103:** 406–414.

18 Imboden J. Psychosocial determinants of recovery. *Adv. Psychosom. Med.* 1972; **8:** 142–155.

19 Stone R. Presentation, investigation and diagnosis of PVFS (ME) in general practice. In Jenkins R, Mowbray J (ed.) *Postviral Fatigue Syndrome.* Chichester, Wiley, 1991: 221–226.

20 Harding T, De Arango M, Balthazar J, *et al.* Mental disorders in four developing countries. *Psychol. Med.* 1980; **19**: 231–241.

21 Wilson D, Widmer R, Cadoret R, Judiesch K. Somatic symptoms; a major feature of depression in a family practice. *J. Affect. Disord.* 1983; **5**: 199–207.

22 Lishman W. Psychogenesis and physiogenesis in the postconcussional syndrome. *Br. J. Psychiatry* 1988; **153**: 460–469.

23 Wessely S. Neurasthenia and chronic fatigue: theory and practice in Britain and America. *Trans. Cult. Psychiat. Rev.* 1994; **31**: 173–209.

24 MacLean G, Wessely S. Professional and popular representations of chronic fatigue syndrome. *Br. Med. J.* 1994; **308**: 776–777.

25 Loudon M. Great expectations. *Br. Med. J.* 1994; **309**: 676.

26 Bandura A. Self efficacy; towards a unifying theory of behavioral change. *Psychol. Rev.* 1977; **84**: 192–215.

27 Klug G, McAuley E, Clark S. Factors influencing the development and maintenance of aerobic fitness: lessons applicable to the fibrositis syndrome. *J. Rheumatol.* 1989; **16(suppl 19)**: 30–39.

28 Edwards C, Bouchier I, Haslett C (ed.) *Davidson's Principles and Practice of Medicine*, 17th edn. Edinburgh, Churchill Livingstone, 1995.

29 Cunha B. The conundrum of chronic fatigue syndrome. *Intern. Med.* 1995; **16**: 92–93.

30 Chalder T, Power M, Wessely S. Chronic fatigue in the community: 'a question of attribution'. *Psychol. Med.* 1996; **26**: 791–800.

31 Helman C. Feed a cold and starve a fever. *Cult. Med. Psychol.* 1978; **7**: 107–137.

32 Mechanic D. The concept of illness behaviour. *J. Chron. Dis.* 1962; **15**: 189–194.

33 Ware N. Suffering and the social construction of illness: the delegitimisation of illness experience in chronic fatigue syndrome. *Med. Anthropol. Q.* 1992; **6**: 347–361.

34 Berrett J. Condemned to live a lonely life. *Guardian* 6 July 1991.

35 Finlay S. Don't listen if your GP says it's 'just nerves'. *Scotsman* 18 August 1986.

36 Marbach J, Lennon M, Link B, Dohrenwend B. Losing face: sources of stigma as perceived by chronic facial pain patients. *J. Behav. Med.* 1990; **13**: 583–604.

37 Basanzger I. Deciphering chronic pain. *Sociol. Health Illness* 1992; **14**: 181–215.

38 Henriksson C. Living with continuous muscle pain—patient perspectives:I Encounters and consequences. *Scand. J. Caring Sci.* 1995; **9**: 67–76.

39 Schweitzer R, Kelly B, Foran A, Terry D, Whiting J. Quality of life in chronic fatigue syndrome. *Soc. Sci. Med.* 1995; **41**: 1367–1372.

40 Shorter E. *From Paralysis to Fatigue: a History of Psychosomatic Illness in the Modern Era.* New York, Free Press, 1992.

41 Evans C. Chronic brucellosis. *J. Am. Med. Assoc.* 1934; **103**: 665.

42 Ballet G. *Neurasthenia*, 3rd edn. London, Henry Klimpton, 1908.

43 Greenberg D. Neurasthenia in the 1980s: chronic mononucleosis, chronic fatigue syndrome, and anxiety and depressive disorders. *Psychosomatics* 1990; **31**: 129–137.

44 Davison K, Pennebaker J. Virtual narratives: illness representations in online support groups. In Petrie K, Weinman J (ed.) *Perceptions of Health and Illness: Current Research and Applications.* London, Harwood Academic Press, 1997.

45 Eland A. ME – not a middle class disease. *Social Work Today* 24 March 1988.

46 Hodgkinson N. Tired and alone, my mind reduced to porridge. *Sunday Times* 21 February 1987.

47 Maros K. Portrait of a plague. *Med. J. Aust.* 1991; **155**: 132.

48 Steincamp J. *Overload: Beating M.E.* London, Fontana, 1989.

49 Bryan J, Melville J. The ME generation. *Observer Magazine* 22 January 1989.

50 Timbs O, Walker I. 'Non diseases' – are you a victim? *Living* August 1991.

51 Willsher K. I beat the disease of the 90s. *Daily Express* 11 April 1990.

52 Askwith R. The ME generation. *Sunday Telegraph Magazine* 22 January 1989.

53 Gaskell R. When it is time for a child to be ill. *The Independent* 27 June 1989.

54 Powell R, Dolan R, Wessely S. Attributions and self-esteem in depression and chronic fatigue syndromes. *J. Psychosom. Res.* 1990; **34:** 665–673.

55 Webb H, Parsons L. Chronic PVFS in the neurology clinic. In Jenkins R, Mowbray J (ed.) *Postviral Fatigue Syndrome.* Chichester, Wiley, 1991: 233–239.

56 Johnson S, DeLuca J, Natelson B. Depression in fatiguing illness: comparing patients with chronic fatigue syndrome, multiple sclerosis and depression. *J. Affect. Disord.* 1996; **38:** 21–30.

57 Katz B, Andiman W. Chronic fatigue syndrome. *J. Pediatrics* 1988; **113:** 944–947.

58 Jacques M. ME and me. *Guardian* 5 October 1996.

59 Ware N, Kleinman A. Culture and somatic experience—the social course of illness in neurasthenia and chronic fatigue syndrome. *Psychosom. Med.* 1992; **54:** 546–560.

60 Fry A, Martin M. Cognitive idiosyncrasies among children with the chronic fatigue syndrome: anomalies in self-reported activity levels. *J. Psychosom. Res.* 1996; **41:** 213–223.

61 Charatan F. Chronic fatigue in the US. *Br. Med. J.* 1990; **301:** 1236.

62 Woodstock S. Belief in ourselves. *Perspectives: The Magazine of the ME Association* 1994, no. 3.

63 Wearden A, Morriss R, Mullis R, *et al.* A double-blind, placebo controlled treatment trial of fluoxetine and a graded exercise programme for chronic fatigue syndrome. *Br. J. Psych.* 1998; **172** 485–490.

64 Bonner D, Butler S, Chalder T, Ron M, Wessely S. A follow up study of chronic fatigue syndrome. *J. Neurol. Neurosurg. Psychiatry* 1994; **57:** 617–621.

65 Shepherd C. *Living with M.E. A Self-help Guide.* London, Cedar, 1989.

66 Smith D. *Understanding ME.* London, Robinson Publishing, 1989.

67 Wilson A, Hickie I, Lloyd A, *et al.* Longitudinal study of the outcome of chronic fatigue syndrome. *Br. Med. J.* 1994; **308:** 756–760.

68 Vercoulen J, Swanink C, Fennis J, Galama J, van der Meer J, Bleijenberg G. Prognosis in chronic fatigue syndrome: a prospective study on the natural course. *J. Neurol. Neurosurg. Psychiatry* 1996; **60:** 489–494.

69 Clark M, Katon W, Russo J, Kith P, Sintay M, Buchwald D. Chronic fatigue; risk factors for symptom persistence in a 2.5-year follow up study. *Am. J. Med.* 1995; **98:** 187–195.

70 Peakman M, Deale A, Field R, Mahalingam M, Wessely S. Clinical improvement in chronic fatigue syndrome is not associated with lymphocyte subsets of function or activation. *Clin. Immunol. Immunopathol.* 1997; **82:** 83–91.

71 Sensky T. Patients' reaction to illness. *Br. Med. J.* 1990; **300:** 622–623.

72 Dainty E. ME and I. *Nursing Standard* 1988; **84:** 49–50.

73 Vadas M. Meditations from an EB woman. *CFIDS Chronicle* Spring/Summer 1990: 66–70.

74 Johnson J. Journey into fear. *Rolling Stone* 30 July 1987.

75 Colby J. *ME: The New Plague.* Peterborough, First and Best in Education, 1996.

76 Cope H, Pernet A, Kendall B, David A. Cognitive functioning and magnetic resonance imaging in chronic fatigue. *Br. J. Psychiatry* 1995; **167:** 86–94.

77 Smith A, Pollock J, Thomas M, Llewelyn M, Borysiewicz L. The relationship between subjective ratings of sleep and mental functioning in healthy subjects and patients with chronic fatigue syndrome. *Hum. Psychopharmacol.* 1996; **11:** 161–167.

78 Field E. Management of the chronic (post-viral) fatigue syndrome. *J. R. Coll. Gen. Pract.* 1989; **39:** 171.

79 Goldstein J. *Chronic Fatigue Syndrome: the Struggle for Health. A Diagnostic and*

Treatment Guide for Patients and their Physicians. Beverley Hills, Chronic Fatigue Syndrome Institute, 1990.

80 Riley J, Ahern D, Follick M. Chronic pain and functional impairment: assessing beliefs about their relationship. *Arch. Phys. Med. Rehab.* 1988; **69:** 579–582.

81 Vlaeyen J, Kole-Snijders A, Boeren R, van Eek H. Fear of movement/(re) injury in chronic low back pain and its relation to behavioral performance. *Pain* 1995; **62:** 363–372.

82 Petrie K, Moss-Morris R, Weinman J. The impact of catastrophic beliefs on functioning in chronic fatigue syndrome. *J. Psychosom. Res.* 1995; **39:** 31–37.

83 Vercoulen J, Bazelmans E, Swanink C, *et al.* Physical activity in chronic fatigue syndrome: assessment and its role in fatigue. *J. Psych. Res.* 1997; **31:**661–673.

84 Hodgkinson L. ME: the mystery disease. *Woman's Journal* November 1988.

85 Ramsay A. More challenges to ME advice. *General Practitioners Weekly Briefing* 20 January 1989: 27.

86 Dawes B, Downing D. *Why M.E? A Guide to Combating Postviral Illness*. London, Grafton, 1989.

87 Colby J. The school child with ME. *Br.J. Special Educ.* 1994; **21:** 9–11.

88 Colby J. *Guidelines for schools*. ME Support Centre, Harold Wood Hospital, 1992.

89 Richards C. People and profiles: Dr E G Dowsett. *Perspectives, The Magazine of the ME Association*, 1991: 24–26.

90 Vercoulen J, Hommes O, Swanink C, *et al.* The measurement of fatigue in patients with multiple sclerosis: a multi-dimensional comparison with patients with chronic fatigue syndrome and healthy subjects. *Arch. Neurol* 1996; **46:** 632–635.

91 Wessely S, Chalder T, Hirsch S, Pawlikowska T, Wallace P, Wright D. Post infectious fatigue: a prospective study in primary care. *Lancet* 1995; **345:** 1333–1338.

92 Eichner E. Chronic fatigue syndrome; how vulnerable are athletes? *Physician Sports Med.* 1989; **16:** 157–160.

93 Riley M, O'Brien C, McCluskey D, Bell N, Nicholls D. Aerobic work capacity in patients with chronic fatigue syndrome. *Br. Med. J.* 1990; **301:** 953–956.

94 Peel M. Rehabilitation in postviral syndrome. *J. Soc. Occup. Med.* 1988;**38:**44–45.

95 Schooley R. Chronic fatigue syndrome: a manifestation of Epstein–Barr virus infection? In Remington J, Swartz M (ed.) *Current Clinical Topics in Infectious Diseases*. New York, McGraw-Hill, 1988: 126–146.

96 Dalrymple W. Infectious mononucleosis: 2. Relationship of bed rest and activity to prognosis. *Postgrad. Med.* 1964; **35:** 345–349.

97 Repsher L, Freebern R. Effects of early and vigorous exercise on recovery from infectious hepatitis. *New Engl. J. Med.* 1969; **281:** 1393–1396.

98 Ray C, Weir W, Stewart D, Miller P, Hyde G. Ways of coping with chronic fatigue syndrome: development of an illness management questionnaire. *Soc. Sci. Med.* 1993; **37:** 385–391.

99 Antoni M, Brickman A, Lutgendorf S, *et al.* Psychosocial correlates of illness burden in chronic fatigue syndrome. *Clin. Infect. Dis.* 1994; **18(suppl 1):** S73–S78.

100 Ray C, Jeffries S, Weir W. Coping with chronic fatigue syndrome: illness responses and their relationship with fatigue, functional impairment and emotional status. *Psychol. Med.* 1995; **25:** 937–945.

101 Moss-Morris R. The role of illness cognitions and coping in the aetiology and maintenance of the chronic fatigue syndrome (CFS). In Weinman J, Petrie K (ed.) *Perceptions of Health and Illness: Current Research and Applications*. Reading, Harwood Academic Publishers, 1997: 411–439.

102 Muris P, van Zuuren F. Monitoring, medical fears and physical symptoms. *Br. J. Med. Psychol.* 1992; **31:** 360–362.

103 Hurry J. The vicious circles of neurasthenia. *Br. Med. J.* 1914; **i:** 1404–1406.

104 Hurry J. *The Vicious Circles of Neurasthenia and their Treatment.* London, Churchill, 1915.

105 Blakely A, Howard R, Sosich R, Murdoch J, Menkes D, Spears G. Psychological symptoms, personality and ways of coping in chronic fatigue syndrome. *Psychol. Med.* 1991; **21:** 347–362.

106 Philips C. Avoidance behaviour and its role in sustaining chronic pain. *Behav. Res. Ther.* 1987; **25:** 273–279.

107 Keefe F, Gill K. Behavioural concepts in the analysis of chronic pain syndromes. *J. Consult. Clin. Psychol.* 1986; **54:** 776–783.

108 David A, Pelosi A, McDonald E, *et al.* Tired, weak or in need of rest: fatigue among general practice attenders. *Br. Med. J.* 1990; **301:** 1199–1122.

109 Pawlikowska T, Chalder T, Hirsch S, Wallace P, Wright D, Wessely S. A population based study of fatigue and psychological distress. *Br. Med. J.* 1994; **308:** 743–746.

110 Euba R, Chalder T, Deale A, Wessely S. A comparison of the characteristics of chronic fatigue syndrome in primary and tertiary care. *Br. J. Psychiatry* 1996; **168:** 121–126.

111 Cope H, David A, Mann A. 'Maybe it's a virus?' Beliefs about viruses, symptom attributional style and psychological health. *J. Psychosom. Res.* 1994; **38:**89–98.

112 Cathebras P, Jacquin L, le Gal M, Fayol C, Bouchou K, Rousset H. Correlates of somatic causal attribution in primary care patients with fatigue. *Psychother. Psychosom.* 1995; **63:** 174–180.

113 Ray C, Jefferies S, Weir W. Coping and other predictors of outcome in chronic fatigue syndrome: a 1-year follow up study. *J. Psychom. Res.* 1997; **43:** 405–15.

13. CFS in children

13.1. Fatigue in childhood

In Chapter 2 we noted that fatigue was one of the commonest symptoms experienced by adults, and one of the most common complaints in the GP's surgery. In contrast, children appear less likely to complain of excessive fatigue, and it is an uncommon reason for consultation before puberty. In Morrell's study of 21 098 consultations in a single general practice, of the 58 that were for a principal complaint of low energy, only four occurred in those under 15. Of the 14 symptoms that he studied, tiredness was the most unusual reason for consultation by a child[1]. In the UK National Morbidity survey the category 'malaise, fatigue, debility, tiredness' was extremely uncommon before adolescence[2]. In a Swedish population study no children under 10, and only 3 per cent of those under 14, reported fatigue[3]. Children tend to complain more of somatic symptoms such as pain or headache, and less of fatigue.

After puberty the prevalence of fatigue-related symptoms starts to rise. In a survey of children in a UK secondary school 18 per cent of boys and 13 per cent of girls responded positively to the question 'have you ever had a lot of trouble walking?'; 13 per cent of both boys and girls reported periods of weakness, and 6 per cent responded to the question 'have you ever been paralyzed?'[4]. In a two-week period 23 per cent of American adolescents reported low energy, and 21 per cent sore muscles[5].

Reporting somatic symptoms increases during adolescence – about 10 per cent experience frequent symptomatic distress[6], and experiencing multiple somatic symptoms becomes by no means unusual[7]. Eleven per cent of adolescent girls and 4 per cent of boys complained of 13 or more somatic symptoms[8]. The complaint of tiredness and low energy increases between the ages of 9 and 12. Eighteen per cent of 9-year-old girls admit to the symptom, and 29 per cent of 12-year-olds. Similar figures for the boys are 13 per cent and 19 per cent[9]. Symptoms in general, including both fatigue and hypersomnia, continue to increase in prevalence during adolescence[4, 10] and early adulthood[11], suggesting that the experience of fatigue is developmentally determined. In the context of depression the symptom 'everything is an effort' ranks fifth among those reported by depressed students, but first amongst depressed adults[12]. Another important factor relating to the experience of symptoms in childhood and adolescence is the person's own illness beliefs; preoccupation with health and illness fears were closely related to the experience of symptoms in a non-clinical population[4].

13.2 CFS in childhood

On 17 May 1994 the *Independent* newspaper carried a full page story on the subject of 'ME' in children. The article concerned one family's battle with ME[13]. First the mother and then her three children had been afflicted for five years. The consequence has been a life of 'complete restriction and isolation. School is a memory'. Mother told the journalist 'each night when I went to bed I hoped I would not wake up in the morning. I even thought at times it would be better for the children if they died'. Even allowing for journalistic hyperbole it is worth quoting the following subsequent paragraph in full:

Andrew will be 21 next month, but has no plans for a party because he has no friends to invite . . . they may read for half an hour or so until they get tired, or listen to music which will be barely audible to most people – their ears are particularly sensitive. Sheena may attempt to write a postcard to a penfriend and then she will have to rest. Jamie (12) may venture out into the garden to look at the pond for 10 minutes but will then sleep for hours.

The rise of ME in children is perhaps the most alarming addition to an already overheated atmosphere. In 1994 the figure of 12 000 child sufferers was quoted[14, 15]; it has risen to 24 000 sufferers one year later[16, 17]. In 1996 one in five schools reported at least one case: 'schools are hotbeds of ME'[18]. What is going on? Is there really an epidemic of CFS in children?

The professional literature offers few answers. Until recently one of the interesting epidemiological observations of CFS was that it is unusual in children. For example, in a survey of Scottish general practitioners 293 cases of CFS were recognized, but only 3 occurred in children under the age of 15[19]. In 1990 the Hospital for Sick Children at Great Ormond Street reported seeing about 10 to 15 cases per year referred from the whole of the country[20]. However, in Andrew Lloyd's epidemiological study in Australia 8 out of 42 cases were under 15[21]. At present the exact dimensions of the problem remain unclear.

Epidemic outbreaks of CFS have also been reported in children, including children as young as 18 months[22]. It is difficult to know what to make of these small, isolated epidemics, and they have perhaps been allocated more importance than may be justified by the quality of the data presented. Some may be outbreaks of infection in which children, often for other reasons, make protracted recoveries. Others may be due to altered perception of the usual level of childhood somatic symptoms or common infections[23].

13.3 Clinical features

The prevalence of CFS in childhood remains unknown, but there is no doubt that children do present with symptoms not dissimilar to those encountered in adults with CFS. The recent consensus document issued by the three UK Royal Colleges considered that the diagnostic criteria developed for adults were equally applicable to children, with the exception of the six-month criterion, considered too long[24].

Chronic fatigue, muscle pain, headache, sore throat, and increased somnolence seem to be typical[25–28]. Many present after an acute infective episode[26, 27]. As in adults, children seen in specialist settings show a bias towards higher socio-economic groups[26, 29]. Also similar to the situation in adults, many children attending specialist centres with a diagnosis of CFS are often 'high achievers'.

Reports from specialist centres emphasize that disability can be profound. Children referred to such centres often have long histories of absence from school, accompanied by impairment in social and leisure activities. Loss of peer relationships is frequent[26–28].

13.4 Aetiology

Psychiatric conditions

The symptoms of CFS in childhood include those of psychological distress. 'In our experience the chief symptoms are psychiatric, consisting of anxiety and a clinging dependency to parents, associated with undisputed fatigue and often incapacitating myalgia'[30]. 'Mood swings and . . . panic attacks are common'[31]. Depression is a very frequent symptom in children presenting with CFS; according to Bell, 60 to 80 per cent of children with CFS report depression[32].

What lies behind such symptoms? Is CFS in children a presentation of childhood depression, for example? Fatigue is certainly a feature of childhood depression[33], and fatigue, especially among boys, is associated with suicidal thoughts[34]. Depression in childhood may also be 'masked' by symptoms of fatigue, weakness, abdominal pain, and school avoidance[35].

There are fewer formal studies of psychiatric disorder in CFS for children than for adults. Wilson and colleagues looked at 39 children in Scotland[29]. Clinically the patients presented with a combination of myalgic and depressive symptoms. Many also had positive serology for recent enteroviral infection (see below). The authors noted the high prevalence of psychological distress, but were non-committal about its origins. Smith and colleagues studied 15 adolescents with chronic fatigue, all of whom would fulfil current criteria for CFS[28]. Despite an intensive series of investigations, little evidence could be found for an infectious cause to their persisting symptoms. Smith and colleagues diagnosed one-third of their subjects as suffering from RDC major depression[28]. Even in the others they noted that the pattern of symptoms was similar to those found in depressed adolescents, with the exception that classic depressive symptoms such as suicidal ideation or anhedonia were uncommon, although fear of dying/preoccupation with death has been reported[29].

Studies comparing children with CFS to normal controls, children with chronic medical conditions, and children with overt psychiatric diagnoses found that children with CFS had more fatigue, and more psychological distress, than those with physical illness, but less than children with specific psychiatric disorders[26, 36–38]. This is identical to the findings in adults (Chapter 10).

A survey of 100 children with so-called 'psychosomatic musculoskeletal pain' showed that only 10 per cent were formally depressed[39]. Instead most had chronic diffuse pain, associated with certain social and family features.

There are now a few accounts appearing in the literature, and even more in the media, in which disability is profound, and the child regressed to a state of immobility and total dependence. These children are usually hospitalized for long periods of time, and may require skilled feeding and physiotherapy to prevent starvation or contractures. Most of these cases cannot be explained on a solely physical basis. Complete immobility in children without neurological cause is a rare, but well recognized, symptom of psychiatric disorder, and identical cases to those now appearing in the media have been described by paediatricians and child psychiatrists as conversion hysteria[40]. Some of these now carry the diagnosis of CFS[20, 41]. In theory hysteria should only be diagnosed when immobility is due to loss of function, rather than fatigue, but in practice the distinction is less clear-cut[42]. Some descriptions of affected children, who 'may have to fed intravenously, be unable to communicate or even sometimes fail to recognise their parents'[43] or 'be unable to cope with light or noise, fed entirely by nasal gastric tube, unable to speak or swallow'[44] overlap with children described with 'pervasive refusal syndrome'[45], in which children refuse to walk, talk, eat, drink, or look after themselves. Those cases have been linked to trauma. So far evidence implicating childhood sexual abuse and childhood CFS has not been presented, with the exception of the small numbers of children with profound disability that proves refractory to standard management[46].

Another important differential diagnosis is school refusal, since persistent non-attendance at school is often a feature of CFS, and affected children can also express anxiety about school. School refusal classically occurs in two situations – one in which there is evidence of separation anxiety from the mother, herself often anxious or depressed, the other associated with difficulties at school, such as bullying or a particular teacher. The child is characteristically well at home, and only develops distress in relation to school attendance. It can also appear in times of change, such as a new school, new class, or new teacher.

Classic school refusal and CFS can thus be distinguished in many cases. However, there are several situations when it is not so easy. First, when the child, particularly in the younger age group, develops physical symptoms rather than more obvious signs of emotional distress. Second, when school refusal complicates a period of physical illness, when the child become anxious about resuming school, but that anxiety is not recognized as such. A wish to resume schooling does not exclude the diagnosis, as some think. Two reports have noted a close connection between symptom exacerbation and the start of the new term, suggesting that anxiety about school was now playing a part[29,47], although others prefer to interpret this as the result of exposure to infection[48]. A Scottish study noted persistent school non-attendance with separation anxiety, again suggestive of school refusal[29]. Some children may be 'high achievers' who often have anxieties about their school performance, which caused them to work excessively hard to achieve at the limits of their ability, and may discourage them from returning after a period of illness. In any child with prolonged absence from school, very careful consideration must always be given to the possibility that school refusal is either a primary or secondary diagnosis.

In conclusion the role of formal psychiatric diagnosis in children remains unclear. It has been argued that CFS in children is associated with somatization[26,49,50], depression[26,28,37,38], and even bipolar disorder[51,52]. Overall we believe that relevant psychological factors contributing to CFS in children are not usually clear-cut psychopathological risk factors such as physical or sexual abuse, but instead may involve a complex family dynamic of involvement, high expectation, limited communication on emotional issues, and previous experience of illness[49,53]. The issue of high expectation is particularly relevant. One study reported that they aspire to an activity level which is higher than either they or their parents actually expect to attain[54].

As in adults, depression may be a sufficient, but not necessary, explanation. Most children are not depressed in the conventional sense[36] but are significantly more psychologically distressed when compared with both normal children and those with physical illness. As in adults, diagnosis alone is probably insufficient to either explain disability or to plan treatment. Nevertheless, the recommendation by Smith and colleagues that routine screening for depressive disorders be undertaken seems sensible[28].

Medical conditions

The possible differential diagnosis of chronic fatigue in childhood is almost as lengthy as that of adults (see Dale and Straus[55], Chapter 3). However, in practice a good history and examination usually reveals most. When 55 children with chronic fatigue were fully evaluated in one centre only one alternative diagnosis (sinusitis) was discovered[27]. In another series no child developed an alternative diagnosis during follow-up[26].

Unlike in adult samples, there have been fewer studies looking for possible virological or immunological abnormalities in children with CFS, other than for the purpose of making alternative diagnoses. Immunoglobulin levels are normal[26], as are serological markers for a range of possible infections, including enterovirus[26-28]. HHV-6 titres do not differ from controls[25,28]. A Scottish study reported that 33 per cent of children were reported as having recent enterovirus infection, on the evidence of the presence of IgM in association with high neutralizing antibody titres[29]. Whether or not this is evidence for active enterovirus infection is now questioned (see Chapter 9). Evidence of past EBV infection is common, but of doubtful significance other than as a possible, indeed probable, trigger. An increased level of circulating immune complexes has been noted by a Czech group[56].

Family factors

To what extent do parents influence chronic fatigue in their children? Even to ask this question is to risk criticism, but nevertheless the issue must be addressed.

There is an wide and uncontroversial literature showing how the symptoms and illness beliefs experienced by parents affect those of their children. Many years of research by paediatricians, sociologists, and psychologists have suggested numerous social and psychological mechanisms to explain these links[57,58]. Particularly well described is the link between symptoms experienced by mothers and those by their daughters[59]. Turning to CFS, both the popular and professional literature frequently draw attention to the observations that children with the illness seem to have an affected parent more often than by chance alone. This could reflect transmission of an infectious agent, but as none has ever been demonstrated this seems unlikely. Genetic factors may be responsible for shared vulnerability, but cannot explain why parent and child should develop symptoms concurrently. Instead, one explanation involves an exaggeration of the normal processes by which parents shape their children's illness experience and beliefs.

Most controversial is the question of whether or not symptoms and/or illness can be directly imposed by the parent onto the child, in its extreme form known as Munchausen's by proxy. Most clinicians who practise in this area will now be able to describe cases in which illness in the child appears strongly linked to the beliefs and behaviours of the parents[60–62]. David Taylor has written of his extensive experience of parents convinced that their children have bizarre medical conditions, often associated with non-existent allergies leading to forced avoidance and severe, often dangerous, dietary restriction. ME has joined that list[63].

Munchausen's by proxy, which implies deliberate deception on the part of the parent, is at the extreme end of the spectrum, and is fortunately exceptionally rare. Such cases do exist, but more common is the imposition of illness on children by parents with the best of intentions. Even in the most outlandish cases we have seen the parents are to be acting in what they perceive to be the best interests of the child, but the outcome is still tragic.

More relevant parental influences are more subtle, and less overt, than implied by labels such as Munchausen's or factitious disorder. Nearly every report on CFS in children makes some mention of the views of the family, usually with some comment to the effect that parents are convinced the child's symptoms are entirely physical, are reluctant to acknowledge any role for psychological mechanisms, or even to permit such an assessment to be made[25, 64]. Authors frequently comment on the strong views often held by the parents about the aetiology of their child's illness, expressed in the familiar 'It's physical, not psychological/all in the mind' dichotomy[25, 27, 47].

13.5 Assessment and investigation

The general principles of assessment do not differ in any substantial manner from good practice in adults (see Chapter 16). It is important to appreciate the validity of the child's complaints. Children are as, if not more, sensitive to any suggestion their ill health might be spurious, or 'all in the mind'. Acknowledging the reality of the child's symptoms reduces the risk of a defensive reaction by either the child or family[27]. Thus although exploration of family and psychosocial issues is always indicated, this must be done with tact and sensitivity[62], especially as many families continue to see the problems as solely 'organic'[27]. It is important to fully assess the family's views on aetiology and management, and where necessary offer appropriate reassurance. Paediatricians are starting to comment on how media information on CFS, often inaccurate and alarmist, can have an adverse impact on doctor–patient communication[65].

As in adults it is essential that a full clinical history and physical examination is performed in every case but the number of physical investigations should be kept to a minimum unless there are specific pointers in the history or examination. Laboratory investigations are usually unhelpful, with the exception of tests for infectious mono-nucleosis[25, 26, 28, 62]. Tests for the heterophile antibody (e.g monospot or Paul Bunnell) may be useful for screening, but do not diagnose either EBV infection or CFS. EBV infection can only be diagnosed by the presence of the VCA IgM antibody. Tests must be kept to a minimum, remembering, however, that they can serve to reassure families about the absence of sinister pathology thus allowing rehabilitation to proceed. Despite the occasional suggestion to the contrary[66] there is no role at the time of writing for complex neuroimaging techniques such as SPECT scan to establish the diagnosis.

13.6 Management

Fortunately, it is our impression that, more than their colleagues dealing with adults, paediatricians are well aware of the psychosocial implications of prolonged fatigue and immobility in childhood. It is likely that the majority of cases of CFS seen by general practitioners and local paediatricians are self-limiting, so long as sensible, balanced management of both child and family takes place[62]. Recent papers in the professional paediatric journals concerning CFS and its treatment in children are notable for their balanced tone (see Lask and Dillon[20], Marcovitch[62], and Katz and Andiman[67]) and the partisan excesses of some of the writings on adults has been absent. Paediatricians with a special interest in the subject emphasize the need to address the problem in 'not just physical, but also in emotional, social and family terms'[32, 62], a point we endorse.

In general the literature endorses an active management approach. By definition CFS in childhood occurs during crucial developmental periods. Every step must be taken to ensure that disruption to education, social, recreational, and peer group progress occurs for as short a period as possible; and unless there is compelling evidence to the contrary (and, as we shall see, there isn't) a 'wait and see' approach is contraindicated.

Active management involves a variety of approaches. The exact choice of approach will depend upon the degree of disability in the child, the views of the family, and the resources available. It will always involve working with all the family to promote increased activity and decrease illness behaviour.

Behavioural activation packages[27, 46, 47, 68–70] have given very encouraging results, often linked with a family therapy approach[53, 71]. As in adults, rest is not contra-indicated, but managed. Hence a child complaining of fatigue might be advised to 'rest for a few minutes' and then encouraged to resume activity[27]. Activities that involve 'bursts' of energy, such as tennis or football, are probably best avoided in favour of more easily monitored activity such as walking[55, 72]. Too rapid mobilization may be counter-productive – instead gradual increases over a period of a few weeks are preferred[41].

Other interventions that remove the child from the normal school or home environment should be used with caution. Home tuition should be avoided except in exceptional circumstances, and again only for a short period[47]. Graded re-integration to school must be encouraged as early as possible[55]. In the largest series to date, if the children were no longer in school immediate return to school was encouraged[27]. We concur that home tuition should be viewed 'as part of the strategy to bring your child back into contact with other children and teachers. Perhaps the next step is a gradual increase in attendance at school with staff and classmates being aware of the situation'[73].

Involvement of the parents in all aspects of treatment is, naturally, vital, because treatment failure may happen when the parents remain convinced that active rehabilitation would be harmful[47,69]. Work is often necessary to assist the parents in broadening their understanding of CFS, just as if they were patients themselves. Family issues are important. Sometimes one member of the family, usually the mother, has given up work to look after the child, leading to a fixed sick role which can be difficult to alter. Existing family characteristics such as overprotectiveness can be exacerbated. The loss of peer group contact reinforces the dependence of the child on the family[49]. Work with the family and liaison between health and education services is almost invariably required[72].

The following paragraph gives some details of practical points that, in the absence of data from randomized controlled trials, are currently considered good practice in rehabilitation[24, 27, 41, 47, 62, 72]:

- Begin by 'demystifying' the problem, giving a firm diagnosis and appropriate reassurance.
- Acknowledge the reality of symptoms and specifically address the 'all in the mind' issue.
- Ascertain current levels of functioning.
- Complete a timetable with child and family to establish clear periods of eating, rest, and activity in the day.
- Start where the child is at, with small increases each week (5 per cent). Stress the need to go at an agreed pace – not too fast and not too slow. As the child's tolerance improves the increases in level of activity can be more substantial.
- Activity might include a graded exercise programme as arranged by physiotherapist or easily monitored exercise (e.g. walking); a mental activity (e.g. reading); school activity; and social activity.
- Identify goals for first week with child and family.
- Review goals at the end of each week, clarifying whether or not they have been achieved, discuss what was difficult for the child and what was easy. Then set goals for the next week.

When dealing with severely affected children it is important that they receive the full range of multidisciplinary input. This is not always possible when children are managed, as sometimes happens, by individual paediatricians who may work in isolation. It is most important not to attempt to manage the complex problem of severely affected children without access to the combined skills of the multidisciplinary team.

13.7 Outcome

The outcome of CFS in children seems generally favourable (see Table 13.1), particularly with appropriate management[74, 75]. The first follow-up study reported that about half the children had improved two years later[28]. In a second natural history study of children seen in a paediatric clinic in 75 per cent symptoms had either

Table 13.1 Prognostic studies of children with fatigue

Study	Setting and definition	Duration of symptoms at outset	Main outcome used	Notes on outcomes
Carter et al.[26]	Paediatric infectious disease clinic, 31 patients under 18 years with 2 months medically unexplained fatigue	median 11 months range 4–37 months	Self-rating of clinical condition at a median of 17 months	100% followed: 24/31 returned to normal or improved with occasional relapse, 2/31 had got worse
Feder et al.[27]	Clinical sample of 54 patients under 21 presenting to a paediatric outpatient department with at least 3-month medically unexplained severely debilitating fatigue	not known	Telephone contact by doctor 24–72 months later	89% followed: 31/48 reported resolution of symptoms; 14/48 had improvement, but continued to have symptoms; 3/48 had no improvement: 1 of these was functioning, the other 2 were house-bound
Marshall et al.[25]	Tertiary care paediatric infectious disease clinic; 23 chronic fatigue patients (aged 4–17) according to clinical referral	median 6 months range 1–60 months	Telephone contact to family – parent or child's assessment of clinical state at 17–10 months	74% followed: 13/17 reported definite improvement, but 6 of these still had periodic episodes of fatigue; 2 reported no change; 1 diagnosed with ulcerative colitis and 1 bedridden with unexplained fatigue
Smith et al.[28]	Secondary care sample of 15 adolescents (aged 13–17) with 6 months medically unexplained fatigue, plus physical symptoms	mean 18.4 months range 6–36 months	Structured telephone interview with patient or parent at 13–32 months	0% followed: 4/15 completely well; 4/15 markedly improved and 7/15 unimproved or worse. 7/15 had mild or no activity restriction and 8/15 had moderate or severe restriction. Median of 15 school days missed in previous six months

improved or resolved over a two-year period, with only two getting worse[26]. Three-quarters of another series had also recovered over a similar time scale[25], with only one child going on to become 'bedridden with debilitating fatigue', that child belonging to a family which had several similarly afflicted members[25].

The outcome after appropriate management is even better. A recent paper reported the outcome of a case series of 50 children with severe chronic fatigue, most of whom recalled a triggering symptomatic infection. A programme beginning with careful assessment and engagement, followed by symptomatic relief, reduction of secondary gain, insisting on regular school attendance, and the gradual resumption of activity despite ongoing fatigue resulted in a good outcome in 94 per cent[27]. Excellent responses to simple occupational and physiotherapy, together with some family work, were noted among the 100 children with unexplained myalgia[39]. Outcome was also favourable in a study of 28 children with fibromyalgia[76], in children a diagnosis difficult to distinguish from CFS[77]. Such findings are uncontrolled and based on selected cases, limiting the conclusions that can be drawn. However, it is precisely such selected cases that are currently referred to paediatricians, and receive so much media attention. The literature therefore does contradict unsupported statements such as 'the average length of illness in teenagers lasts about four and a half years'[78].

13.8 Conclusion

When assessing a child with CFS it is difficult to fault Bell's advice that 'it is essential to examine family functioning and emotional risk factors objectively'[32]. Unfortunately not everyone agrees; a fact sheet prepared for children with ME advises that 'if your GP tries to send you to a psychiatrist, refers you to social workers or prescribes graded exercise programmes, refuse and change doctors immediately' (Undated Fact Sheet; Advice for Young ME Sufferers, ME Action Campaign). The sensible conclusion of Smith and colleagues that screening for psychological disorders was worthwhile was similarly labelled 'superficial and sceptical' by a physician sufferer[79].

We are unable to complete this chapter without some comment on these last quotes, and the general atmosphere surrounding the subject of children and ME at the time of writing. There can be no dispute that the subject of ME and children has been particularly prominent in the last few years, and that those who campaign to increase awareness of the condition have recently tended to concentrate their efforts on the subject of children who may be considered, in the unpleasant jargon, 'more newsworthy'.

There seems to have been little or no recognition of the possible adverse consequences of this campaign. Those of us clinically involved in the care of CFS have noted a dramatic increase in the number of referrals of severely disabled children in the last four years, views echoed by paediatricians of our acquaintance. Such children have been seen before, but not in such numbers. Given the severity of disability, and the educational/legal implications, it is difficult to accept that such children have been overlooked in the past, and that all we are seeing is a change in referral patterns. We think that there has been a true increase in the incidence of such presentations recently. We also think that this is the consequence, and not the cause, of the increasingly fevered atmosphere of the publicity in this area.

Psychiatrists have long been aware of the dangers of labelling – once someone has been given a label of a particular disorder they take on the characteristics of the disorder. There is no reason to disbelieve, and every reason to accept, that children are particularly sensitive to such issues. American paediatricians recently wrote that dangers exist in labelling children with a disease which 'has profound implications for their level of functioning in society, especially when the disease is not well defined in childhood and when there are no irrefutable laboratory markers for it'[80]. Another American neurologist, with a strong record of support and advocacy for adult CFS patients, likewise cautioned strongly against the same label in children[81]. If children or their parents are told that 'the average length of illness in teenagers lasts about four and a half years'[31,78] then it is possible that such observations become self-fulfilling prophecies, particularly as some of those who make such observations espouse management strategies that both differ from and occasionally contradict those reported in the literature, and endorsed in this chapter. We conclude that anyone contemplating the diagnosis in a child should be aware of the many difficulties that might follow, and should not do so without reflection[20,81].

We therefore hope that the media publicity surrounding the subject of CFS and children will show some much-needed restraint, and consider the possible consequences. The tragic story related in the newspaper article that introduced this section is, we believe, a warning of what can happen when these restraints are not observed. CFS does exist in children, but the devastating accounts of illness that we have encountered in our clinical work appear more understandable when considered in their wider cultural context, and should be preventable.

References

1 Morrell D. Symptom interpretation in general practice. *J.R.Coll.Gen.Pract.* 1972; **22:** 297–309.

2 OPCS. *Morbidity Statistics from General Practice; Third National Morbidity Survey*, 3rd edn. London: HMSO, 1985.

3 Essen-Moller E. Individual traits and morbidity in a Swedish rural population. *Acta Psych. Scand.* 1956 **(suppl 100):**1–160.

4 Eminson M, Benjamin S, Shortall A, Woods T, Faragher B. Physical symptoms and illness attitudes in adolescents: an epidemiological study. *J. Child Psychol. Psychiatry* 1996; **37:** 519–528.

5 Garber J, Walker L, Zeman J. Somatoform symptoms in a community sample of children and adolescents: further validation of the children's somatization inventory. *Psychol. Assessment* 1991; **3:** 588–595.

6 Aro H, Paronen O, Aro S. Psychosomatic symptoms among 14–16 year old Finnish adolescents. *Social Psychiatry* 1987; **22:** 171–176.

7 Campo J, Fritsch S. Somatization in children and adolescents. *J. Am. Acad. Child. Adolesc. Psychiatry* 1994; **33:** 1223–1235.

8 Offord D, Boyle MH, Szatmari P, *et al.* Ontario Child Health Study: II. Six-month prevalence of disorder and rates of service utilization. *Arch. Gen. Psychiatry* 1987; **44:** 832–836.

9 Carskadon MA, Acebo C. Parental reports of seasonal mood and behavior changes in children. *J. Am. Acad. Chil. Adolesc. Psychiatry* 1993; **32:** 264–269.

10 Kovacs M. Presentation and course of major depressive disorder during childhood and later years of the life span. *J. Am. Acad. Child. Adolesc. Psychiatry* 1996; **35**: 705–715.

11 Hagnell O, Grasbeck A, Ojesjo L, Otterbeck L. Mental tiredness in the Lundby study; incidence and course over 25 years. *Acta Psychiat. Scand. 1993;* **88**: 316–321.

12 Wells VE, Klerman GL, Deykin EY. The prevalence of depressive symptoms in college students. *Social Psychiatry* 1987; **22**: 20–28.

13 Hunt L. Despair in a doll's house. *The Independent* 17 May 1994.

14 Reilly H. Luke is 9 years old. *Daily Mirror* 10 July 1994.

15 Colby J. Study finds 12,000 pupils may be suffering from ME. *Sunday Times* 5 June 1994.

16 Illman J. Cry of the ME generation. *Guardian* 1 March 1995.

17 Pearson D. Unwilling to school. *Sunday Times* 20 August 1995.

18 Woodham A. Sick at school. *Good Housekeeping* May 1996: 82.

19 Ho-Yen D. General practitioners' experience of the chronic fatigue syndrome. *Br. J. Gen. Pract.* 1991; **41**:324–326.

20 Lask B, Dillon M. Postviral fatigue syndrome. *Arch. Dis. Child.* 1990; **65**: 1198.

21 Lloyd A, Hickie I, Boughton R, Spencer O, Wakefield D. Prevalence of chronic fatigue syndrome in an Australian population. *Med. J. Aust.* 1990; **153**: 522–528.

22 Bell K, Cookfair D, Bell D, Reese P, Cooper L. Risk factors associated with chronic fatigue syndrome in a cluster of pediatric cases. *Rev. Infect. Dis.* 1991; **13(suppl 1)**: S32–S38.

23 May P, Donnan S, Ashton J, Ogilvie M, Rolles C. Personality and medical perception in benign myalgic encephalomyelitis. *Lancet* 1980; **ii**: 1122–1124.

24 Anon. *Chronic Fatigue Syndrome: Report of a Committee of the Royal Colleges of Physicians, Psychiatrists and General Practitioners.* London, Royal College of Physicians, 1996.

25 Marshall G, Gesser R, Yamanishi K, Starr S. Chronic fatigue in children: clinical features, Epstein–Barr virus and human herpesvirus 6 serology and long term follow up. *Pediatr. Inf. Dis. J.* 1991; **10**: 287–290.

26 Carter B, Edwards J, Kronenberger W, Michalczyk L, Marshall G. Case control study of chronic fatigue in pediatric patients. *Pediatrics* 1995; **95**: 179–186.

27 Feder H, Dworkin P, Orkin C. Outcome of 48 pediatric patients with chronic fatigue; a clinical experience. *Arch. Fam. Med.* 1994; **3**: 1049–1055.

28 Smith M, Mitchell J, Corey L, McCauley E, Glover D, Tenover F. Chronic fatigue in adolescents. *Pediatrics* 1991; **88**: 195–201.

29 Wilson P, Kusumaker V, McCartney R, Bell E. Features of coxsackie B virus (CBV) infection in children with prolonged physical and psychological morbidity. *J. Psychosom. Res.* 1989; **33**: 29–36.

30 Behan PO, Bakheit AM. Clinical spectrum of postviral fatigue syndrome. *Br. Med. Bull.* 1991; **47**: 793–808.

31 Colby J. The school child with ME. *Br. J. Special Educ.* 1994; **21**: 9–11.

32 Bell D. Chronic fatigue syndrome in children. *J. Chronic Fatigue Syndrome* 1995; **1**: 9–33.

33 Angold A, Weissman MM, John K, Wickramaratne P, Prusoff B. The effects of age and sex on depression ratings in children and adolescents. *J. Am. Acad. Child. Adolesc. Psychiatry* 1991; **30**: 67–74.

34 Choquet M, Menke H. Suicidal thoughts during early adolescence: prevalence, associated troubles and help-seeking behavior. *Acta Psychiat. Scand.* 1990; **81**: 170–177.

35 Sturtz G. Depression and chronic fatigue in children. A masquerade ball. *Primary Care* 1991; **18**: 247–257.

36 Carter B, Kronenberger W, Edwards J, Michalczyk L, Marshall G. Differential diagnosis of chronic fatigue in children: behavioral and emotional dimensions. *Develop. Behav. Pediatrics* 1996; **17**: 16–21.

37 Walford G, McCNelson W, McCluskey D. Fatigue, depression and social adjustment in children with chronic fatigue syndrome. *Arch. Dis. Child.* 1993; **68:** 384–388.

38 Pelcovitz D, Septimus A, Friedman S, Krilov L, Mandel F, Kaplan S. Psychosocial correlates of chronic fatigue syndrome in adolescent girls. *J. Develop. Behav. Paediatrics* 1995; **16:** 333–338.

39 Sherry D, McGuire T, Mellins E, Salmonson K, Wallace C, Nepom B. Psychosomatic musculoskeletal pain in childhood: clinical and psychological analyses of 100 children. *Pediatrics* 1991; **88:** 1093–1099.

40 Goodyer I. Hysterical conversion reactions in childhood. *J. Child. Psychol. Psychiatry* 1981; **22:** 179–188.

41 Lask B. What does ME mean to me? The psychiatrist's view. *Maternal Child Health* 1991; **16:** 6–9.

42 Grattan-Smith P, Fairley M, Procopis P. Clinical features of conversion disorder. *Arch. Dis. Child.* 1988; **63:** 408–414.

43 Bassindale C. The ME generation. *Evening Standard* 23 April 1996.

44 Carpenter R. Why ME isn't a myth. *Daily Express* 16 November 1995.

45 Lask B, Britten C, Kroll L, Magagna J, Tranter M. Children with pervasive refusal. *Arch. Dis. Child.* 1991; **66:** 866–869.

46 Cox D, Findley L. Chronic fatigue syndrome in adolescence. *Br. J. Hosp. Med.* 1994; **51:** 614.

47 Vereker M. Chronic fatigue syndrome: a joint paediatric–psychiatric approach. *Arch. Dis. Child.* 1992; **67:** 550–555.

48 Colby J. *Guidelines for Schools.* ME Support Centre, Harold Wood Hospital, 1992.

49. Garralda M. Severe chronic fatigue syndrome in childhood; a discussion of psychopathological mechanisms. *Eur. J. Child. Adolesc. Psychiatry* 1992; **1:** 111–118.

50 Baetz-Greenwalt B, Jensen U, Lee A, Saracusa C, Goldfarb J. Chronic fatigue syndrome (CFS) in children and adolescents; a somatoform disorder often complicated by treatable organic disease. *Clin. Infect. Dis.* 1993; **17:** 571.

51 Sharpe M, Johnson B, McCann J. Mania and recovery from chronic fatigue syndrome. *J. R. Soc. Med.* 1991; **84:** 51–52.

52 Giannopoulou J, Marriott S. Chronic fatigue syndrome or affective disorder? Implications of the diagnosis on management. *Eur. J. Child. Adolesc. Psychiatry* 1994; **3:** 97–100.

53 Pipe R, Wait M. Family therapy in the treatment of chronic fatigue syndrome in adolescence. *ACPP Rev. Newslett.* 1995; **17:** 9–16.

54 Fry A, Martin M. Cognitive idiosyncrasies among children with the chronic fatigue syndrome: anomalies in self-reported activity levels. *J. Psychosom. Res.* 1996; **41:** 213–223.

55 Dale J, Straus S. The chronic fatigue syndrome; considerations relevant to children and adolescents. *Adv. Pediatric Infect. Dis. 1992;* **7:** 63–83.

56 Kminek A, Simunek I, Janatkova I. Chronic fatigue syndrome, complement and infection with Epstein–Barr virus in children. *Complement Inflamm.* 1990; **7:** 125.

57 Mechanic D. The influence of mothers on their childrens health, attitudes and behaviors. *Pediatrics* 1964; **33:** 444–453.

58 Pennebaker J. *The Psychology of Physical Symptoms.* New York, Springer, 1982.

59 Garralda M. Somatisation in children. *J. Child. Psychol. Psychiatry* 1996; **37:** 13–33.

60 Harris F, Taitz L. Damaging diagnosis of myalgic encephalomyelitis in children. *Br. Med. J.* 1989; **299:** 790.

61 MacDonald T. Myalgic encephalomyelitis by proxy. *Br. Med. J.* 1989; **299:** 1030–1031.

62 Marcovitch H. Chronic fatigue states in children. In Jenkins R, Mowbray J (ed.) *Postviral Fatigue Syndrome.* Chichester, Wiley, 1991: 335–344.

63 Taylor D. Outlandish factitious illness. In David T (ed.) *Recent Advances in Paediatrics.* Edinburgh, Churchill Livingstone, 1992: 63–76.

64 Kennedy J, Pearce J. Chronic fatigue syndrome in childhood. *Curr. Opinion Psychiatry* 1995; **8:** 231–234.

65 Hickson G, Clayton E. Are you and your waiting room's televised 'expert' saying the same thing? *Clin. Pediatrics* 1993: 172–174.

66 Anon. *Report from the National Task Force on Chronic Fatigue Syndrome (CFS), Post Viral Fatigue Syndrome (PVFS), Myalgic Encephalomyelitis (ME)*. Bristol, Westcare, 1994.

67 Katz B, Andiman W. Chronic fatigue syndrome. *J. Pediatrics* 1988; **113:** 944–947.

68 Wachsmuth J, MacMillan H. Effective treatment for an adolescent with chronic fatigue syndrome. *Clin. Pediatrics* 1991; **30:** 488–490.

69 Rikard-Bell C, Waters B. Psychosocial management of chronic fatigue syndrome in adolescence. *Aust. NZ J. Psychiatry* 1992; **26:** 64–72.

70 Sidebotham P, Skeldon I, Chambers T, Clements S, Culling J. Refractory chronic fatigue syndrome in adolescence. *Br. J. Hosp. Med.* 1994; **51:** 110–112.

71 Graham H. Family interventions in general practice: a case of chronic fatigue. *J. Fam. Therapy* 1990; **13:** 225–230.

72 Quinn L, Titcomb J, Silvera M, Thompson M, Rolles C. The treatment of chronic fatigue syndrome in a paediatric population: the Burlesdon House experience. *Submitted.*

73 Anon. *Guidelines for Parents of Children with ME*. Stanford-le-Hope, Essex, ME Association, 1988.

74 Arav-Boger R, Spirer Z. Chronic fatigue syndrome: pediatric aspects. *Israeli J. Med. Sci.* 1995; **31:** 330–334.

75 Joyce J, Hotopf M, Wessely S. The prognosis of chronic fatigue and chronic fatigue syndrome: a systematic review. *Q. J. Med.* 1997; 90: 223–233.

76 Buskila D, Neumann L, Hershman E, Gedalia A, Press J, Sukenik S. Fibromyalgia syndrome in children – an outcome study. *J. Rheumatol.* 1995; **22:** 525–528.

77 Bell D, Bell K, Cheney P. Primary juvenile fibromyalgia syndrome and chronic fatigue syndrome in adolescents. *Clin. Infect. Dis.* 1994; **18(suppl 1):** S21–S23.

78 Franklin A. *Children with ME: Guidelines for School Doctors and General Practitioners.* Stanford-le-Hope. Essex, ME Association, 1995.

79 Van Aerde J. Chronic immune dysfunction syndrome: an epidemic? *Pediatrics* 1992; **89:** 802–803.

80 Carter B, Edwards J, Marshall G. Chronic fatigue in children: illness or disease? *Pediatrics* 1993; **90:** 163.

81 Plioplys A. Chronic fatigue syndrome should not be diagnosed in children. *Pediatrics* 1997: **100:** 270–1.

14. Other chronic fatigue syndromes

14.1 Introduction

This book is about chronic fatigue and chronic fatigue syndrome (CFS). However, CFS is not the only chronic fatigue syndrome. We have already made frequent reference to other disorders characterized by similar symptoms. When bowel symptoms are prominent in a subject with chronic fatigue, irritable bowel syndrome is a likely diagnosis; when muscle pain is prominent, the result may be fibromyalgia; and when chest pain and breathlessness are important complaints, effort syndrome may be diagnosed.

All these syndromes share various features[1]. All are 'medically unexplained', in the sense that no clear-cut biomedical explanation has ever been accepted as underlying the symptoms, although many have been proposed. As we shall show in this chapter, all show considerable overlap and all show considerable psychiatric comorbidity, especially in specialist clinics. Women appear to be more vulnerable to all of them.

The choice of fatigue syndrome can be arbitrary. Receiving any particular diagnosis is also related to the speciality of the doctor consulted; faced with a patient whose symptoms are otherwise identical, a cardiologist is more likely to diagnosis effort syndrome or hyperventilation than a rheumatologist. The choice of specialist may also relate to beliefs about aetiology – if the same person, with the same symptoms, now gives a history of a non-specific viral precipitating illness, then referral to an infectious disease specialist might result in the label of post-viral fatigue. The final label given to the patient may depend upon the particular symptom emphasized by the patient and/or idiosyncratic local referral practices.

There are also important differences. Despite the overlap between the various syndromes, there is little uniformity between management practices. The mainstay of the treatment of fibromyalgia is graded activity and/or antidepressants. Diet plays a considerable role in the management of irritable bowel, whilst maximizing rest is still the most common strategy advocated for CFS. The social context of the conditions also differs. Irritable bowel syndrome is an accepted part of gastroenterological practice, and gastroenterological journals are a rich source of scholarly articles on the subject. Fibromyalgia is not regarded with the same degree of acceptance within mainstream rheumatology, but is not a particularly controversial subject either. The suggestion that psychological factors and/or treatments might be effective in either condition would be met with equanimity by most gastroenterologists or rheumatologists. Neither condition has much presence in the media or sociopolitical arena. In contrast CFS and chronic Lyme disease are far from accepted in mainstream professional and academic circles and, perhaps in consequence, maintain a strong presence in the media. Unlike the other syndromes, those who recognize the disorder can often strongly reject the relevance of psychological models in understanding or treating the disorders.

We believe that the nosological similarities between these various fatigue syndromes are greater than any differences. We are unaware of any fundamental abnormalities that allow firm divisions to be drawn between the conditions. In previous chapters we have used references from the literature on other fatigue syndromes where it highlights various aspects of knowledge concerning CFS. In this chapter we will briefly review the salient features of other fatigue syndromes.

14.2 Fibromyalgia

In Chapter 6 we noted the parallel history of fibromyalgia and CFS. Both grew out of a Victorian concept – former from fibrositis, the latter from neurasthenia. Both disappeared from mainstream medicine, only to reappear, the former in the 1970s, the latter in the 1980s. The re-emergence of both was triggered by new scientific findings, for fibromyalgia related to the anatomy of tender points and the description of a particular sleep disturbance, for CFS the apparent link with EBV.

Fibromyalgia has been defined by the American College of Rheumatology (ACR) as a history of widespread pain and pain in 1 out of 18 tender point sites on digital examination[2]. These ACR criteria have been widely adopted, just as the CDC criteria have been adopted for CFS. In addition, it is accepted that patients also have very frequent complaints of sleep disturbance, mood disturbance, and fatigue. Unlike CFS, fibromyalgia appears to be diagnosed on the basis of not only self-reported symptoms, but also an objective sign, the tender point. However, the status of tender points has been vehemently attacked[3,4], and is probably better understood as a marker of patient distress and abnormal perception of pain rather than a 'hard' physical sign[3,5].

There is considerable overlap between fibromyalgia and CFS. Seventy per cent of those with debilitating fatigue for more than six months also had persistent diffuse muscle pain[6]. Between 85 per cent and 95 per cent[7–9] of fibromyalgia patients complain of general fatigue. Myalgia, enshrined in the term 'myalgic encephalomyelitis', is part and parcel of CFS. Tender points, the hallmark of fibromyalgia, are also common in CFS[10,11]. Sleep disorder is common to both[12]. No essential differences emerged in a comparison of two groups labelled as CFS or fibromyalgia respectively[13,14]. Like CFS, most fibromyalgia sufferers seen in clinics are female, the commonest age group is between 18 and 45, depression is common and the prognosis in that setting is poor (see Buchwald[12] and Chapter 8).

Formal studies confirm this overlap. Of 33 patients with primary fibromyalgia 14 (42 per cent) met full CDC CFS criteria, and 9 (27 per cent) were only one item short[15]. Several authors have already commented on the comorbidity between fibromyalagia and CFS[6,7,16–18]. Even in adolescents, CFS and primary juvenile fibromyalgia syndrome are remarkably similar[19]. Current authorities now emphasize the similarities between CFS and fibromyalgia[6,8,10].

Even the presumed infectious links, thought by some to be specific to CFS, are found in fibromyalgia. Of one series of fibromyalgia patients 55 per cent confirmed that their illness had started with a viral illness[14,20]. A substantial minority report symptoms such as sore throats, cough, swollen lymph nodes, and low-grade fevers[13]. Don Goldenberg, an academic rheumatologist practising in Boston, has been one of the most prolific authors on, and supporters of, fibromyalgia. His model of how infections might be associated with the subsequent development of fibromyalgia is very similar to those proposed in this text (Chapter 12). He suggests that infection is 'one of many events that promote a maladaptive behaviour pattern which secondarily leads to fibromyalgia. . . . The anxiety caused by, and preoccupation with, chronic infections such as Lyme Disease may lead to avoidant behaviour and inactivity, sleep disturbances, mood disturbances, tense muscles and decreased exercise tolerance. . . . Societal focus on undetected agents, potential cures, new serological tests and disability . . . would foster a loss of self control over one's illness'[20].

Fibromyalgia appears to be a common feature of hospital practice – fibromyalgia and fibrositis syndromes make up a considerable proportion of the workload of a rheumatologist, perhaps 30 per cent[21]. In the United States the diagnosis is made in 16 per cent of new referrals, and is second only to osteoarthritis as a reason for consulting a rheumatologist[22].

The epidemiology of fibromyalgia in the population has started to be clarified. Chronic muscle pain is common. A community study from the north of England found that the prevalence of chronic widespread muscle pain was 13.2 per cent, which represents a prevalence of 11.3 per cent when standardized to the adult population of England and Wales[23]. Twenty per cent of the population in an American community survey complained of chronic regional pain, with a further 10 per cent complaining of chronic widespread pain[24]. Fibromyalgia is less common. In a population study of 50- to 70-year-olds in Sweden, primary fibromyalgia had a prevalence of 1 per cent[25]. In a Norwegian study 10.5 per cent of women aged 20 to 49 met criteria for fibromyalgia, implying both widespread muscle pain and also muscle tenderness[26,27]. Some 3.4 per cent of American women and 0.5 per cent of men met the full criteria for fibro-myalgia[24].

As with CFS, these figures depend upon the exact criteria employed, and may represent arbitrary boundaries where none exist in nature. There is convincing evidence that fibromyalgia is not a discrete entity, but is instead part of a continuum from no muscle pain to severe pain with tender points[28,29]. Indeed, the authors of a large Finnish population study[30] found little evidence for a discrete disorder called fibromyalgia, concluding instead that it represented the extreme end of 'the different (though correlated) dimensions of illness, pain and mental distress'. As we discussed in Chapter 7, new epidemiological studies from both Britain and the United States continue to produce evidence against the existence of a discrete disorder labelled fibromyalgia[5,23,24,31].

One interesting difference between fibromyalgia and the popular perception of CFS is its social class distribution. In one population study one of the strongest associations of fibromyalgia was social class. However, this was in the opposite direction to that so often claimed for CFS, the disorder being almost absent in the higher socio-economic groups[30]. However, this difference is more a matter of public perception, since epidemiological evidence has failed to confirm the alleged upper social class excess for CFS (see Chapter 7).

Some of the suggested aetiologies of fibromyalgia are similar to those advanced for CFS. In this book we have drawn attention to relevant research on fibromyalgia where it adds to our understanding of CFS. Thus in Chapter 8 considerable use was made of the literature looking at muscle structure and function in both conditions, concluding that despite the prominence of muscle symptoms, fibromyalgia, like CFS, was unlikely to be the result of primary muscle disease in anything other than a small minority. Infective and immunological theories have been less popular for fibromyalgia than CFS, but no convincing evidence for either a virological or immunological origin to fibromyalgia has been presented.

We do not intend to discuss the literature on psychiatric disorder and fibromyalgia in any depth. Suffice it to say that a series of studies show that in clinical samples seen in rheumatological settings psychiatric disorders such as depression are very common. These diagnoses are less prevalent in primary and community samples (see Chapter 10), but depressive symptoms remain closely associated with the 'typical' symptoms of fibromyalgia, namely muscle pain and sleep disturbance. Just as with CFS, fibromyalgia overlaps with, but is not the same as, disorders such as depression. Just as with CFS, there are also intriguing neurobiological differences between the two disorders (see Chapter 11).

One study is particularly worthy of comment, because, to date, it has not been performed in CFS. Ahles and colleagues studied psychological disorder in fibromyalgia using a particularly rigorous methodology, including blinding of the researcher, to try and reduce observer bias[32]. They found no excess of psychiatric disorder in the fibromyalgia cases, but, as in both irritable bowel syndromes and CFS, fibromyalgia patients reported increased rates of somatic symptoms, as observed by others[33].

14.3 Irritable bowel syndrome

Irritable bowel syndrome (IBS) is a condition characterized by altered bowel function, associated with pain and a feeling of abdominal distension. However, IBS is also more than just bowel symptoms. IBS patients are frequent consulters with other non-gastroenterological symptoms such as fatigue, weakness, and headache[34]. Fatigue is a prominent part of irritable bowel syndrome[35–37]: in one study 96 per cent of IBS sufferers complained of constant lethargy, and ranked it as the third worst symptom after abdominal pain and altered bowel habit[38].

Just as with fibromyalgia, there is an increasing body of opinion that groups IBS within the spectrum of fatigue syndromes, and it is not surprising that others have found considerable overlap between IBS and fibromyalgia[5,7,39,40], between IBS and CFS[41], and between all three[42]. Like CFS, it is more common in women, with rates of between two and four times that in men[34]. This is part due to referral bias, since hospital samples of IBS in India and Sri Lanka show an over-representation of males[43]. However, even in community samples, the female excess remains, albeit less marked.

IBS is one of the commonest fatigue syndromes. In a secondary analysis of several large American community surveys self-reported 'irritable bowel' or 'spastic colon' had a prevalence of 2.9 per cent[34]. The symptoms of IBS are commoner, with a prevalence between 8 and 22 per cent[44]. Of those responding to an American household survey, 11 per cent fulfilled criteria for IBS[45], whilst a British community study concluded that 22 per cent of the population had symptoms consistent with the diagnosis[46]. As with chronic fatigue, few seek professional help, hence studies based on referrals to gastroenterology clinics report a selected sample. Nevertheless, even if only a few of those affected seek help, these form a considerable part of the workload of gastroenterologists, in one survey constituting nearly half of all referrals[47].

The mechanism of IBS remains unknown. Claims have been made for the influence of diet, abnormal gut motility, and for both psychiatric and psychophysiological disorder. Psychological distress predicts the development of IBS after acute gastro-enteritis, in much the same manner as it predicts the development of CFS after other viral infections[48]. Another similarity is the role played by perception. The most convincing explanation for the symptoms of IBS suggests a role for the perception of gastrointestinal function – although opinion is divided as to whether the disorder is based on an abnormal perception of normal gut function, or a normal perception of abnormal function[43]. The irritable bowel is abnormally sensitive to stimuli, ranging from gut distension, food, cholecystokinin, caffeine, or psychosocial stress.

As with all the fatigue and myalgia syndromes, it is important to remain aware of the role of help-seeking behaviour. As we noted in Chapter 10, the close association between psychological distress and IBS found in clinical samples does not extend to community samples of those not seeking help. The hypothesis that psychological distress in functional syndromes is associated with consulting a doctor and demanding help, rather than being an intrinsic factor of the condition itself, has been largely confirmed in IBS.

14.4 Effort syndrome (Da Costa's syndrome, neurocirculatory asthenia, soldier's heart, mitral valve prolapse)

Irritable bowel may be the commonest fatigue syndrome, but effort syndrome has the most distinguished history[49]. The first recognized description was that of Da Costa in American Civil War soldiers[50]. Originally labelled as 'soldier's heart', partly because of the prominence of cardiac symptoms such as breathlessness and chest pain, and also because one of the earliest proposed aetiologies was the pressure of soldier's back-packs on the chest. Weir Mitchell's Civil War experience in treating exhausted soldiers played an important part in forming his views on the nature of neurasthenia.

What was effort syndrome? It was 'that condition of ill-health in which the symptoms and signs produced in normal subjects by excessive exercise are called forth in patients by lesser amounts and in which no definite physical signs of structural disease are anywhere discovered'[51]. A pattern of frequent relapse, often associated with minor exertion, was also common[49].

The importance of heart disease declined over the years, reflected by the shift from the term 'soldier's heart' to 'effort syndrome' in Britain or 'neurocirculatory asthenia' in America[51]. The change in title reflected an increasing consensus that symptoms were the result of an exaggerated physiological response to exercise[52]. Three major causes were identified. The first were common infections and febrile illnesses[49, 50, 52, 53]; effort syndrome was thus an acquired neurasthenia. The second were constitutional factors such as weakness or bad nerves, sometimes simplified as constitutional neurasthenia. The third was the stress of active service.

The apogee of the effort syndromes was reached during the First World War, when the problems of soldiers unable to undertake active duties, but without any clear-cut diagnosis or injury, reached epidemic proportions. Both the British and American governments instituted programmes for research and treatment of the conditions, leading to a large and often impressive literature. In 1916 the British Association for the Advancement of Science issued an influential report on the condition, and many others followed. The best treatments involved some form of graded activity and/or exercise – rest was originally tried, but as Sir Thomas Lewis wrote 'rest in bed has been found to be detrimental rather than beneficial'[52]. Sir Thomas Lewis, Sir James Mackenzie, and Sir William Osler all endorsed proposals, soon implemented, that systematic exercise programmes be introduced into all large military hospitals.

Effort syndrome, now usually called neurocirculatory asthenia, was again recognized, studied and treated in the Second World War. In Chapter 8 we drew attention to the important work on the subject of effort syndrome and exercise response performed by Maxwell Jones at the Mill Hill Hospital during that war. This literature continues to grow (see Chapter 8).

Of the three factors – infection, constitutional weakness, and stress – it was the third that increased in importance over the years. From the time when authorities such as Sir Thomas Lewis affirmed the role of emotional shock and trauma in precipitating the condition, the importance attached to psychological factors continued to grow. Cohn vigorously argued that patients with effort syndrome should be distinguished from those make slow recoveries from infections[54]. The former condition was a 'neurosis, dependent upon anxiety and fear'[54], the latter the forerunner of the modern post-viral fatigue syndromes. It was observations such as these, and those concerning the overlapping condition of shell shock, that played a crucial role in drawing attention to the psychological casualties of modern warfare[55], and a direct line of descent can be traced from effort syndrome to the modern condition of post-traumatic stress disorder[56].

By the Second World War effort syndromes were seen as largely psychological conditions with secondary overbreathing and sympathetic overdrive[57]. No one was more associated with the diagnosis than the eminent cardiologist Paul Wood. The change in his views mirrored the changing views of not just effort syndrome, but all the fatigue syndromes, between the wars. Originally seeing it as a distinct disorder his views shifted over the years, until in the final edition of his influential text book he was grouping effort syndrome under the anxiety disorders, the latter having primacy[58]. Giovanni Fava and his colleagues at the University of Bologna have provided modern systematic confirmation of Wood's observation, namely the majority of a sample of patients with 'neurocirculatory asthenia' fulfilled criteria for psychiatric disorder, most prominently anxiety[59].

In recognition of these similarities, some have argued that effort syndromes and CFS are one and the same[60]. Nowadays effort syndrome and Da Costa's seem to be losing their popularity, but have been replaced by terms such as 'hyperventilation syndrome'[57] or 'mitral valve prolapse'. The latter, seen by many as the successor to effort syndrome, neurocirculatory asthenia, and so on[49, 61], is diagnosed by a history of atypical chest pain, palpitations, and fatigue, with a clinical finding of a mid-systolic click with or without a mid-systolic murmur. In one study 96 per cent of cases had fatigue, 95 per cent palpitations, 92 per cent chest pain, 87 per cent dizziness, 87 per cent headache, and so on[62]. It is commoner in women. Another similarity is the high frequency of psychological symptoms; 95 per cent of the same sample had mood swings and 90 per cent were anxious. There is also an increased rate of panic disorder[63]. The day-to-day unpredictability of symptoms experienced by sufferers is also reminiscent of CFS. Not surprisingly, investigators are starting to notice the overlap between mitral valve prolapse and the fatigue/myalgia syndromes[64].

Cardiologists differ in the importance they attach to the auscultatory findings, and the syndrome is controversial[65]. Similar echocardiographic abnormalities have been found in 21 per cent of normal female students. Many have argued that the syndrome of mitral valve prolapse is a non-specific one, and that cardiac factors are not responsible for the associated chest pain[65-67]. No consensus has yet emerged on the nosological status of mitral valve prolapse, but it seems likely to share at least some common links with fatigue syndromes.

Effort syndrome, neurocirculatory asthenia, and mitral valve prolapse are thus *bona fide* fatigue syndromes. They have a similar heritage to CFS, in that both first emerged in Victorian medicine, the one from soldier's heart, the other from neurasthenia. Both have considerable overlaps with psychiatric diagnoses; CFS with depression, effort syndromes with anxiety disorders. Another area of overlap is their neurobiological basis. In Chapter 8 we drew attention to some new work on autonomic dysfunction in CFS, whilst pointing out the debt that such research owes to the many years of similar investigations into the role of the sympathetic nervous system and effort syndrome.

14.5 Chronic brucellosis and chronic Lyme disease

The suggestion that symptoms of fatigue, malaise, pain, and depression could be attributed to persistence of *Brucella abortus* first surfaced in 1903[68]. By the 1930s a condition known as chronic brucellosis was recognized, if not universally accepted[69]. In Chapter 6 we introduced the public health specialist, Alice Evans, who campaigned for the recognition of chronic brucellosis and its differentiation from neurasthenia and psychiatric disorders[70]. Despite her efforts, and unlike neurasthenia, chronic brucellosis never entered common medical usage: Evans also commented that physicians often did not make the correct diagnosis until the possibility had been pointed out, after which they tended to notice other cases. In Chapter 6 we described the demise of chronic brucellosis, as researchers noted both the lack of any evidence of chronic infection, linked to the presence of substantial psychological morbidity[71-73]. Researchers concluded that chronic brucellosis was a psychoneurosis.

An interesting parallel with brucellosis is the case of chronic Lyme disease. First recognized as an arthritis in the United States, but also as a cause of a particular rash (erythema migrans), it was linked to the spirochaete *Borrelia burgdorferi* in 1982. It can cause neurological disease of both the peripheral and central nervous system[74], usually associated with evidence of meningoencephalitis and/or peripheral neuropathy, together with characteristic skin lesions. It has been claimed that it can give rise to long-term neuropsychological sequelae, most particularly involving disturbances of memory function[75,76], but the specificity of this association is disputed[77].

A combination of the sudden rise to prominence of Lyme disease, linked with recognition of its capacity for neurological involvement, triggered a period of intense public and media interest in America in the late 1980s[78]. The link with chronic brucellosis is because of the emergence of 'chronic Lyme disease' as a label frequently applied to chronically fatigued patients in the USA. In a survey of 100 referrals to a clinic specializing in Lyme disease, it was only relevant in 37 per cent, and 25 per cent were diagnosed as fibromyalgia[79]. A later study surveyed 800 patients with non-specific musculoskeletal and neurological symptoms, all of whom had received the label of chronic Lyme disease. Ten per cent fulfilled criteria for fibromyalgia[80]. Similar misdiagnoses have been observed in paediatric populations[81]. Active infection is an unusual cause of persistent symptoms, particularly after a course of appropriate antibiotics[82]. Despite that, it remains true that many patients labelled as having chronic Lyme disease continue to take long-term antibiotics for little benefit but with possible adverse consequences. 'Lyme disease patients may gradually withdraw from their usual activities and wait for the antibiotics to cure them'[80, 82], in keeping with similar observations on the development of chronicity in CFS (Chapter 12).

It is now agreed that the symptoms of fatigue and headache are not particularly associated with chronic Lyme disease, representing non-specific constitutional symptoms rather than evidence for central nervous system infection. 'In other individuals, particularly those seronegative for Lyme disease, Lyme encephalopathy is an unlikely explanation for a chronic fatigue state'[83]. As one might expect, those who believe, or have been told, that chronic Lyme disease is the cause of their ill health react angrily to such suggestions[84]. This is one of the many parallels between the social and political history of chronic Lyme disease and that of CFS[78].

14.6 Burnout

Although not usually considered as a medically unexplained syndrome, largely because it is assumed that the cause is psychological, the so-called 'burnout syndrome' is another relatively recent fatigue syndrome. Burnout is a syndrome described in carers, providers, and health care workers. It is characterized by exhaustion, loss of interest in work, and diminished personal and professional accomplishment[85]. It is a concept derived by occupational psychologists and frequently discussed in the lay press. Unlike the familiar end of the day tiredness, linked to exertion and physical load, burnout is closely related to psychosocial factors such as job conflict and loss of enjoyment rather than workload *per se*[86, 87]. Other factors producing burnout and exhaustion include shift work, poor sleep, and domestic work[88, 89].

Despite considerable research from the field of social psychology, the relationship of burnout to more conventional measures of depression and anxiety, let alone CFS, remains uncertain. Burnout in nurses has been linked to both conventional measures of depression and also personality factors[90, 91]. Another interesting observation is that burnout is associated with low early morning cortisol[92], a finding of potential relevance to understanding chronic fatigue (see Chapter 11).

The concept of burnout has been developed from studies of the 'caring professions', such as teaching, nursing, and medicine. It is assumed that these are professions particularly high in both workload and emotional demands, although we are unaware if this has ever been formally confirmed. Nevertheless, teachers, nurses, and doctors are assumed to be particularly vulnerable, and dominate the literature. The similarities between those apparently at risk of burnout and those claimed to be at risk of CFS are intriguing.

References

1 Nimnuan T, Sharpe M, Wessely S. Functional somatic syndromes are expressions of the same process. **submitted**.

2 Wolfe F, Smythe H, Yunus M, *et al.* The American College of Rheumatology 1990 criteria for the classification of fibromyalgia: report of the multicenter criteria committee. *Arth. Rheumat.* 1990; **33:** 160–173.

3 Cohen M, Quintner J. Fibromyalgia syndrome, a problem of tautology. *Lancet* 1993; **342:** 906–909.

4 Bohr T. Problems with myofascial pain syndrome and fibromyalgia syndrome. *Neurology* 1996; **46:** 593–597.

5 Wolfe F, Ross K, Anderson J, Russell I. Aspects of fibromyalgia in the general population: sex, pain threshold and fibromyalgia symptoms. *J. Rheumatol.* 1995; **22:** 151–156.

6 Goldenberg D, Simms R, Geiger A, Komaroff A. High frequency of fibromyalgia in patients with chronic fatigue seen in a primary care practice. *Arth. Rheumat.* 1990; **33:** 381–387.

7 Yunus M, Masi A, Aldag J. A controlled study of primary fibromyalgia syndrome: clinical features and association with other functional syndromes. *J. Rheumatol.* 1989; **16(suppl 19):** 62–71.

8 Buchwald D, Sullivan J, Komaroff A. Frequency of 'chronic active Epstein–Barr virus infection' in a general medical practice. *J. Am. Med. Assoc.* 1987; **257:** 2303–2307.

9 Buchwald D, Garrity D. Comparison of patients with chronic fatigue syndrome, fibromyalgia, and multiple chemical sensitivities. *Arch. Intern. Med.* 1994; **154:** 2049–2053.

10 Komaroff A, Goldenberg D. The chronic fatigue syndrome: definition, current studies and lessons for fibromyalgia research. *J. Rheumatol.* 1989; **16(suppl 19):** 23–27.

11 Ramsay M. *Postviral Fatigue Syndrome: The Saga of Royal Free Disease*. London, Gower Medical, 1986.

12 Buchwald D. Fibromyalgia and chronic fatigue syndrome: similarities and differences. *Rheum. Dis. Clin. N. Am.* 1996; **22:** 219–243.

13 Buchwald D, Goldenberg D, Sullivan J, Komaroff A. The 'chronic active Epstein–Barr virus infection' syndrome and primary fibromyalgia. *Arth. Rheumat.* 1987; **30:** 1132–1136.

14 Goldenberg D. Fibromyalgia and other chronic fatigue syndromes: is there evidence for chronic viral disease? *Sem. Arth. Rheumat.* 1988; **18:** 111–120.

15 Hudson J, Pope H, Goldenberg D. Chronic fatigue syndrome. *J. Am. Med. Assoc.* 1991; **265:** 357–358.

16 Norregaard J, Bulow P, Prescott E, Jacobsen S, Danneskiold-Samsoe B. A four-year follow-up study in fibromyalgia: relationship to chronic fatigue syndrome. *Scand. J. Rheumatol.* 1993; **22:** 35–38.

17 Wysenbeek A, Shapira Y, Leibovici L. Primary fibromyalgia and the chronic fatigue syndrome. *Rheumat. Int.* 1991; **10:** 227–229.

18 Prescott E, Jacobsen S, Kjoller M, Bulow P, Danneskiold-Samsoe B, Kamper-Jorgensen F. Fibromyalgia in the adult Danish population: II. A study of clinical features. *Scand. J. Rheumatol.* 1993; **22:** 238–242.

19 Bell D, Bell K, Cheney P. Primary juvenile fibromyalgia syndrome and chronic fatigue syndrome in adolescents. *Clin. Infect. Dis.* 1994; **18(suppl 1):** S21–S23.

20 Goldenberg D. Do infections trigger fibromyalgia? *Arth. Rheumat.* 1993; **36:** 1489–1492.

21 Treadwell E, Metzger W. Chronic fatigue: psyche or sleep? *Arch. Intern. Med.* 1990; **150:** 1121.

22 Marder WD, Meenan RF, Felson DT, *et al.* The present and future adequacy of rheumatology manpower. A study of health care needs and physician supply. *Arth. Rheumat.* 1991; **34:** 1209–1217.

23 Croft P, Schollum J, Silman A. Population study of tender point counts and pain as evidence of fibromyalgia. *Br. Med. J.* 1994; **309:** 696–699.

24 Wolfe F, Ross K, Anderson J, Russell IJ, Hebert L. The prevalence and characteristics of fibromyalgia in the general population. *Arth. Rheumat.* 1995; **38:** 19–28.

25 Jacobsson L, Lindgarde F, Manthorpe R. The commonest rheumatic complaints of over six weeks duration in a twelve-month period in a defined Swedish population. *Scand. J. Rheumatol.* 1989; **3:** 353–360.

26 Forseth K, Gran J. The prevalence of fibromyalgia among women aged 20–49 in Arendal, Norway. *Scand. J. Rheumatol.* 1992; **21:** 74–78.

27 Forseth K, Gran J. The occurrence of fibromyalgia-like syndromes in a general female population. *Clin. Rheumatol.* 1993; **12:** 23–27.

28 Masi A, Yunus M. Concepts of illness in populations as applied to fibromyalgia syndromes. *Am. J. Med.* 1986; **81:** 19–25.

29 Kolar E, Hartz A, Roumm A, Ryan L, Jones R, Kirchdoerfer E. Factors associated with severity of symptoms in patients with chronic unexplained muscular aching. *Ann. Rheumat. Dis.* 1989; **48:** 317–321

30 Makela M, Heliovaara M. Prevalence of primary fibromyalgia in the Finnish population. *Br. Med. J.* 1991; **303:** –219.

31 Croft P, Burt J, Schollum J, Thomas E, Macfarlane G, Silman A. More pain, more tender points: is fibromyalgia just one end of a continuous spectrum? *Ann. Rheumat. Dis.* 1996; **55:** 482–485.

32 Ahles T, Khan S, Yunus M, Spiegel D, Masi A. Psychiatric status of patients with primary fibromyalgia, patients with rheumatoid arthritis, and subjects without pain: a blind comparison of DSM-III diagnoses. *Am. J. Psychiat.* 1991; **148:** 1721–1726.

33 Robbins J, Kirmayer L, Kapista M. Illness worry and disability in fibromyalgia. *Int. J. Psychiat. Med.* 1990; **20:** 49–64.

34 Sandler R. Epidemiology of irritable bowel syndrome in the United States. *Gastroenterology* 1990; **99:** 409–415.

35 Whorwell P, McCallum M, Creed F, Roberts C. Non colonic features of the irritable bowel syndrome. *Gut* 1986; **27:** 37–40.

36 Watson W, Sullivan S, Corke M, Rush D. Globus and headache: common symptoms of the irritable bowel syndrome. *Can. Med. Assoc. J.* 1978; **118:** 387–388.

37 Nyhlin H, Ford M, Eastwood J, *et al.* Non-alimentary aspects of the irritable bowel syndrome. *J. Psychosom. Res.* 1993; **37:** 155–162.

38 Maxton D, Morris J, Whorwell P. Ranking of symptoms by patients with the irritable bowel syndrome. *Br. Med. J.* 1989; **299:** 1138.

39 Veale D, Kavanagh G, Fielding J, Fitzgerald O. Primary fibromyalgia and the irritable bowel syndrome. *Br. J. Rheumatol.* 1991; **30:** 220–222.

40 Triadafilopoulos G, Simms R, Goldenberg D. Bowel dysfunction in fibromyalgia syndrome. *Digest. Dis. Sci.* 1991; **36:** 59–64.

41 Gomborone J, Gorard D, Dewsnap P, Libby G, Farthing M. Prevalence of irritable bowel syndrome in chronic fatigue. *J. R. Coll. Physicians* 1996; **30:** 512–513.

42 Hudson J, Goldenberg D, Pope H, Keck P, Schlesinger L. Comorbidity of fibromyalgia with medical and psychiatric disorders. *Am. J. Med.* 1992; **92:** 363–367.

43 Drossman D, Thompson W. The irritable bowel syndrome; review and a graduated, multicomponent treatment approach. *Ann. Intern. Med.* 1992; **116:** 1009–1016.

44 Sandler RS, Drossman DA, Nathan HP, McKee DC. Symptom complaints and health care seeking behavior in subjects with bowel dysfunction. *Gastroenterology* 1984; **87:** 314–318.

45 Drossman D, Li Z, Andruzzi E, *et al.* U.S. householder survey of functional gastrointestinal disorders. Prevalence, sociodemography, and health impact. *Digest. Dis. Sci.* 1993; **38:** 1569–1580.

46 Jones R, Lydeard S. Irritable bowel syndrome in the general population. *Br. Med. J.* 1992; **304:** 87–90.

47 Sammons M, Karoly P. Psychosocial variables in irritable bowel syndrome: a review and proposal. *Clin. Psychol. Rev.* 1987; **7:** 187–204.

48 Gwee K, Graham J, McKendrick M, Collins S, Walters S, Read N. Psychometric scores and persistence of irritable bowel after infectious diarrhoea. *Lancet* 1996; **347:** 150–153.

49 Paul O. Da Costa's syndrome or neurocirculatory asthenia. *Br. Heart J.* 1987; **58:** 306–315.

50 Da Costa J. On irritable heart: a clinical study of a form of functional cardiac disorder and its consequences. *Am. J. Med. Sci.* 1869; **61:** 17–52.

51 Grant R. Observations on the after histories of men suffering from the effort syndrome. *Heart* 1926; **12:** 121–142.

52 Lewis T. Report on neuro-circulatory asthenia and its management. *Military Surg.* 1918; **42:** 409–420.

53 Mackenzie J. Soldier's heart. *Br. Med. J.* 1916; **i:** 117–120.

54 Cohn A. The cardiac phase of the war neuroses. *Am. J. Med. Sci.* 1919; **158:** 453–470.

55 Hyams K, Wignall S, Roswell R. War syndromes and their evaluation: from the U.S. Civil War to the Persian Gulf War. *Ann. Intern. Med.* 1996; **125:** 398–405.

56 McFarlane A, Atchison M, Rafalowicz E, Papay P. Physical symptoms in post traumatic stress disorder. *J. Psychosom. Res.* 1994; **38:** 715–726.

57 Nixon PG. An appraisal of Thomas Lewis's effort syndrome. *Q. J.Med.* 1995; **88:** 741–747.

58 Wood P. *Diseases of the Heart and Circulation.* Philadelphia, Lippincott, 1968.

59 Fava G, Magelli C, Savron G, *et al.* Neurocirculatory asthenia: a reassessment using modern psychosomatic criteria. *Acta Psychiat. Scand.* 1994; **89:** 314–319.

60 Rosen SD, King JC, Wilkinson JB, Nixon PGF. Is chronic fatigue syndrome synonymous with effort syndrome? *J. R. Soc. Med.* 1990; **83:** 761–764.

61 Wooley C. Where are the diseases of yesteryear? Da Costa's syndrome, soldier's heart, the effort syndrome, neurocirculatory asthenia – and the mitral valve prolapse syndrome. *Circulation* 1976; **53:** 749–751.

62 Scordo K. Effects of aerobic exercise training of symptomatic women with mitral valve prolapse. *Am. J. Cardiol.* 1991; **67:** 863–868.

63 Alpert M, Mukerji V, Sabeti M, Russel J, Beitman B. Mitral valve prolapse, panic disorder and chest pain. In Richter J, Beitman B, Cannon R (ed.) *Unexplained Chest Pain. Medical Clinics of North America,* 1991: 1119–1134.

64 Pellegrino M. Atypical chest pain as an initial presentation of fibromyalgia. *Arch. Phys. Med. Rehab.* 1990; **71:** 526–528.

65 Chambers J, Bass C. Chest pain with normal coronary anatomy: a review of natural history and possible etiologic factors. *Prog. Cardiovasc. Dis.* 1990; **33:** 161–184.

66 Gottlieb S. Mitral valve prolapse: from syndrome to disease. *Am. J. Cardiol.* 1987; **60:** 53–58.

67 Arfken C, Lachman A, McLaren M, Schulman P, Leach C, Farrish G. Mitral valve prolapse: associations with symptoms and anxiety. *Pediatrics* 1990; **85:** 311–315.

68 Bassett-Smith P. Duration of Mediterranean fever. *Br. Med. J.* 1903; **ii:** 1589.

69 Evans C. Chronic brucellosis. *J. Am. Med. Assoc.* 1934; **103:** 665.

70 Evans C. Brucellosis in the United States. *Am. J. Pub. Health* 1947; **37:** 139–151.

71 Spink W. What is chronic brucellosis? *Ann. Intern. Med.* 1951; **35:** 358–374.

72 Cluff L, Trever R, Imboden J, Canter A. Brucellosis: II. Medical aspects of delayed convalesence. *Arch. Intern. Med.* 1959; **103:** 398–405.

73 Imboden J, Canter A, Cluff L. Brucellosis: III. Psychologic aspects of delayed convalescence. *Arch. Intern. Med.* 1959; **103:** 406–414.

74 Halperin JJ, Krupp LB, Golightly MG, Volkman DJ. Lyme borreliosis-associated encephalopathy. *Neurology* 1990; **40:** 1340–3.

75 Krupp LB, Masur D, Schwartz J, *et al.* Cognitive functioning in late Lyme borreliosis. *Arch. Neurol.* 1991; **48:** 1125–9.

76 Benke T, Gasse T, Hittmair Delazer M, Schmutzhard E. Lyme encephalopathy: long-term neuropsychological deficits years after acute neuroborreliosis. *Acta Neurol. Scand.* 1995; **91:** 353–7.

77 Ravdin L, Hilton E, Primeau M, Clements C, Barr W. Memory functioning in Lyme borreliosis. *J. Clin. Psychol.* 1996; **57:** 282–286.

78 Aronowitz R. Lyme disease: the social construction of a new disease and its social consequences. *Millbank Q.* 1991; **69:** 79–112.

79 Sigal LH. Summary of the first 100 patients seen at a Lyme disease referral center. *Am. J. Med.* 1990; **88:** 577–81.

80 Hsu V, patella S, Sigal L. 'Chronic lyme disease' as the incorrect diagnosis in patients with fibromyalgia. *Arth. Rheumat.* 1993; **36:** 1493–1500.

81 Sigal LH, Patella SJ. Lyme arthritis as the incorrect diagnosis in pediatric and adolescent fibromyalgia. *Pediatrics* 1992; **90:** 523–528.

82 Sigal LH. Persisting complaints attributed to chronic Lyme disease: possible mechanisms and implications for management. *Am. J. Med.* 1994; **96:** 365–74.

83 Schoen R. Lyme disease. *Curr. Opin. Infect. Dis.* 1990; **4:** 609–614.

84 Barinaga M. Furore at Lyme disease conference. *Science* 1992; **256:** 1384–1385.

85 Leiter M, Durup J. The discriminant validity of burnout and depression; a confirmatory factor analytic study. *Anxiety, Stress & Coping* 1994; **7:**357–373.

86 Jackson S, Schwab R, Schuler R. Towards an understanding of the burnout phenomenon. *J. Appl. Psychol.* 1986; **71:** 630–640.

87 Murtomaa H, Haavio Mannila E, Kandolin I. Burnout and its causes in Finnish dentists. *Commun. Dent. Oral. Epidemiol.* 1990; **18:** 208–212.

88 Tierney D, Romito P, Messing K. She ate not the bread of idleness: exhaustion is related to domestic and salaried working conditions among 539 Quebec hospital workers. *Women's Health* 1990; **16:** 21–42.

89 Kandolin I. Burnout of female and male nurses in shiftwork. *Ergonomics* 1993; **36:** 141–147.

90 Glass D, McKnight D, Valdimarsdottis H. Depression, burnout and perceptions of control in hospital nurses. *J. Consul. Clin. Psychol.* 1993; **61:** 147–155.

91 Piedmont R. A longitudinal analysis of burnout in the health care setting: the role of personal dispositions. *J. Personal Assessment* 1993; **61:** 457–473.

92 Prubner J, Kirschbaum C, Hellhammer D. Burnout, pain and early morning free cortisol levels in teachers. *International Society of Psychoneuroendocrinology.* 18–22 August 1996, Cascais, Portugal: 87.

15. CFS: a social history of twentieth-century illness

15.1 The world of fiction

To introduce the social context of CFS we will use two fictional examples to set the scene for the remainder of this chapter. The device of fiction is particularly useful, since it can portray the symbolic elements of CFS/ME without being encumbered by facts – fiction can deal entirely in perception.

The most widely viewed fictional portrayal of CFS came from the USA when the illness was featured in a popular television series, 'Golden Girls', in September 1989, and greeted as a 'landmark event' by the main US patients' group. In 'Golden Girls' we first see the image of the 'bad' doctor, who is rude to the patient, keeps her waiting, finds all her tests normal, and tells her to pull herself together, before finally diagnosing her condition as one of loneliness – an emotional problem. Another neurologist pronounces her well, and recommends that she see a psychiatrist. However, she has already done so, and produces two letters saying her problems are physical, not psychological (the psychiatrist who pronounces the patient normal is one of the few positive roles accorded psychiatry*). In an ironic reversal of the usual script, it is the neurologist who pronounces the verdict that 'what the hell do they know – psychiatry's not a science'. The second neurologist is even more dismissive than the first – Dorothy's problems are growing old, and would be cured by taking a cruise or changing the colour of her hair.

In the second episode we meet the other side of the coin – described in a review as 'every CFIDS [chronic fatigue and immune dysfunction syndrome, favoured by the patient's organization in the USA] patient's wildest dream come true' – a good doctor

---

*A frequent figure in the literature is the good psychiatrist who declares the sufferer psychologically normal. For example, one non-fictional neurologist, unable to find anything physically wrong with a sufferer, became 'beside himself with wrath, and suggested that I see a psychiatrist. . . . The psychiatrist told me that I was no madder than the rest of the population and sent me back to the by now quivering and speechless neurologist'[73]. It is only when they act in this fashion that psychiatrists can be confident of receiving favourable mention in the CFS literature. Pleas are often made for a multidisciplinary approach to CFS, although this rarely extends to psychiatrists. One exception was provided by an epidemiologist who told a journalist that 'there is need for multidisciplinary approaches. We are talking about a disease, the investigation of which requires epidemiologists, virologists, psychologists'. However, 'Why the psychologist? To prove you're not all crazy' (Grufferman, cited in Feiden[48]).

who refers her to a virologist, after assuring her she is sane. The virologist tells her she has CFS, and that he 'believes she is really sick and not merely depressed'. Dorothy observes with relief 'I really have something real'. In the final scene Dorothy celebrates that her disease finally has a name, even though the doctor told her he could do nothing about it. The denouement is reached when the previous unsympathetic neurologist enters the same restaurant, and she is able to voice all her resentment towards him. The favourable reaction to these episodes should be contrasted with the opposite reaction to a single unflattering reference to 'ME' in the British television series 'EastEnders', which led to the BBC issuing an apology.

A second fictional treatment of ME occurs in Clare Francis' recent ecological thriller, *Requiem*[1]. Clare Francis, round the world yachtswoman and best selling author, is also well known as an ME sufferer, and founder of the campaigning group 'Action on ME'. Although *Requiem* is not ostensibly about ME, it is dedicated to fellow sufferers, and reviewers were not slow to grasp the connection. One scene exemplifies some of the sophisticated dynamics at the heart of ME. The main character's wife has developed a mysterious but devastating illness, a combination of ME, multiple allergy, and chemical sensitivity. Eventually he and his wife consult a medical toxicologist, who, like the neurologist in 'Golden Girls', exemplifies all that is viewed as bad in the medical profession. The tests are all normal, so the consultant turns to the psychiatrist, who is present in the same room (possible in fiction). This psychiatrist is no longer the Viennese psychoanalyst with his couch, attempting to explain symptoms in terms of previous psychic trauma. Instead he is much of his times, very English, well dressed and articulate. He takes a biopsychosocial model, describing how all illnesses have both physical and psychological components, and invokes the example of chronic pain. He explains antidepressants in biochemical terms, and uses terms such as 'cognitive therapy'.

But it doesn't work. Throughout the psychiatrist is apologetic, as if he does not believe his own explanations. The husband sees it as a way of making the psychological acceptable, and only confirms his fears. His wife was perfectly healthy before. Why should she have succumbed? The husband accepts the psychiatrist's explanation that stress can affect the immune system, but she wasn't stressed. He rejects the psychiatrist, whilst his wife rejects all the doctors.

The psychiatrist appears once more. The wife has died in odd circumstances, and the psychiatrist is called to the Coroner's Court. Now the psychiatrist is able to twist all the previous evidence into the diagnosis of depression. The psychiatrist was worried about the wife's mental state, felt her to be depressed, argued against her discharge, and now insinuates that she killed herself. However, the Coroner delivers an open verdict. The chapter concludes with the husband's relief on the verdict. He feels that it was his wife on trial, and that she has only now been acquitted. 'The charge – mental instability'.

'Golden Girls' and *Requiem* provide several examples of what we identity as the crucial themes of the social history of CFIDS/ME:

- the reaction to a psychiatric diagnosis
- the imputation of malingering
- the need for a name

- the absence of validating evidence, such as physical signs or tests
- the newness of the disease
- the disease as a medical mystery or controversy
- the need for political action
- the changing relationship of doctor and patient.

15.2 Chronic fatigue and the fear of mental illness

Why do patients with chronic fatigue believe they have ME, and why does that belief take the form it does? First the results of primary care studies show that most don't. Despite their prominence, the labels of CFIDS/ME are not common. Few of those in primary care with chronic fatigue consider they have ME – of the order of 1 per cent[2]. In a primary care survey only a third of those who fulfilled the most rigorous criteria for CFS thought that their problem was ME/CFIDS or another synonym, and only 10 per cent were members of a self-help group[3]. In contrast virtually everyone referred to our specialist clinic already attributes their illness to CFS, and a third are members of one of the self-help groups[3].

For those who do, the answers are complex. First of all, we must consider the alternatives. Most sufferers from chronic fatigue believe, whether rightly or wrongly, that the explanation for their ill health lies in the particulars of their psychological and social lives. However, for some this is unacceptable.

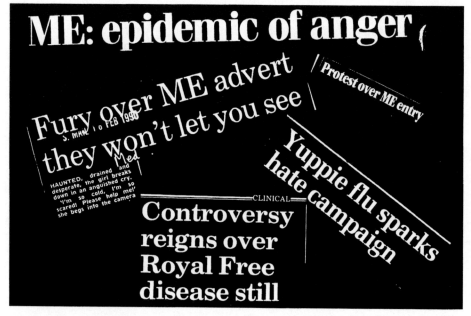

Fig. 15.1 'The relationship between CFS and psychological disorder: a source of bitterness'.

Underneath the ME/CFIDS movement is a strong and passionate antipsychiatry rhetoric. This has not arisen as a result of the interest shown by psychiatrists in the topic (few have much knowledge of, or contact with, sufferers). The first wave of publicity surrounding ME in the UK already showed the suspicion of psychological medicine that would become its hallmark. This publicity lead to the formation of the most radical of the patient's organizations in this country, the ME Action Campaign. In its first newsletter Claire Francis, the President of the Campaign and probably the most famous sufferer in Britain, wrote 'psychiatry is the dustbin of the medical profession'[4] (a not inaccurate perception, see below). Eight years later psychiatry was still 'opinion dressed up as science, stupid and hypocritical'[5]. Those who watched the 'Ranzten Report' on ME will need no persuading of the contempt in which psychiatry is held.

At the heart of the ME/CFIDS movement is the rejection of any form of psychological causation or treatment. Being referred to a psychiatrist is 'being blackballed'[6], 'being on trial'[7] or 'imprisoned for a crime I didn't do'[8]. Courtroom analogies are apt, since the atmosphere surrounding the condition is now an adversarial one. The accusation is not just that the sufferer is guilty of being depressed, or of having a psychiatric disorder, but of not being ill at all – of being a malingerer, of having an imaginary disease. A recent analysis of the writings of CFS patients on the Internet noted that 'contributors' posts indicate that they are familiar with the latest research and discussions of chronic fatigue: authors who include in their writings suspected psychological factors or psychosocial treatments are viewed as anathema, 'practically subhuman in their callous and ignorant statements'[9]. It would be tedious to list the number of variations on the theme of 'ME exists. It is not a psychological illness'[10] that can be found in the media and popular literature.

Believing that illness has an external cause protects the patient from the stigma of being labelled 'psychiatrically disordered'[11] Viruses are the commonest attribution encountered in the specialist setting, partly because they are so common, partly because some infections are indeed associated with increased risk[12], but also because, as we have already pointed out, 'the victim of a germ infection is . . . blameless'[13]. In the context of CFS 'to attribute the continuing symptoms to persistence of a "physical" disease is a mechanism that carries the least threat to a person's self-esteem'[14]. The reviewer of one self-help book for a British newspaper wrote 'an infection is respectable. It has none of the stigma of a psychologically induced illness, which implies weakness or lack of moral fibre'[15]. 'Patients who suffer from unrelenting fatigue fear they have a serious, occult medical problem and worry that people will think they had a mental problem or a blameworthy characterological weakness of will'[16]. One sufferer put it at its simplest – 'increasingly convinced that I had contracted some kind of "bug" that was steadily destroying my health, I determined to identify and eliminate the evil foreign agent'[17]. Note that we make no comment on the accuracy or otherwise of the chosen belief – that has been addressed elsewhere – we are now instead concerned with the psychological and social meanings of the explanations.

The popular literature on ME is suffused with the underlying message that psychological disorders in general, and depression in particular, are diagnoses to be avoided[18]. A variety of strategies are used to counter the threat posed by psychological disorder, this includes insulting or discrediting psychiatric research and researchers, denying the available evidence, altering the meaning of psychological or psychiatric terms (antidepressants are thus immunomodulators, or effective against food allergy), seeing psychological disorders as solely organic conditions, or only as the consequence of CFS.

Such efforts are necessary because of the connotations of psychological and psychiatric disorders. Sometimes such conditions are seen as unreal or non-existent, 'all in the mind'. At other times they are viewed as a moral judgement on the sufferer – reflecting qualities such as lack of effort, poor motivation, and so on. Hence when a chronically fatigued patient is diagnosed as depressed, this can be equated with the message that the sufferer is not really ill, but malingering, shirking their duties, and so on.

An interview with a sufferer, herself a counsellor, contained a telling exchange. She described the reaction of her physician as 'this illness doesn't exist, what you've got is not organic'. The interviewer interjected 'It's in the mind', to which the sufferer/counsellor's response was 'That's it. It's depression, for example'[19].

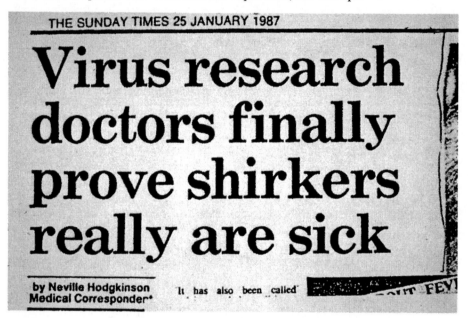

THE SUNDAY TIMES 25 JANUARY 1987

Virus research doctors finally prove shirkers really are sick

by Neville Hodgkinson
Medical Correspondent

It has also been called

Fig. 15.2 Shirking or sick? Not a difficult choice.

Such impressions are by no means inaccurate on two levels. The denigration of the reality of psychiatric disorder, which to a practising psychiatrist seems ill informed and naive, are all too often shared by the medical profession. Some doctors do equate psychological disorder with unreal disorder. A consultant physician who specialises in the disorder told a newspaper that 'People with PVFS often have to put up with a lot of disbelief – there were many doctors who diagnosed this as a psychiatric disorder although on the whole it is taken much more seriously now'[20]. A doctor agreed that it is important that psychiatric patients are separated from ME because 'some neurotic patients devalue the tales of genuine sufferers'[21]. Another is quoted as telling a medical conference that 'ME is an imaginary disease . . . for which the best treatment is psychiatric'[22].

Writing about the rise, and subsequent fall, of psychosomatic explanations for ulcerative colitis, Aronowitz and Spiro[23] note that an uncomfortable attribute of the psychosomatic concept is the potential it has for blaming the patient for the disease. According to anthropologist Norma Ware who has conducted a study of CFIDS patients in Boston, it 'places the responsibility for illness on the shoulders of patients and, consequently, increases their suffering'[24]. A recent article on chronic Lyme disease talked about the difficulties faced by patients in their dealing with doctors – some were even considered malingerers. Many were referred to psychiatrists when their medical physicians lost faith in the validity of their patients' complaints'[25]. Doctors thus share many of the prejudices of the ME/CFIDS sufferer: psychiatrists treat imaginary, malingered, or non-existent diseases. When physicians are felt to have attributed the origins of the patient's symptoms to psychological causes, patients feel stigmatized[26] – an accurate perception.

This is nothing new. Going back to Beevors, Allbutt, and Alvarez[27] we have seen how one of the uncomfortable accompaniments of the rise of modern diagnostic and scientific medicine has been the tendency to denigrate those who fall outside its scope. Thus a social historian might conclude that whilst our Freudian century has seen the general, and indeed uncritical, acceptance of psychological explanations for health and disease, the story of ME, CFIDS, and MCS (multiple chemical sensitivity) shows the limitations of such claims.

Another reason for the vehement rejection of psychiatry is because it is perceived as dealing only with the insane: 'psychiatrists decided ME is a psychiatric disorder – i.e. we are mad'[28]. Again, this too is becoming an increasingly accurate perception of modern psychiatry. Many of the recent trends in psychiatry are consistent with that observation[29]. For those rejected by medicine, and who are clearly not suffering from a major mental disorder such as a psychosis, modern psychiatry is not an attractive home. Whilst we bitterly regret this, there is little denying its accuracy.

The consequences of this lack of validation are many and grievous. There is little doubt that those who later receive a diagnosis of ME/CFIDS recall the previous lack of a diagnosis which they could accept as a source of distress, and react with relief when the label of ME is given[30], even if they are also told that the disorder is untreatable. 'The day Nomi Antelman learned she had an incurable disease, she rejoiced'[31]. Another sufferer was first told she had a virus that would go away. Later this optimistic prognosis was altered, as she learnt she had ME which would, as she described, take away her independence, regress her to being a baby, and in which progress would be minimal. She 'felt fantastic'[32]. For another, even if the prognosis was uncertain 'the mental relief was phenomenal'[33]. The same has been observed in fibromyalgia[34]. Even then, such relief is not always sustained, since despite all efforts the diagnosis of ME still has an ambiguous status in the eyes of outsiders[35].

Psychological diagnoses are unacceptable for a variety of reasons, both emotional and practical. One sufferer was refused sickness insurance benefit because his policy excluded depression, of which he had a past history. His claim to be now suffering from ME was rejected, although he was informed that this decision would be changed if a test for ME were to be developed and he tested positive[36]. Hence sufferers cannot afford to be depressed, both symbolically and literally.

CFIDS/ME began with the rejection of psychiatry. Over the years the reputation of psychiatry within ME circles has not increased. In 1994, in response to a fairly standard piece of newspaper misreporting, columnist and critic Alison Pearson wrote that because doctors do not know the cause of ME they 'decide it doesn't exist. Far less embarrassing to say people presenting the symptoms are nutters than to admit to being baffled yourself'. She concluded that 'one day ME will have a satisfactory medical definition. In the meantime we can always hope that the . . . psychiatrists contact a really vicious fictional virus'[37]. In the same month the press officer for one self-help group wrote that a psychological explanation for CFS was 'demonising the patient'[10], echoing numerous similar letters to newspapers and magazines in the last few years. The intensity of such reactions led one medical journalist to describe the actions of *aficionados* of ME as 'attempting to censure the encephalomyelitically incorrect'[38].

15.3 The media and CFS

Commentators frequently draw attention to the influence of the media on modern illness beliefs in general, and CFS in particular, and some go as far as blaming the media for the entire phenomenon. We think this is simplistic, and the role played by the media is rather more complex.

Media coverage must have influenced the choice of labels made by chronically fatigued patients; in other words rather than creating the problem, media coverage may have influenced whether or not the person believed he or she was suffering from CFS, candida, irritable bowel syndrome, food allergy, or others. Many patients attending CFS clinics explicit remark on how they were finally able to make sense of their symptoms and give their illness a name after hearing media coverage[39]. There can also be no doubting the crucial role the media has played in the increasing concern about the role played in our lives by toxins, chemicals, pollutants, and others, which in turn influences the nature and pattern of symptom reporting[40,41].

In both epidemic and non-epidemic CFS, media and professional attention may have led to a gradual relabelling of existing morbidity as a new disease. Journalists need to make a living and are likely to respond to novelty in illness as much as elsewhere. This has been well described in the United States[42] and mirrors the experience of many infectious disease and neurological specialists in the UK. The same process is observed in other countries such as Spain[43], and no doubt many others.

We can see some of these forces operating in the story of the Lake Tahoe epidemic, which occupies a similar symbolic place in the modern history of CFS to those taken by the Los Angeles and Royal Free episodes in the early history of ME. Here media attention may have lead to a spurious epidemic. The investigators sent by the Centers for Disease Control to investigate the outbreak at Lake Tahoe reported that media attention had led large numbers of subjects from outside the area to refer themselves to the interested doctors for testing[44], whilst other doctors in the area were not seeing anything unusual[45]. It seems unlikely that the media created these cases of CFS, but could have influenced a distorted perception of a local increase in rates.

We believe that the extensive media coverage of ME/CFS must have facilitated the spread of interest in and the diagnosis of CFS; after all, to achieve that was the stated aim of the media campaign promoted by the patient organizations. It is, however, naive to suggest that the rise of CFS was created by the media. Instead, it may be more accurate to note the role played by the media in polarizing the debate on the subject. In the UK we have noted that whereas the professional literature has a preponderance, albeit slight, of research articles taking a psychosocial approach to the problem, the opposite is true of the newspaper and magazine coverage[46]. There seems to be a general tendency of the media and lobbyists to promote polarization and division whenever considering unexplained symptoms and syndromes, areas which by their nature are grey and uncertain[47].

The media has also played a part in the changing relationship between doctor and patient, and assisted in the rise of consumer activism. Journalists interviewed about ME/CFS stated that they explicitly saw the subject in the context of the reaction against medical paternalism, and hence a valid topic for reporting[46].

15.4 ME/CFIDS as a political movement

'Censuring the encephalomyelitically incorrect'[38] introduces another strand, the rise of politically active patient groups. The extraordinary prominence accorded ME or CFIDS, and the speed with which it occurred, owes much to the sufferers themselves. One book began 'Without the commitment of a loyal cadre of patient activists, it is uncertain when CFS . . . would have gained the attention of the national press and the scientific community'[48].

What are the aims of the patient organizations? Some are straightforward, such as increasing public awareness of the condition. It was an article in the local newspaper in Portland, Oregon that led to the founding of the first self-help group for CFS in the USA in 1985[48]. A similar role is often given to a campaigning article by American sufferer Hiliary Johnson in *Rolling Stone* in 1987[49]. Media coverage increased public awareness in both the United Kingdom and the United States – increasing media coverage is an acknowledged task of the CFS organizations.

Patient support groups soon noted that the absence of medical research was one obstacle to the legitimization of CFS, and used their lobbying skills to reverse this. In 1990 the influential *Washington Post* columnist Jack Anderson praised the crucial role of 'constant grass roots action' and 'heavy lobbying' that forced doctors to carry out research in CFS. Unlike most medical research, the impact and benefit of CFS research accrue before any results appear. The Centers for Disease Control Study[50], described by the *Wall Street Journal* as having 'one major goal . . . to replicate experiments showing that people with the condition suffer from immune system irregularities and not psychiatric troubles'[51], gave 'an official stamp of legitimacy to the syndrome' before a single patient was seen. When studies do report physical abnormalities the results have a political significance; recent research on immune abnormalities was further described by the *Wall Street Journal* as lending credibility to CFIDS patients in their struggle to confront reluctant politicians[51]. In the United Kingdom a series of Parliamentary Questions have urged the Department of Health to 'fund research into physical causes . . . of ME'[52]. Not all research is helpful, since if funding is given to research considered to be psychiatric, then considerable harm is seen to be done. In consequence some activists lobby (sometimes using such devices as anonymous denunciations and allegations) medical research charities, government institutions, and medical journals to prevent the funding, execution, and publication of research felt to be inimical to the cause.

Another goal of the patients' organizations is to overcome perceived medical ignorance on the subject. Ramsay[53], the founding father of ME in the UK, described his difficulties in convincing the Department of Health that ME was a real disease, just as William Playfair had failed to convince the British Medical Association likewise in the previous century (see Chapter 5). One of the objectives of the patients' organizations is to increase medical awareness of the disease. Information packs are freely circulated to general practitioners and speakers supplied for postgraduate meetings. Medical 'ignorance' must represent a failure of medical education. George Beard campaigned against the neglect of neurasthenia in the medical schools[54], whilst William Playfair made a similar complaint about the medical texts[55]. Similarly, ME has 'bizarre symptoms about which doctors are not taught at medical school'[56]. In the alternative sector this can be further extended to incorporate views about the changing nature of the environment, and hence illness – commenting on the reluctance of the profession to accept the role of allergies, pollution, etc in the genesis of CFS one doctor stated that 'Ordinary medical texts and training are geared to treat people who no longer exist' (Levin, cited in Steincamp[22]).

Political action by patients' organizations has polarized the context in which CFS is seen. The atmosphere surrounding the condition is now an adversarial one, accompanied by a rhetoric of struggle and injustice: a typical headline is 'Justice for the neglected and maligned sufferers of ME'[57]. Paul Cheney, one of the most prominent doctors on the CFIDS scene in the United States says that 'we who believe that this is a real disease are almost in a death grip with those forces who would stifle debate, trivialize this problem, and banish patients who suffer from it beyond the edges of traditional medicine'[58]. A leading ME campaigner compared the plight of ME sufferers in Britain to the 27 years incarceration of Nelson Mandela and the ordeal of the Beirut hostages[59]. Such analogies leave little doubt about the passions involved. Bitterness and anger permeate both the public writings on CFS, and the more private exchanges found on the Internet[9].

The arrival of patient activism is not, of course, unique to ME/CFIDS, and must be placed within the context of the rise of consumerism within medicine during the 1980s. One marker of this wider change in the relationship between patients and modern medicine is the general distrust of medical care so frequently expressed by sufferers[35,60,61]. A physician sufferer attending a CFS conference wrote that 'the most startling observation was the widespread animosity and lack of faith of most of the participants in the medical profession'[62]. The first editorial produced by the most radical of the patient's organizations active in the UK noted that 'doctors know all the answers . . . to maintain their mystique and authority, doctors have had to rely increasingly on heavy drugs and less and less on listening to their patients'[4], often allied with alternative or 'green' beliefs (see below). As historian Edward Shorter notes, physicians are frequently described as 'heartless ignoramuses, blinkered in the cul-de-sac of mainline medicine'[63]. One of the many reasons why media coverage of CFS has been extensive is that journalists often explicitly agree with this consumer agenda, supporting the validity of the patient's subjective experience against the limitations of the doctor's 'expert' knowledge.

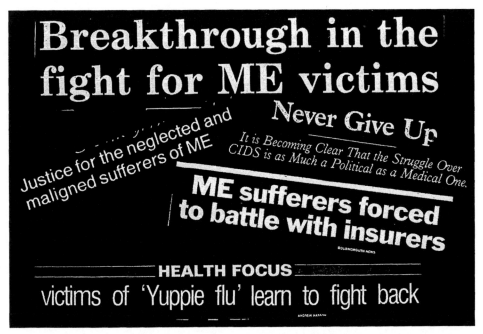

Fig. 15.3 CFS and the rhetoric of struggle.

The attitudes shown towards medicine is also paradoxical: the same literature that is so critical of the medical profession also espouses a touching faith in the ultimate success of medical science in unlocking the enigma of CFS. The medical literature is followed in detail (all the self-help groups produce regular updates of medical research). As one physician noted: 'it is ironic that millions of patients have learned to analyze the significance of medically arcane findings about natural killer cells and interleukin-2, while many physicians are still debating whether the illness exists at all' (Bell, quoted in Feiden[48]). Papers are analysed less on their merit but on how they help 'the cause'[64], and something similar can be observed in the writings of individual patients on the Internet[9]. One of the British patients' organizations announces the best and worst papers of the year; a paper from the Institute of Psychiatry was the worst. This is not, of course, unique to CFS – much the same has been noted in the struggle to establish the legitimacy of chronic Lyme disease[65].

The self-help literature combines both a general suspicion of modern medicine (regarded as impersonal, reliant on tests, and distant from the patient) with a belief that medicine possesses the answer, and that a test will be found. The relationship between ME/CFIDS and the medical profession is paradoxical, since one can see both 'a vigorous attack on medical authority and the desire for its approval'[64].

The rise of ME/CFIDS, with its unique political dimension, is reflected in the changing nature of the medical consultation. It is this new aspect of the medical consultation that can so easily catch doctors off guard, and can contribute to mutual antagonism between patient and physician. Patients have experienced chronic fatigue since medical records began. What is new is that some modern patients present to the doctor not with symptoms, but with a diagnosis already made. 'What is your position or view on ME?' is not an uncommon start to a consultation. The British self-help organizations maintain lists of doctors who are known to be sympathetic to the cause, their American counterparts have 'Physician Rolls of Honour'. There is a considerable popular literature on what to do if your doctor seems ill informed on the subject – advice ranging from presenting him or her with the latest research, changing doctors, or making a complaint. Shorter suggests it is this process, the fixity of belief and the rise of consumerism, which gives ME its peculiar flavour[63]. Whereas in the past sufferers were open to medical counter-suggestion, this is no longer possible: the balance of power between professional and lay models of illness is changing, no matter how much the former resist the change[66].

15.5 CFS is a twentieth-century disease

At an early stage CFS was characterized as a new disease. One of the first papers on sporadic CFS began 'A "new disease" is spreading in the civilised world'[67], incidentally reinforcing the message that CFS is also restricted to Western settings. By 1987 'the diagnosis of the year' in the United States was chronic Epstein–Barr virus[68]; the following year and on the other side of the Atlantic 'there is no doubt that *the* illness of the year is ME'[69]. In order to maintain this 'newness' it is necessary to update the period, so that from the 'malaise of the 80s'[70], CFS has become the 'disease of the 90s'[71, 72] and even 'disease of the fast paced 21st century'[73]. The single most common headline chosen for newspaper articles on ME is 'The ME Generation'[5, 74–79].

If this is a new disease, then some new cause must be found to explain its sudden appearance. Another article entitled 'the ME Generation' opened with the words 'What is modern life doing to us?'[76]. The most frequent answer to that question invokes the concept of the immune system in trouble, weakening under the assault of late twentieth-century life. 'ME is very much a disease of our time – an attack on the immune system exacerbated by stress, pressure and the demands of twentieth century life'[80].

There is a scientific literature on immune dysfunction in CFS (Chapter 9), but it is inconsistent and unclear with little evidence of any substantial immune deficiency. In contrast the popular literature on ME/CFIDS makes much of the immune system, which provides a link with most of the other twentieth-century diseases. 'Weakening' of the immune system is at the heart of the popular models of CFIDS – this can be the result of viral infections, nutritional deficiencies, chemicals, candida, and so on[81] – indeed, one of the ways in the popular literature acknowledges a role for psychological factors and even depression is via their alleged effect on the immune system. Some 77 per cent of the members of a New Zealand self-help group believed that immune system dysfunction caused their illness, with 69 per cent also blaming a virus, and 30 per cent agreeing that pollution was also a cause[82].

As a result of this onslaught ME is 'an overload disease unique to this century'[12], since 'the body can tolerate so much stress from whatever source, but at some point the bucket gets full'[83]. One frequently encountered modern source of this 'overload' is the alleged over-prescription of antibiotics causing altered immunity (see, for example, Askwin[76] and Bradford[84]). Another regular culprit is immunization. Claire Francis traces her illness to childhood when she 'was given her first polio vaccine injection' from which 'she never really recovered'[85]. On another occasion she has labelled ME 'an immune dysfunction disease, possibly caused by pollution'[86]. From whatever source, the resulting strain on the immune system destroys the ability to resist infections such as viruses (hence post-viral fatigue) or candida, and also food allergies and intolerances that have previously been 'hidden'[22]. Another 'overload' causing ME is the deteriorating quality of the air we breath, the water we drink, and the food we eat[87], all of them contributing to our 'toxic lifestyle'[88].

David Dowson, a leading alternative medicine practitioner, gave his explanation of ME to London's *Evening Standard*[77]. The virus leads to depression of the immune system. He used a frequent immune analogy in which the body is a boat with a hole in its side. The immune system is trying to pump the water out, but the boat, overloaded with toxic products, continues to sink. Complementary medicine removes these loads, of which Dr Dowson identified the following: persistent infection, candida, magnesium deficiency, electromagnetic radiation, liver toxicity (due to solvents or pesticides), and depression. Lest anyone be alarmed by the last mentioned, 'depression, and he is adamant about this, is the *result* rather than the cause' (italics in original).

One can already see how these explanations are not mutually exclusive – indeed, the opposite is true. 'Never in history have people been exposed to greater assaults on their bodies by environmental pollution. Food additives and drugs may also harm the body and adversely affect the immune system. Certain doctors even claim that long term antibiotics depress the immune system'[89].

What are the cultural sources of these explanations? HIV is one. 'Who had heard of AIDS or ME . . . 10 years ago?'[84]. Some of the popular literature makes explicit a link between CFS and AIDS. CFS is 'AIDS minor' or a 'sister illness to AIDS'[90]. According to the President of the CFIDS Association in the USA 'you would have to be blind not to make the connection' (Iverson, cited in Regush[90]). Others have speculated that CFS is caused by a variant of HIV, or why the illness appears to be commoner in areas with high rates of HIV[91]. A complete issue of a New York magazine was devoted to making the links between AIDS and CFIDS: CFS was 'the bottom of the AIDS iceberg'. If that was so, then why did the medical 'establishment' persist in denying this link? The answer was not just a cover up, but 'the medical cover up of the century'[92]. 'If it weren't for the emergence of AIDS, chronic fatigue syndrome would be the disease of the decade'[93], and, just in case we have failed to get the message, we are told that 'Doctors at Harvard Medical School have gone so far as to question whether AIDS is actually a chronic and fatal form of ME'[94]. Thus when it was announced that researchers had identified a retrovirus in patients with CFS the storm of publicity was predictable. The subsequent failure of other researchers to confirm this finding went largely unnoticed by the press (see Chapter 9).

The term 'CFIDS' has been adopted by the largest patients' organization in the United States. This has led to the ironic situation of a scientific paper being published under the title of CFIDS in which no patient had any observed immune deficiency[95]. Part of the decision to adopt this name has been a conscious and stated attempt to draw upon the awareness, publicity, and political activism that surrounds AIDS. Another reason lies in the popular grasp of the HIV metaphor – the invisible but deadly virus destroying the immune system. Abbey and Garfinkel note that 'CFS built upon two of the most interesting themes in modern medicine, infectious disease and immunology'[96]. The result of the HIV epidemic is that the concept of a mysterious yet deadly virus that infects the immune system is now firmly in the popular consciousness, and provides a scientific framework for what are other concerns.

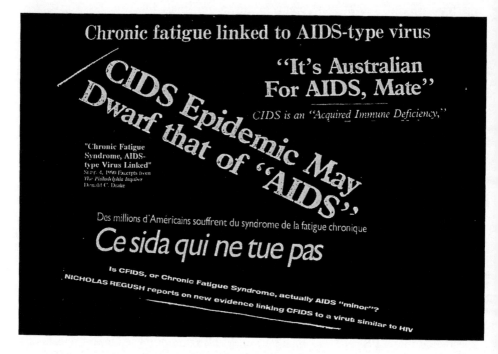

Fig. 15.4 CFS and AIDS: a popular link?

Another source for the assault on the immune system comes from modern views on internal purity and pollution. These concerns appear in the literature linking candida infection of the gut, altered immunity, and CFIDS. The latter may be due to a 'persistent and slight infection of intestines'[97]. The candida infection itself, or the 'toxins' it produces, or even simply the products of digestion, leak into the body and cause autointoxication[98], affecting, inevitably, the immune system. Thus 'yeast toxins weaken your immune system'[81], but a weakened immune system causes yeast infections, illustrating the essential circularity of these models. For the ME patient, candida is one more addition to the climate of fear; after all, the infection spreads to the 'digestive tract, the lungs, the brain, the toenails. It was feasting on me'[77]. In consequence colonic lavage is one treatment for ME in the United Kingdom, because it 'is the best way to flush viruses out of the system'[169].

15.6 CFS is not a twentieth-century illness

The range of aetiologies visible in the popular literature on CFIDS and ME thus superficially reflect a variety of modern concerns, but just how modern are they? The answer is, not very. Even the claim to be modern is far from modern. The parent of CFS, neurasthenia, was also a 'disease of our time'. The phrase 'disease of the century' was frequently used in the context of neurasthenia[99–101], also described as 'a bitter comment on 19th century life'[102]. Neurasthenia too was the consequence of modern civilization, and hence was inevitably becoming more common[103].

What about aetiologies? The modern popular explanations of 'overload' from viruses, pollution, stress all have strong resonances with the mechanisms and causes advanced for neurasthenia during the last century[96, 104]. One popular characterization of neurasthenia was of the body giving way under attack from outside, becoming, as Beard described it, 'overloaded'[105]. Contemporary observers ascribed this overload to the deteriorating quality of life, to new organisms, new stresses, new ways of working, the decline of leisure, and the increasingly decadent and acquisitive nature of society. The idea that neurasthenia could also be the result of acute or chronic infection was the subject of numerous papers (see Wessely[106] and Chapter 6).

Even the idea that we are slowly poisoning our bodies from our intestines is far from new. As Shorter has pointed out, thousands of women lost various intestinal organs during the vogue of autointoxication and focal infection. The former idea, that the products of the colon can leak into the bloodstream causing toxic symptoms, was part of late Victorian medical culture[107]. Guy's Hospital surgeon Willie Lane made his reputation removing such colons at the start of this century[108], ending his career as a surgeon baronet. Medications to stimulate or purify the system and to rid the body of the products of autointoxication (including colonic lavage)[109] were used by most neurasthenia physicians[110]. Even in the 1930s Walter Alvarez at the Mayo Clinic commented that his management of the patient who was 'tired, weak and toxic' included a period of colonic lavage, if only to convince the patient it was useless[27].

Colonic lavage and autointoxication is one the few examples in which the historical continuity so visible in the ME literature is formally acknowledged: Willie Lane's 1920 *Lancet* paper was reprinted in detail in one of the first publications of the ME Action Campaign, where it was called the 'ME Hypothesis'. Nevertheless, few of those modern ME sufferers who currently undergo colonic lavage or other treatments for candida will be aware of the historical basis of the treatment[107].

We have shown how the concept of ME arising from overwork either at the start of illness, or alternatively excessive activity during illness, is central to the modern popular view of aetiology. But overwork, stress, and strain are not unique to our time either. The neurasthenia experts were equally preoccupied with the deleterious consequences of overwork, which they too blamed on a variety of contemporary changes in society. Medical authorities viewed emotional strain and overwork, the agent by which the nervous system became exhausted (which could be purely physical, mental, or a mixture of both) as the inevitable consequence of a host of new social ills. George Beard, the father of neurasthenia, with his facility for similes, joined together a number of discontents into an explanatory model for his disease. For example, Beard, and many others, ascribed neurasthenia to the new, acquisitive nature of society, singling out wireless telegraphy, science, steam power, newspapers, and the education of women, all the product of 'modern civilisation'[105]. Much of this was conveyed by similes drawn from business life (the exhausted businessman overdrawn on his nervous capital, overspent nervous resources, and others) or from technology (the flat battery, the overspent dynamo, the battery that could not give its charge).

The dramatic rise of neurasthenia seemed to confirm its status as a disease of modern civilization[103] – its increasing frequency was 'as certain as the fact of civilization itself'[111]. Just as CFS today is the price paid for pollution, exhaust fumes, food additives, aerosols, antibiotics, and so on, neurasthenia was the price to be paid for industrialization, the rise of capitalism, and the consequent strains to which the business and professional classes were exposed[112].

The system giving way under the strains of modern living thus unites both neurasthenia and CFS. The cause of this overload has changed in some particulars, but not in the general tendency to blame unwelcome features of modern existence – new organisms, new stresses, new ways of working, and the deteriorating quality of the environment. Those who described neurasthenia and now CFS are using the prevailing scientific discourse to express what are wider social concerns, but as cultural historian Peter Gay observed, 'the symptoms of contemporary culture they liked to adduce in proof were, though plausible villains, not easily demonstrated agents of nervousness'[113]. Similarly, although many of us may agree with the frequently voiced dissatisfaction with the state of our environment and society encountered in the popular literature on CFS, it does not follow that such factors are the cause of our unexplained ills.

15.7 CFS and other modern illness

Such views also link CFS to other illnesses of chronic fatigue, characterized by multiple unexplained syndromes, and rarely accepted by conventional physicians. Professional studies frequently refer to the overlap between CFS and candida[114], multiple chemical sensitivity[115], sick building syndrome[116,117], and between each other. If one ignores the scientific aridity of consensus conferences and operational criteria and moves into the world of patient literature, then the similarities are overwhelming. The list of symptoms held to be typical of CFS reappears in texts on yeast infections, food allergies, electromagnetic sensitivity, hypoglycaemia, sick building syndrome, dental amalgam, chemical sensitivity, and others. Stewart[118] has shown how these conditions overlap in the same patients. Of 50 patients diagnosed with environmental hypersensitivity disorder, 38 (76 per cent) had also sought treatment for food allergy, 32 (64 per cent) for CFS, 29 (58 per cent) candidiasis, and 23 (46 per cent) for hypoglycaemia.

The explanations for these conditions are similar, and overlap. CFS causes candida, candida is a cause of CFS. William Crook sold nearly a million copies of his book *The Yeast Connection*[119]. In 1992 he then published *Chronic Fatigue Syndrome and the Yeast Connection*[81]. Dental amalgam disease is due to the mysterious toxic properties of mercury amalgam, leaking into our bodies and poisoning our immune system. It is a cause of CFS – some of our patients have had all their dental fillings removed at considerable pain and expense. Shorter has already traced the history of multiple chemical sensitivity, which depends upon the concept of immune system dysfunction, as does food allergy. Few of the popular self-help books on the subject fail to include some mention of themes such as food allergy, environmental sensitivity, hypoglycaemia, candida, and so on[28,87,120,121]. Similar preoccupations are a regular theme of the magazines and newsletters of patients' groups. These are seen partly as aetiological factors for CFS, partly as overlapping diagnoses, and partly as complications.

Nowhere is this clearer than in the overlap between ME/CFIDS and allergy. ME is a form of severe allergy for many[122], and most self-help books include large sections on allergy. One sufferer from ME relates how he became a total allergic: 'this is a slightly dramatic state because if anyone walked into our house wearing aftershave, bang, I'd pass out'[59]. A doctor with ME proved to be allergic to over 100 different foods[123]. A young farmer with ME was tested by a clinical ecologist, and found to be 'seriously allergic' to every one of 120 different substances. He subsequently committed suicide[124].

The conclusion of such explanatory models is to combine them into what might almost be called a 'General Theory'. The New York magazine *Christopher Street* has published a series of articles under the banner 'The Age of Chronic Immune Dysfunction'. CFS, AIDS, and multiple chemical sensitivity are part of a 'unified syndrome of immune dysregulation'[125]. This article takes the familiar line of that these new illnesses are 'being noted in ever greater numbers around the world, but particularly so in the "civilised" First World'. From this the author describes a syndrome in which the immune system is both 'up' and 'down' regulated. The key elements responsible include the Western diet, which consists of too many additives and not enough vitamins, the use of antibiotics leading to candida overgrowth, virtually any infective agent, metal toxicity from pesticides, pollution, and insecticides, mercury amalgam in our teeth, immunization, radiation including electromagnetic emissions from power lines but also computers, word processors and hair dryers, and the ubiquitous stress[125]. A popular magazine echoed this risk factors, as well as introducing many more, in a recent feature on the hazards of daily life[88], and included over 40 different suggestions about how to reduce this risk, such as placing the television against an outside wall, avoiding barbecues, not walking near the kerb, avoiding canned food, and not talking for hours on your mobile phone. In another typical article the author explains how viruses alter the immune system making the body susceptible to the effects of bacteria, toxins, candida, chemicals, stress, and so on[126]. A combination of new fears of the general environment linked to age-old concerns that are an inevitable accompaniment of the introduction of new technology lie behind the epidemic of reported sensitivity to electrical fields that swept across Sweden, the Scandinavian equivalent of American chemical sensitivity. No pathological or immunological basis could be found for the symptoms, which could not be reproduced in double-blind conditions[127].

The logical conclusion of this general theory is to see ME or CFIDS as a 'signal of the sickness of the planet'[128], hence the solution can be nothing less than 'improving the total environment'[129].

ME/CFS/CFIDS is better understood not as the result of any unique or specific aspect of late twentieth-century life, but as a *'fin de siècle'* illness, just as neurasthenia was itself a *fin de siècle* illness of the nineteenth century. Their apparent modernity may be understood as another manifestation of the perennial theme linking changes in society with unwelcome illness.

15.8 CFS as narrative

Explanations and descriptions of ME/CFIDS are thus not always be to taken as literal truths, but as metaphorical descriptions. The use of metaphors is inescapable; one sufferer, himself a priest, admitted that ME is 'hard to describe in neat non-metaphorical language'[130]. Take the following example: a sufferer related the following story. She 'was married to an actor who was often away on tour making the relationship very difficult and she was left to cope with a toddler, breast-feed a young baby and run a house'. Looking back she told the journalist that all the above left her 'unable to fight off the viral infection which gave her ME'[131]. Another sufferer who worked as a publisher described her life before ME as living a constant battle against stress, feeling a great deal of anxiety, and suffering from a range of nervous symptoms[132]. However, when she finally became ill, this was not a simple continuation of those problems, but a new virus which 'set in' to her body, and led to ME. The previous anxiety had acted to weaken her immune system.

The author of a self-help book on CFS included a chapter on the immune system, and introduced one section with a quote from herself saying 'My immune system is not what it used to be, and it never was'[133]. Other subsequent quotations were used to illustrate a series of histories from ME patients. Many of them told of lifetimes of illness, vulnerability to infections, and multiple symptoms – 'I have had something in my system all my life: periodically it flares up. I've had diphtheria three times, Legionnaire's disease, viral pneumonia twice and cancer. I get sick after stressful events'.

One can see these stories as telling a narrative. CFS allows the sufferer to make sense of his or her past, and to explain previous inabilities to meet expectations or fulfil cherished goals. The same argument has been made for Victorian neurasthenia, allowing individuals to make sense of rapidly changing times and often to explain their own individual crises and disappointments[134]. It is also an accepted fact of social psychology that people constantly reconstruct their personal history to be consistent with their present goals and needs – 'alike with the person and the group, the past is being continuously remade, reconstructed in the interests of the present' (Bartlett 1932, cited in Lees-Haley and Brown[40]).

CFS allows sufferers to incorporate outside events into their own narratives, but without challenging their self-esteem. It can be a 'cry for help' as the sufferer struggles with overwhelming stress[135]. CFS may permit this to be expressed in suitable terms; stress, therefore, is acceptable in so much as it weakens the immune system. In Norma Ware's series the commonest explanation provided by sufferers was of stress weakening the immune system and leaving it vulnerable to a virus, the final cause of the CFIDS[24]. The attack of the virus presumably signals the point at which the previous disorder, manifested as symptoms, gives way to disability and the inability to maintain such roles as work or home. Experiencing stress is acceptable, succumbing to stress less so, and must be explained by a linking biological mechanism.

Some readers may prefer to see these narratives as an accurate account of the pathogenesis of illness. As we have discussed in Chapter 9 there is a rich literature on the links between mind, brain, and immunity, but the literature is inconclusive, and cannot be interpreted in such a literal way. Instead we suggest these stories show the immune system as a narrative device, a cultural explanation, and a method of linking mind and body that preserves self-esteem.

CFS thus serves as a conduit for the expression of social concerns and social ills. Concerns about the quality of the environment become expressed as an assault on our immunity, concerns about diet reappear in theories of intestinal intoxication, concerns about the threat of HIV reappear as mysterious viruses also destroying our immune system, even concerns about the quality of education can be translated into the cognitive effects of CFS. Just as spontaneous hypoglycaemia 'more actively medicalizes and biologizes social issues than even orthodox medicine'[136], so does CFS.

Indeed, at the extremes of language CFS can assume metaphysical properties. CFS is 'demonic'[48], a 'devil illness'[137]. It is a modern pestilence, 'another illness that makes up part of the sign Jesus said would mark the last days'[89].

15.9 CFS and modern science

What has also emerged in this chapter is the manner in which writings on CFS are a reflection of the prevailing scientific discourse. This has been a theme since the time of neurasthenia. When George Beard constructed his illness, he consciously drew on the current scientific discourses. These included Marshall Hall's discovery of the spinal reflex arc, Edison's electricity, Du Bois Reymond's electrical nervous impulse, Spencer's Social Darwinism, and so on[138], which he then mixed in with his own social theories. Beard's neurasthenia parodied the science of the day. Some of his contemporaries noted this and ridiculed him in consequence, but most accepted his writings at face value (i.e. neurasthenia was a modern problem understood using the most up-to-date scientific concepts available).

For example, it seemed logical that if neurasthenia was due to overwork, then the solution was rest. Rest conserved energy, the quantity which neurasthenics lacked. This was given the necessary scientific respectability by reference to the new laws of thermodynamics, and institutionalized in the rest cure (see Chapter 5). Now that nervous energy was being understood in electrophysiological terms, it seemed logical that energy could also replaced by electrical methods. George Beard was as well known for his writings on the therapeutic uses of electricity as on neurasthenia. Few articles on neurasthenia failed to refer to galvanic or faradic treatment, and several dealt with nothing else[139].

Once again electrical treatments and diagnoses flourish for ME. One sufferer is diagnosed by a 'biotron', a machine which 'tests the flow of energy through the acupuncture points'[140]. An English doctor uses 'galvanic currents' in treatment, another uses faradism[141], whilst a New Zealand doctor treats ME with electromagnetic therapy, 'a small pad giving off a low electrical field on her back'[22]. Beard's explanations would, however, now be seen as archaic – in order to appeal to the modern patient the jargon must correspondingly keep up with the times. This can be illustrated by the story of one particular treatment device (Novagen) currently marketed for the treatment of ME in the United Kingdom. A few of our patients have appeared in clinic wearing a small device, costing over £100, clipped to their shirts. Readers of an ME journal were told by one of the best known alternative medicine practitioners in Britain that the device begins by analysing the subject's brain waves, which are recorded and displayed on a computer. 'The device to detect these waves is in a small head set . . . which sits on the head of the patient. The detector is a quartz crystal, and through this light is shone'[142]. A sufferer takes up the story – the therapeutic part of the device 'emits pulses of magnetism which are picked up by the nerves in the skin', transmitted to the brain, where they 'stimulate certain areas which recent research has shown do not function properly in ME patients'.

This passage illustrates our point. The non-scientific reader is likely to be impressed by such words as quartz crystal or laser. There is a reference to recent research about brain waves. All CFS patients complain bitterly of such symptoms as poor concentration, impaired memory, and so on, so it seems plausible that 'brain waves' do not function in ME. Sufferers lack energy, so replacing it with magnetic energy does not seem far-fetched. It did not seem far fetched to George Beard and legions of Victorian doctors who treated neurasthenics with galvanic, magnetic, or electrical stimulation either. The modern neurophysiological researcher whose work was being parodied did find it far-fetched, and was moved to write in another patients' magazine that the 'scientific' principles behind Novagen were 'fallacious at every step', indeed, he traced another source for the device: 'Fans of Flash Gordon will recognise the influence of Dr Zarkov here'[143]. The Victorians would have recognized the central themes of lack of energy, and the need to replace this precious commodity from some source or other, what has altered is simply the language in which this is expressed. What has not altered is the way in which that language is a parodic representation of the medical science of the day.

15.10 CFS as protest

We have suggested how the literature on modern CFS is suffused with the language of conflict and struggle. CFS is as much about protest as it is about illness. As we have suggested, this protest is about many things. On the individual level CFS can be a personal protest about the prevailing ethos of success and achievement. Many sufferers blame the pressure to be 'successful', marked by overcommitted, overactive 'have it all' lifestyles[24] for their illness. Some write that out of illness comes something positive, a reappraisal of their life and priorities, and an implicit, and often explicit, protest against the type of pressures they blame for their illness. Recovery from neurasthenia likewise involved 'a return to the simple life . . . a war against the desire of money'[144].

A frequent theme of the literature is that modern society no longer allows people to convalesce after periods of illness; personal accounts often include a statement that if only the sufferer had been permitted a period of convalescence, and not forced (either by external pressures or their own personality) to resume work, then they would not have developed the illness. CFS writings offer an eloquent critique of the pace of current life, and the perceived depersonalization of modern medicine, although whether or not there ever was such a golden age in which life was lived at a more leisurely pace and doctors had more time for you is questionable.

Medical anthropologist Arthur Kleinman, famous for his studies of neurasthenia in Communist China, makes similar observations about that illness as a form of social protest. He argues that neurasthenia was one response to the extraordinary political pressures of the time, in which individuals felt powerless to control what was happening to themselves or their families, but unable to be seen as psychologically (i.e. morally) vulnerable[145]. Kleinman sees neurasthenia in Communist China as an expression of individual protest that developed when other political or social channels were blocked. Perhaps CFS similarly allows individuals to make a statement about the conditions and pressures of modern life without losing self-respect, to opt out of the prevailing social ethic of the 1980s and 1990s without being exposed to the hurtful charge or insinuation of failure.

'With hard work went the belief we were indestructible. Any sign of weakness, of an inability to cope with being a workaholic was interpreted as a sign of failure, as an indication we couldn't hack it in the new competitive society. To work all hours was macho, to flunk it was to be a wimp'[146]. Respect, both self and from others, is another key theme of CFS, and lack of it is a potent cause of protest. For many CFS sufferers it is the medical profession who are the most prominent offenders. We have suggested that the turbulent rise of CFS has been inspired by this perceived injustice. The changing balance of power between doctor and patient now allows the latter to voice their protest at what they consider maltreatment. Such protests permeate the culture of CFS, but how justified are they? In a fascinating but little known paper, using the instruments derived from the Midtown Manhattan study, a classic piece of psychiatric epidemiology, Dohrenwend and Crandell looked at both professional and non-professional attitudes to common symptoms[147]. Doctors and patients were found to regard different symptoms with differing degrees of concern. 'Feeling weak all over for much of the time' was regarded as 'very serious' by only 6 per cent of psychiatrists and 9 per cent of physicians, making it one of the least important of 43 listed symptoms. In contrast, the same symptom was one of the most important symptoms listed by non-professional samples. These differences are understandable – doctors, well aware of the non-specificity of fatigue, focus more on specific complaints such as haemoptysis or self-harm. On the other hand patients experience it as disabling, distressing, and of possible sinister significance.

Given the prevailing medical disposition to regard 'physical' illness as their rightful business, and hence worthy of respect, in contrast to 'psychological' disorders, this division is also mirrored in the diagnostic practices of most doctors facing a patient with chronic fatigue. Whereas doctors working in primary care are most likely to record psychological diagnoses in patients presenting with new episodes of fatigue, the same episodes are most likely to be viewed by patients as of physical origin[148]. We feel this lack of congruence between both the importance placed on fatigue, and the diagnoses made in fatigued patients, is one of many reasons why so much misunderstanding, and even hostility, results from the interaction between the exhausted patient and his or her doctor. CFS is a forceful avenue of protest against this state of affairs.

CFS is also a natural protest against the organization of medical services. There is some literature on whom people chose to consult with symptoms. In an American study of a community sample of subjects with depression, sleep and energy disturbances predicted those who consulted a doctor. Having decided to seek help, the same factor was associated with consultation with a physician, whereas a factor representing guilt and suicidal ideation was, not surprisingly, associated with consultation with a mental health professional[149]. CFS patients who, for whatever reason, frequently experience depression but rarely exhibit abnormal guilt or lowered self-esteem (see Chapter 10) and who proceed to consult a physician rather than a psychiatrist, are not aberrant or abnormal in this choice. When doctors attempt to reverse this situation by either suggesting a psychiatric referral to a particular patient, or indicate their views in the public arena on the importance of psychiatric factors, CFS patients protest with vigour either in the consulting room or the press.

Finally, CFS is a protest against medical power. The first modern 'first person' account of ME of which we are aware already called on sufferers to dispense with the need for doctors, and find their own solutions. 'We must keep our friends among gentle people. Not among the powerful. Why delude ourselves it was possible to have an honest relationship with such people?'[150].

15.11 The practical consequences

As we will show (Chapter 18) and contrary to the oft expressed opinion, CFS and related disorders are not untreatable. The converse nihilistic attitude comes from both sides of the CFS controversy. Those who regard it as little more than a disguise for hysteria or work avoidance feel that such people are beyond help, whilst those devoted to the cause feel their main job is one of support and loyalty. For a long time perhaps the commonest advice that patients received was from a variety of sources is to rest, avoid activity, and wait for nature to take its course. An American self-help book[48] heads a section with the title 'Rest, Rest and More Rest', and discusses 'aggressive rest therapy', as does an English self-help title[120]. The following quote again serves as an illustration of a considerable literature, although we have also chosen it because it is a direct, albeit inadvertent, quotation from George Beard, the founder of neurasthenia: 'The treatment is rest, and plenty of it . . . the sufferer should always treat her energy resources as if they were money in the bank and be careful not to overdraw'[151].

We have already described why we think that CFS patients can adopt rest as a primary coping strategy (Chapter 12), and what we see as the long-term consequences of that (Chapters 8 and 12). However, we also think that rest has a cultural salience. Overwork was the scourge of the 1980s, ME the hubristic result, so rest is both the solution to ME, and a symbol of a kinder, gentler, more environmentally aware 1990s[146].

15.12 Conclusion

Understanding modern illness ideas is relevant not only to our understanding of CFS, but to all who are interested in the social and cultural history of medicine. In this chapter we have attempted to use the example of CFS in its popular idiom of ME and CFIDS to draw attention to several themes. These have included the modern preoccupation with the immune system, itself linked to the appearance of HIV; the belief that this system is being compromised by various features of modern life; the concept of 'overload'; the themes of toxicity and purity; the general increasing fascination with medicine; the increased promise of medical science but also the reaction against modern medical science and the rise in medical consumerism. We suggest that the fear and stigma of mental illness, and the need for explanations that are both protective of self-esteem and in keeping with modern views on sickness and health, are also important. Finally, we believe that unless the practitioner has an understanding of the range of beliefs encountered in the world of chronic fatigue and allied conditions, and the reasons why such beliefs are held, then the business of management will prove difficult. It is to that business that we now turn.

References

1 Francis C. *Requiem*. London, Pan, 1992.
2 Pawlikowska T, Chalder T, Hirsch S, Wallace P, Wright D, Wessely S. A population based study of fatigue and psychological distress. *Br. Med. J.* 1994; **308:** 743–746.
3 Euba R, Chalder T, Deale A, Wessely S. A comparison of the characteristics of chronic fatigue syndrome in primary and tertiary care. *Br. J. Psychiatry* 1996; **168:** 121–126.
4 Francis C. A beginning. *Interaction*, 1988; **1:** 1.
5 Francis C. Out to lunch. *Sunday Express Magazine* 1 October 1995.
6 Conant S. *Living with Chronic Fatigue*. Dallas, Taylor, 1990.
7 Hartnell L. Personal view. *Br. Med. J.* 1989: 1577–1578.
8 Gardner K. *Interaction: The Journal of the ME Action Campaign* 1988; **I**, i.
9 Davison K, Pennebaker J. Virtual narratives: illness representations in online support groups. In Petrie K, Weinman J (ed) *Perceptions of Health and Illness: Current Research and Applications*. London, Harwood Academic Press, 1997, 463–486
10 Anon. The ME controversy. *Yorkshire Post*, 2 November 1994.
11 Abbey S. Somatization, illness attribution and the sociocultural psychiatry of chronic fatigue syndrome. In Kleinman A, Straus S (ed.) *Chronic Fatigue Syndrome*. Chichester, Wiley, 1993: 238–261.
12 White P, Thomas J, Amess J, Grover S, Kangro H, Clare A. The existence of a fatigue syndrome after glandular fever. *Psychol. Med.* 1995; **25:** 907–916.
13 Helman C. Feed a cold and starve a fever. *Cult. Med. Psychol.* 1978; **7:** 107–137.
14 Katz B, Andiman W. Chronic fatigue syndrome. *J. Pediatrics* 1988; **113:** 944–947
15 Seagrove J. The ME generation. *Guardian* 19 May 1989.
16 Greenberg D. Neurasthenia in the 1980s: chronic mononucleosis, chronic fatigue syndrome, and anxiety and depressive disorders. *Psychosomatics* 1990; **31:** 129–137.
17 Miller P. My healing journey through chronic fatigue. *Yoga Journal*, 1992: 61–124.
18 Wessely S. Neurasthenia and chronic fatigue: theory and practice in Britain and America. *Trans. Cult. Psychiat. Rev.* 1994; **31:** 173–209.

19 Dryden W. The counsellor and ME. In Dryden W (ed.) *The Dryden Interviews: Dialogues on the Psychotherapeutic Process*, 1992: 100–109.

20 Anon. Watchdog to look into ME resources. *Dundee Courier and Advertiser* 11 November 1994.

21 Timbs O. Postviral puzzle. *Observer* 2 August 1987.

22 Steincamp J. *Overload: Beating M.E.* London, Fontana, 1989.

23 Aronowitz R, Spiro H. The rise and fall of the psychosomatic hypothesis in ulcerative colitis. *J. Clin. Gastrol.* 1988; **10**: 298–305.

24 Ware N. Society, mind and body in chronic fatigue syndrome: an anthropological view. In Kleinman A, Straus S (ed) *Chronic Fatigue Syndrome*. Chichester, Wiley, 1993: 62–82.

25 Burrascano J. The overdiagnosis of Lyme disease. *J. Am. Med. Assoc.* 1993; **270**: 2682.

26 Marbach J, Lennon M, Link B, Dohrenwend B. Losing face: sources of stigma as perceived by chronic facial pain patients. *J. Behav. Med.* 1990; **13**: 583–604.

27 Alvarez W. What is wrong with the patient who feels tired, weak and toxic? *New Engl. J. Med.* 1935; **212**: 96–104.

28 Macintyre A. *M.E. Postviral Fatigue Syndrome: How to Live With It.* London, Unwin, 1989.

29 Wessely S. The rise of counselling and the return of alienism. *Br. Med. J.* 1996; **313**: 158–160.

30 Woodward R, Broom D, Legge D. Diagnosis in chronic illness: disabling or enabling – the case of chronic fatigue syndrome. *J. R. Soc. Med.* 1995; **88**: 325–329.

31 Ames M. Learning to live with incurable virus. *Chicago Tribune* 9 June 1985; Section 5: 3.

32 Forna A. A real pain. *Girl About Town* 21 May 1987.

33 Brodie E. Understanding M.E. *Nursing Times* 1988; **84**: 48–49.

34 Henriksson C. Living with continuous muscle pain—patient perspectives.: Encounters and consequences. *Scand. J. Caring Sci.* 1995; **9**: 67–76.

35 Weinberg M, Louw J, Schomer H. Myalgic encephalomyelitis and the personal construction of self. *S. African J. Psychol.* 1994; **24**: 21–26.

36 Stopp C. ME sufferers forced to battle with insurers. *Independent on Sunday* 27 June 1993.

37 Pearson A. Pain on the non-believers. *Evening Standard* 22 November 1994.

38 Delamothe T. Look at ME. *Br. Med. J.* 1994; **308**: 798.

39 Clements A, Sharpe M, Borrill J, Hawton K. Illness beliefs of patients with chronic fatigue syndrome: a quantitative investigation. *J. Psychosom. Res.* 1997: **42**: 615–62.

40 Lees-Haley P, Brown R. Biases in perception and reporting following a perceived toxic exposure. *Percept. Motor Skills* 1992; **75**: 531–544.

41 Roht L, Vernon S, Weir F, Pier S, Sullivan P, Reed L. Community exposure to hazardous waste disposal sites: assessing reporting bias. *Am. J. Epidemiol.* 1985; **122**: 418–433.

42 Jones J, Straus S. Chronic Epstein–Barr virus infection. *Ann. Rev. Med.* 1987; **38**: 195–209.

43 Digon A, Goicoechea A, Moraza M. Chronic fatigue syndrome. *J. Neurol. Neurosurg. Psychiatry* 1992; **55**: 85.

44 Holmes G, Kaplan J, Stewart J, Hunt B, Pinsky P, Schonberger S. A cluster of patients with a chronic mononucleosis-like syndrome: is Epstein–Barr virus the cause? *J. Am. Med. Assoc.* 1987; **257**: 2297–2303.

45 Boly W. Raggedy Ann town. *Hippocrates*, 1987: 31–40.

46 MacLean G, Wessely S. Professional and popular representations of chronic fatigue syndrome. *Br. Med. J.* 1994; **308**: 776–777.

47 Spurgeon A, Gompertz D, Harrington J. Modifiers of non-specific symptoms in occupational and environmental syndromes. *Occup. Environ. Med.* 1996; **53**: 361–366.

48 Feiden K. *Hope and Help for Chronic Fatigue Syndrome: The Official Guide of the CFS/CFIDS Network*. New York, Prentice Hall, 1990.

49 Johnson J. Journey into fear. *Rolling Stone*, 3 August 1987: 42–57.

50 Gunn W, Connell D, Randall B. Epidemiology of chronic fatigue syndrome: the Centers for Disease Control Study. In Kleinman A, Straus S (ed.) *Chronic Fatigue Syndrome.* Chichester, Wiley, 1993: 83–101.

51 Anon. CDC to study illness derided as 'Yuppie flu'. *Wall Street Journal* 19 November 1990.

52 Hood J. 10 Minute Rule Bill on myalgic encephalomyelitis. *Hansard* 23 February 1988.

53 Ramsay M. *Postviral Fatigue Syndrome: The Saga of Royal Free Disease.* London, Gower Medical, 1986.

54 Beard G. *A Practical Treatise on Nervous Exhaustion (Neurasthenia): its Symptoms,* Nature, Sequences, Treatment. New York, William Wood, 1880.

55 Playfair W. The systematic treatment of functional neuroses. In Tuke D (ed.) *Dictionary of Psychological Medicine.* London, Churchill, 1892: 850–857.

56 Field E. A neurologist's view of M.E. *Interaction.* 1988: No.2.

57 Field E. Justice for the neglected and maligned sufferers of ME. *Guardian* 7 August 1990.

58 Ostrom N. It's a dirty little war: proponents of a 'psychoneurotic' cause of CFIDS try again. *Christopher Street* 1989; **1:** 32–33.

59 Masefield P. *Link to Life. M.E.* London, Boxtree, 1994: 1–29.

60 Millon C, Salvato F, Blaney N, *et al.* A psychological assessment of chronic fatigue syndrome/chronic Epstein–Barr virus patients. *Psychol. Health* 1989; **3:** 131–141.

61 Jenkins M. Thoughts on the management of myalgic encephalomyelitis. *Br. Homeopathic. J.* 1989; **78:** 6–14.

62 Lopis R. CFS sufferers lose faith in medicine. *Australian Doctor* 19 July 1996.

63 Shorter E. Sucker-punched again! Physicians meet the disease-of-the-month syndrome. *J. Psychosom. Res.* 1995; **39:** 115–188.

64 Aronowitz R. From myalgic encephalitis to yuppie flu: a history of chronic fatigue syndrome. In Rosenberg C, Golden J (ed.) *Framing Disease.* New Brunswick, Rutgers University Press, 1992: 155–181.

65 Aronowitz R. Lyme disease: the social construction of a new disease and its social consequences. *Millbank Q.* 1991; **69:** 79–112.

66 Arksey H. Expert and lay participation in the construction of medical knowledge. *Sociol. Health Illness* 1994; **16:** 448–468.

67 Holt G. Epidemic neuromyasthenia: the sporadic form. *Am. J. Med. Sci.* 1965: 124–138.

68 Hales D. The fatigue diseases: why are you so tired? *American Health* May 1987: 54–57.

69 Hodgkinson L. ME: the mystery disease. *Woman's Journal* November 1988.

70 Anon. Malaise of the 80s. *Newsweek* 27 October 1986.

71 Willsher K. I beat the disease of the 90s. *Daily Express* 11 April 1990.

72 Cowley G, Hager M, Joseph N. Chronic fatigue syndrome: a medical mystery. *Newsweek* 12 November 1990.

73 Anon. Craig faces two year battle to beat 21st-century disease. *Today* 13 March 1989.

74 Monckton C. The ME generation. *Evening Standard* 25 July 1988.

75 Bryan J, Melville J. The ME generation. *Observer Magazine* 22 January 1989.

76 Askwith R. The ME generation. *Sunday Telegraph Magazine* 22 January 1989.

77 Cleave M. The ME generation. *Evening Standard* 1 September 1993.

78 Illman J. Cry of the ME generation. *Guardian* 1 March 1995.

79 Bassindale C. The ME generation. *Evening Standard* 23 April 1996.

80 Flett K. Why ME? *Arena* March 1990.

81 Crook W. *Chronic Fatigue Syndrome and the Yeast Connection.* Jackson, Professional Books, 1992.

82 Moss-Morris R, Petrie K, Weinman J. Functioning in chronic fatigue syndrome: do illness perceptions play a role? *Br. J. Health Psychol.* 1996; **1:** 15–25.

83 Jacobs G. *Candida albicans: Yeast and Your Health.* London, Optima, 1990.

84 Bradford N. How to beat the new bugs. *Good Housekeeping* March 1992.

85 Francis C. Mad cow disease. *Evening Standard* 3 April 1992.

86 Fletcher M, Francis C. Why I have to fight this living death. *Sun* 17 February 1988.

87 Dawes B, Downing D. *Why ME? A Guide to Combating Postviral Illness.* London, Grafton, 1989.

88 Dickson J. Beating your toxic lifestyle. *Options* June 1995.

89 Anon. In search of a cause. *Awake* 22 August 1992.

90 Regush N. AIDS: words from the front. *Spin* 1990: 69–70, 79–80.

91 Blaugrund A. Now you have it, now you don't. *7 Days* 28 June 1989.

92 Ostrom N. The chronic fatigue story: the medical cover-up of the century. *Christopher Street*, 1989: 11.

93 Donald P. Chronic Epstein–Barr syndrome. *Head Neck Surg.* 1988; **7:** 11–12.

94 Chaitow L. Postviral fatigue syndrome: fact or fantasy? *Women's Journal* March 1988.

95 Sandman C, Barron J, Nackoul K, Goldstein J, Fidler F. Memory deficits associated with chronic fatigue immune dysfunction syndrome. *Biol. Psychiat.* 1993; **33:** 618–623.

96 Abbey S, Garfinkel P. Neurasthenia and chronic fatigue syndrome: the role of culture in the making of a diagnosis. *Am. J. Psychiat.* 1991; **148:** 1638–1646.

97 Garrison J. Chronic fatigue: an ancient ill? *San Francisco Examiner* 17 March 1991.

98 Dawson C. ME and my shadow. *Guardian* 11 January 1989.

99 Ballet G, Proust A. *The Treatment of Neurasthenia.* London, Henry Kimpton, 1902.

100 Rankin G. Neurasthenia; the wear and tear of life. *Br. Med. J.* 1903; **i:** 1017–1020.

101 Ash E. Nervous breakdown: the disease of our age. *Medical Times* 1909; **37:** 35–54.

102 Paul C. The treatment of neurasthenia. *J. Ment. Sci.* 1894; **40:** 134–135.

103 Jewell J. Influence of our present civilization in the production of nervous and mental disease. *J. Nerv. Ment. Dis.* 1881; **8:** 1–24.

104 Wessely S. The history of chronic fatigue syndrome. In Straus S (ed.) *Chronic Fatigue Syndrome.* New York, Dekker, 1994: 41–82.

105 Beard G. American nervousness. New York, GP Putnam's, 1881.

106 Wessely S. History of the postviral fatigue syndrome. *Br. Med. Bull.* 1991; **47:** 919–941.

107 Loblay R. What's in a name? The 'yeast connection' and 'chronic fatigue syndrome'. *Patient Management*, 1992: 15–20.

108 Lane A. Reflections on the evolution of disease. *Lancet* 1921; **ii:** 1117–1123.

109 McGrew F. Neurasthenia and the rest cure. *J. Am. Med. Assoc.* 1900; **34:** 1466–1468.

110 Stea J, Fried W. Remedies for a society's debilities: medicines for neurasthenia in Victorian America. *NY State Med. J.* 1993; **93:** 120–127.

111 Ely T. Neurasthenia as modified by modern conditions, and their prevention. *J. Am. Med. Assoc.* 1906; **47:** 1816–1819.

112 Haller J. Neurasthenia: the medical profession and urban 'blahs'. *NY State Med. J.* 1970; **70:** 2489–2497.

113 Gay P. *The Bourgeois Experience. Victoria to Freud. Volume II: The Tender Passion.* Oxford University Press, 1986.

114 Renfro L, Feder H, Lane T, Manu P, Matthews D. Yeast connection among 100 patients with chronic fatigue. *Am. J. Med.* 1989; **86:** 165–168.

115 Buchwald D, Garrity D. Comparison of patients with chronic fatigue syndrome, fibromyalgia, and multiple chemical sensitivities. *Arch. Intern. Med.* 1994; **154:** 2049–2053.

116 Shefer A, Dobbins J, Fukuda K, Steele P, Koo D, Nisenbaum R, Rutherford G. Fatiguing stress among employees in three large state office buildings. California, 1993, was there an outbreak? *J. Psychiat. Res.* 1997; **31:** 31–43.

117 Chester A, Levine P. Concurrent sick building syndrome and chronic fatigue syndrome: epidemic neuromyasthenia revisited. *Clin. Infect. Dis.* 1994; **18(suppl 1):** S43–S48.

118 Stewart D. The changing face of somatisation. *Psychosomatics* 1990; **31:** 153–158.

119 Crook W. *The Yeast Connection*, 3rd edn. Jackson, Professional Books, 1989.

120 Franklin M, Sullivan J. *The New Mystery Epidemic. M.E. What is it? Have you got it? How to get Better.* London, Century, 1989.

121 Wookey C. *Myalgic Encephalomyelitis: Post-viral Fatigue Syndrome and How to Cope With it.* London, Croom Helm, 1986.

122 Wilson C. Myalgic encephalomyelitis: an alternative theory. *J.R. Soc.Med.* 1990; **83:** 481–483.

123 Fairley J. Will my life ever be normal again? *Woman's Journal* March 1995: 116–117.

124 Dunn E. Too ill to live, not ill enough to die. *Daily Telegraph* 21 March 1989.

125 Culbert M. Chronic and acute elements of a syndrome of immune dysregulation: Part 1. *Int. J. Alt. Complement Med.* 1994: 25–32.

126 Allen J. Myalgic encephalomyelitis. *Homeopathy* 1992; **42:** 152–154.

127 Andersson B, Berg M, Arnetz B, Melin L, Langlet I, Liden S. A cognitive-behavioural treatment of patients suffering from 'electric hypersensitivity'. Subjective effects and reactions in a double-blind provocation study. *J. Occup. Environ. Med.* 1996; **38:** 752–758.

128 Griffin S. The internal athlete. *Ms* May/June 1992: 37–38.

129 Steincamp J. M.E. Mystery epidemic. *NZ Listener* 19 May 1984.

130 Hadley J. What kind of angel? *Tablet* 25 June 1994.

131 Holmes P. ME and you. *Cosmopolitan* June 1988.

132 Abercrombie B. Living with ME. *Which Way to Health?* June 1992: 84–85.

133 Berne K. *Running on Empty: Practical Strategies for Coping with ME.* London, Bloomsbury, 1992.

134 Kalfus M. *Frederick Law Olmsted: The Passion of a Public Artist.* New York University Press, 1990.

135 Lewis S. Personality, stress, and chronic fatigue syndrome. In Cooper C (ed.) *Handbook of Stress, Medicine, and Health* London, CRC Press, 1996: 233–249.

136 Singer M, Arnold C, Fitzgerald M, Madden L, von Legat C. Hypogylcaemia: a controversial illness in U.S. Society. *Med. Anthropol.* 1984; **8:** 1–35.

137 Hope J. My battle with 'devil' illness by Bergerac star Sean. *Daily Mail* 8 September 1990.

138 Rosenberg C. The place of George M. Beard in nineteenth-century psychiatry. *Bull. Hist. Med.* 1962; **36:** 245–259.

139 Leduc S. Electrical treatment of neurasthenia. *Practitioner* 1911: 151–165.

140 Cleave M. My doctor doesn't believe in ME. *Evening Standard* 14 May 1993.

141 Daneff T. Could your back hold the clue to 'Yuppie flu'? *Daily Mail* 2 December 1992.

142 Dowson D. Novagen – a new treatment for ME? *Interaction: The Journal of the ME Action Campaign* Autumn 1992: 26–27.

143 Butler S. Novagen and myalgic encephalomyelitis. *Perspectives: The Journal of the ME Association,* 1994: No. 52, viii-ix.

144 Oppenheim H. *Text-book of Nervous Diseases for Physicians and Students,* 5th edn. London, Foulis, 1908.

145 Ware N, Kleinman A. Culture and somatic experience-the social course of illness in neurasthenia and chronic fatigue syndrome. *Psychosom. Med.* 1992; **54:** 546–560.

146 Jacques M. ME and me. *Guardian* 5 October 1996.

147 Dohrenwend B, Crandell D. Psychiatric symptoms in community, clinic and mental hospital groups. *Am. J. Psychiat.* 1970; **126:** 1611–1621.

148 Ridsdale L, Evans A, Jerrett W, Mandalia S, Osler K, Vora H. Patients who consult with tiredness: frequency of consultation, perceived causes of tiredness and its association with psychological distress. *Br. J. Gen. Pract.* 1994; **44:** 413–416.

149 Dew M, Dunn L, Bromet E, Schulberg H. Factors affecting help-seeking during depression in a community sample. *J. Affect. Disord.* 1988; **14:** 233–234?

150 Jeffreys T. *The Mile-high Staircase.* Auckland, Hodder and Stoughton, 1982.

151 Anon. Post viral fatigue syndrome. *Manual of Family Health.* London, Royal College of Nursing, 1992: 489–490.

Section IV:

Assessment and management of chronic fatigue and chronic fatigue syndrome

16. Assessment of the chronically fatigued patient

16.1 Introduction

We now turn our attention to clinical management. We begin with the patient for whom the diagnosis of chronic fatigue syndrome is being considered. Two types of presentation may raise this possibility. One is the patient who complains of severe fatigue or exhaustion. The other is the patient who arrives already equipped with a diagnosis (whether by a doctor or self-made) of chronic fatigue syndrome (CFS), chronic fatigue and immune dysfunction syndrome (CFIDS), or myalgic encephalomyelitis (ME). It is important to note that although these groups of patients overlap, they are not identical.

Clinical example. A typical patient will be found in the infectious disease or neurological department of the hospital. Their principal complaint is of fatigue, poor concentration, and muscle pain. These symptoms are reported to be exacerbated by physical and mental exertion, and have led to a substantial reduction in daily activities. The history is of an fairly acute onset of symptoms after a 'viral illness'. Appropriate enquiry may reveal symptoms suggestive of depression or anxiety, but without prominent guilt or suicidal ideation. The patient believes the illness to be 'medical' rather than 'psychiatric'.

What is the clinician to do when presented with this clinical problem? We will suggest an approach to assessment in this chapter, review evidence for the efficacy of treatments in Chapter 17, and outline practical management in Chapter 18.

16.2 Aims of the assessment

Aims of the assessment are listed in Table 16.1. and its components in Table 16.2.

Table 16.1 The aims of the assessment of a patient with possible CFS

Establish a working relationship with the patient
Exclude alternative medical diagnosis
Consider alternative/additional psychiatric differential diagnosis

Make a positive diagnosis of CFS if appropriate
Elaborate the diagnosis with a biopsychosocial assessment

Create an initial management plan

Table 16.2 Components of the assessment

Establishing a positive relationship with the patient
History
Mental status examination
Physical examination
Investigations
Diagnosis
Biopsychosocial formulation
The initial management plan

Establishing a working relationship with the patient

The first task is the establishment of a positive relationship with the patient. This is more likely to occur if the physician adopts the strategies listed in Table 16.3. These strategies are, of course, common to all illness, but in CFS special attention must be paid to both the patient's and one's own beliefs about the illness. Although patients' illness beliefs vary, in specialist settings most believe that their symptoms are the result of an organic disease process, and resent any suggestion that they are psychological or psychiatric in nature (see Chapters 12 and 15). Correspondingly, any suggestion by the clinician that the symptoms are imagined, psychogenic, or psychiatric is likely to be perceived as an insult and may cause irretrievable damage to the doctor–patient relationship[1].

Table 16.3 Establishing a positive working relationship

Take the patient's physical complaints seriously
Respect the patient's illness beliefs (without necessarily agreeing with them)
Empathize with experiences of being 'disbelieved' by others
Empathize with effects of illness and express willingness to help
Allow plenty of time, and allow the option of breaks/rest periods if needed.

The doctor's beliefs and attitudes are also important [2]. He or she may believe that complaints in the absence of demonstrable disease are imaginary, or be as resolutely and irrationally wedded to the idea that they are psychological in origin as the patient is to them being physical. Even if the assessing doctor holds sympathetic attitudes, the patient may have previously encountered others who did not. We therefore routinely ask if the patient has ever experienced such 'illness disconfirmation' from professionals ('there's nothing wrong with you' or 'this illness doesn't exist') in order to permit them to ventilate dissatisfaction with previous medical care. Patients say that such experience is common [3–5]. We also emphasize how difficult it must be to face directly the limits of medicine – 'it must have been difficult for you, since no one has given you a simple cure, or even an adequate explanation, for your illness' [6] or 'no doubt you have received many conflicting messages from other doctors about what is wrong'. Once these potential stumbling blocks have been negotiated, it is usually possible to establish a therapeutic alliance.

Identifying diagnosable organic disease

Most physicians who are interested in this subject can recount stories of patients with recognized physical disorders which were missed, and mislabelled as CFS [7–9]. The list of possible medical causes of CFS is long (see Chapter 3). Table 16.4 lists conditions relatively frequently confused with CFS. In practice, however, excluding alternative diagnoses is usually straightforward [10].

Table 16.4 Medical differential diagnosis

General conditions
    Occult malignancy
    Autoimmune disease
    Endocrine disease (e.g. Addison's's disease, hypothyroidism)
    Organ failure: cardiac, respiratory, or renal

Neurological
    Disseminated sclerosis
    Myasthenia gravis
    Parkinson's disease
    Myositis

Infectious
    Chronic active hepatitis (B or C)
    Lyme disease
    Human immunodeficiency virus

Respiratory
    Nocturnal asthma

Chronic toxicity
    Alcohol
    Solvents
    Heavy metals
    Irradiation

Sleep disorders
    Narcolepsy
    Obstructive sleep apnoea

Identify treatable psychiatric syndromes

It is important to identify those syndromes conventionally regarded as 'psychiatric' when these have implications for treatment. This is a more difficult task than excluding organic disease because CFS and psychiatric disorder are both syndromes defined only in terms of symptoms. The precise relationship between 'psychiatric' syndromes and CFS is problematic (see Chapter 10). However, rather than becoming bogged down in unresolved nosological difficulties we would encourage the assessing clinician to be pragmatic and to make psychiatric diagnoses when the requisite symptoms are present, if such diagnoses suggest specific treatment strategies. These may be considered as either alternative or additional to CFS depending on how well they explain the illness. The main principal psychiatric diagnoses to be considered are listed in Table 16.5.

Table 16.5 Psychiatric differential diagnosis

Depressive disorder
  Major depression (including depressive phase of bipolar disorder)
  Dysthymia

Anxiety disorder
  Generalized anxiety disorder
  Panic and agoraphobia

Somatoform disorder
  Hypochondriasis
  Somatization disorder

Others
  Eating disorder
  Substance dependence
  Psychotic disorder

Adopt a broad perspective on the illness

Both the available evidence and our clinical experience indicates the need to go beyond simple diagnosis. Management is most likely to be effective if the clinician takes a broad 'multidimensional' view of the patient's complaints encompassing the physiological, cognitive, behavioural, and social aspects of their presentation [11–14]. It is particularly important to focus on factors that may be *perpetuating* the illness, irrespective of what caused it (see Table 16.8).

16.3 The history

The components of the history are listed in Table 16.6.

Table 16.6 Elements of the history

---

1. *Presenting problems*:
   List all problems (somatic, psychological, and social)
   Clarify nature of symptoms, especially fatigue
   Enquire into changes in life, activity, and sleep and associated distress

2. *The history of the illness*:
   Onset and course
   Patient's understanding of the illness
   Coping strategies used
   Previous and current treatment for this illness

3. *Current situation*:
   Family context
   Employment and financial benefits

4. *Background*:
   Family and personal history
   Past medical and psychiatric history
   Personality

Presenting complaints

The complete problem list

Before encouraging patients to elaborate a detailed account we find it useful to obtain an exhaustive list of their presenting problems. The list should include all their symptoms (somatic, cognitive, and emotional) as well as any other difficulties (interpersonal, occupational, or social) that they are facing. The interest in the full range of the patient's symptoms is more than looking for diagnostic clues. The patient usually views physical symptoms as the core to their condition, and the prime reason for seeking the attention of a health professional. It is therefore essential that the doctor shows a clear and unequivocal interest in these symptoms and the associated disability.

It can be helpful to prompt the patient to produce more symptoms (e.g. 'are there any other symptoms you have not yet told me about?') Our experience is that other doctors have actively attempted to discourage the patient from doing just that. The doctor should also be aware of differences between patients and the medical profession in the perceived importance of certain symptoms, including fatigue [15].

The interest in the full range of their problems is to prevents a premature narrowing of the field of enquiry, and to get difficulties other than symptoms 'on the table'.

Fatigue

It is particularly important to obtain a clear description of the symptom of fatigue. The word 'fatigue' may have many meanings [16]. One particularly important distinction is between sleepiness and lack of energy. Although these complaints commonly coexist, very prominent sleepiness is more suggestive of a sleep disorder (see Chapter 3) [17]. Another important distinction is between an intolerance of effort, which has long been the hallmark of chronic fatigue states [18] (Chapter 8), and fatigue that reflects a reluctance to do anything which is more characteristic of depressive states. In order to meet current criteria for CFS the fatigue must not only be chronic (more than six months) but must also impair activities. It is therefore important to determine just how much the fatigue interferes with activity. This information will be useful later in treatment when determining appropriate short and long term behavioural goals (see Chapter 18).

Sleep

Sleep disturbance is common in patients with CFS, and may play a role in the development of symptoms (see Chapter 11). A detailed sleep history, including periods of daytime rest or sleep, is therefore always indicated as it may offer a target for treatment intervention.

Cognitive symptoms

Cognitive symptoms, such as poor concentration and memory, are often as prominent as complaints of physical fatigue. Characteristically patients describe frequent cognitive errors, such as making slips of the tongue or being unable to find the correct word. Recent memory may also appear impaired. Formal studies, however, do not confirm any particular disorder of memory, and impairment on standard neuropsychological tests rarely matches the severity of the subjective complaints (see Chapter 11). Instead, the most consistent pattern observed is an impairment of selective attention leading to a problem with effortful cognition. Just as the sense of exercise and exertion is altered, so is the sense of cognitive effort. This observation may be used as evidence to convince the patients of the role of the central nervous system in the illness and consequently of the relevance of treatments aimed at modifying central nervous system functioning.

Effect of illness and emotional distress

In order to assess disability it is essential to identify how the illness has changed the patient's life. Once the range and intensity of physical and cognitive difficulties have been detailed, it is natural to move on to how this has affected the patient in terms of mood, coping and so on, the implication being that these symptoms might be understandable, albeit important, reactions to the illness. Although the relationship between mood and chronic fatigue is complex, this approach is least likely to make the patient think that the physician is reinterpreting their illness experience as 'merely psychiatric'.

The history of the illness

Onset

Some patients seen in specialist settings report that their illness began with an acute viral infection (see Chapter 9), and offer no other precipitants. It is important, however, that the physician maintains a broad 'biopsychosocial' perspective; enquiry into the period preceding onset often reveals that psychosocial stressors has been present *prior* to the apparent triggering infection[19]. Some clinicians report that a period of severe stress or loss prior to onset is extremely common, or that stress exacerbates already existing symptoms. Whilst the precise role that stress plays in triggering CFS remains uncertain (Chapter 10), it is a concept that most patients find both understandable and acceptable, particularly if linked with what is known about stress and immunity[20] (see Chapter 9). If the patient is reluctant to identify such stressors we have found it helpful to remind them that they have inevitably experienced viral infections in the past which did not lead to long term ill health, and then to ask 'what was different this time?' Stresses and events occurring after the onset of illness also need elucidation. Many sufferers report that their illness was exacerbated by a premature return to work. This concern can provide a useful introduction to the concepts of gradual rehabilitation outlined below.

Course

By the time patients present to a specialist clinic the illness has often lasted many months. It is important therefore to obtain a longitudinal perspective. In particular patients may have suffered from depressive disorder at other points in their illness, even if they do not currently meet diagnostic criteria[21]. We also routinely ask about factors which make symptoms better or worse. Patients may report that a variety of factors have adverse effects, such as alcohol, exercise, or stress. Any possible adverse effects of activity will need to be addressed in detail later when planning treatment. Adverse effects of stress may provide an avenue for exploring relevant psychological issues in a non-confrontational fashion.

Patients' understanding of their illness

We regard exploring the patients' own understanding of their illness as a fundamental part of assessment. This is best done by asking open ended questions such as 'what do you think is wrong?' and 'what do you think causes the symptoms?'. An appreciation of a patient's understanding of their illness is an essential starting point for the formulation and treatment plan agreed between physician and patient. It is important to gain an impression of the strength in which the patient holds their illness beliefs. Conviction in a *solely* physical cause for symptoms is at present the single most consistent association of poor prognosis[22-24]. We have suggested possible explanations for this finding (Chapter 12), and now we note it may be an important target for therapy (see below).

Coping strategies

Patients have often spent considerable time thinking about their illness and trying out different ways of coping[20]. An enquiry into the strategies they have adopted may not only reveal potential illness-perpetuating factors such as excessive rest, but also set the scene for an examination of alternatives. To this end it is important to establish how the patient arrived at their current strategy. For example previous attempts to be active may have been too sudden, and have resulted in severe exhaustion, which the patient attributed to exacerbation of disease and as result adopted persistent rest and avoidance.

Previous and current treatment for this illness

An enquiry into the patient's previous treatment experience should be made. There are two main reasons for this: first, it may help to avoid repeating previous failed treatments, such as trials of particular antidepressants; second, it may reveal why previous therapies failed (e.g. an antidepressant may have been discontinued too early).

Patients may be currently consulting other physicians and non-medical therapists. In our experience agreement between those treating the patient – or suspension of competing models of treatment – is more likely to lead to a successful outcome. We usually explain to the patient the dangers of competing therapies and therapeutic models, as well as pointing out that mixing treatments makes it impossible to know whom to credit for any successes (and also whom to blame for any failures).

Current situation

Family context

It is a mistake to neglect the patient's family in the assessment. Families of patients with CFS, may, like the families of patients with chronic pain[25], have strong ideas about the illness and about what should be done. This is nowhere more important than in the case of children[26] (see Chapter 13). As well as asking the patient about the views and behaviour of the family it is valuable to interview them directly, and, if appropriate, to involve them in the patient's rehabilitation.

Employment and financial benefits

The patient's current employment (if any) and attitude to it are important factors to be considered in their rehabilitation. Having a job to return to was an independent predictor of treatment success in an outpatient chronic pain rehabilitation programme[27], and our experience suggests that these factors also predict outcome in patients with CFS. The attitude of employers toward appropriate changes of duties and/or a gradual return to work are also important[28]. Finally, we would suggest that, when sufficient trust is established, the physician asks the patient whether they really *want* to return to their previous job – if not the motivation for rehabilitation is likely to be poor[1].

Financial benefits and payments may also be of relevance, especially if their payment is contingent on the patient remaining unwell. Although it may be difficult, and probably unhelpful, to know whether these payments are perpetuating the illness, the implications of losing them must be anticipated in rehabilitation plans. The negotiation of a graduated tapering of benefits after employment has begun may help to overcome this obstacle.

Background

Family and personal history

A family history of depression may indicate both a genetic vulnerability and experience of illness that may have shaped the patient's attitudes. Recollections of childhood may occasionally reveal evidence of early trauma and unhelpful parenting, both may be used to help the patient to see current difficulties in context and to avoid self-blame. Long absences from school, or a history of 'grumbling appendix', repeated episodes of 'glandular fever' or 'hypoglycaemia' may be pointers to recurrent depression or somatization disorder.

The previous occupational and relationship history will indicate the level of pre-illness functioning; it is unrealistic to expect the patient to exceed these with treatment for CFS. It is also said that certain professions such as medicine, teaching, and nursing predispose to CFS either by virtue of particular stressors, or by frequent exposure to viral infection. There is, however, as yet no systematic evidence to support this contention (see Chapters 5 and 8).

Past medical and psychiatric history

Enquiry into previous history should include a systematic enquiry about the symptoms of previous depression, previous unexplained complaints, and previous episodes of similar illness. The patient's account may be usefully supplemented by obtaining all the relevant records. Previous episodes of depression, and of unexplained symptoms, may offer useful clues, both to the current diagnosis and to the treatments that are likely to be effective.

Personality

An attempt should be made to assess premorbid personality. The role of personality in the genesis of CFS is controversial. Clinically many patients report that prior to the onset of illness, they were particularly active in both work and leisure (Chapter 10). Obtaining such a history, if present, can aid understanding the background to the current illness (vulnerability), previous failed attempts at rehabilitation (either undertaking too much too soon or frustration leading to inconsistent activity), as well as suggesting some lifestyle modifications after recovery to prevent a similar pattern repeating itself. The account of an informant should be obtained whenever possible.

16.4 The mental status examination

This should *always* be performed. Much of the information necessary to determine the presence or absence of psychiatric syndromes can be obtained during normal history taking, and in particular when asking about the effects of the illness. It is important additionally to specifically enquire about certain symptoms with a view to excluding important alternative diagnoses. Psychotic disorders, eating disorders, and substance misuse are clearly distinguishable diagnoses with important implications for treatment. Depression and anxiety syndromes are more difficult to diagnose with confidence because the symptoms are similar to those of CFS, but are important alternative/additional diagnoses (see below).

Depression

Patients with CFS frequently describe report 'mood swings' (which on further enquiry are typically episodic low mood), but they rarely report the more *pervasive* depressed mood typical of depressive disorder. In order to make a diagnosis of major depression it is therefore important to also enquire about *anhedonia*, the feeling of inability to experience pleasure. This key symptom can sometimes be difficult to differentiate from a physical inability to perform a previously enjoyed task. Enquiry may therefore focus on not only whether the activity (e.g. playing football) has ceased, but also whether the patient is still interested in it (e.g. watching football on television). The greater the duration of fatigue, the more assiduously should the doctor enquire about the symptoms of mood disorder – two studies have shown that the longer the period of fatigue, the greater the risk of depression[29,30], although there are exceptions[31].

The importance of a complete mental state assessment is hard to overstate. 'Failure to diagnose depression is usually due to failure to seek it rather than any confusion in diagnostic terms'[32]. As Hickie and colleagues showed in Australian primary care, general practitioners regularly fail to detect the presence of depressive disorder in patients presenting with fatigue[33].

Suicide is the only cause of death in CFS. Suicidal thoughts and feelings of hopelessness should therefore be routinely enquired about.

Anxiety

Although many of the somatic symptoms complained of by patients with CFS are similar to those listed under generalized anxiety disorder, CFS patients rarely describe the psychological phenomenon of *worry* that is characteristic of generalized anxiety disorder. If they do, it is worry about the effect of the illness, making it hard to judge its diagnostic importance. If an anxiety disorder is suspected further enquiry should therefore focus on the anxiety-associated feelings of tension, apprehension, and exaggerated startle responses.

Phobic anxiety with avoidance may be missed if the examiner is not vigilant to the possibility of this diagnosis. The cessation of activities such as shopping or socializing may be attributed solely to loss of stamina; careful enquiry, however, may reveal a possible phobic basis to such symptoms. For example patients who report being able to enter anxiety-provoking situations such as supermarkets *only* in the presence of a spouse may have agoraphobia. Similarly, marked sensitivity to noise or light may be a clue to agoraphobia with panic; particular if a sensitivity to artificial rather than natural light is encountered. Where patients report episodic severe symptoms (especially breathlessness, palpitations, and paraesthesia) panic disorder should be considered. In our experience the associated catastrophic thought content is frequently fear of collapse.

Somatoform disorders

Although the treatment implications of a diagnosis of somatoform disorder are fewer than that of depression or anxiety, the diagnoses of hypochondriasis and somatization disorder require special consideration. At a simplistic level these diagnoses would seem to be applicable to many patients with CFS. The situation is in fact more complex. This is because the diagnosis of somatoform disorder required that the somatic symptoms be unexplained by a medical condition; a judgement hard to make conclusively in the current climate of controversy surrounding CFS[34]. In practice, however, we would suggest following our general rule of erring on the side of making diagnoses such as hypochondriasis and somatization which have implications for management.

Hypochondriasis is a syndrome based on the fear of having, or idea that one has, a serious disease, based on a misinterpretation of bodily symptoms. In cases where the patient is preoccupied with fears of diverse and terrible physical diseases such as cancer and multiple sclerosis the diagnosis of hypochondriasis may be appropriate. For the majority who are, in our experience, more concerned with symptoms than anxious about disease the appropriateness of this diagnosis is more doubtful.

Somatization disorder is a syndrome of multiple, recurrent *medically unexplained* symptoms over a prolonged period of time. A few patients with CFS seen in a specialist clinic have a sufficient number and variety of symptoms to qualify for this diagnosis, if the symptoms are regarded as unexplained by a medical condition. If the diagnosis is valid in the patients with CFS it implies a poor prognosis (see Chapter 10).

Dementias

These are conditions characterized by multiple cognitive disorders due to a patho-physiological process affecting the brain. Although patients with CFS complain of cognitive impairment the deficits revealed on cognitive testing are subtle (see Chapter 11). Evidence of marked cognitive impairment should prompt consideration of an alternative diagnosis.

16.5 The physical examination

Physical examination is always appropriate but often neglected. Abnormal physical signs should not be accepted as compatible with a diagnosis of CFS. For example, although many patients complain of swollen or tender lymph nodes, this is a symptom, not a sign. Clinically significant lymphadenopathy needs investigation. Similarly, patients may experience a sensation of feeling feverish, but true pyrexia ($>38°C$) also indicates the need for investigation.

Physical abnormalities which reflect the consequence of chronic ill health and inactivity may be found. Muscle wasting may be the result of prolonged bedrest, and indicates that rehabilitation is an urgent priority, but will be prolonged. Postural hypotension may also be a consequence of chronic inactivity[35]. We routinely test for this, since if present it can explain, and hence help the patient to understand, symptoms such as dizziness. In our experience it usually resolves with increased activity.

16.6 Investigations

We have already alluded to the protean nature of chronic fatigue, which can be the presentation of a number of illnesses, both medical and psychiatric. It is the clinical history that is most relevant, as it is across medicine[36]. In Table 16.7 we list our strategy. This is based on systematic research[30, 37, 40] and the suggestions of other clinicians[41, 42]. Some authors in the specialist setting have shown statistically increased rates of abnormal results on tests for parameters such as antinuclear factor, immune complexes, cholesterol, immunoglobulin subsets, and so on. These are encountered only in a minority, and are rarely substantial[43]. Their significance is for researchers rather than clinicians, and we feel that routine testing for such variables is more likely to result in iatrogenic harm than good. There is no diagnostic test or pattern of tests that can assist in the diagnosis of CFS, as is sometimes claimed.

If an adequate history has been taken, screening investigations are relatively unfruitful: the report with highest number of alternative diagnoses found after further investigation is 5 per cent[44]; most studies report lower rates. A study in a specialist fatigue clinic found that detailed physical examination and laboratory testing contributed to the diagnosis in only 8.5 per cent of chronically fatigued patients; this was considerably lower than the yield of a psychiatric interview[38].

Table 16.7 Recommended investigations

All patients
  Full blood count
  Erythrocyte sedimentation rate or C-reactive protein
  Urea and electrolytes
  Thyroid function tests
  Urine protein and glucose

Can be helpful in selected cases
  Epstein–Barr virus serology
  Toxoplasmosis serology
  Cytomegalovirus serology
  Human immunodeficiency virus serology
  Chest X-ray,
  Creatinine phosphokinase
  Rheumatoid factor
  Cerebral MRI (for demyelination)

Not helpful
  Enteroviral serology
  VP-1 test
  Cerebral blood flow assessment

16.7 Specialist referral

The problem of when or if to ask a specialist physician for help in the assessment of the chronically fatigued patient often concerns primary care physicians. We do not believe that such referral should be routine, as the primary care physician remains the mainstay of effective management[45, 46]. We do suggest that referral to a specialist physician should be considered when there is an increased probability of an alternative diagnosis. These could be circumstances such as the very young or old, patients reporting recent foreign travel, weight loss, any neurological signs, difficulty walking, pyrexia of unknown origin (objectively confirmed), or in any case when a second opinion is needed in respect of a possible alternative diagnosis.

16.8 Diagnosis

Should the diagnosis be made at all?

Many doctors are reluctant to make the diagnosis of CFS. Interestingly primary care physicians are less reluctant than specialists[47, 48]. Many physicians may, with good reason as the reader of this book will be aware, harbour doubts about the nosological status of CFS and be wary of the potential negative effect of disease labels on patients[49]. The absence of any pathognomic symptom or diagnostic test for CFS serves only to make the decision of whether or not to make a diagnosis more difficult.

Such high-minded scepticism is, in our opinion, rarely beneficial in the clinical situation. Patients need a label in order to make sense of their own experience[50, 51]. Without such it is almost impossible for them to organize their dealings with the world of work and financial benefits[14]. We therefore advise that if a patient with fatigue already believes that their diagnosis is CFS or one of its variants, that belief should not be challenged unless an alternative diagnosis is available. We also believe that a new diagnosis of CFS has a place in clinical practice, providing it is made clear clear to the patient that in the current state of knowledge this is a descriptive term, that no discrete pathological process has so far been identified, recovery is possible and treatment is available. In these circumstances we are happy to make a firm, positive diagnosis of CFS (see Chapter 18).

Which diagnosis should be made?

We do not use the term 'myalgic encephalomyelitis' (ME). This is because both its literal and implicational meaning is of a sinister disease process. An admission of ignorance is better than misguided certainty[46, 52].

16.9 Biopsychosocial formulation

Important though diagnosis is, for a condition as heterogenous as CFS it is inadequate as the sole basis guide to choice of treatment. We favour the supplementation of diagnosis with a multidimensional description of the illness that expands the biomedical perspective and deconstructs it into understandable components. Thus biological psychological and social influences are identified and categorized as predisposing, precipitating, and perpetuating factors. The general format is illustrated in Table 16.8. The use of this approach is illustrated by returning to a further examination of the case example described above.

Table 16.8 Outline grid of possible factors and estimate of their relative importance (based on literature and clinical experience) for use in aetiological formulation

	Predisposing	*Precipitating*	*Perpetuating*
Biological			
Genetic	+		
Acute illness		+ + +	
Effects of inactivity			+ + +
Sleep disorder		+	+ + +
Specific CFS pathophysiology		+	+
Psychological			
Early experience	+		
Life events	+	+ +	+
Chronic conflicts	+	+	+ +
Mood disorder	+ +	+ +	+ +
Attitudes	+ +	+	+ + +
Illness beliefs	+	+	+ + +
Avoidance behaviour		+	+ + +
Social			
Attitude of family	+		+ +
Social stigma	+	+	+ +
Iatrogenesis	+	+	+ + +
Misinformation	+	+	+ + +
Occupational issues	+ +	+ +	+ + +
Benefits of sick role			+

+ = possible role; + + = probable role; + + + = important role.

Clinical example. The further assessment of the patient described at the beginning of this chapter revealed that she believed that her symptoms were caused by an ongoing virus infection and was worried about making them worse. These ideas had been reinforced by books her mother had bought for her about the illness. She consequently avoided activity and had been profoundly inactive for over a year, often lying in bed and sleeping for long periods. She was therefore likely to be physiologically de-conditioned. She was frustrated with her inability to do things and often felt low in mood about her predicament.

Her job as a teacher had been very stressful but since becoming ill she had been unable to work – she did not want to return and was in disputed medical retirement. She was cared for by her mother who also believed she had permanent disability. Her friends sometimes implied that she was not really ill. Her doctor said that the best thing for her was prolonged rest.

Her family were very achievement oriented and regarded depression as weakness. She had a previous history of recurrent 'glandular fever' her symptoms during which were consistent with major depressive episodes.

A biopsychosocial assessment was made and is illustrated in Table 16.9. The most likely illness perpetuating factors are highlighted – these are potential targets for intervention.

Table 16.9 Summary grid for factors of possible relevance in the clinical example

	Predisposing	Precipitating	Perpetuating
Biological			
Genetic	?		
Acute illness		+ +	
Effect of inactivity			+ + +
Sleep disorder		+	+ + +
Specific CFS pathophysiology	?	?	?
Psychological			
Early experience	?		
Life events		+ +	
Chronic conflicts		+	+
Mood disorder	+ + +	+	+
Attitudes		+	+ + +
Illness beliefs	+	+	+ + +
Avoidance behaviour		+	+ + +
Social			
Attitude of family	+	+	+ +
Iatrogenesis	+	+	+ +
Social stigma			+ +
Misinformation		+	+ + +
Occupational issues		+ +	+ + +
Benefits of sick role			+

+ = possible role; + + = probable role; + + + = important role.

16.10 Management plans

The management of patients with CFS must be based on the available evidence of what has been shown to be effective for patients who meet the criteria for this diagnosis. It also makes clinical sense that treatment be tailored as far as possible to the individual. This can be achieved by targeting one or more of the most likely illness-perpetuating factors identified in the individual assessment. In the case summarized in Table 16.9 the initial intervention could be focused on the patient's understanding of their situation and how they might be able to escape from this predicament. It is important the patient 'own' the treatment plan. One way to achieve this is to ask them to 'brainstorm' possible interventions. In any case it is desirable to outline the management plan to the patient before the end of the first meeting if time permits. This conveys an appropriately positive message, allows them time to think about what is being suggested and sets the scene for future treatment.

16.11 Special issues

The hostile patient

Occasionally, despite careful attention on engagement, patients arrive with a pre-conception that the assessment will be unhelpful and even destructive of their well-being. This is a bad start, but not insurmountable. It may be necessary to defer the detailed information collection, and to focus entirely on understanding the reasons for their hostility. Once identified appropriate reassurance can be given and the practicalities of assessment negotiated. Never underestimate the power of simple compassion.

The insurance assessment

The issue of benefits and insurance payments is exceptionally difficult in this area, and likely to lead to confrontation unless carefully handled. Disability systems and insurance agencies are sceptical concerning CFS – the combination of a disorder based entirely on self-report, without any agreed diagnostic test, yet also apparently associated with long term often profound disability, understandably causes some concerns in such quarters[53]. Much of the self-help literature on both sides of the Atlantic concerns the iniquities of the various benefits systems, and both personal and political strategies to overcome them. We have adopted a pragmatic approach to this problem. When asked to comment on benefits or insurance claims we support the patient as much as is possible, but do not support claims for permanent disability or medical retirement until all reasonable efforts at rehabilitation have been tried.

The 'difficult' family

It is wise to see family members as part of the assessment. This is especially the case for children. Although time consuming if there is evidence that the beliefs, attitudes, and behaviour of the family are important it is a false economy to avoid seeing them, individually if possible. If it is felt that either partners or parents are encouraging disability, albeit inadvertently, it will be as important to try and engage them in treatment as the individual patient[26,54].

16.12 Conclusion

The assessment may be completed on one long session or spread over several shorter ones. The exact duration of these sessions should, if possible, be determined by the patient rather than the clinic timetable. Once complete, detailed treatment plans can be made. In order to do this the physician should be aware of the evidence for the relative effectiveness of the large number of treatments claimed to be of use in CFS and how to implement practical management. These are the topics of the next two chapters.

References

1 Butler C, Rollnick S. Missing the meaning and provoking resistance: a case of myalgic encephalomyelitis. *Fam. Pract.* 1996; **13**: 106–109.
2 Scott S, Deary I, Pelosi A. General practitioners' attitudes to patients with a self-diagnosis of myalgic encephalomyelitis. *Br. Med. J.* 1995; **310**: 508.
3 Henriksson C. Living with continuous muscle pain—patient perspectives.: Encounters and consequences. *Scand. J. Caring Sci.* 1995; **9**: 67–76.
4 English T. Skeptical of skeptics. *J. Am. Med. Assoc.* 1991; **265**: 964.
5 Ware N. Suffering and the social construction of illness: the delegitimisation of illness experience in chronic fatigue syndrome. *Med. Anthropol. Q.* 1992; **6**: 347–361.
6 House A. The patients with medically unexplained symptoms: making the initial psychiatric contact. In Mayou R, Bass C, Sharpe M (ed.) *The Treatment of Functional Somatic Symptoms*. Oxford University Press, 1995: 89–102.
7 Gray J, Bridges A, McNeill G. Atrial myxoma: a rare cause of progressive exertional dyspnoea. *Scot. Med. J.* 1992; **37**: 186–187.
8 Hurel S, Abuiasha B, Bayliss P, Harris P. Patients with a self diagnosis of myalgic encephalomyelitis. *Br. Med. J.* 1995; **311**: 329.
9 Mesch U, Lowenthal R, Colemen D. Lead poisoning masquerading as chronic fatigue syndrome. *Lancet* 1996; **347**: 1193.
10 Matthews D, Manu T, Lane T. Evaluation and management of patients with chronic fatigue. *Am. J. Med. Sci.* 1991; **302**: 269–277.
11 Demitrack M, Greden J. Chronic fatigue syndrome; the need for an integrative approach. *Biol. Psychiat.* 1991; **30**: 747–752.
12 Vercoulen J, Swanink C, Fennis J, Galama J, van der Meer J, Bleijenberg G. Dimensional assessment of chronic fatigue syndrome. *J. Psychosom. Res.* 1994; **38**: 383–392.
13 Mayou R, Bass C, Sharpe M. Overview of epidemiology, classification and aetiology. In Mayou R, Bass C, Sharpe M (ed.) *Treatment of Functional Somatic Symptoms*. Oxford University Press, 1995: 42–65.
14 Mayou R, Sharpe M. Diagnosis, illness and disease. *Q. J. Med.* 1995; **88**: 827–831.
15 Dohrenwend B, Crandell D. Psychiatric symptoms in community, clinic and mental hospital groups. *Am. J. Psychiat.* 1970; **126**: 1611–1621.
16 Berrios G. Feelings of fatigue and psychopathology. *Comp. Psychiatry* 1990; **31**: 140–151
17 Horne J. Dimensions to sleepiness. In Monk T (ed.) *Sleep, Sleepiness and Performance*. New York, Wiley, 1991: 169–195.
18 Waller A. The sense of effort: an objective study. *Brain* 1891; **14**: 179–239.
19 Gunn W. In Kleinman A, Straus S (ed.) *Chronic Fatigue Syndrome*. Chichester, Wiley, 1993: p288.
20 Clements A, Sharpe M, Simkin S Borrill J, Hawton K. Illness beliefs of patients with chronic fatigue syndrome: a quantitative investigation. *J. Psychosm. Res.* 1997: **42**: 615–24.
21 Manu P, Matthews D, Lane T, *et al.* Depression among patients with a chief complaint of chronic fatigue. *J. Affect. Disord.* 1989; **17**: 165–172.
22 Sharpe M, Hawton K, Seagroatt V, Pasvol G. Follow up of patients with fatigue presenting to an infectious diseases clinic. *Br. Med. J.* 1992; **302**: 347–352.
23 Wilson A, Hickie I, Lloyd A, *et al.* Longitudinal study of the outcome of chronic fatigue syndrome. *Br. Med. J.* 1994; **308**: 756–760.
24 Vercoulen J, Swanink C, Fennis J, Galama J, van der Meer J, Bleijenberg G. Prognosis in chronic fatigue syndrome: a prospective study on the natural course. *J. Neurol. Neurosurg. Psychiatry* 1996; **60**: 489–494.

25 Benjamin S, Mawer J, Lennon S. The knowledge and beliefs of family care givers about chronic pain patients. *J. Psychosom. Res.* 1992; **36:** 211–217.

26 Vereker M. Chronic fatigue syndrome: a joint paediatric–psychiatric approach. *Arch. Dis. Child.* 1992; **67:** 550–555.

27 Cott A, Anchel H, Goldberg W, Fabich M, Parkinson W. Non-institutional treatment of chronic pain by field management: an outcome study with comparison group. *Pain* 1990; **40:** 183–194.

28 Peel M. Rehabilitation in postviral syndrome. *J. Soc. Occup. Med.* 1988; **38:** 44–45.

29 Morrison J. Fatigue as a presenting complaint in family practice. *J. Fam. Pract.* 1980; **10:** 795–801.

30 Ridsdale L, Evans A, Jerrett W, Mandalia S, Osler K, Vora H. Patients with fatigue in general practice: a prospective study. *Br. Med. J.* 1993; **307:** 103–106.

31 Cathebras P, Robbins J, Kirmayer L, Hayton B. Fatigue in primary care: prevalence, psychiatric comorbidity, illness behaviour and outcome. *J. Gen. Intern. Med.* 1992; **7:** 276–286.

32 Havard C. Lassitude. *Br. Med. J.* 1985; **i:** 299.

33 Hickie I, Koojer A, Hadzi-Pavlovic D, Bennett B, Wilson A, Lloyd A. Fatigue in selected primary care settings: socio-demographic and psychiatric correlates. *Med. J. Aust.* 1996; **164:** 585–588.

34 Johnson S, Deluca J, Natelson B. Assessing somatization disorder in the chronic fatigue syndrome. *Psychosom. Med.* 1996; **58:** 50–57.

35 Sharpe M, Bass C. Pathophysiological mechanisms in somatization. *Int. Rev. Psychiat.* 1992; **4:** 81–97.

36 Hampton J, Harrison M, Mitchell J, Pritchard J, Seymour C. Relative contribution of history-taking, physical examination, and laboratory investigation in diagnosis and management of medical outpatients. *Br. Med. J.* 1975; **ii:** 486–489.

37 Kroenke K, Wood D, Mangelsdorff D, Meier N, Powell J. Chronic fatigue in primary care: Prevalence, patient characteristics and outcome. *J. Am. Med. Assoc.* 1988; **260:** 929–934.

38 Lane T, Matthews D, Manu P. The low yield of physical examinations and laboratory investigations of patients with chronic fatigue. *Am. J. Med. Sci.* 1990; **299:** 313–318.

39 Valdini A, Steinhardt S, Feldman E. Usefulness of a standard battery of laboratory tests in investigating chronic fatigue in adults. *Fam. Pract.* 1989; **6:** 286–291.

40 Cope H, Mann A, Pelosi A, David A. Psychosocial risk factors for chronic fatigue and chronic fatigue syndrome following presumed viral infection: a case control study. *Psychol. Med.* 1996; **26:** 1197–1209.

41 Walls R. How to investigate the patient with chronic fatigue. *Mod. Med. Aust.* 1995: 115–120.

42 Anfinson T. Diagnostic assessment of chronic fatigue syndrome. In Stoudemire A, Fogel B (ed.) *Medical–Psychiatric Practice.* Washington, DC, American Psychiatric Press, 1995: 215–256.

43 Bates D, Buchwald D, Lee J, *et al.* Clinical laboratory test findings in patients with chronic fatigue syndrome. *Arch. Intern. Med.* 1995; **155:** 97–103.

44 Swanink C, Vercoulen J, Bleijenberg G, Fennis J, Galama J, Van Der Meer J. Chronic fatigue syndrome: a clinical and laboratory study with a well matched control group. *J. Intern. Med.* 1995; **237:** 499–506.

45 Wessely S, David A, Butler S, Chalder T. The management of chronic 'post-viral' fatigue syndrome. *J. R. Coll. Gen. Pract.* 1989; **39:** 26–29.

46 Anon. *Chronic Fatigue Syndrome: Report of a Committee of the Royal Colleges of Physicians, Psychiatrists and General Practitioners.* London, Royal College of Physicians, 1996.

47 Ho-Yen D. General practitioners' experience of the chronic fatigue syndrome. *Br. J. Gen. Pract.* 1991; **41:** 324–326.

48 Denz-Penhey H, Murdoch J. General practitioners acceptance of the validity of chronic fatigue syndrome as a diagnosis. *NZ Med. J.* 1993; **106:** 122–124.

49 Hadler N. The dangers of the diagnostic process. Iatrogenic labelling as in the fibrositis paralogism. In Hadler N (ed.) *Occupational Musculoskeletal Disorders.* New York, Raven Press, 1993: 16–33.

50 Woodward R, Broom D, Legge D. Diagnosis in chronic illness: disabling or enabling-the case of chronic fatigue syndrome. *J. R. Soc. Med.* 1995; **88:** 325–329.

51 Sutton G. 'Too tired to go to the support group': a health needs assessment of myalgic encephalomyelitis. *J. Publ. Health Med.* 1996; **18:** 343–349.

52 Scadding J. Essentialism and nominalism in medicine: logic of diagnosis in disease terminology. *Lancet* 1996; **348:** 594–596.

53 Lechky O. Life insurance MDs sceptical when chronic fatigue syndrome diagnosed. *Can. Med. Assoc. J.* 1990; **143:** 413–415.

54 Feder H, Dworkin P, Orkin C. Outcome of 48 pediatric patients with chronic fatigue; a clinical experience. *Arch. Fam. Med.* 1994; **3:** 1049–1055.

17. Treatment of CFS: the evidence

17.1 Introduction

It is hard to imagine any illness for which more unproven remedies have been advocated with greater enthusiasm than CFS. Contemplating the extensive popular literature[1-6] one is struck by the range of treatments advocated: from aspirin to aromatherapy, antidepressants to acupuncture, and magnesium to massage. It is striking how often these books plead for a holistic approach, rightly complaining that modern medicine often focuses too much on diseases instead of the individual, but then falling into the same trap. Many of the treatments recommended are based only on anecdotal improvements some sufferers have made, or on unproven theories of immune dysfunction, candida infestations, dietary deficiencies, and so on. Very little treatment advice is based on the results of randomized controlled trials. Much the same could also be said about the medical management of CFS.

Our clinical experience suggests that the advice offered by these books does not go unheeded. Indeed, many patients are taking multiple treatments, some of which may be harmless, others merely expensive, and still others which are potentially hazardous. For example, the most consistently recommended treatment for CFS is rest. Thus one book states that rest should be a 'positive, constructive treatment'[3] another states 'the one clear thing we do know is that any exercise will make people worse'[6] and a third advocates 'aggressive rest therapy'[7]. This is surprising because there are very few indications for rest in modern medicine, and because we have seen in Chapter 3 how profoundly damaging long periods of rest can be. Furthermore there is no good evidence for its effectiveness in patients with CFS.

We believe strongly that before any treatment can be widely recommended it should have been submitted to rigorous testing using the methodology of the randomized controlled trial (RCT) in order to assess both its benefits and disadvantages. This approach is probably the only ethical means of ensuring patients are not unnecessarily submitted to ineffective or dangerous treatments. This chapter will review the evidence available from RCTs of treatment for CFS and related conditions such as fibromyalgia. The next chapter will describe our usual clinical management of patients with CFS which is based on this literature.

17.2 The randomized controlled trial: strengths and weaknesses

The evidence of treatment efficacy reviewed here will be almost exclusively from randomized controlled trials (RCTs). The process of randomization of patients to alternative treatments has become the gold standard for the evaluation of new therapies[8,9]. RCTs have several important advantages over other study designs. First, they abolish selection bias: whereas in clinical practice, choice of treatment may depend upon the clinician's views of the patient's likelihood of responding to it – and this would lead to bias in the assessment of clinical outcome – this cannot happen in an RCT since treatment group is allocated randomly. Neither patient nor doctor have any say in allocation. Second, provided sample sizes are large enough, RCTs are capable of abolishing confounding, even when it is due to *unknown* confounders. In other words, with a large randomized controlled trial one can be reasonably confident that differences detected in improvements between treatment groups are not due to differences in the patients in these two groups: a randomized controlled trial allows one to compare like with like more reliably than any other research methodology. Third, if properly designed and blinded, they are able to separate the non-specific effects of medical attention and the optimism new treatments lead to, from specific actions of the treatment to be studied.

These advantages mean that RCTs are far more robust than any other form of evaluation of treatment. Anecdotal reports, case series, and open trials can only ever be considered as suggestive evidence which should encourage further research. Despite the advantages of RCTs many of the trials are not without their problems[8,10]. The following general observations tie together some of the common themes which will appear in the discussion of trials.

Sample size and power

RCTs are expensive and time consuming for both investigators and patients. It is therefore not surprising that many of the studies reported here are small. This means that even quite impressive differences between treatments may be missed (so-called type II error). Imagine, for example, if 30 patients (15 per group) were recruited to a trial, and one expected recovery in 20 per cent of those given a placebo: such a trial would be incapable of detecting important clinically significant differences at conventional statistical power. In fact one would have to see recovery in approximately 75 per cent of those on active treatment to achieve statistical significance. Hence a small difference in treatment effects would be hard to distinguish from a chance association. Such large treatment effects are unrealistic in chronic conditions of uncertain aetiology, yet sample sizes of 30 are not uncommon in the trials reviewed in this chapter.

Measurement of outcome and 'blinding'

CFS is diagnosed on the basis of subjective complaints. Whilst many of the trials report immune function or other laboratory measures as outcomes, the only outcomes which are likely to matter to patients are how they feel and how much they can do. These outcomes usually rely on self-reporting of symptoms and levels of activity. Because of this it is important to maintain blindness to treatment. It is very simple to check whether clinicians and patients in RCTs have correctly guessed which treatment they were allocated to, but only one of the trials reported here did this. On the other hand, some of the trials report invasive treatments which are associated with specific side effects, and which may very well lead to the subjects and investigators guessing which treatment they are on. This then leads to the possibility of bias being introduced. This problem is also of relevance where the treatment is such that the patient cannot be blind: as in psychotherapy and exercise trials.

Subgroup analyses

The temptation of a researcher to report any statistically significant finding is great, and it is perhaps not surprising in these early studies to find that *post hoc* subgroup analyses are very common. A typical example is where some measure of disease activity (e.g. an immunological measure) at baseline is used to subdivide subjects[11]. Readers should always beware of studies which conclude: 'treatment X is effective in that subgroup of patients with Y'. It is more likely that the conclusions are based on secondary analyses of the data than any *a priori* scientific theory. Subgroup analyses are more appropriate if the study has been designed to address a specific issue and the randomization has been designed accordingly. For example the study by Vercoulen *et al.*[12] performed a stratified randomization on the basis of depressive symptoms. Analysis according to that subgroup is acceptable since it suggests there was an *a priori* hypothesis. The most rigorous way to deal with subgroup analyses is to present them as treatment–subgroup interaction terms. Such analyses were not performed in any of the studies which did subgroup analyses.

Duration of trials

Many of the individuals included in these trials had been unwell for some years. If treatments are to become widespread it is necessary that they should be assessed over reasonable periods of time. Many of the RCTs reported here followed patients for short periods of a few weeks. Treatments should be evaluated for longer periods if they are to be widely used.

Publication bias

A well recognized problem in attempting any synthesis of a collection of RCTs is publication bias. Publication bias occurs when 'positive' trials of a new treatment are published more readily than 'negative' ones. There is compelling evidence that publication bias exists for many new treatments[13–15], and unless all RCTs are registered at outset, it is likely to remain an important limitation.

Generalizability

If a treatment is shown to be efficacious in an RCT, can this result be generalized to a wider population of sufferers? One of the key problems for studies which advocate behavioural change is that some sufferers may not be prepared to attempt the treatment, and refuse to be randomized. Thus RCTs may be selecting a group of patients with better prognosis.

Special problems for psychotherapy/exercise trials

Trials which assess the effects of a psychotherapeutic intervention or some other form of behaviour change have additional problems. First, they often cannot be adequately blinded. Second, as psychotherapies rely on an individual therapist administering the therapy in a standard way, negative results are often more difficult to interpret as they may simply suggest that the therapist is not very good at his or her job. Third, it is often difficult to extract an 'active ingredient' out of a psychotherapy trial. For example in the trials of cognitive behaviour therapy (CBT) is it behavioural change or changes in cognitions which are important? The simplest way to overcome these sorts of dilemmas is to view therapy as a 'black box'. Finally, psychotherapy trials are particularly dependent on the compliance of the patient which is harder to assess in this situation than in trials of drug treatments.

Intention to treat analyses

Another frequent problem in RCTs relates to their analysis and the approach taken to subjects who drop out of treatment. Two approaches are widely used: intention-to-treat analysis and completer analysis. Completer analysis, as its name suggests, only analyses the results of subjects who stay in the trial up to completion. Thus the analysis ignores patients who drop out of treatment for one reason or another. Intention-to-treat analysis deals with data from these patients in one of two ways: if possible they are reassessed as though they were still in the trial. Alternatively, an assumption is made that since stopping treatment they have remained unchanged and the results of their last assessment are carried forward to the endpoint analysis. Either way, intention-to-treat analysis has an important advantage over completer analysis: it retains the full benefit of randomization in eliminating bias. For example, tolerating treatment is associated with a good outcome: thus in a trial of lipid-lowering agents[16], patients who completed treatment were found to do better than those who stopped treatment *irrespective* of whether they were on placebo or active treatment! Thus staying on treatment *per se* may be associated with a good prognosis. If one imagined an RCT where an ineffective treatment which had many side effects was being compared with placebo, the drop-out rate is likely to be different between groups. Indeed only those who are especially compliant (and therefore have the best prognosis) will complete the active treatment. The placebo completer will be a less selected group and therefore there is likely to be a selection bias in favour of the treatment if a completer analysis was performed. Such bias would not happen in an intention-to-treat analysis. The majority of the studies reported here report completer analyses, and hence may exaggerate the benefits of active treatment.

With these provisos in mind we shall now review all the available RCTs of physical and psychological treatments in CFS and other fatigue syndromes, especially fibromyalgia.

17.3 Anti-inflammatories and analgesics

Given that CFS is characterized by muscle pain, it is not surprising that anti-inflammatory agents are frequently used by patients and prescribed by doctors. We are not aware of any RCTs assessing their use in CFS, but there are a few which have looked at them in fibromyalgia.

A study by Yunus *et al.*[17] compared the non-steroidal anti-inflammatory drug (NSAID) ibuprofen with placebo in fibromyalgia. Follow-up was over three weeks, and of nine outcomes only one, morning fatigue, was shown to improve on ibuprofen. There was a large placebo effect. Another study of ibuprofen also failed to give consistent results in support of the treatment[18]. Goldenberg *et al.*[19] randomized patients in a comparison of naproxen and placebo. The design was factorial and the other contrast was between low-dose amitriptyline and placebo. They did not report any significant benefit of naproxen, but speculated that the group with naproxen and amitriptyline did best. A similar design has been used to compare ibuprofen and alprazolam with placebo[20] with unclear results which indicated those on combined therapy did best. There were more responders in the group which received both drugs simultaneously, but little evidence for an independent effect of ibuprofen. Another study[21] compared a combination of paracetamol, cariosprodol (a muscle relaxant), and caffeine in female patients with fibromyalgia. Some improvement in overall symptoms and pain for those in the active treatment group were reported, although it is unclear which component of the compound was responsible.

Overall these trials suggest that non-steroidal anti-inflammatory agents are ineffective in fibromyalgia. Whilst these drugs have an important role in the management of other rheumatological complaints, they have well documented and potentially dangerous side effects such as gastric erosions. On the available evidence there is no case to make NSAIDs widely available in the treatment of CFS.

17.4 Antidepressants

Rationale for the use of antidepressants in CFS

We have seen elsewhere in this volume (Chapters 4 and 10) that fatigue is common in depression and depression is common in CFS. There are several strands to the rationale of antidepressant use in CFS. First, irrespective of the role of depression in the *aetiology* of CFS it might be reasonable to assume that antidepressants are effective in patients with CFS who have comorbid depression. After all, there is good evidence to suggest that they are an effective treatment of depression when it accompanies a number of defined organic diagnoses. In a review of the literature[22] we identified 11 placebo controlled trials of antidepressant use in medically ill depressed patients, of which eight showed a benefit for those treated with active medication. Thus if antidepressants are effective in treating depression accompanying heart disease[23], cancer[24], chronic obstructive pulmonary disease[25], multiple sclerosis[26], Parkinson's disease[27], stroke[28, 29], and HIV infection[30], it seems reasonable to give depressed patients with CFS the opportunity to benefit from them.

Secondly, antidepressants have proven benefit in the management of some of the commonest symptoms of CFS. These include pain[31] and sleep disorders[32]. Such symptomatic management, whilst not necessarily changing the underlying condition, might be expected to lead to improvements in function.

Finally, it has been suggested that antidepressants, by virtue of their action on central monoaminergic transmission, might have a direct effect on the core features of CFS. There is certainly some support for the notion that abnormalities of central neurotransmitters such as serotonin are seen in CFS (see Chapter 11).

Randomized controlled trials of antidepressants in CFS

We are aware of three RCTs which have treated CFS with antidepressants. The first by Vercoulen *et al.*[12] compared fluoxetine and placebo in the treatment of 96 patients diagnosed according to the Oxford criteria. Randomization was stratified such that patients were subdivided according to whether or not they had depression. Treatment was over eight weeks, and patients were then followed for another eight weeks after stopping treatment. Outcomes used included the Beck Depression Inventory[33] and the Sickness Impact Profile (a quality of life measure)[34]. Surprisingly, fluoxetine did not appear to have any significant effect on either of these two outcomes, either at the point where treatment was terminated, or at the final follow-up.

Wearden *et al.*[35] used a factorial design to examine the effects of fluoxetine and an exercise regime on the symptoms of CFS. Patients were diagnosed according to the Oxford criteria. A total of 136 patients were randomized and 96 completed the six-month period of treatment. Fluoxetine did not make a statistically significant difference in the primary outcome measure (a fall in fatigue score to below the threshold for CFS), but it did cause some improvement on fatigue and depression. The overall implication of this study was that fluoxetine may be beneficial in the treatment of CFS irrespective of depression status.

Natelson *et al.*[36] compared the monoamine oxidase inhibitor phenelzine in 24 patients with CFS diagnosed by the CDC criteria. The treatment was given over four weeks after which a range of measures including a modified Karnofsky scale[37], a fatigue severity scale, a symptom profile, profile of mood states, and functional status questionnaires were used to assess recovery. The randomization was unbalanced leaving 15 patients in the phenelzine group and the remainder on placebo. Six patients dropped out of phenelzine treatment suggesting it is not well tolerated. The somewhat unorthodox analysis suggested a pattern of improvement in patients given phenelzine. Given the small numbers of patients included in this study it would be surprising if any clear answers were forthcoming, and it would be premature to prescribe phenelzine on the basis of such a study.

The only other RCT we are aware of compared treatment with sertraline and clomipramine[38] in 40 patients. The two drugs were equally well tolerated but sertraline seemed to produce more of an improvement in depression scale. Without a placebo group it is hard to draw firm conclusions from these findings.

How should these results be interpreted? One reason for the difference between Vercoulen's study and that of Wearden is that the former used a relatively short duration of treatment, and the main outcomes were assessed after antidepressants had been discontinued. Another may be that the patients in the first study had a longer duration of illness and were more based in tertiary care, indicating that they may have been a severe and chronic group. Another possibility is that an interaction between exercise and fluoxetine treatment exists and it is this, rather than fluoxetine *per se* which was responsible for the result of Wearden *et al.*

If the situation for antidepressants is unclear in CFS what about the related disorder, fibromyalgia? Table 17.1 summarizes the RCTs which have used antidepressants to treat this condition. The most widely used antidepressant has been the tricyclic amitriptyline. This has been used in low doses of 10–50 mg which most psychiatrists would consider ineffective as a treatment of depression[39]. These trials are reasonably consistent in their results: a *small* proportion of patients with fibromyalgia (about 20 per cent) do have important clinical gains on amitriptyline. These results may be due to amitriptyline acting on sleep disturbance and as a muscle relaxant, rather than through a specific antidepressant action. This is borne out by the observation that another tricyclic compound, cyclobenzaprine, which is not an antidepressant may improve symptoms of fibromyalgia[40–42] possibly due to its muscle relaxant and analgesic properties. Furthermore studies of fluoxetine and citalopram in fibromyalgia do not show any benefit for these drugs[43–45], which have well recognized antidepressant action but does not appear to be so effective in the management of neuropathic pain[31]. The reason for this difference in antidepressants is unclear but may relate to the tricyclics' action on central noradrenaline, their blockade of histamine receptors, or their alpha-adrenergic action[31].

What can be recommended on the basis of this evidence? We do not think there is sufficient evidence to use antidepressants widely as a first line treatment of CFS. We suggest that their use is restricted to the following situations: (1) where there is clear-cut evidence of depression accompanying CFS, and (2) as an empirical treatment in patients who have severe problems with myalgia or sleep disturbance. In this setting it is reasonable to use a low dose of a tricyclic antidepressant such as amitriptyline.

17.5 Immune modulators

Rationale for use of immunotherapies

We have discussed the perplexing range of immune changes purported to occur in CFS elsewhere (Chapter 9). Immune therapies have been proposed on the basis that that CFS is a disease of the immune system and should therefore be amenable to treatment with therapies which aim to correct immune dysfunction.

Trials of immunoglobulin IgG

Two early studies gave conflicting results. Peterson *et al.*[46] described an RCT of 30 patients with CFS diagnosed according to CDC criteria, 13 of whom were depressed.

Table 17.1 A summary of randomized control trials of antidepressants in the treatment of fibromyalgia

Trial	Drug	Duration of treatment	No.	Main outcomes	Notes
Norregaard et al.[44]	Citalopram	8 weeks	43	No improvement in any symptoms	
Wolfe et al.[43]	Fluoxetine	6 weeks	42	No improvement in any symptoms	
Caruso et al.[100]	5-Hydroxytryptophan	30 days	50(45)	19/23 treated had a good outcome vs 5/22 of placebo	Some problems with the reporting of statistics
Goldenberg et al.[19]	Amitriptyline 25 mg	6 weeks	62	Amitriptyline group had improved sleep, global ratings of symptoms, physical global ratings, fatigue score, and pain	Factorial design which compared naproxen with placebo simultaneously. Naproxen probably not effective
Carette et al.[101]	Amitriptyline 50 mg	9 weeks	70	Improvement of sleep, patient global ratings, and physical ratings, but most ratings did not reach statistical significance at 9 weeks.	
Scudds et al.[102]	Amitriptyline 10–50 mg	4 weeks	36	27/36 patients reported improvement on amitriptyline vs 8/37 on placebo	Crossover study
Carette et al.[103]	Amitriptyline	4 weeks	22	27% reported improvement on amitriptyline vs none on placebo	Crossover study
Carette et al.[40]	Amitriptyline	6 months	208	At 1 month 36% of amitriptyline improved vs none on placebo. By 6 months 36% and 19% respectively. Non-significant	Also compared cyclobenzaprine which showed similar rate of improvement at one and 5 months

Patients were randomized to receive six infusions of either IgG or albumin 1 per cent (placebo) given over a period of 150 days at 30-day intervals. One patient in each group withdrew due to adverse effects. Apart from a slight advantage for the placebo on social functioning there were no differences over the period of the study.

A similar study from Australia produced rather different results. Lloyd et al.[47] administered infusions of IgG or placebo to CFS patients. Outcome was assessed three months after the end of therapy. Most of the outcomes were based on clinician ratings and they included the Hamilton Depression Rating Scale (HRSD)[48] and visual analogue scales of quality of life: 10/23 of the active versus 3/26 of the placebo group responded according to the physician based interview.

Why were these studies different? In an editorial of the same issue of the *American Journal of Medicine*[49] several reasons were given. First, chance: both studies were relatively small, so a genuine benefit of IgG could have been missed in the American study (type II error: see above). Second, the treatment schedules differed, and only half the dose was given in the American study. Third, the inclusion criteria differed and finally the outcome for the Australian study was three months after the end of treatment, and the differences seem to have been based mainly on clinician based measures. We suspect another problem may account for these findings: the Australian study reported a very high rate of phlebitis among those given IgG, suggesting that the blindness may have been broken. The editorial concluded that whilst it was possible that IgG was associated with some benefit, more research was required before it became more widely available. The treatment was costly, and there were considerable adverse effects. A subsequent trial from the Australian group[50] has failed to replicate their earlier finding, and this group no longer advocate immunoglobulins as a treatment for CFS.

Dialysable leucocyte extract

Another trial by Andrew Lloyd and colleagues[51] assessed the effect of dialysable leucocyte extract on symptoms in patients diagnosed according to Australian criteria. The trial had a factorial design and the other treatment comparison was cognitive behaviour therapy versus clinic attendance (see below for results of this). The rationale used was that dialysable leucocyte extract was effective in the treatment of conditions with defective cell-mediated immunity such as leprosy and the authors claimed similar defects in CFS. Treatment involved eight intramuscular injections over a four-month period. Follow-up was seven months after randomization. The treated group showed no benefits on any of the measures used.

Interferon-α

See and colleagues from the University of California assessed interferon-α in CFS[52]. Patients were given interferon over a period of 12 weeks. At the end of the trial there was no overall difference in outcomes. Four patients were withdrawn from treatment with interferon, two of whom had developed a neutropenia (a potentially fatal reduction in the number of circulating white blood cells). Much was made of a subgroup analysis which showed that for the seven patients with isolated NK cell dysfunction interferon was effective. Unfortunately such subgroup analyses are likely to be unhelpful and lead to type I errors. Given the seriousness of side effects reported, and the cost of interferon, the evidence given in this trial does not support the use of this drug for CFS.

Antihistamines

The reportedly high levels of allergy seen in patients with CFS led to the assessment of the antihistamine, terfenadine[53]. Patients with CFS were randomized to terfenadine or placebo. No difference in any outcome was noted over the study period. A subgroup analysis of those with clinically proven allergy also failed to show any benefit, although the numbers in this group were very small.

Taken as a whole, these results indicate that immune therapies should not be used in the treatment of CFS.

17.6 Corticosteroids

We have seen elsewhere that CFS may be associated with a down-regulated hypothalamic–pituitary–adrenocortical axis. Corticosteroids have been assessed in the treatment of CFS. Hydrocortisone has been compared with placebo in the treatment of CFS (Straus *et al.* 1998). This study showed only a modest and statistically nonsignificant benefit in patient rated 'wellness'. The study used relatively high doses of corticosteroids and this led to significant adrenal suppression, which is potentially much more hazardous than the improvement in clinical symptoms. At the time of writing another study using lower doses of hydrocortisone is under way at King's College Hospital. Preliminary analysis suggests some benefit for active treatment. In fibromyalgia, another study[54] used a crossover design to assess the efficacy of the steroid prednisolone. There was no evidence of improvement on prednisolone, and in fact it seemed to make patients somewhat worse. These results suggest that corticosteroids are likely to do more harm than good in the doses they have been used in.

17.7 Antiviral agents

We have seen elsewhere in this book that viral illness has been suggested as one of the main causes of CFS. The use of antiviral agents is based on the view that the symptoms of CFS are caused by *active* viral infection. Two RCTs have assessed antiviral treatments.

Strayer *et al.*[55] assessed the effect of a new anti-RNA virus drug (poly(1) poly(C_{12}U)) against placebo in 92 patients. Treatment was over a 24 week period, and outcome was measured on Karnofsky[37] performance score. There was a significant benefit for those given the active drug, but no difference in side effects, leading the investigators to suggest this effect was not due to inadvertent unblinding of subjects.

The antiviral agent acyclovir was compared with placebo in a crossover design by Straus *et al.*[56]. Each patient received a spell on acyclovir and another spell on placebo with a six-week washout period in between. Outcome was based on self-assessment by the patient of their overall health. There were no differences in treatments in terms of symptoms. Of considerable concern was the fact that three developed reversible renal failure on acyclovir. A subgroup analysis on those patients who had positive Epstein–Barr virus serology showed no benefit in this particular group. The conclusion was that acyclovir was not beneficial in the treatment of CFS.

As with so many other treatments in CFS, there appears to be no consistent pattern of response to these antiviral infections. There are several possible reasons for this. Antiviral agents are specific treatments for specific viral infections. Unless they possess some unconnected and essentially non-specific antifatigue action (note that the first antidepressants were recognized serendipitously) their action must depend on their effect on a specific pathogen. Patients who are not infected with that pathogen would not be expected to respond to the corresponding antiviral agent. Another problem with using antiviral agents relates to the pathophysiology of fatigue when caused by previous infection. Whilst the literature reviewed in this book suggests that some severe viral infections may be associated with subsequent chronic fatigue and CFS, there is less evidence that this is due to viral persistence. Antiviral agents are not indicated in the treatment of CFS.

17.8 Dietary supplements

Several RCTs have assessed the role of the constituents of a normal diet in the treatment of CFS. The rationale for such treatments is not compelling. Although there is one uncontrolled study showing that a proportion of patients with CFS appear to have low serum folate concentrations[57] and other studies have looked at red blood cell magnesium (see below), a small case–control study found no difference between CFS sufferers and normal controls in either intake or blood levels for a range of vitamins and minerals[58]. Dietary deficiencies usually only occur in conditions of excessive loss (as in iron deficiency anaemia associated with bleeding from an occult carcinoma, or menorrhagia) or inadequate intake (either due to dietary deficiency, which is rare in industrialized countries, or malabsorption). Cox *et al.*[59] reported an RCT of magnesium for CFS. The rationale was based on the findings of a case–control study reported in the same paper which demonstrated low magnesium levels in the red blood cells. The RCT involved 32 patients diagnosed according to Australian criteria, who were given six intramuscular injections of magnesium or placebo over at weekly intervals for six weeks. Patients were assessed for six weeks, and 12/15 of the active group improved as opposed to 3/17 of those on placebo – a statistically and clinically significant difference.

This remarkable result had not been replicated[60,61]. Nor has the finding that most patients in the trial had low baseline levels of magnesium[58,61–64]. It has also been pointed out that the amount of magnesium used in this trial is less than one-tenth of the weekly recommended allowance[65]. This implies that there would have to be a gross deficiency in CFS for there to be a response to such modest doses. The biological basis of this treatment is therefore in doubt and confirmation of the results of this trial are necessary before the treatment can be recommended.

Behan *et al.*[66] reported a trial of high dose essential fatty acids (evening primrose oil) in patients with a clinical diagnosis of post-viral fatigue syndrome. Randomization was based on the toss of a coin. Outcome was based on a five-symptom questionnaire and was assessed at one and three months. A global assessment of outcome was based on clinician rating. At one month 74 per cent of the active group were reported to be improved as opposed to 23 per cent of those receiving placebo. At three months this difference had grown to 85 per cent versus 17 per cent. These dramatic results were not replicated in another trial[67].

Essential fatty acids (evening primrose oil) have been widely used in many different conditions ranging from cancer to premenstrual syndrome. The results of many of the trials of the treatment remain controversial[68], and further studies are required before this can be recommended as a widespread treatment for CFS. Professor Behan's group now regard the treatment as of little value[104]

A general practice based study in Scotland[69] used a vitamin, mineral, and amino acid supplementation to treat patients with chronic fatigue and past evidence of coxsackie B virus infection. The trial used a crossover design. Patients were crossed over at three months. The study showed no significant advantage for the active preparation, although there was a trend towards improvement in those receiving it. Unfortunately only 19 patients completed the study, and the results are based on this sample of completers. The treatment consisted of a combination of 33 minerals, vitamins, and amino acids so the biological mechanism, if any, remains obscure. The use of a crossover design in this study is inappropriate, because if the active treatment was correcting a dietary deficiency one would anticipate a very powerful continuation of the effect when the patients were receiving placebo.

In the 1980s one popular treatment in parts of the USA was a bovine liver extract which contained high concentrations of folic acid and cyanocobalamin, a treatment which emphasizes the historical continuity between the treatment of neurasthenia and that of CFS (see Chapter 5). This was assessed in a randomized crossover trial of 15 patients by Kaslow *et al.*[70]. The treatment consisted of self-administered daily injections of placebo or active substance. The 'active' preparation appeared to have no advantage over placebo, but overall scores in both groups improved indicating a strong placebo effect. Again the use of crossover design is questionable.

These dietary supplements are probably unlikely to do any major harm, although some are expensive. In the absence of a clear dietary deficiency or malabsorption we remain sceptical about their biological plausibility and suggest that larger trials are necessary before recommending such treatments.

17.9 RCTs of exercise in CFS

We suspect the most widely followed treatment for CFS is rest. The model espoused by much of the self-help literature views the body as a machine with a flat battery or empty petrol tank which is refuelled by rest. This metaphor is flawed: we saw in Chapter 3 how fatigue in many physical illnesses may be improved by exercise. This section reviews the literature on exercise as a treatment for CFS fatigue. We start, however, with a discussion of some of the literature on exercise in fibromyalgia.

Burckhardt *et al.*[71] studied the effect of education and exercise in patients with fibromyalgia. Patients were randomized to receive either education, education and exercise, or no treatment. The exercise consisted of one hour weekly. No differences were detected between the active groups, but they both did better than the no-treatment group. Another essentially negative trial compared aerobic dance twice weekly over 20 weeks in women with fibromyalgia[72]. Exercise was not associated with any improvement in pain, but did lead to improved muscular strength.

We are aware of two other trials of exercise in fibromyalgia which found more positive evidence of benefit. McCain *et al.*[73] compared a supervised cardiovascular fitness training programme with flexibility exercises. Those receiving aerobic training had improved cardiovascular fitness, a higher pain threshold and a non-significant trend to improvement in pain ratings. There was also a trend towards more people in exercise group getting better by patient and physician ratings. Another study[74] compared exercise with relaxation. Exercise was associated with improvements in the number of tender points, total myalgia scores, and aerobic fitness, although the effect size was not reported.

The evidence for exercise in fibromyalgia is therefore mixed. Perhaps the clearest point that can be made is that exercise does not seem to cause *harm* in these trials. What about exercise in CFS?

A study by Kathy Fulcher and Peter White at St Bartholomew's Hospital used a graded exercise programme in 66 non-depressed patients diagnosed according to the Oxford criteria[75]. Patients were randomized to participate either in aerobic exercises or flexibility training. Aerobic exercise was postulated to be the active ingredient in this trial, with flexibility training forming a control group. Subjects were seen once weekly over the 12-week programme and told to exercise at least five days per week, building up their level of activity by one to two minute increments each week until they were exercising for 30 minutes per day, at which point exercise intensity was increased up to a maximum of 60 per cent VO_{2max}. Flexibility training consisted of stretching and relaxation exercises which the subjects were encouraged to do at home as well. The main outcome was the self-rated clinical global impression scale.

The results of this trial were impressive. Of those who completed aerobic training, 55 per cent reported feeling much better or very much better as opposed to 27 per cent of the comparison group. One patient in each group felt worse at the end of treatment. As a group, those on the aerobic treatment had significantly better outcome in terms of physical fatigue, global ratings of health on the SF-36, and better physical functioning on the SF-36. Anxiety and depression measures did not much differ between groups and were not markedly improved (although subjects were by definition non-depressed at baseline). The investigators allowed those given flexibility training to cross over to aerobic training following the end of the trial, and they were also able to show significant improvements in this group. It is worth noting that self-rated improvement was not correlated with improvements in VO_{2max} reinforcing the point made elsewhere in this book, that subjective fatigue is not synonymous with exercise capacity.

A key finding in the Fulcher and White study is that objective measures of physical fitness were *not* associated with outcome (i.e. clinical improvement was not related to improving physical fitness). Instead we suspect that the benefits were linked to confidence, predictability, and overcoming avoidance, lending support to our view that disability is more related to behavioural avoidance and confidence than simple physical fitness.

Similar results have been reported by a group in Manchester[35]. In the factorial design described above (see Section 17.4) CFS patients were randomized to receive fluoxetine or placebo *and* exercise or no exercise. The exercise group were instructed to do graded exercise for 20 minutes three times a week up to 75 per cent of VO_{2max}. No instructions were given regarding what to do if symptoms worsened. There was no 'placebo' to exercise as in the Fulcher and White study. There were more drop-outs among those prescribed exercise, and the compliance with the full six-month programme was incomplete in all but one-third. None the less, exercise produced a significant improvement in fatigue, functional work capacity, and health perception, and despite the differential drop-out rates, this result held when an intention to treat analysis was performed.

These two studies demonstrate that a relatively simple strategy of exercise may lead to a significant and lasting improvement in some patients with CFS. The results of these studies beg two questions: first, is it a placebo effect? We have seen elsewhere that patients' drug treatments are often accompanied by a placebo effect and here it is difficult to blind patients regarding the treatment condition. The Fulcher and White study overcame this by using two active treatments, thus there would have been therapeutic optimism in both treatment groups. Another argument against a placebo effect is that the placebo effect tends to rely on the anticipation of improvement. We have seen previously that many patients with CFS actively avoid exercise due to a belief that it will cause a deterioration in their condition, making these results more striking.

The second key question is how acceptable this treatment is. The two studies did report that only a relatively small proportion of eligible patients were not prepared to take part. In our experience many patients with CFS, especially those with a long history, avoid exercise because in their experience it is inextricably linked with relapse. These beliefs are frequently reinforced by the lay literature where the advice is often to rest at all costs. This implies that a large proportion of patients with CFS require more than simply the experience of gradual exercise programmes to persuade them that exercise may be beneficial.

17.10 Cognitive behaviour therapy

Elsewhere in this book we have emphasized the importance of beliefs and attributions in CFS (Chapter 12). In our clinical experience patients hold a wide variety of beliefs such as viral persistence, immune dysfunction, candida infestations, and many others (see Chapter 15). However, as we have seen elsewhere in this book the scientific evidence for these beliefs is weak. Furthermore, such beliefs are not merely benign if inaccurate ideas, but have profound consequences for patients who hold them. A belief in viral persistence, some unknown agent sitting in nerves or muscles and always ready to flare up, leads to rest and avoidance. These beliefs have been shown to be indicators of a poor prognosis in CFS in every study in which they have been examined[76,77] (see Chapter 12).

Cognitive behavioural therapy (CBT) rests on the assumption that beliefs people hold about themselves and their future are powerful predictors of mood and behaviour. The approach was first used in the treatment of depression, but now has demonstrated efficacy in treating a wide variety of neurotic disorders including anxiety states and post-traumatic stress disorder, as well as medically unexplained physical symptoms and in a range of physical illnesses[78]. Chapter 11 describes the cognitive behavioural formulation of CFS. This chapter describes the RCTs.

An open study showed early promise for CBT[79]. Patients who were able to tolerate the treatment did considerably better than those who dropped out, and the cohort of treated patients showed significant improvements in a number of outcomes including measures of functioning and symptoms. These results were contradicted in another open study[80] which compared outcome in two groups of CFS patients those offered CBT and those not offered it. It suggested that CBT was only effective in treating the depressive symptoms of CBT, but not fatigue itself. However, the model used in the latter study was of allowing the patients to accept the disability caused by the illness (i.e. allowing them to cope with the symptoms), rather than attempting to use behavioural activation or cognitive reattribution.

Another 'negative' result came from the Australian group headed by Andrew Lloyd which reported the first RCT of a psychological treatment for CFS[51]. The study design has been described in the section on immunotherapies, but briefly consisted of a factorial design of CBT versus no treatment and immunotherapy versus placebo. Ninety patients with Australian criteria CFS were randomized and followed up seven months after randomization. The psychological treatment consisted of six sessions of CBT given biweekly, each session lasting 30–60 minutes. The therapy consisted of encouragement for the patient to exercise at home and an attempt to shift beliefs that the patient was helpless. The results of this trial were disappointing. Neither treatment group showed any additional benefit over standard medical management on the visual analogue scale report of symptoms or thre Karnofsky scale[37] measures at seven months.

Sharpe et al.[81] reported a study of CBT in 60 patients with CFS seen in secondary care. Patients met Oxford criteria for CFS. CBT was given in weekly sessions over a 16-week period. The comparison was normal care by the patient's general practitioner. CBT consisted of an assessment of the patient and an individualized cognitive formulation of their symptoms, accompanied by explanation and education. The therapy involved behavioural experiments, collaborative re-evaluation of thoughts and beliefs inhibiting return to normal functioning- and problem solving activities. Patients were assessed at five months, eight months, and one year following randomization. The main outcome was improvement on the Karnofsky scale[37]. Although the CBT group showed an advantage in terms of the Karnofsky score, these were not significant until 12 months, when 73 per cent of those treated had improved satisfactorily compared with 27 per cent on standard care. Other measures such as distance walked, days in bed per week, subjective assessment of effect of illness, fatigue severity showed a significant advantage for CBT at five and eight months.

Deale et al.[82] at King's College Hospital in London have replicated Sharpe's results. They randomized 60 patients with CFS to received either CBT or relaxation. CBT was given over 13 sessions at weekly to fortnightly intervals. The model of CBT was similar to that used in Sharpe's study, although the emphasis was more behavioural, involving earlier activity scheduling. The first three sessions aimed at engaging the patient, and explaining the treatment rationale. At the fourth session a schedule of activities was prescribed. The activity scheduling continued, and cognitive strategies were gradually introduced, to address fears about symptoms, perfectionism, and performance expectations. Relaxation involved progressive muscle relaxation and visualization. The main outcome was physical functioning on the MOS short form[83]; other measures of symptoms and activities were rated at six months follow-up. The study reported a good outcome in 63 per cent of those treated with CBT as opposed to 17 per cent with relaxation, a highly statistically significant result. CBT showed a particular benefit for measures of fatigue and disability, whereas it did not have a significant effect on depression.

Do these conflicting results suggest that CBT is only effective in the Northern Hemisphere? The intensity of the treatment offered in Australia was considerably less than in the British studies, whilst the intensity of the comparison treatment, standard care, was far greater. All patients improved, but the improvement was similar in both groups. It may be that the support offered for the CBT comparison group was good enough to bring about some change in itself. Furthermore, in the Australian study it is unclear precisely what behavioural interventions occurred, and there was no attempt to alter fundamental illness beliefs. The treatment rationale may have been compromised by the presence of an immunological trial involving regular injections of active or placebo immunotherapy. The rationale that was used for CBT in Oxford and London is based on the model that although immune and/or infective factors are responsible for illness onset, other factors are responsible for symptom perpetuation. It would be hard to reconcile the two approaches being tested. The strong correlation between the patients' belief (albeit erroneous) at the end of the trial that they had received active immunotherapy and symptomatic improvement, suggests that the patient group found it similarly hard. The authors themselves wonder if the number of sessions was adequate. Hence the differences between the Australian and British studies may relate to the different models of illness used – those that involved some form of gradual return to activity combined with some form of cognitive reatribution were successful, whilst those that did not offer adequate alternative explanations for symptom maintenance, or address illness and symptom beliefs were less successful.

Cognitive behaviour therapy requires skilled personnel, who are only likely to be available in a few specialist centres. A study by Chalder *et al.* from King's College Hospital[84] looked at using certain elements of the therapy in a self-help package in primary care. The study used sampling from a large epidemiological study to identify GP attenders who on follow-up had significant fatigue lasting at least six months (chronic fatigue). Patients were randomized to receive a self-help book or no treatment. Those randomized to self-help were seen briefly by a nurse and the basic details of the book were described. The book described information about the nature of fatigue, and a series of self-help strategies based on cognitive and behavioural techniques. Outcome was based on scores from a fatigue questionnaire[85] and measures of functional capacity. The intervention group were less fatigued than controls and at three months 37 per cent of the experimental versus 61 per cent of the comparison group met criteria for fatigue, a result which met statistical significance.

It is important to note that the patients selected into this study were not necessarily CFS cases, and some would have been excluded from other studies on the basis of psychiatric or medical disorder. On the other hand it does suggest that relatively simple psychosocial treatments in primary care could be effective in managing fatigue.

Summarizing the results of the last two sections we suspect that the trials of exercise and CBT have much in common. CBT involves many behavioural interventions which would include activity scheduling, and challenging patients' avoidance of exercise. One commonly used device in CBT is the behavioural experiment where the patient is asked to increase exercise slightly and witness its effects, thereby challenging beliefs about relapse. Exercise treatment must to some extent address the fears of patients otherwise they will not participate, and therefore involves a similar process of testing the fears.

These therapies have been widely used in other illnesses: so for example CBT has shown to be helpful in fibromyalgia[86] and for patients presenting with a range of medically unexplained symptoms[87]. CBT and exercise have also been shown to be useful in physical illnesses. We have stressed the importance of psychosocial factors in perpetuating the symptoms of CFS, but this does not mean that the use of exercise and CBT imply a solely psychogenic model for CFS. Similar techniques have been used in managing fatigue, improving quality of life, and assisting in the rehabilitation of patients with heart disease[88, 89], cancer[90, 91], and neuromuscular disorders[92] – an important message for patients when attempting to engage them into a treatment programme.

17.11 Alternative medicine

Alternative medicine describes treatments which are usually not available through orthodox medical settings. The terms covers a broad ranges of treatments, some of which have considerably more credibility with the medical establishment than others. Whilst treatments like acupuncture and hypnotherapy could conceivably involve mechanisms which have a sound physiological basis, for example through relaxation or higher perception of pain, it is hard to imagine any mechanism for homeopathy, faith healing, or aromatherapy other than placebo effects. Alternative medicines have been widely advocated in CFS, but we are aware of only one randomized controlled trial. In fibromyalgia a wider range of treatments have been assessed.

Deluze et al.[93] reported a trial of electroacupuncture in fibromyalgia. Patients were randomized to receive either electroacupuncture, which involves pulsing low-voltage electrical currents at various sites, or a sham procedure, which used electric currents, but at the wrong sites. The active treatment group reported improvements in seven out of eight outcomes (which included measures of pain, analgesia use, sleep, and global ratings), whereas the placebo group showed no improvement.

Hypnotherapy has been assessed in fibromyalgia[94]. The therapy consisted of relaxation exercises, and patients were taught strategies to control muscle pain and sleep. A comparison group received massage and muscle relaxation from a physiotherapist. The assessor was blinded to treatment allocation. Those receiving hypnotherapy reported significantly greater improvement in sleep, pain, and fatigue than the comparison group, although the physician's global assessment of outcome was no different between the two groups.

Homeopathy has been assessed in fibromyalgia[95] and CFS[96]. In the study of fibromyalgia there was some evidence that the homeopathy group had fewer tender points, and better sleep and pain scores at follow-up, although the analysis of the results was somewhat unclear. The study in CFS compared homeopathic remedies prescribed on an individual basis with placebo remedies. Patients with undefined 'ME' were randomized, and followed over one year with diaries. The outcomes were based on patient assessed recovery. About one-third of those treated with homeopathic remedies were rated as 'recovered' or 'greatly improved' as opposed to 3 per cent of the placebo group. No statistical tests of significance were performed, but our own analysis suggests that these results would be statistically significant. The authors of the study conceded that many of the patients on homeopathic remedies did not improve and they were suitably circumspect in their interpretation of their results. The lack of placebo response is surprising.

Clearly the alternative therapies are a heterogeneous group, and whilst we maintain a healthy scepticism for those (like homeopathy) whose mechanisms contradict our knowledge of the natural sciences, the results of the trials of electroacupuncture and hypnotherapy seem encouraging. Indeed it some of the methods used in hypnotherapy do not differ very much from those we advocate in cognitive behaviour therapy, and may well act by improving self-efficacy, and using problem solving techniques. Sadly though, the message is yet again 'more research needed'.

17.12 Conclusion

What conclusions may be drawn from this review of the treatments for CFS and other fatigue states? Three of Bradford Hill's factors[97] which suggest causation are relevant to this debate. First, the consistency of the evidence. To widely accept a treatment one requires reasonably consistent evidence which, given the dangers of publication bias and all the other factors which may lead to undue optimism in the evaluation of new treatments[98], means that basing treatment on single small trials is not acceptable. Conversely, a weak treatment effect may not be detected in small studies so a single negative finding does not necessarily imply the treatment is useless. Second, he pointed to biological plausibility. Treatments where no clear biological mechanism can be proposed will tend to have less credibility in medicine than those which have a sound mechanism. This is not to suggest that biological plausibility is *essential* (some of the earliest achievements of modern medicine involved giving poorly understood treatments, as in Lind's intervention for scurvy[99]), but treatments which are plausible have a distinct advantage. Third, the strength of an association. We have seen that some treatments appear to have a strong benefit, and these are more likely to be useful.

Using these criteria we see that most of the drug treatments tend to satisfy at best one of these criteria. Antidepressants in CFS are plausible but do not look especially promising. There is some consistency for a weak effect in improving the pain and sleep disorder associated with fibromyalgia. Magnesium supplementation and gamma linoleic acid and some of the alternative remedies appear to give reasonably strong effects, but we are not impressed by the biological basis of these, and they are based on single small studies. The two studies of exercise in CFS both show a strong improvement and we would argue have a biological basis, similarly the studies of cognitive behaviour therapy, whilst not showing unanimity, do show a more favourable pattern.

Our recommendations are, then:

- One widely recommended treatment, rest, is likely to be actively harmful.
- Many of the treatments reviewed here had serious side effects.
- There is some evidence for dietary supplementation including magnesium and essential fatty acids, but these are without any sound biological basis, and the evidence is based on single trials. We do not believe these therapies are indicated at present.
- Alternative remedies are often popular with patients. We have reservations regarding their usefulness. We believe some therapies reinforce maladaptive beliefs and behaviours and are therefore harmful. On the other hand treatments which are cheap, free from side effects, and do not promote maladaptive illness beliefs may help.
- There is good evidence that a majority of patients with CFS benefit from a programme of graded exposure to exercise and/or cognitive behavioural therapy.
- Antidepressants are not clearly indicated in CFS. They should be reserved for the following situations: patients with a clear history of depression, where therapeutic doses of tricyclic or selective serotonin re-uptake inhibitors (SSRIs) should be given; and as a symptomatic treatment of pain and sleep disturbance. Small doses of tricyclics are probably worth trying.

CBT with exercise appears to be the most promising treatment of CFS. We would argue that aside from the issue of efficacy these treatments have other advantages. Firstly, they do not presuppose any (as yet) unproven causality, but do consider perpetuating factors. This may avoid the need to be drawn into an unhelpful discussion about the initial cause of symptoms. It is often very helpful to mention to the patient that similar approaches are widely used in other groups of patients with illnesses with clear organic aetiology, for example in cardiac rehabilitation. Secondly, these treatments favour a model of the illness which includes psychological and physical factors, and consequently represent the holistic approach which so many sufferers yearn for, and which many commentators have complained is missing in the reductionist world of late twentieth-century medicine[5].

The next chapter will describe practical details of the treatment of patients with CFS.

References

1 Goldstein JA. *Chronic Fatigue Syndromes: the Limbic Hypothesis.* New York, Haworth Medical Press, 1993.
2 Williams X. *Fatigue: the Secrets of Getting your Energy Back.* London, Cedar, 1996.
3 Macintyre A. *M.E.: Postviral Fatigue Syndrome how to live with it.* London, Unwin, 1989.
4 Franklin M, Sullivan J. *M.E. What is it? Have I got it? How to get Better.* London, Century, 1989.
5 Steincamp J. *Overload: Beating ME, the Chronic Fatigue Syndrome.* London, Fontana, 1989.

6 Dawes B, Downing D. *Why ME?* London, Grafton, 1989.

7 Feiden K. *Hope and Help for the Chronic Fatigue Syndrome: the Offical Guide of the CFS/ CFIDS Network*. New York, Prentice Hall, 1990.

8 Hotopf MH, Lewis G, Normand C. *The Treatment of Depression: Evaluation and Cost-effectiveness*. London, London School of Hygiene and Tropical Medicine, 1996.

9 Sharpe M, Gill D, Strain J, Mayou R. Psychosomatic medicine and evidence-based treatment. *J. Psychosom. Res.* 1996; **41**: 101–107.

10 Hotopf MH, Lewis G, Normand C. The evaluation of antidepressants: a critique of current literature. *Psychol. Med.* (in press)

11 Pocock SJ, Hughes MD, Lee RJ. Statistical problems in the reporting of clinical trials. A survey of three medical journals. *New Engl. J. Med.* 1987; **317**: 426–432.

12 Vercoulen J, Swanink C, Zitman F. Fluoxetine in chronic fatigue syndrome: a randomized, double-blind, placebo-controlled trial. *Lancet* 1996; **347**: 858–861.

13 Lauritsen K, Havelund T, Laursen LS, Rask-Madsen J. Withholding unfavourable results in drug company sponsored clinical trials. *Lancet* 1987; **i**: 1091

14 Spector TD, Thompson SG. The potential and limitations of meta-analysis. *J. Epidemiol. Commun. Health* 1991; **45**: 89–92.

15 Egger M, Davey Smith G. Misleading meta-analysis. *Br. Med. J.* 1995; **310**: 752–754.

16 The Coronary Drug Research Project. Influences of adherence to treatment and response to cholesterol on mortality in the coronary drug project. *New Engl. J. Med.* 1980; **303**: 1038–1041.

17 Yunus MB, Masi AT, Aldag JC. Short term effects of ibuprofen in primary fibromyalgia syndrome: a double blind, placebo controlled trial. *J. Rheumatol.* 1989; **16**: 527–532.

18 Kravitz HM, Katz RS, Helmke N, Jeffriess H, Bukovky J, Fawcett J. Alprazolam and ibuprofen in the treatment of fibromyalgia – report of a double blind placebo-controlled study. *J. Musculoskeletal Pain* 1994; **2**: 3–27.

19 Goldenberg DL, Feelson DT, Dinerman H. A randomized, controlled trial of amitriptyline and naproxen in the treatment of patients with fibromyalgia. *Arthritis Rheumatism* 1986; **29**: 1371–1377.

20 Russell IJ, Fletcher EM, Michalek JE, McBroom PC, Hester GG. Treatment of primary fibrositis/fibromyalgia syndrome with ibuprofen and alprazolam: a double-blind, placebo-controlled study. *Arthritis Rheumatism* 1991; **34**: 552–560.

21 Vaeroy H, Abrahamsen A, Forre O, Kass E. Treatment of fibromyalgia (fibrositis syndrome): a parallel double blind trial with carisoprodol, paracetamol and caffeine (Somadril comp) verus placebo. *Clin. Rheumatol.* 1989; **8**: 245–250.

22 Hotopf MH, Wessely S. Treatment of depression in physical illness. In Checkley SA (ed.) *The Management of Depression*. Oxford University Press, 1997.

23 Veith RC, Raskind MA, Caldwell JH, Barnes RF, Gumbretch G, Ritchie JL. Cardiovascular effects of tricyclic antidepressants in depressed patients with chronic heart disease. *New Engl. J. Med.* 1982; **306**: 954–959.

24 Costa D, Mogos I, Toma T. Efficacy and safety of mianserin in the treatment of depression of women with cancer. *Acta Psychiatrica Scand.* 1985; **72(suppl 320)**: 85–92.

25 Borson S, McDonald GJ, Gayle T, Deffebach M, Lakshiminarayan S, Van Tuinen C. Improvement in mood, physical symptoms, and function with nortriptyline in patients with chronic obstructive airways disease. *Psychosomatics* 1992; **33**: 190–201.

26 Schiffer RB, Wineman NM. Antidepressant pharmacotherapy of depression associated with multiple sclerosis. *Am. J. Psychiatry* 1990; **147**: 1493–1497.

27 Anderson J, Aabro E, Gulmann N, Hjelmsted A, Pederson HE. Anti-depressive treatment in Parkinson's disease. *Acta Psychiat. Scand.* 1980; **62**: 210–219.

28 Reding MJ, Orto LA, Winter SW, Fortuna IM, Di Ponte P, McDowell FH. Antidepressant therapy after stroke. *Arch. Neurol.* 1986; **43:** 763–765.

29 Lipsey JR, Robinson RG, Pearlson GD, Rao K, Price TR. Nortriptyline treatment of post-stroke depression: a double blind study. *Lancet* 1984; **1:** 297–300.

30 Rabkin JG, Rabkin R, Harrison W, Wagner G. Effect of imipramine on mood and enumerative measures of immune status in depressed patients with HIV disease. *Am. J. Psychiatry* 1994; **151:** 516–523.

31 Max MB, Lynch SA, Muir J, Shoaf SE, Smoller B, Dubner R. Effects of desipramine, amitriptyline, and fluoxetine on pain in diabetic neuropathy. *New Engl. J. Med.* 1992; **326:** 1250–1256.

32 Sharpley AF, Cowen PJ. Effect of pharmacologic treatments on the sleep of depressed patients. *Biol. Psychiatry* 1995; **37:** 85–98.

33 Beck AT, Ward CH, Mendelson M. An inventory for measuring depression. *Arch. Gen. Psychiatry* 1961; **4:** 561–571.

34 Bergner M, Bobbitt RA, Cartner WB, Gilson BS. The sickness impact profile: development and final revision of a health status measure. *Med. Care* 1981; **19:** 787–805.

35 Wearden A, Morriss R, Mullis R, *et al.* A double-blind, placebo controlled treatment trial of fluoxetine and a graded exercise programme for chronic fatigue syndrome. *Br. J. Psychiat.* 1998; **172:** 485–490.

36 Natelson BH, Cheu J, Pareja J, Ellis SP, Poliscastro T, Findley TW. Randomised, double blind, controlled placebo-phase in trial of low dose phenelzine in the chronic fatigue syndrome. *Psychopharmacology* 1996; **124:** 226–230.

37 Karnofsky DA, Burchenal JH. The clinical evaluation of chemotherapeutic agents in cancer. In MacLeod CM (ed.) *Evaluation of Chermotherapeutic Agents: Symposium. Microbiology Section, New York Academy of Medicine.* New York, Columbia University Press, 1949; 191–206.

38 Behan PO, Hannifah H. 5-HT reuptake inhibitors in CFS. *J. Immunol. Immunopharmacol.* 1995; **15:** 66–69.

39 Paykel ES, Priest RG. Recognition and management of depression in general practice: consensus statement. *Br. Med. J.* 1992; **305:** 1198–1202.

40 Carette S, Bell MJ, Reynolds WJ, *et al.* Comparison of amitriptyline, cyclobenzaprine, and placebo in the treatment of fibromyalgia. *Arthritis Rheumatism* 1994; **37:** 32–40.

41 Bennett RM, Gatter RA, Campbell SM, Andrews RP, Clark SR, Scarola JA. A comparison of cyclobenzaprine and placebo in the management of fibrositis. *Arthritis Rheumatism* 1988; **31:** 1535–1542.

42 Quimby LG, Gratwick GM, Whitney CD, Block SR. A randomized trial of cyclobenzaprine for the treatment of fibromyalgia. *J. Rheumatol.* 1989; **16(suppl 19):** 140–143.

43 Wolfe F, Cathey MA, Hawley DJ. A double-blind placebo controlled trial of fluoxetine in fibromyalgia. *Scan. J. Rheumatol.* 1994; **23:** 255–259.

44 Norregaard J, Volkmann H, Danneskiold-Samsoe B. A randomized controlled trial of citalopram in the treatment of fibromyalgia. *Pain* 1995; **61:** 445–449.

45 Cortet B, Houvenagel E, Forzy G, Vincent G, Delcambre B. Evaluation of the effectiveness of serotonin (fluoxetine hydrochloride) treatment. Open study in fibromylagia. *Rev. Rheum. Mal. Osteoarthritis* 1992; **59:** 497–500.

46 Peterson PK, Shepard J, Macres M, *et al.* A controlled trial of intravenous immunoglobulin G in chronic fatigue syndrome. *Am. J. Med.* 1990; **89:** 554–560.

47 Lloyd A, Hickie I, Wakefield D, Boughton C, Dwyer J. A double-blind, placebo-controlled trial of intravenous immunoglobulin therapy in patients with chronic fatigue syndrome. *Am. J. Med.* 1990; **89:** 561–568.

48 Hamilton M. A rating scale for depression. *J. Neurol. Neurosurg. Psychiatry* 1960; **23:** 56–62.

49 Straus SE. Intravenous immunoglobulin treatment for the chronic fatigue syndrome. *Am. J. Med.* 1990; **89:** 551–553.

50 Vollmer-Conna V, Hickie I, Hadzl-Pavlovic D, Tymms K, Wakefield D, Dwyer J, Lloyd A. Intravenous immunoglobulin is ineffective in the treatment of chronic fatigue syndrome. *Am. J. Med.* 1997; **103:** 38–43.

51 Lloyd A, Hickie I, Boughton R, *et al.* Immunologic and psychological therapy for patients with chronic fatigue syndrome. *Am. J. Med.* 1993; **94:** 197–203.

52 See DM, Tilles JG. Alpha interferon treatment of patients with chronic fatigue syndrome. *Immunol. Invest.* 1996; **25:** 153–164.

53 Steinberg P, McNutt BE, Marshall P, *et al.* Double-blind placebo-controlled study of efficacy of oral terfenadine in the treatment of chronic fatigue syndrome. *J. Allergy Clin. Immunol.* 1996; **97:** 119–126.

54 Clark S, Tindall E, Bennett RM. A double blind crossover trial of prednisone versus placebo in the treatment of fibrositis. *J. Rheumatol.* 1985; **12:** 980–983.

55 Strayer DR, Carter WA, Brodsky I, *et al.* A controlled clinical trial with a specifically configured RNA drug, poly(1).poly(C12U), in chronic fatigue syndrome. *Clin. Infect. Dis.* 1994; **18(suppl 1):** S88–S95.

56 Straus SE, Dale JK, Tobi M, *et al.* Acyclovir treatment of the chronic fatigue syndrome. *New Engl. J. Med.* 1988; **319:** 1692–1698.

57 Jacobson W, Saich T, Borysiewicz LK, Behan WMH, Behan PO, Wreghitt TG. Serum folate and chronic fatigue syndrome. *Neurology* 1993; **43:** 2645–2647.

58 Grant JE, Veldee MS, Buchwald D. Analysis of dietary intake and selected nutrient concentrations in patients with chronic fatigue syndrome. *J. Am. Dietetic Assoc.* 1996; **96:** 383–386.

59 Cox IM, Campbell MJ, Dowson D. Red blood cell magnesium and chronic fatigue syndrome. *Lancet* 1991; **337:** 757–760.

60 Clague JE, Edwards RHT, Jackson MJ. Intravenous magnesium loading in chronic fatigue syndrome. *Lancet* 1992: **340:** 124–5.

61 Hinds G, Bell NP, McMaster D, McCluskey DR. Normal red cell magnesium concentrations and magnesium loading tests in patients with chronic fatigue syndrome. *Ann. Clin. Biochem.* 1994; **31:** 459–461.

62 Swanink CM, Vercoulen JH, Bleijenberg G, Fennis JF, Galama JM, van der Meer JW. Chronic fatigue syndrome: a clinical and laboratory study with a well matched control group. *J. Intern. Med.* 1995; **237:** 499–506.

63 Gantz NM. Magnesium and chronic fatigue. *Lancet* 1991; **338:** 66.

64 Deulofeu R, Gascon J, Gimenez N, Corachon M. Magnesium and chronic fatigue syndrome. *Lancet* 1991; **338:** 641.

65 Young IS, Trimble ER. Magnesium and chronic fatigue syndrome. *Lancet* 1991; **337:** 1094–1095.

66 Behan PO, Behan WMH, Horrobin D. Effect of high doses of essential fatty acids on the postviral fatigue syndrome. *Acta Neurol. Scand.* 1990; **82:** 209–216.

67 McCluskey DR. Pharmacological approaches to the therapy of chronic fatigue syndrome. In: Bock GR, Whelan J. (ed.) *Chronic Fatigue Syndrome. Ciba Foundation No. 177.* Chichester, Wiley, 1993: 280–287.

68 Kleijnen J. Evening primrose oil. *Br. Med. J.* 1994; **309:** 824–825.

69 Martin RWY, Ogston SA, Evans JR. Effects of vitamin and mineral supplementation on symptoms associated with chronic fatigue syndrome with coxsackie B antibodies. *J. Nutrit. Med.* 1994; **4:** 11–23.

70 Kaslow JE, Rucker L, Onishi R. Liver extract–folic acid–cyanocobalamin vs placebo for chronic fatigue syndrome. *Arch. Intern. Med.* 1989; **149:** 2501–2503.

71 Burckhardt CS, Mannerkorpi K, Hedenberg L, Bjelle A. A randomized, controlled clinical trial of education and physical training for women with fibromyalgia. *J. Rheumatol.* 1994; **21:** 714–720.

72 Mengshoel AM, Komnaes HB, Bobre O. The effects of 20 weeks of physical fitness training in female patients with fibromyalgia. *Clin. Exp. Rheumatol.* 1992; **10:** 345–349.

73 McCain GA, Bell DA, Mai FM, Halliday PD. A controlled trial of the effects of a supervised cardiovascular fitness training program on the manifestations of primary fibromyalgia. *Arthritis Rheumatism* 1988; **31:** 1135–1141.

74 Martin L, Edworthy SM, MacIntosh B, Nutting A, Butterwick D, Cook J. Is exercise helpful in the treatment of fibromyalgia? *Arthritis Rheumatism* 1993; **36:** S251

75 Fulcher KY, White PD. A randomised controlled trial of graded exercise therapy in patients with the chronic fatigue syndrome. *Br. Med. J.* 1997; **314:** 1647–52.

76 Sharpe M, Hawton K, Seagroatt V, Pasvol G. Follow up of patients presenting with fatigue to an infectious diseases clinic. *Br. Med. J.* 1992; **305:** 147–152.

77 Vercoulen JHMM, Swanink CMA, Fennis JFM, Galama JMD, van der Meer JWM, Bleijenberg G. Prognosis in chronic fatigue syndrome (CFS): a prospective study on the natural course. *J. Neurol. Neurosurg. Psychiatry* 1996; **60:** 489–494.

78 Sensky T. Patient's reaction to illness. *Br. Med. J.* 1990; **300:** 622–623.

79 Butler S, Chalder T, Ron M, Wessely S. Cognitive behaviour therapy in chronic fatigue syndrome. *J. Neurol. Neurosurg. Psychiatry* 1991; **54:** 153–158.

80 Friedberg F, Krupp LB. A comparison of cognitive behavioural treatment for chronic fatigue syndrome and primary depression. *Clin. Infect. Dis.* 1994; **18(suppl 1):** S105–S110.

81 Sharpe M, Hawton K, Simkin S, *et al.* Cognitive therapy for chronic fatigue syndrome: a randomized controlled trial. *Br. Med. J.* 1996; **312** 22–26.

82 Deale A, Chalder T, Marks I, Wessely S. A randomized controlled trial of cognitive behaviour versus relaxation therapy for chronic fatigue syndrome. *Am. J. Psych.* 1997; **154:** 408–414.

83 Stewart AD, Hays RD, Ware JE. The MOS short-form General Health Survey. *Med. Care* 1988; **26:** 724–732.

84 Chalder T, Wallace P, Wessely S. Self-help treatment of chronic fatigue in the community: a randomised controlled trial. *Br. J. health. Psychol.* 1997; **2:** 189–97.

85 Chalder T, Berelowitz C, Pawlikowska T. Development of a fatigue scale. *J. Psychosom. Res.* 1993; **37:** 147–154.

86 Goldenberg DL, Kaplan KH, Nadeau MG, Brodeur C, Smith S, Schmid CH. A controlled study of a stress-reduction, cognitive behavioral treatment program in fibromyalgia. *J. Musculoskeletal Pain* 1994; **2:** 53–65.

87 Speckens AEM, Van Hemert AM, Spinhoven P, Hawton KE, Bolk JH, Rooijmans GM. Cognitive behavioural therapy for medically unexplained physical symptoms: a randomised controlled trial. *Br. Med. J.* 1995; **311:** 1328–1332.

88 Koch M, Douard MD, Broustet J. The benefit of graded physical exercise in chronic heart failure. *Chest* 1992; **101(suppl):** 231S–235S.

89 Coats AJS, Adamopoulos A, Meyer TE, Conway J, Sleight P. Effects of physical training in chronic heart failure. *Lancet* 1990; **335:** 63–66.

90 Questad KA. An empirical study of a rehabilitation program for fatigue related to cancer. *Dissertation Abstr. Int.* 1983; **44:**

91 MacVicar M, Winningham M. Effect of aerobic training on functional status of women with breast cancer. *Oncol. Nursing Forum* 1991 **(suppl:)** 62.

92 McCartney N, Moroz D, Garner SH, McComas AJ. The effects of strength training in patients with selected neuromuscular disorders. *Med. Sci. Sports Exercise* 1988; **20:** 362–368.

93 Deluze C, Bosia L, Zirbs A, Chantraine A, Vischer TL. Electroacupuncture in fibromyalgia: results of a controlled trial. *Br. Med. J.* 1992; **305:** 1249–1252.

94 Haanen HCM, Hoenderdos HTW, van Romunde LKJ, *et al.* Controlled trial of hypnotherapy in the treatment of refractory fibromyalgia. *J. Rheumatol.* 1991; **18:** 72–75.

95 Fisher P, Greenwood A, Huskisson EC, Turner P, Belon P. Effect of homeopathic treatment on fibrositis (primary fibromyalgia). *Br. Med. J.* 1989; **299:** 365–366.

96 Awdry R. Homeopathy may help ME. *Int. J. Altern. Complement. Med.* 1996; 12–21.

97 Hill AB. The environment and disease: association or causation? *Proc. R. Soc. Med.* 1965; **58:** 295–300.

98 Gotzsche PC. Methodology and overt and hidden bias in reports of 196 double-blind trials of nonsteroidal antiinflammatory drugs in rheumatoid arthritis. *Controll. Clin. Trials* 1989; **10:** 31–56.

99 Lind J. An inquiry into the nature, causes and cure of the scurvy. In Buck C, Llopis A, Najera E, Terris M (ed.) *The Challenge of Epidemiology.* Washington, Pan American Health Organisation, 1989.

100 Caruso I, Sarzi Puttini P, Cazzola M, Azzolini V. Double-blind study of 5-hydroxytryptophan versus placebo in the treatment of primary fibromyalgia syndrome. *J. Int. Med. Res.* 1990; **18:** 201–209.

101 Carette S, McCain GA, Bell DA, Fam AG. Evaluation of amitriptyline in primary fibrositis. *Arthritis Rheumatism* 1986; **29:** 655–659.

102 Scudds RA, McCain GA, Rollman GB, Harth M. Improvements in pain responsiveness in patients with fibrositis after successful treatment with amitriptyline. *J. Rheumatol.* 1989; **16 (suppl 19):** 98–103.

103 Carette S, Oakson G, Guimont C, Steriade M. Sleep electroencephalography and the clinicial response to amitriptyline in patients with fibromyalgia. *Arthritis Rheumatism* 1995; **38:** 1211–1217.

104 Chaudhuri A, Behan W, Behan P. Chronic fatigue syndrome. *Proc. R. Coll. Physician Edin.* 1998; **28:** 150–163.

105 Mackenzie R, O'Fallon A, Dale J et al. Low-dose hydrocortisone for treatment of chronic fatigue syndrome *J. Am. Med. Assoc.* 1998; **280:** 1061–66.

18. Treatment of the patient with CFS

18.1 Introduction

The management of the patient with CFS is in many ways the culmination of this book. Treatment of the individual patient is based on the findings of the assessment outlined in Chapter 16, the knowledge of the efficacy of treatments reviewed in Chapter 17, and on an awareness of the biological, psychological, and social issues discussed in the other chapters. We hope that this penultimate chapter will add to those that have gone before, by providing the reader with additional guidance on the practical administration of treatment. We will do this by posing the questions: who should give the treatment, what should it be, and where should it be given?

18.2 Who should treat patients with CFS?

We are of the opinion that all patients with possible CFS should be assessed by a medical doctor. In reality, many do not have either the time or interest to undertake detailed assessment and treatment of patients with CFS. In these cases a substantial contribution from other disciplines such as nursing and clinical psychology is advantageous. However, probably more important than professional discipline is the possession of appropriate knowledge, skills, and attitudes.

Practitioner knowledge, skills, and attitudes

Our clinical experience suggests that the effective management of the patient with CFS, requires specific knowledge, a certain level of skill, and also certain attitudes[1]. We have outlined these below in the hope that awareness of them will help others avoid repeating our own errors.

Knowledge

If you have read this book from the beginning we hope that you now possess an up-to-date knowledge of CFS, combined with a healthy scepticism about the 'latest' paper, theory, or news bulletin. However, if forced to summarize the necessary minimum knowledge we think practitioners should acquire we suggest those listed in Table 18.1.

Table 18.1 Knowledge required for effective treatment of patients with CFS

A. *Essential*

    Know how to make an adequate biopsychosocial assessment

    Know that there is no convincing current evidence for a specific disease cause (such as persistent viral infection)

    Know that several potentially reversible factors play a perpetuating role (unhelpful illness beliefs, depression, anxiety, sleep disorder, inactivity, low cortisol, personal and occupational problems)

    Know that there is some evidence to support the use of antidepressant agents

    Know that cognitive behaviour therapy is of demonstrated value

B. *Desirable*

    Know biological, psychological, and social theories of CFS

    Know of overlap between CFS, depression, and other functional somatic complaints

    Know how social security and insurance benefits work

    Know current popular views of CFS and 'ME'

Skills

Knowledge needs to be put into practice, and that may require specific skills. These are a combination of the basic skills of the physician with those of the psychotherapist[2]. Clinical skills we have found to be of particular relevance to the management of CFS are listed in Table 18.2. Training in cognitive behaviour therapy is especially useful, but rarely available.

Table 18.2 Skills required for effective treatment of patients with CFS

The ability to empathize with the patient's predicament

The ability to 'sell' specific treatments

The ability to negotiate illness beliefs

The ability to convey realistic optimism

Attitudes

Knowledge and skills are not everything. In our view there are some attitudes (including some that are sadly relatively common in the medical profession) that are incompatible with the effective treatment of patients suffering from poorly understood illnesses such as CFS. Our experience suggests that fixed and narrow ideas about the nature of the illness and a rigid approach to treatment are more likely to achieve conflict than cure. The effective practitioner accepts a degree of humility and acknowledges that whilst he or she possesses a 'map' of scientific information about CFS and its treatment, the patient is the expert on the 'territory' of their own illness. This approach, which exponents of cognitive therapy refer to as 'collaborative empiricism'[3], is particularly helpful useful in avoiding the disputes (centring on 'who is the real expert here?') that all too often arise within a more traditional doctor–patient relationship. Helpful practitioner attitudes are listed in Table 18.3.

Table 18.3 Attitudes required for effective treatment of patients with CFS

Unqualified acceptance of the validity of patients' illness experience
Willingness to listen to their views and take them seriously
A positive attitude to therapy
Ability to tolerate slow progress and setbacks
Willingness to let the patient take the credit for success

18.3 How should patients with CFS be treated?

The management of patients with CFS follows the same principles as that of other poorly understood or functional illnesses[4,5]. Authoritative guides to the management of CFS are now available[6,7]. However, despite a multitude of claims, the only specific treatment that has been convincingly shown in randomized trials to be of long-term benefit to unselected groups of patients with CFS is cognitive behaviour therapy (CBT)[6,8,9] (see also Chapter 17). This form of treatment is based on a biopsychosocial conceptualization of the patient's problems[10] as outlined in Chapter 16. It is sufficiently flexible to be tailored to the needs of the individual, and includes psychotherapeutic, informational, behavioural, and problem solving components[11].

It is our view, however, that the formal administration of such an intensive and 'broad spectrum' treatment is neither a necessary requirement, nor indeed a realistic expectation, for all patients with CFS. Rather our clinical experience suggests that in many cases a common-sense approach to treating patients using simpler therapies that are, in effect, components of CBT may be effective[12–14]. We must point out, however, that although there is evidence to support the effectiveness of the specific treatments of information-giving, exercise, and the use of antidepressant drugs in a proportion of patients with CFS (see Chapter 17), further trials are needed before the general effectiveness of, and predictors of response to, these simpler interventions is firmly established.

Despite these limitations we have decided for pragmatic reasons to outline these simpler therapies as well as complex cognitive behaviour therapy. How should one choose which treatment to give? At present we suggest that the choice of treatment be based on two principles: tailoring interventions to the individual patient and stepped care.

Tailoring of treatment

The biopsychosocial assessment described in Chapter 16 offers the possibility of targeting therapy at specific illness-perpetuating factors. Thus the patient who does not understand their illness may be given information; the patient with depression is prescribed antidepressant medication; and the patient with marked physiological deconditioning is encouraged to embark on graded exercise. Examples of such tailoring are given in Table 18.4.

Table 18.4 Targets for treatment

Important misunderstandings about the illness	Education
Depression/anxiety disorders	Antidepressant drugs
Major disturbance in activity/rest/sleep pattern	Behavioural therapy
Psychological conflicts and problems	Practical psychotherapy
Physical deconditioning	Graded activity

Stepped care

The major reason for suggesting that simple interventions may have a role in the treatment of CFS is efficiency. Efficient therapy requires that the 'cost' of treatment (in terms of time, effort, and money) to patient, practitioner, and health service is kept to a minimum. A stepped care approach is one away to achieve this. By 'stepped care' we mean that the administration of treatments is planned in such a way that patients only receive more 'costly' treatments if they have not responded to less 'costly' ones[15]. This chapter is organized to reflect this approach. We therefore begin this chapter by describing the simplest of treatments – sympathetic advice – and end with outlining intensive individual CBT. This treatment hierarchy is illustrated in Table 18.5.

Table 18.5 Hierarchy of interventions for a stepped care approach

1. Give simple education and advice
2. Prescribe an antidepressant drug
3. Provide supervision for behavioural change
4. Offer outpatient cognitive behaviour therapy
5. Offer inpatient multidisciplinary rehabilitation

18.4 Education and advice

Almost all patients require education about CFS and how to cope with it. Many are grateful for a positive and demystifying explanation for the illness and are receptive to practical advice. Others come to the consultation with strongly held specific illness beliefs and are antagonistic to alternatives. For such patients new ways of thinking about the illness must be put forward in a fashion that both avoids conflict and encourages curiosity.

What to say

The main points that we suggest be conveyed to all patients are listed in Table 18.6. For patients who disagree with these, or find the information difficult to accept, suggestions of what to say are outlined below.

Table 18.6 Education and advice: main points

Nature of the illness
   Illness is real but probably not a specific disease such as viral infection
   Changes in brain function are present but probably reversible
   Activity induced symptoms do not indicate damage
   People can improve and recover

Advice about coping
   The patient has a major role to play in their recovery (but is not to blame for being ill)
   Prolonged complete rest is harmful
   Regularity of sleep, rest, and activity is important
   Gradual increases in activity are possible
   Antidepressant drugs may be helpful in some cases
   Changes in lifestyle and personal goals may be necessary

Mental versus physical

If the patient insists that their illness is 'entirely physical – not mental' the point can be made that the findings of modern medical research question this distinction; traditionally 'mental' diseases are being linked to changes in the brain; and traditionally 'organic disease', such as ischaemic heart disease, is being found to be influenced by psychological factors. In the case of CFS there is evidence both for changes in brain function and for psychological factors playing an important role in determining outcome.

Rather than asking whether the illness is 'organic' or 'mental' it can be suggested that the more important question is 'reversible' or 'irreversible'? Some illnesses such as cancer are relatively irreversible; others such as depression are largely reversible. Current evidence suggests that the majority of cases of CFS fall into the latter category. This is good news. The next question is how can the pathophysiology of the illness be reversed?

Rest, activity, and sleep

The role of activity is central to a discussion of how to reverse pathophysiology. Excessive rest, excessive or chaotic sleep, and excessive bursts of unsustainable physical exertion should all be discouraged (see Chapter 3). The suggestion that the pathophysiology of the illness may be reversible by gradual increases in activity may then follow.

Proposed increases in activity may be met by two main objections. First 'I have already tried that – it didn't help and made me worse'. Second, 'I try as hard as I can – I am not lazy'. These objections can be anticipated and countered by acknowledging the patient's efforts, pointing out that they may be, in fact, trying *too* hard, and that a very gradual increase from a comfortable baseline is what you had in mind. What have they to lose?

Life problems, conflicts, and stressors

Education about the condition should also include a recognition that stresses of various kinds may have contributed to the patient becoming ill and may now stand in the way of recovery. In our experience an overcommitted lifestyle and excessive occupational stress are particularly common problems[16]. Many who have left their previous employment may be in two minds about returning; on the one hand they may feel they ought to, on the other that they do not want to return to the demands that contributed to their illness. In all these cases it is essential to get the issue of occupation 'on the table'. A practical problem-solving approach[17] in which alternative plans of action are generated, considered, and tried out is of great value and offers a more constructive alternative to avoidance than refuge in chronic 'illness behaviour'[18].

How to convey it

Information giving is most effective if it takes into account the patient's existing beliefs[19]. New information can then be framed and targeted accordingly. It may also be helpful to provide the patient with a cassette tape of the consultation[20]. Written materials can also save time and can reinforce verbal advice. We have produced our own information sheets. A slim and inexpensive book by Trudie Chalder contains similar material[21].

18.5 Pharmacological interventions

No pharmacological agent has been convincingly shown to be helpful to patients diagnosed as having CFS (see Chapter 17). There does, however, appear to be some role for antidepressant drugs and their use will therefore be described below.

Antidepressant agents

There is a very large body of evidence indicating the effectiveness of the antidepressant drugs in relieving depressive disorder. The evidence for patients with CFS with or without associated depressive disorder is more equivocal. None the less in the current state of knowledge it seems reasonable to (and indeed perhaps negligent not to) treat depressive disorder associated with CFS. For patients without good evidence of depressive disorder, the position is less clear. In such cases antidepressants may be prescribed on an empirical basis, with potential beneficial effects for sleep, reduction in pain, and increased energy as well as improvement of mood[22,23].

Choice of agent

There is no convincing evidence to suggest the superiority of any of the main categories of antidepressant drugs over another in CFS; each has certain specific advantages and disadvantages as listed in Table 18.7.

Table 18.7 Antidepressant drugs: advantages and disadvantages of common classes

Agent	Advantages	Disadvantages
Tricyclic (e.g. amitriptyline)	Sedative that aids sleep	Side effects may limit dose
SSRI (e.g. sertraline)	Easily tolerated	May exacerbate sleep disturbance.
MAOI (e.g. moclobamide)	May be 'energizing'	Patients concerned about 'toxicity'

SSRI, selective serotonin, re-uptake inhibitor; MAOI, monoamine oxidase inhibitor.

Justifying the use of antidepressants to the patient

It is usually possible to persuade the patient with CFS to try antidepressants on an 'experimental basis', provided that the doctor is aware of the potentially negative implications of taking drugs with this name ('antidepressants are for psychological illness – my problem is different'). We commonly (and truthfully) justify their use by describing them as 'broad spectrum' agents that can improve pain, sleep, and energy, as well as mood[22,23]. Research that has identified a possible cerebral serotonergic abnormality in patients with CFS provides an additional argument to support their use[24].

Achieving patient adherence

Patients with CFS are very sensitive to the side effects of antidepressant drugs. The reason for this is uncertain. Possible mechanisms include the focusing of attention on and amplification of somatic sensations, and changes in cerebral responses to these agents. In either case an adequate explanation of the purpose of the drug, the anticipated side effects, and the likely delay of benefit being perceived is essential. The drug should be started in the lowest possible dose and increased gradually; the ongoing encouragement and support of the prescribing doctor is important in maintaining adherence[25]. We suggest that even if initially prescribed in low dose, an antidepressant should be given in a 'therapeutic dose' for at least six weeks before being deemed ineffective. The risk of not doing this is that potentially effective agents may be wrongly dismissed and their potential benefit lost.

Other pharmacological agents

No other drugs are recommended. It is desirable to wean patients off the large range of conventional and alternative remedies suggested for CFS, although a flexible approach is appropriate if these appear to be affording the patient some symptomatic relief and are harmless.

18.6 Behavioural interventions

By behavioural intervention is meant offering patients practical help to implement the advice they have been given about sleep, rest, and activity.

Sleep

Problems with sleeping of an insomnia type are almost the rule in patients with CFS[26] (see Chapter 11). Poor sleep at night is often associated with chaotic sleep–wake patterns and long periods of daytime sleep[27]. Although we do not have direct evidence about the importance of treating such sleep problems in CFS, there is sufficient circumstantial evidence[28,29] to make the 'regularization' of sleep a worthwhile aim. Excessive sleeping and a chaotic sleep pattern may be treated by the setting and monitoring of getting up times, and avoidance of daytime napping[30]; insomnia may be treated using established 'sleep hygiene' methods[31], or by prescribing a sedative antidepressant agent such as trazodone[32].

Activity, rest, and exercise

In implementing changes in activity and rest, the first step is to find out the patient's current pattern. One method is for the patient to keep an hour-by-hour diary. This often reveals an oscillating pattern of 'bursts' of vigorous activity interspersed with prolonged rest. Before any overall increase in activity is contemplated, it is essential to stabilize such fluctuations. This may be done by agreeing a 'desirable' current level of *sustainable* activity to nocturnal period of reasonable duration (*which may actually be less than the current level*), highlighting discrepancies between the desirable and current pattern, and then reducing these discrepancies by successive approximation[33–35]. This process may require several weeks.

Once reasonable stability has been achieved, gradual increases in activity can be planned. Targets must be appropriate. That means they should be realistically achievable in the light of the patient's disability, and activities that the patient currently avoids, but wishes to resume[33–35]. Graded activity programmes can be carried out by the patient alone, perhaps with the guidance of a spouse. Formal supervision of exercise may also be helpful in providing patients with ongoing guidance and encouragement as well as physiological monitoring[36]. However, the evidence suggests that many patients require more than simple exercise. The combination of exercise with an antidepressant agent may be better than exercise alone – especially for patients who have evidence of depression. Even then, compliance with increased activity is likely to be limited unless the patient also receives psychological treatment to help them to reappraise their fears and beliefs about the illness[37].

Nearly all patients can be managed in the outpatient setting. However, a period of inpatient admission to a multi-disciplinary unit may be necessary for patients confined to bed or wheelchair. Such programmes are not surprisingly costly, but the results more than justify the expense[34,35].

18.7 Cognitive behaviour therapy

Cognitive behaviour therapy (CBT) is an integration of the education and behavioural interventions described above. For patients who have not responded to the simpler and less 'costly' individual treatments, CBT is the treatment of choice. For the interested reader more detailed accounts of CBT in general[3,11,38,39] and its application to CFS in particular[35,40–42] are available.

A cognitive behavioural model of CFS

The cognitive behavioural model of CFS[43] was introduced in Chapter 12. It assumes (1) that the individual illness-perpetuating factors interact together and (2) that cognitive factors are especially important in those interactions. A simple diagram to illustrate how the illness-perpetuating factors may interact is illustrated in Fig. 18.1, and the way in which factors interact to inhibit increases in activity is shown in Table 18.8. This model and example illustrate the limitation of single treatment interventions and highlight the need for a strategic approach.

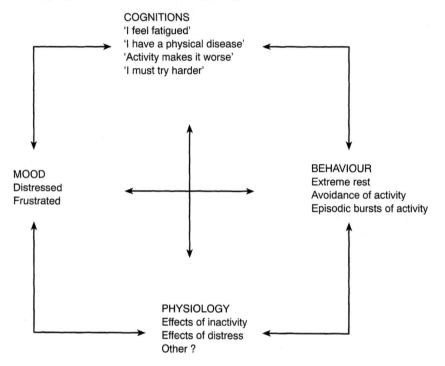

Fig. 18.1 A simple cognitive behavioural model of the perpetuation of CFS.

Table 18.8 Increases in activity: interaction of illness-perpetuating factors

Illness-perpetuating factor	Influence of illness-perpetuating factors on attempts to increase activity
Physiology: Deconditioning	Initial increase in fatigue and pain
Mood: Demoralized	Lack motivation
Cognitions: Can't do anything about illness	No confidence
Will make illness worse	Fear – avoidance
Environment: Overprotective others	Discourage attempts

Advantages of CBT

CBT therefore embodies a treatment strategy based on the cognitive behavioural model. The model illustrates how by targeting intervention at a specific perpetuating factor, change can be produced in others. This strategic approach consequently offers greater *power* for changing mutually the reinforcing illness-perpetuating factors than simpler therapies described above. This process is illustrated in Table 18.9.

Table 18.9 Increases in activity: effect on illness-perpetuating factors

Illness-perpetuating factor	Influence of increased activity
Physiology: Deconditioning	Reduces
Mood: Demoralized	Gain motivation
Cognitions: Can't do anything about illness	'Yes I can' – increased self-efficacy
Will make illness worse	'No I haven't' – reduced fear of symptoms
Environment: Overprotective others	Others observe change; modify their attitudes

The advantages of CBT over simpler treatments

CBT has several advantages over the less 'costly' and simpler treatments described above. First, it can treat multiple illness-perpetuating factors in the same patient; second, it can be strategically targeted at the most important factors; and third, the multiple interventions that comprise CBT can be combined in a way that enhances the effectiveness of each.

The form of therapy

Both the course of therapy and the individual treatment sessions are structured. Most courses of CBT are of relatively brief duration and consist of 10–20 one-hour treatment sessions, in addition to which patients carry out homework assignments. Table 18.10 outlines the stages of treatment.

Table 18.10 The five main stages of treatment: approximate session numbers

Stage of therapy		Sessions
1.	Assessment, formulation, and goal setting	1–3
2.	Stabilize activity/rest/sleep	4–10
	Re-evaluation of illness beliefs	
	Experiment of gradual increase inactivity	
3.	Reviewing unhelpful attitudes	8–12
4.	Problem solving practical difficulties	10–14
5.	Review and planning for future	12–16

Assessment, formulation, and goal setting

Basic assessment should have been completed before embarking on any form of treatment. The individualized biopsychosocial assessment[42] (as described in Chapter 16) provides the information necessary to outline an initial cognitive model as shown in Fig. 18.1 above. Additional information may be obtained from diaries, questionnaires, and further interviews. The goals of therapy are negotiated with the patient as described in the section on behavioural interventions above.

Re-evaluation of illness beliefs

CBT offers an intensive and highly flexible approach to helping the patient learn about their illness. The collaborative empirical approach implies that rather than simply being expected to accept what the doctor says, the patient is encouraged to actively test their beliefs against evidence – a powerful approach that avoids argument between patient and practitioner.

The first step in this process is to help the patient to clarify exactly what their current thoughts and beliefs about the illness are. This may be done by asking the patient to record their thoughts in writing (either as homework or within a treatment session). Those occurring prior to and during activity are particularly important in preventing increases in activity.

The second step is for the patient, with the therapist's guidance, to generate possible alternatives to thoughts that appear to be preventing changes in behaviour. One method for doing this is the so-called 'double-column technique', in which patients write their thoughts and beliefs in one column, and then list possible alternatives in another. An example is shown in Table 18.11.

Table 18.11 The double-column technique

Column 1: original thought	Column 2: alternative thought
It's hopeless, I will never get better	How do I know? I haven't given this new approach a try yet. I do know that some people do recover
Thus therapy will make me worse	It might, but I don't know that it will and if I don't try I won't find out. It has helped others

Evidence is then sought to enable the patient to choose whether the original thought or the alternative is the most accurate. Sometimes, as with 'it's hopeless, I will never get better' simple scrutiny may reveal that the original thought was negatively biased. In other cases as with 'this treatment will make me worse', the inaccuracy may not be so obvious, and the patient should be encouraged to seek new evidence. A potent way of doing this is to 'suck it and see' – that is, conduct an experiment (see below).

Behavioural experiments: gradual increases in activity

The basic principles of behaviour change are described above. When behaviour change is used as a 'behavioural experiment' it is important, as with all experiments, to set up precise predictions and to carefully measure the results. For example, if the patient has the belief 'activity will make me worse' a specific testable prediction is derived such as 'increases in activity will produce persistent increases in symptoms'. The patient's general impression of symptoms is not good enough because it is subject to a range of potential biases. Systematic recording on rating scales is preferable.

The therapist must also make sure that such experiments are 'no-lose' exercises. Thus if the patient is able to increase activity, this is evidence for the benefit of this approach; if not it provides valuable information about the obstacles to doing so and offers further targets for intervention. In this context it is important to anticipate that the patient is likely to experience a *transient* exacerbation in symptoms with each increase in activity. These represent physiological not pathological processes (see Chapter 8). None the less such increases in symptoms may be catastrophically interpreted by the patient as 'this is making me worse'. Cautious target setting and careful design of the experiment can avoid this pitfall, and as the new, increased level of activity is maintained the symptoms will gradually subside to the original level.

Persistent and repeated recording of thoughts and challenging of these may be required to dispel fully dispel the patient's illness fears. A positive outcome is for the patient to come to regard transient increases in symptoms as welcome evidence that they are challenging the pathophysiological processes that are impeding recovery.

Reviewing of unhelpful attitudes

More general beliefs and attitudes may emerge as difficulties in carrying out the behavioural experiment. A common example is perfectionism with an 'all or nothing' approach to tasks. If such problems are severe the patient may be encouraged to review the advantages and disadvantages of holding this attitude. An example is shown in Table 18.12. A revised version of the attitude, such as 'it is more important strike a balance than to try to do everything' may then be discussed and the patient encouraged to change his or her behaviour accordingly.

Table 18.12 Reviewing attitudes such as perfectionism

Attitude:	I must do everything perfectly
Advantages:	Motivates me (but does it really?)
	I feel good if I think I've done something right (but only briefly)
Disadvantages:	I never get things finished
	It makes me self-critical
	My work always disappointments me
	I never feel that I've finished
	I find it difficult to plan gradual increasing activity

Attitude change is a potentially difficult and long term task. If time is short a simpler method is to repeatedly encourage the patient and their partner or parent to make the rehabilitation programme the highest priority task in their daily life rather than the meeting of external demands or unrealistic standards,

Problem solving of practical difficulties

As behaviour change progresses, external obstacles to recovery often become apparent. For example, a patient who has been chronically disabled, off work, and perhaps receiving financial benefits, has to cope with the financial and social transition from sickness to health. This may involve potential 'loss of face' and practically may mean loss of financial benefits without the guarantee of remunerative employment. Issues that were present when the patient first became ill, such as difficulties at work, may also remain unresolved. These problems are best dealt with using a problem solving approach as described above

Consolidating gains and planning for the future

By the end of therapy, the therapist and patient should have a final and agreed formulation of the illness. It is useful at this point for the patient to produce a written document including both the formulation and a list of the things that they have learnt from the therapy. This document can also include practical guidelines for themselves on how to continue their rehabilitation and how to cope with 'relapse'. It is our experience that patients often refer to these documents subsequently. The fact that the patient can continue the work of therapy on his or her own, by being 'their own therapist', may be important in producing continuing improvement after formal treatment has ended[8,9].

Administration of therapy

Individual or group

Our own personal experience is almost entirely with 'one-to-one' CBT. The advantage of this form of administration is that it can be closely tailored to the individual. Cognitive behaviour therapy can also be given in group form, however[44]. On the one hand group therapy has the potential advantages of greater efficiency and the added therapeutic factor of the group process; on the other hand groups also require careful patient selection and are very demanding of the therapist. At present we prefer an individual approach.

How many sessions?

A reasonable average number for most patients would be 10 to 20 individual sessions over a four- to six-month period, perhaps with one or two follow-up or 'booster' sessions. Some patients may require more than this.

18.8 Potential problems

Several issues may complicate the management of patients with CFS.

Hostile and reluctant patients

Many patients are initially hostile to the idea of a further referral, particularly to any unit with a perceived 'psychological' orientation. We have found it best to confront such feelings immediately on seeing the patient, and to openly sympathize with their plight. 'Did you think that seeing us meant that doctors weren't taking your symptoms seriously?' can lead to questions directly about the experience of disconfirmation and perceived stigmatization implicit in referral to a psychological or general hospital psychiatry service.

Reluctance to try a cognitive behavioural approach should be explored. If it is fear of the effects of increased activity it can be helpful to lay out the alternatives facing the patient in stark fashion: if they are right in avoiding activity they will prevent a transient worsening of their illness by the treatment; but if they are wrong they are depriving themselves of a major increase in quality of life. It is emphasized that whilst the therapist can outline the potential benefits and risks, but the choice is theirs.

Patients with poor prognosis

For patients who have been identified as having a poor prognosis because of a long history of severely impaired functioning, or poor response to treatment, regular if infrequent long term follow-up may be the best approach[45]. This is at least likely to limit iatrogenic harm from unnecessary investigations and ineffective treatments, and may actually improve the patient's functioning in the longer term[46]. No treatment is ever successful for everyone – for some patients long term support is the best option.

Spouse/parent problems

If family members hold very strong views about the nature of the illness that interfere with treatment, such as insisting that the patient persists with rest, the techniques of examining alternatives described above may help them to 'give the treatment a try'. In a very small number of cases, especially children, the patient's family may strongly resist their efforts to rehabilitate[47,48] (see also Chapter 13). It may then appear that the patient's sick role is necessary for the stability of the family. Such cases can be very difficult to manage but may benefit from family therapy[49].

Benefits and insurance payments

Some benefits and insurance payments require that the patient repeatedly demonstrate their state of ill health. As with chronic pain, such systems may be considered to be disincentives for recovery[50]. In these cases we encourage a frank discussion of the advantages and disadvantages of remaining disabled. It must be admitted, however, that such powerful extrinsic forces can be difficult to overcome.

Conflict with alternative therapists

Patients with CFS often turn to alternative medicine[51]. Some complementary therapies may be continued in parallel with rehabilitative management. If, however, they interfere with that treatment, the need to pursue one approach at a time should be explained to the patient, and the use of the competing therapy deferred until the current management plan has been completed.

18.9 The future

We need both a brief treatment for more widespread use in primary care and more powerful treatment for resistant cases. We also need to know more about the predictors of response to brief therapy. At present we have to be guided largely by clinical impression. This experience suggests that some patients can benefit from simple interventions; these require evaluation in randomized trials. Experience also suggests that patients who have never coped well or who are in difficult occupational circumstances do not do well. The new 'schema-based' therapies[52] may be appropriate for this group. All these issues require empirical evaluation. There will always be more to learn about the treatment of CFS.

Services

Chronic fatigue is just one example of the large range of medically unexplained syndromes that are poorly managed by existing services. This is part of the wider problem created by a split of specialist service provision into psychiatry devoted to 'mental health' and medical services that focus on 'organic disease'[53]. As in Victorian times, some patients with fatigue prefer to see their problem as physical and to use medical rather than psychiatric services. Who wouldn't? Although the general principles of cognitive behavioural treatment can in principle be applied by any clinician, more complex or difficult cases require the skills of a trained cognitive behaviour therapist. Unfortunately such persons are rare and this may be a major impediment to the development of effective services. The provision of appropriately skilled therapists and the development of integrated medical–psychiatric services presents a considerable challenge to existing health services[54].

References

1 House AO. The patient with medically unexplained symptoms: making the initial psychiatric contact. In Mayou R, Bass C, Sharpe M (ed.) *Treatment of Functional Somatic Symptoms*. Oxford University Press, 1995: 89–102.

2 Frank JD. Therapeutic factors in psychotherapy. *Am. J. Psychother.* 1971; **25**: 350–361.

3 Beck AT, Rush AJ, Shaw BF, Emery G. *Cognitive Therapy of Depression*. New York, Guilford Press, 1979.

4 Sharpe M, Peveler R, Mayou RA. The psychological treatment of patients with functional somatic symptoms: a practical guide. *J. Psychosom. Res.* 1992; **36**: 515–529.

5 Sharpe M. An overview of the treatment of functional somatic symptoms. In Mayou R, Bass C, Sharpe M (ed.) *Treatment of Functional Somatic Symptoms.* Oxford University Press, 1995: 66–88.

6 Joint Working Party of the Royal Colleges of Physicians, Psychiatrists and General Practitioners. *Chronic Fatigue Syndrome.* London, Royal College of Physicians, 1996.

7 National Institutes of Allergy and Infectious Diseases. *Chronic Fatigue Syndrome: Information for Physicians.* Bethesda, MD, NIAID, 1996.

8 Sharpe M, Hawton KE, Simkin S, *et al.* Cognitive behaviour therapy for chronic fatigue syndrome: a randomized controlled trial. *Br. Med. J.* 1996; **312:** 22–26.

9 Deale A, Chalder T, Marks IM, Wessely S. A randomized controlled trial of cognitive behaviour therapy versus relaxation therapy for chronic fatigue syndrome. *Am. J. Psychiatry* 1997: **154:** 408–14.

10 Engel GL. The need for a new medical model: a challenge for biomedicine. *Science* 1977; **196:** 129–196.

11 Clark DM, Fairburn CG (ed.) *Science and Practice of Cognitive Behaviour Therapy.* Oxford University Press, 1996.

12 Pemberton S, Hatcher S, Stanley P, House A. Chronic fatigue syndrome: a way forward. *Br. J. Occup. Therapy* 1994; **57:** 381–383.

13 Denman AM. The chronic fatigue syndrome; a return to common sense. *Postgrad. Med. J.* 1990; **66:** 499–501.

14 Cox DL, Findlay L. Is chronic fatigue syndrome treatable in an NHS environment? *Clin. Rehab* 1994; **8:** 76–80.

15 Fairburn CG, Peveler RC. Bulimia nervosa and a stepped care approach to management. *Gut* 1990; **31:** 1220–1222.

16 Ware NC. Society, mind and body in chronic fatigue syndrome: an anthropological view. In Bock GR, Whelan J (ed.) *Chronic Fatigue Syndrome: CIBA Foundation Symposium No. 173.* Chichester, Wiley, 1993: 62–73.

17 Hawton KE, Kirk J. Problem-solving. In Hawton K, Salkovskis PM, Kirk J, Clark DM (ed.) *Cognitive Behaviour Therapy for Psychiatric Problems.* Oxford Medical Publications, 1989: 406–427.

18 Mechanic D. The concept of illness behaviour. *J. Chron. Dis.* 1962; **15:** 189–194.

19 Helman CG. Communication in primary care: the role of patient and practitioner explanatory models. *Soc. Sci. Med.* 1985; **20:** 923–931.

20 Tattersall MH, Butow PN, Griffin AM, Dunn SM. The take-home message: patients prefer consultation audiotapes to summary letters. *J. Clin. Oncol.* 1994; **12:** 1305–1311.

21 Chalder T. *Coping with Chronic Fatigue.* London, Sheldon Press, 1995.

22 Lynch SP, Seth R, Montgomery S. Antidepressant therapy in the chronic fatigue syndrome. *Br. J. Gen. Pract.* 1991; **41:** 339–342.

23 Goodnick PJ, Sandoval R. Psychotropic treatment of chronic fatigue syndrome and related disorders. *J. Clin. Psychiatry* 1993; **54:** 13–20.

24 Bakheit AM, Behan PO, Dinan TG, O'Keane VO. Possible upregulation of hypothalamic 5-hydroxytraptamine receptors in patients with postviral fatigue syndrome. *Br. Med. J.* 1992; **304:** 1010–1012.

25 Katon WJ, Robinson P, VonKorff M, *et al.* A multifaceted intervention to improve treatment of depression in primary care. *Arch. Gen. Psychiatry* 1996; **53:** 924–932.

26 Sharpe M, Hawton KE, Seagroatt V, Pasvol G. Patients who present with fatigue: a follow up of referrals to an infectious diseases clinic. *Br. Med. J.* 1992; **305:** 147–152.

27 Sharpley AL, Clements A, Hawton KE, Sharpe M. Do patients with 'pure' chronic fatigue syndrome (neurasthenia) have abnormal sleep? *Psychosom. Med.* 1997; **59:** 592–596.

28 Silva AB, Bertorini TE, Lemmi H. Polysomnography in idiopathic muscle pain syndrome (fibrositis). *Arg. Neuropsiquiatr.* 1991; **49:** 437–441.

29 Chambers MJ, Alexander SD. Assessment and prediction of outcome for a brief behavioral insomnia treatment program. *J. Behav. Ther. Exp. Psychiatry* 1992; **23:** 289–297.

30 Horne J. *Why We Sleep.* Oxford University Press, 1988.

31 Sloan EP, Hauri P, Bootzin R, Morin C, Stevenson M, Shapiro C. The nuts and bolts of behavioural therapy for insomnia. *J. Psychosom. Res.* 1993; **37(suppl 1):** 19–37.

32 Nierenberg AA, Adler LA, Peselow E, Zornberg G, Rosenthal M. Trazodone for antidepressant-associated insomnia. *Am. J. Psychiatry* 1994; **151:** 1069–1072.

33 Sharpe M, Chalder T. Management of the chronic fatigue syndrome. In Illis LS (ed.) *Rehabilitation of the Neurological Patient*, 2nd edn. Oxford; Blackwell, 1992: 282–294.

34 Chalder T, Butler S, Wessely S. In-patient treatment for chronic fatigue syndrome. *Behav. Cogn. Psychotherapy* 1996; **24:** 351–365.

35 Sharpe M. Cognitive behaviour therapy. In Demitrack M, Abbey S (ed.) *Psychiatric Aspects of Chronic Fatigue Syndrome.* New York, Guilford Press, 1996: 240–262.

36 Cully KK, Sisto SA, Natelson BH. Use of exercise for treatment of chronic fatigue syndrome. *Sports Med.* 1996; **21:** 35–48.

37 Wearden A, Morriss RK, Mullis R, Appleby L, Campbell I. A double blind, placebo controlled trial of fluoxetine and a graded exercise programme for chronic fatigue syndrome. *Br. J. Psychiat.* 1998; **172:** 485–490.

38 Salkovskis PM. The cognitive-behavioural approach. In Creed F, Mayou R, Hopkins A (ed.) *Medical Symptoms not Explained by Organic Disease.* London, Royal College of Psychiatrists and Royal College of Physicians of London, 1992: 70–84.

39 Persons JB. *Cognitive Therapy in Practice: a Case Formulation Approach.* New York, W W Norton, 1989.

40 Wessely S, David AS, Butler S, Chalder T. Management of chronic (post-viral) fatigue syndrome. *J. R. Coll. Gen. Pract.* 1989; **39:** 26–29.

41 Deale A, David AS. Chronic fatigue syndrome: Evaluation and management. *J. Neuropsychiatry Clin. Neurosci.* 1994; **6:** 189–194.

42 Sharpe M, Chalder T, Palmer I, Wessely S. Chronic fatigue syndrome: a practical guide to assessment and management. *Gen. Hosp. Psychiatry* 1997: **19:** 185–99.

43 Surawy C, Hackmann A, Hawton KE, Sharpe M. Chronic fatigue syndrome: a cognitive approach. *Behav. Res. Ther.* 1995; **33:** 535–544.

44 Bennett RM, Burckhardt CS, Clark SR, O'Reilly CA, Wiens AN, Campbell SM. Group treatment of fibromyalgia: a 6 month outpatient program. *J. Rheumatol.* 1996; **23:** 521–528.

45 Smith GR, Monson RA, Ray DC. Psychiatric consultation in somatization disorder – a randomized controlled study. *New. Eng. J. Med.* 1986; **314:** 1407–1413.

46 Smith GR, Rost KM, Kashner TM. A trial of the effect of a standardized psychiatric consultation on health outcomes and costs in somatizing patients. *Arch. Gen. Psychiatry* 1995; **52:** 238–243.

47 Rikard-Bell CJ, Waters BGH. Psychosocial management of chronic fatigue syndrome in adolescence. *Aust. NZ J. Psychiatry* 1992; **26:** 64–72.

48 Vereker MI. Chronic fatigue syndrome: a joint paediatric-psychiatric approach. *Arch. Dis. Child.* 1992; **67:** 550–555.

49 Graham H. Family interventions in general practice: a case of chronic fatigue. *J. Fam Ther.* 1990; **13:** 225–230.

50 Main CJ, Benjamin S. Psychological treatment and the health care system: the chaotic case of back pain. Is there a need for a paradigm shift? In Mayou R, Bass C, Sharpe M (ed.) *Treatment of Functional Somatic Symptoms.* Oxford University Press, 1995: 214–230.

51 Bass C, Mayou RA. Alternative and complementary treatments. In Mayou R, Bass C, Sharpe M (ed.) *Treatment of Functional Somatic Symptoms.* Oxford University Press, 1995: 428–438.

52 Young JE. *Cognitive Therapy for Personality Disorders: a Schema Focussed Approach.* Florida, Professional Resource Exchange Inc., 1990.

53 Kirmayer LJ. Mind and body as metaphors: hidden values in biomedicine. In Lock M, Gordon D (ed.) *Biomedicine Examined.* Dordrecht, Kluwer, 1988: 57–92.

54 Royal Colleges of Physicians and Royal College of Psychiatrists. *Joint Working Party Report: the Psychological Care of Medical Patients; Recognition of Need and Service Provision.* London, Royal College of Physicians, 1995.

55 Essame C, Phelan S, Aggett P, White P. Pilot study of a multidisciplinary inpatient rehabilitation of severely incapacitated patients with the chronic fatigue syndromes. *J. Chronic Fat. Syndrome* 1998; **4**: 51–58.

Section V:

Overview

19. Conclusions

19.1 What is fatigue?

We all recognize fatigue when we experience it, but establishing a satisfactory definition has not proven easy. We consider 'fatigue' to be a general term covering a range of phenomena that are often, but not necessarily, associated with exertion. The meaning of the term is therefore both intuitively obvious, based on one's own experience, but also elusive. We propose that this ambiguity is inevitable and irreducible – instead it must simply be acknowledged. We can retain the concept, but must operationalize our definitions. In particular we must first distinguish between fatigue in performance and the feeling of fatigue.

The feeling of fatigue

Even a report of a feeling of fatigue may refer to a range of perceptions including exhaustion, lack of motivation, and sleepiness. Again, we have suggested that like depression the term is rooted in language. The feeling of fatigue is common, and is continuously distributed in the population. For many it is part of life, but when severe or combined with another factor, such as depression, disability, illness fears or personal problems, it becomes a focus for medical consultation.

The clinical problem

In clinical practice we are faced not with fatigue but with a patient complaining of fatigue. We have suggested that the best approach is to consider not only symptoms and pathophysiology but also mood, cognition, behaviour, and circumstance. Each of these is not mutually exclusive but are contributors to the clinical problem.

We have seen that fatigue as a symptom is common in the population and may be associated with a wide range of illness. It is a crucial part of the illness experience of the patient, but is less helpful when the doctor considers the most likely diagnosis. When no clear-cut cause can be identified it becomes a source of frustration to the doctor and dissatisfaction and even disaffection for the patient. This is now the problem of CFS.

19.2 What is chronic fatigue syndrome?

What, then, is CFS? The research reviewed above suggests that the closer one gets, the less one understands it. Are the psychiatrists, virologists, and immunologists all seeing different conditions, or different aspects of the same illness?

Overall, we doubt that there is a single cause of CFS, any more than there is a single cause of high blood pressure. We doubt that one factor, be it psychosocial, viral or immunological, will satisfactorily explain anything other than a minority of cases. We believe that a number of factors contribute to the syndrome. We assume it has a genetic basis, albeit almost entirely unexplored. There remains a strong clinical case for assuming that exposure to certain infections play a role in initiating symptoms. Certainly infections such as EBV, hepatitis, and viral meningitis have been confirmed as risk factors. Differences in the way in which the body deals with such agents, and the ability to mount and control an efficient immune response may play a part. We suspect that the current upsurge of interest in the links between infection, the immune response to infection, and central neurotransmitter activity will lead to significant insights. We are less certain that the current activity surrounding the function of the HPA axis will lead to fundamental insights – it is possible that the reason why it has been so intensively studied is because it presents fewer methodological problems than more direct measures of central activity. The advent of new radiolabels for some of the serotonin receptors may result in more profitable lines of inquiry.

Regardless of the results of further neurobiological inquiries, there can be no doubting the important role played by psychological, social, and cultural factors. Previous experience clearly increases vulnerability to CFS. Whether or not coincident life stress also plays a part remains uncertain, but it would be surprising if it did not. Subsequent events certainly play a crucial role in determining the eventual outcome. The person's own emotional make up and coping strategies are important, but perhaps the reactions of family, friends, and particularly the medical profession, may add the final element to the illness we call CFS.

In integrating these risk factors into a model for CFS, we predict that it will be necessary to make distinctions between the expression of symptoms, and the development of disability. We suggest that agents such as EBV or viral meningitis can lead to the experience of abnormal symptoms, such as fatigue, malaise, and myalgia. However, the transition from symptoms to disability may be more closely linked to cognitive and behavioural factors. Hence interventions such as CBT designed to reduce disability and counteract maladaptive coping strategies ought to be more effective in reducing disability than symptoms. The evidence so far supports this model – many patients do show considerable improvements in disability and everyday functioning, but are not rendered symptom free by cognitive or behavioural interventions.

If we were to point to one area which might unite at least some of these disparate observations it would the field of perception. One theme that emerges from the literature of all the fatigue syndromes is the possibility of a general disorder of perception, perhaps of both symptoms and disability. At the heart of this misperception lies the sense of effort[1]. CFS patients clearly experience increased effort in everyday physical and mental tasks, reflected in sense of painful muscle exertion, and painful cognitive processing. This increased effort is the not the result of increased neuromuscular or metabolic demands (a Victorian concept), nor does it result in any substantial decline in actual muscle or cognitive performance. The result is a mismatch between patients' evaluation of their physical and mental functioning and the external evidence of any consistent deficits. The basis of this disorder of effort must remain speculative, particularly since the perception of effort is a complex topic[2]. We presume it is because the sufferer needs to devote more attention, or even energy, to processes that the rest of us find automatic, be it muscular exertion or mental concentration. Why that should be remains very unclear, but must be a priority for research[1]. Similarly, the perception of pain has been relatively neglected, but we believe studies of the activation of peripheral pain systems and their central control may be another fruitful line of inquiry.

From this fundamental problem flow other problems identified in CFS, such as increased symptom monitoring, decreased tolerance, increased anxiety, and so on. These are not unique to CFS. Fibromyalgia patients appear abnormally sensitive to muscle-derived stimuli[3]. IBS patients may more be sensitive to gastrointestinal discomfort from a variety of sources[4]. Thus some centrally mediated disorder of perception of information may underlie the experience of fatigue syndromes, and explain the widespread discrepancies between the intensity of symptoms and disability, and objective testing of a number of different parameters, both physiological and neuropsychological.

When we began to pursue our clinical and research interests in CFS we expected to find high rates of affective disorder. This indeed turned out to be correct, but with the passage of time it is our impression that the dramatic over-representation of major affective disorder, reported in those initial studies of chronic selected hospital samples, seems to be declining. Perhaps referring doctors are become more aware of the need to routinely screen for mood disorder. We have likewise noted less reluctance on the part of both doctors and patients to contemplate antidepressant therapy. Perhaps also samples are becoming less chronic, as patients are referred earlier. Perhaps researchers tend to find what they expect – certainly the role of anxiety disorders has been underestimated.

Whatever the reason, CFS is certainly not simply the somatic presentation of affective disorder. Such a view is both simplistic and inaccurate, and runs counter to our own view of the heterogeneity of the condition. The concept of affective spectrum disorder[5] may still be relevant to all the fatigue and myalgia syndromes, but even there one must resist the temptation to see all such conditions as variants of the old concept of masked depression. Depression itself brings with it many conceptual problems similar to those we have noted in CFS – it includes much, but explains little.

Instead, we have become more convinced of the links between CFS and the area of chronic pain. The analogies are many: the increased rates of affective and somatic symptoms, the role of avoidance behaviour in sustaining symptoms, the role of physical factors as precipitants, the need for rehabilitation rather than cure, and the role of social and economic factors in perpetuating disability and causing conflict both with and between doctors.

19.3 CFS as a final common pathway

Researchers have struggled to identify a single cause of CFS, known in the United States as the 'smoking gun'. We doubt these efforts will be successful. Other researchers have conceded, often willingly, that a single discrete cause cannot be identified, and instead accepted the concept of heterogeneity, assuming that a number of different causes are operative, and that their identification will in turn lead to a division of CFS. It has been suggested that CFS is rather like assuming the existence of a chronic abdominal pain disorder before it is reclassified into diseases of the gall bladder, colon, appendix, and so on. Such arguments often carry the subtext that this division will fall neatly into physical and psychological causes, with the implicit, and sometimes explicit, assumption that alongside the psychological chaff will be found the physical wheat. It is also interesting how some of those who advance this argument assume that their condition (either the one they suffer from, the one they research, or the one they treat) will inevitably fall on the physical side of the divide.

We see the merits of assuming heterogeneity. *Post hoc* subgroup analysis is notoriously prone to error, but in the last year or so some evidence has started to surface suggesting that dividing subjects by mode of onset has merit[6,7]. We are also impressed with the evidence presented by the Australian group suggesting that differences exist between the minority of cases with long illness histories and ill defined onset compared to the majority with less disability and shorter illness durations, whom they label 'acquired neurasthenia'[8]. However, it remains premature to shift at this stage from being ardent 'lumpers' to passionate 'splitters'.

Likewise, of course, some discrete causes of CFS will be identified, just as, as we noted in Chapters 2 and 7, hypertension is sometimes causes by renal artery stenosis or Conn's disease. But such rare aetiologies add little to our understanding of the commoner problem of essential hypertension.

Instead, if pushed, we admit to seeing CFS as the final common pathway of a number of risk factors. The analogy we prefer is that of ischaemic heart disease. We know that a number of risk factors exist for the condition – smoking, high blood pressure, stress, genetics, diet, and so on. However, a heart attack is a heart attack, regardless of the pattern of risk factors involved. CFS too we see as a final common pathway, to which a number of risk factors contribute. Throughout this book we have enthusiastically propagated the concept of predisposing, precipitating, and perpetuating factors, all of which may operate in the individual patient, and none of which may on their own be sufficient to explain the disorder.

Thus we doubt that at some future time clinicians will be able to enforce a rigorous and valid subclassification of CFS, based upon some putative biological or psychological marker. Nor do we think that efforts to come up with some reliable way of splitting CFS into those with a physical, and those with a psychological, disorder, the ultimate aim of some CFS researchers, will ever be attained. Instead we think that in each individual patient it will be necessary to consider the contribution of genetic, biological, behavioural, and emotional factors. Each sufferer may show different contributions from each set of variables, just as in some patients with heart attacks obesity plays a lesser role to smoking, or vice versa.

To support this view we draw attention to the non-specificity of the CFS concept. We see patients in whom a chronic fatigue syndrome has developed after glandular fever. Such a patient will be diagnosed as having post-viral fatigue syndrome, or CFS. But we also know that similar, indeed identical, syndromes develop after a large number of other viral agents, such as CMV, viral meningitis or hepatitis, claims which are all supported by well designed studies. Bacterial and protozoal agents are also implicated. Moving from the infectious field, a different literature describes illnesses that are also indistinguishable from our patient with EBV post-infectious fatigue syndrome, but receive other labels, and often researchers apply fundamentally different explanatory models. Post-concussional syndromes are one example. Chronic whiplash is another. We have also seen papers describing the alleged consequences of ingestion of toxic oil or pesticides, or the long term consequences of receiving a silicone breast implant, all of which are identical to the descriptions of the patients we encounter in the CFS clinic.

Similarly, the role of psychological stress seems to be a general, rather than a specific one. We described in detail the study performed by one of the authors and his colleagues in which a large cohort of subjects who attended general practice with a viral infection were studied both before and after presenting with the index infection[9]. Those with prior symptoms and/or previous psychological disorders were at greater risk of developing chronic fatigue and/or CFS.

This model, in which pre-exposure psychological or social variables explain some of the post-exposure outcome[9, 10], is not unique to the relationship between common viral infections and CFS. We found the same for viral meningitis, in which the contribution of the precipitating infection was more substantial, but the combination of previous psychiatric disorder and viral meningitis was particularly associated with the onset of CFS[11]. Similar results have been presented to explain the transition from acute to chronic back pain[12], from herpes zoster to post-herpetic neuralgia[13], from acute gastroenteritis to irritable bowel syndrome[14], from head injury to the post-concussional syndrome[15], from trauma to PTSD[16], and to explain the development of post-surgical fatigue[17]. Similarly, the role of avoidance behaviour in perpetuating symptoms is not unique to CFS either[18 19 20].

We thus assume CFS to be a multifactorial process, rather than a collection of discrete disorders yet to be identified. We feel that some risk factors may be specific to CFS, but the majority are themselves general risk factors for the development of long term symptomatic outcomes after acute insults.

19.4 Why does it matter? – the significance of CFS

Clinical

The clinical significance of CFS is twofold. First and most obviously, anyone who has attended a CFS clinic, or spent time with those who carry the label of CFS, can be in no doubt as to the importance of the problem in terms of individual suffering, family disruption, and economic impact, even if the source of that suffering is unclear. Second, CFS is an important reminder of the limitations of the narrow biomedical approach to illness, and the consequent limitations of medical thinking and practice. The lessons that CFS can teach are applicable in many other areas of medicine.

Biological

CFS provides many opportunities for furthering our understanding of fundamental neurobiological processes, and for adding to our fledgling knowledge of the inter-action between biological, social, and psychological factors. We already note the growth of interest in CFS by those who specialize in interdisciplinary research – such as the new discipline of psychoimmunology, or behavioural medicine. Unidisciplinary approaches that dominated the first wave of interest and research into CFS have now given way to more broadly based and intellectually stimulating approaches, some-thing that must be welcome.

Social

In this book we have devoted considerable attention to the role played by wider social forces in the shaping of CFS. We do not consider that CFS is fundamentally a social construction, but we do think that CFS exists in the real world, where patients experience real and quantifiable suffering. In this world patients encounter wider attitudes towards suffering and ill health, and bring their own views as well. All too frequently these world views collide, most often in the setting of the doctor's surgery. Understanding these interactions, and the difficulties that often result, is not an intriguing footnote to the question of CFS. It is as much as part of the condition as we see it today as any putative neurobiological, psychological, or virological process.

The importance of a sociocultural perspective is twofold. First, because without it one cannot hope to comprehend the extraordinary passions and disputes that accompany the condition, and which, while not unique to CFS, are certainly more prominent there than elsewhere. Second, because the very uncertainty of CFS provides a window into modern ideas of illness, which would not be open in illnesses with a more defined pathophysiological basis[21][22]. This is the perspective we adopted in Chapter 15.

Historical

In this book we make no apologies for our frequent references to the historical record. We also make no apologies for giving in to the temptation to draw lessons from the past that we propose have relevance for the future. Perhaps the strongest observation that can be made from the historical evidence is humility – we have been here before. Many of the problems that confront both patients suffering from fatigue syndromes and the doctors attempting to both understand and heal them have been addressed in the past, and some might say more successfully than in the present, even without the benefits (and occasional hindrance) of modern technology.

The second lesson is the continuing importance of social factors in the fatigue syndromes. Historians such as Anton Rabinbach[23] and Tom Lutz[24,25] have drawn attention to the economic metaphors that imbued neurasthenia. We have extended this to show how CFS, when viewed through the mirror of popular writings, provides similar metaphors to express the concerns of our age. One cannot also fail to note the similarities between late Victorian England and the America of the 1890s and the period of the late 1980s in both countries, which saw the re-emergence of chronic fatigue as modern CFS.

Neurasthenia alerts us to the relevance of social factors in the construction of new diseases, as neurasthenia was then and CFS is now. The historical record also shows how the tension between organic and psychological aetiological models is nothing new. Neurasthenia flourished when both doctors and patients alike viewed it as an organic diagnosis free from blame, and indeed almost praiseworthy in its causes. Such simplistic models naturally gave way to medical disillusionment, followed by a turn to psychological models. This proved to be no panacea for two reasons. First, psychologization, in the form it took of doctrinaire psychogenesis, was accompanied by polarization, distrust, and polemic. Pure psychogenic theories were, and still are, untenable in the clinical setting. The Freudian revolution, which hastened the dismantling of neurasthenia, continues to have a malign influence on the management of fatigue syndromes to this day. The second reason why psychologization will not provide a simple solution to the problem of fatigue is also pragmatic – the Freudian revolution is now in reverse, but not as we would wish. From believing that psychiatry deals with psychogenic problems, we have now shifted to the equal extreme. Psychiatry is once again returning to its pre-Freudian alienism roots. Severe mental illness, falsely viewed as synonymous with the psychoses, viewed from a firmly organic perspective, is now its business. Modern psychiatry is no more welcoming to the patient with chronic fatigue than in the days of the Freudian ascendancy.

History therefore teaches us to avoid any simplistic somatic/psychological polarization if one wishes to understand chronic fatigue, or to help those who suffer with it. History also teaches us just how a delicate a path we have to tread to achieve those objectives. In this book we have tried to do just that – others will judge how successfully.

References

1 Lawrie S, MacHale S, Power M, Goodwin G. Is the chronic fatigue syndrome best understood as a primary disturbance of the sense of effort? *Psychol. Med.* 1997; **27**: 995–9.

2 Mihevic P. Sensory cues for perceived exerion: a review. *Med. Sci. Sports Exer.* 1981; **13:** 150–163.

3 Mikkelsson M, Latikka P, Kautiainen H, Isomeri R, Isomaki H. Muscle and bone pressure pain threshold and pain tolerance in fibromyalgia patients and controls. *Arch. Phys. Med. Rehabil.* 1992; **73:** 814–818.

4 Drossman D, Thompson W. The irritable bowel syndrome; review and a graduated, multicomponent treatment approach. *Ann. Internal Med.* 1992; **116:** 1009–1016.

5 Hudson J, Pople H. The concept of affective spectrum disorder: relationship to fibromyalgia and other syndromes of chronic fatigue and chronic muscle pain. *Baillières Clin. Rheumatol.* 1994; **8:** 839–856.

6 Mawle A, Nisenbaum R, Dobbins J, *et al.* Immune responses associated with chronic fatigue syndrome: a case-control study. *J. Infect. Dis.* 1997; **175:** 136–141.

7 Deluca J, Johnson S, Ellis S, Natelson B. Sudden vs gradual onset of chronic fatigue syndrome differentiates individuals on cognitive and psychiatric measures. *J. Psych. Res.* 1997; **31:** 83–90.

8 Hickie I, Lloyd A, Hadzi-Pavlovic D, Parker G, Bird K, Wakefield D. Can the chronic fatigue syndrome be defined by distinct clinical features? *Psychol. Med.* 1995; **25:** 925–935.

9 Wessely S, Chalder T, Hirsch S, Pawlikowska T, Wallace P, Wright D. Post infectious fatigue: a prospective study in primary care. *Lancet* 1995; **345:** 1333–1338.

10 Imboden J. Psychosocial determinants of recovery. *Adv. Psychosom. Med.* 1972; **8:** 142–155.

11 Hotopf M, Noah N, Wessely S. Chronic fatigue and minor psychiatric morbidity after viral meningitis: a controlled study. *J. Neurol. Neurosurg. Psychiatry* 1996; **60:** 504–509.

12 Burton A, Tillotson K, Main C, Hollis S. Psychosocial predictors of outcome in acute and subchronic low back trouble. *Spine* 1995; **20:** 722–728.

13 Dworkin R, Hartstein G, Rosner H, Walther R, Sweeney E, Brand L. A high-risk method for studying psychosocial antecendents of chronic pain: the prospective investigation of Herpes Zoster. *J. Abnorm. Psychol.* 1992; **101:** 200–205.

14 Gwee K, Graham J, McKendrick M, Collins S, Walters S, Read N. Psychometric scores and persistence of irritable bowel after infectious diarrhoea. *Lancet* 1996; **347:** 150–153.

15 Jacobson R. The post concussional syndrome: physiogenesis, psychogenesis and malingering: an integrative model. *J. Psychosom. Res.* 1995; **39:** 675–693.

16 Blanchard E, Hickling E, Taylor A, Loos W, Forneris C, Jaccard J. Who develops PTSD from motor vehicle accidents? *Beh. Res. Ther.* 1996; **34:** 1–10.

17 Aarons H, Forester A, Hall G, Salmon P. Fatigue after major joint arthroplasty: relationship to pre operative fatigue and postoperative emotional state. *J. Psychosom. Res.* 1996; **41:** 225–233.

18 Philips C. Avoidance behaviour and its role in sustaining chronic pain. *Behav. Res. Ther.* 1987; **25:** 273–279.

19 Salkovskis P. The importance of behaviour in the maintaince of anxiety and panic: a cognitive account. *Behav. Psychother.* 1991; **19:** 6–19.

20 Bryant R, Harvey A. Avoidant coping style and post-traumatic stress following motor vehicle accidents. *Behav. Res. Ther.* 1996; **33:** 631–635.

21 Mayou R, Sharpe M. Diagnosis, illness and disease. *Quart. J. Med.* 1995; **88:** 827–831.

22 Scadding J. Essentialism and nominalism in medicine: logic of diagnosis in disease terminology. *Lancet* 1996; **348:** 594–596.

23 Rabinbach A. *The Human Motor: Energy, Fatigue and the Origins of Modernity.* New York, Basic Books, 1990.

24 Lutz T. *American Nervousness: 1903.* Ithaca, Cornell University Press, 1991.

25 Lutz T. Neurasthenia and fatigue syndromes. In Berrios G, Porter R, (ed) *A History of Clinical Psychiatry: The Origin and History of Psychiatric Disorders.* London, Athlone, 1996: 532–544.

Index